DIAGNOSTIC IMAGING TECHNIQUES

Farid Ezat

ALLIED HEALTH PRESS

Diagnostic Imaging Techniques

Author: **Farid Ezat**

Allied Health Press
4164 Lakeshore Road
Burlington ON L7L 1A4
Canada
www.alliedhealthpress.com
Email: orders@arclereducation.com

ISBN: 978-1-77956-775-8

ABOUT THE AUTHOR

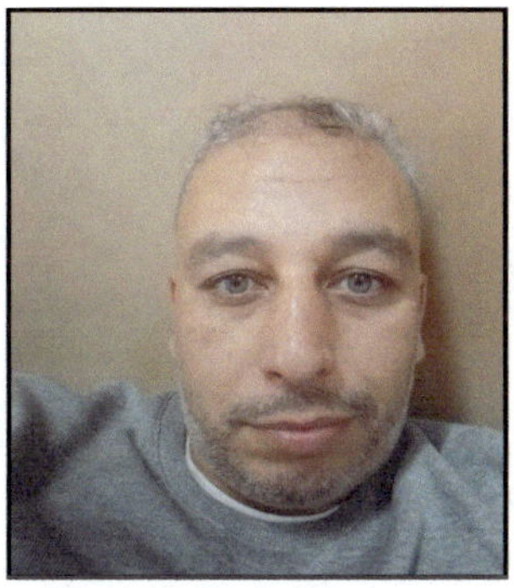

Farid ezat is a dedicated medical doctor with a diverse background in radiology, general practice, and research. Currently serving as a consultant teleradiologist for teleradiology solution , Bangaluru , India , He meticulously analyzes radiological images and engages in research. Previously, Farid honed his clinical skills as a General Practitioner in Alexandria main university hospitals. Farid's academic journey includes earning his Master degree from the Alexandria university ", Faculty of Medicine in Egypt. Committed to continuous learning, Farud actively participates in extracurricular activities and preparing for final FRCR exam.

Brief Table of Contents

Getting Started with This Book

Chapter Openers

A list of Chapter Outline is presented providing a brief Introduction to what will be covered in the chapter.

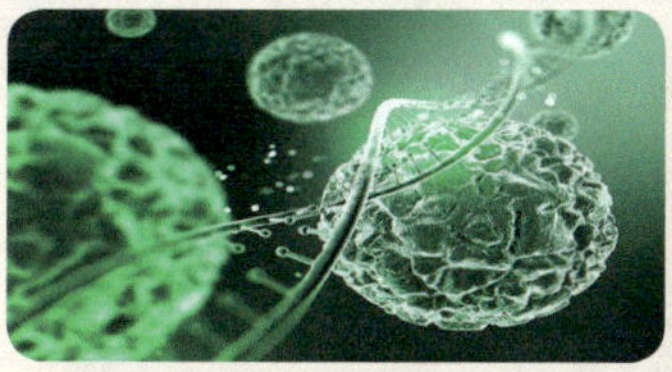

Introduction

Often referred to as the science of life, biology is a broad field of study aimed at comprehending the several kinds of life on Earth, from tiny creatures to sophisticated multicellular entities. Comprising several subfields, including molecular biology, ecology, and evolutionary biology, each of which advances our knowledge of living systems, this field clarifies the mechanisms controlling life events, including development, reproduction, and interaction with the surroundings, which is the central goal of biology. Moreover, biology fills in the void between the natural sciences and medicine by offering a necessary understanding of health, illness, and the interactions between organisms and their environments. Dealing with urgent global issues such as climate change, biodiversity loss, and new diseases depends on an awareness of these complex biological interactions, therefore highlighting the critical part biology plays in modern civilization. Fundamentally, biology explores and tests ideas about the living world using the scientific method. Through methodical observation and experimentation,

LEARNING OBJECTIVES

After studying this chapter, you will be able to:

1. Discuss the scientific method in biology;
2. Explain the cell theory;
3. Discuss the genetics and heredity;
4. Evolution and natural selection;
5. Focus on ecology and ecosystems;
6. Learn about human biology;
7. Evaluate the plant biology;
8. Explain the microbiology;
9. Focus on current trends in biology.

1.1. The Scientific Method in Biology

Learning Outcome

1. Describe the steps of the scientific method;
2. Focus on hypothesis formation;
3. Learn about experimental design.

Learning Outcomes

The beginning of each section of every chapter contains a set of Learning Outcomes that inform students of concepts they should understand. These outcomes help students understand what they should be able to do if they have mastered the material in that section.

Test Your Knowledge

Throughout each chapter, Test Your Knowledge cues you to note which topics have been covered and to self-test your understanding of the material presented.

Test Your Knowledge

1. Explain why correlation does not imply causation in scientific experiments.
2. How does the scientific method help reduce the influence of personal opinions in research?

Chapter Summary

The Summary Section appear at the end of each chapter and summarize main concepts covered throughout the chapter. These points provide key concepts in an engaging and meaningful way.

Summary

The investigation of biological principles highlights the importance of a comprehensive view of life by reflecting the intricate interactions that occur within living systems. The complexity of biology goes beyond individual species or systems, as this essay highlights; it also includes the interactions that mold ecosystems and affect biodiversity. Researchers can conduct in-depth analyses of metabolomic data using sophisticated technologies like MetaboAnalyst, which offer insights into the molecular mechanisms underlying these interactions. As demonstrated by the developments in MetaboAnalyst, for example, the integration of diverse omics data promotes a thorough understanding of metabolic pathways and helps identify important biological markers necessary for research on development and disease (Chong et al., 2018). Additionally, the phenomenon of ecological invasions is a key component of biological research and a vital field of study. The introduction of non-native species into unfamiliar habitats has significant ramifications and calls for multidisciplinary management strategies. Examining the origins and effects of these biological incursions, invasion science has become a crucial field that highlights the need to comprehend ecological dynamics and community interactions. As interest in biological invasions increases, new findings are emerging that put conventional ecological theories and practices to the test. The importance of incorporating various scientific viewpoints is shown by this developing discipline, which also highlights how invasive species shape ecosystems and advances our knowledge of ecological resilience (David et al., 2013). When taken as a whole, these discoveries from invasion science and metabolomics highlight the value of multidisciplinary biology research. Fostering cross-disciplinary collaboration and utilizing technological breakthroughs to improve our comprehension of intricate biological interactions are crucial as we look to the future of biological research. In addition to deepening our understanding of the complexities of life, this method lays the groundwork for tackling urgent environmental issues. Future studies can ensure the continued relevance of biology in a world that is constantly changing by acknowledging the interconnection of biological systems and opening the door to creative solutions that support sustainability and biodiversity conservation. We might imagine a thorough comprehension of life that serves both academia and society at large through ongoing investigation and integration of scientific knowledge.

Knowledge Assessment

The chapter includes material designed to review and reinforce each content. It includes Critical Thinking Questions to help test of your understanding of information presented in the chapter and Short answer Questions to review your understanding of the key concepts presented in the chapter.

Critical Thinking Questions

1. **Who is known as the "Father of Modern Biology"?**
   a. Aristotle
   b. Charles Darwin
   c. Gregor Mendel
   d. Louis Pasteur
2. **What is the basic unit of life?**
   a. Atom
   b. Molecule
   c. Cell
   d. Organism
3. **Which branch of biology studies the interaction of organisms with their environment?**
   a. Genetics
   b. Ecology
   c. Physiology
   d. Botany
4. **Which macromolecule is the main source of energy for living organisms?**
   a. Proteins
   b. Lipids
   c. Carbohydrates
   d. Nucleic acids
5. **DNA is primarily responsible for which function in living organisms?**
   a. Energy production
   b. Protein synthesis
   c. Storing genetic information
   d. Regulating body temperature

Short Answer Questions

1. What is biology, and why is it important to study biology?
2. What are the three main domains of life, and how are they different from one another?
3. Define homeostasis and give an example of how it works in living organisms.
4. What is the cell theory, and why is it fundamental to biology?
5. How do autotrophs and heterotrophs differ in the way they obtain energy?
6. What is the scientific method, and how is it applied in biological research?
7. Discuss how biology helps address global challenges such as climate change, disease, and food security.
8. Explain the levels of biological organization from the smallest unit to the largest. Provide examples at each level.
9. Describe the relationship between structure and function in biology, giving specific examples from cells or organs.
10. How has the discovery of genetics shaped our understanding of inheritance and variation among organisms?

Supplementary Materials

Key Terms: A list of key terms is given for quick reference

KEY TERMS FROM THIS CHAPTER

Annotation enrichment analysis	Biological structure	Cell
Cell theory	Cellular structure	Ecology
Ecosystems	Genetics	Human biology
Microbiology	Natural selection	Organism
Plant biology		

Further Resources: Recommendations for additional readings, websites, and multimedia resources.

References

1. Argelaguet, R., Velten, B., Arnol, D., Dietrich, S., Zenz, T., Marioni, J. C., Buettner, F., et al. (2018). Multi-omics factor analysis—A framework for unsupervised integration of multi-omics data sets. *Molecular Systems Biology, 14*. https://doi.org/10.15252/msb.20178124.
2. Bacher, S., Blackburn, T. M., Essl, F., & Genovesi, P. (2017). *Socio-Economic Impact Classification of Alien Taxa (SEICAT).* https://core.ac.uk/download/286567949.pdf (accessed on 8th March 2025).
3. Barnett, R., Brace, S., Cucchi, T., & Dobney, K. (2013). *Divergent Evolutionary Processes Associated with Colonization of Offshore Islands.* https://core.ac.uk/download/20664364.pdf (accessed on 8th March 2025).

Detailed Table of Contents

CHAPTER 11

Dental and Maxillofacial Imaging 311

CHAPTER 12

Pediatric Imaging 341

CHAPTER 13

Musculoskeletal Imaging 373

LIST OF FIGURES

PREFACE

Modern healthcare has been improved by diagnostic imaging which offers clear and noninvasive views of the body. After X-rays were discovered over a century ago, imaging has advanced to show things in the body that were not visible before. Using ionizing radiation, magnetic fields, sound waves or radioactive tracers gives each modality its own set of advantages. Radiography lets us see bones and lungs, CT gives clear cross-sectional pictures, MRI shows soft-tissue contrast without radiation, ultrasound allows us to observe blood flow and organ action in real time and nuclear medicine reveals activities at the molecular level. All of these tools allow clinicians to diagnose, plan treatment, guide care and monitor the patient's condition with as little discomfort as possible.

Better detector designs, improved image reconstruction methods and better integration of software have helped speed up the process and make images clearer which has boosted confidence in diagnosis. Because of digital storage and transmission, studies can be instantly transferred across different locations, making it possible for remote consultation and review by various specialists. Also, using PET/CT or PET/MRI allows doctors to get both anatomical and functional images at the same time which is useful for tumor staging, planning treatments and checking if the therapy is working. Because new technologies are being developed such as AI for images and portable imaging devices, it is important for practitioners and technologists to understand the details and benefits of each technique to benefit their patients.

The aim of this volume, Diagnostic Imaging Techniques, is to present the essentials and practical advice in a straightforward way. The book combines information about theory with real cases, pointing out major imaging parameters, protocols, safety issues and how to interpret images. The book links the science of each modality to its use in daily diagnostic situations.

The chapters take the reader from basic concepts to more advanced uses of statistics. Chapter 1 explains the physics of images and provides a summary of choosing the right imaging modality. Chapter 2 goes over radiographic imaging, including how beams are made, the use of film and digital receptors, image contrast and ways to optimize the dose. Chapter 3 focuses on computed tomography, looking at spiral and multi-detector systems, image reconstruction and the main clinical uses. Chapter 4 talks about magnetic resonance imaging, covering nuclear spin, pulse sequences, safety measures and tips for making soft tissues easier to see. Chapter 5 explains the physics of ultrasound, the equipment used, Doppler techniques and procedures that use guidance. Chapter 6 examines nuclear medicine, talking about radiopharmaceuticals, gamma cameras, SPECT and PET systems and quality control. Chapter 7 explains how mammography is done, including screening, tomosynthesis and other additional methods. Chapter 8 discusses fluoroscopic studies which include dynamic imaging of the gastrointestinal tract, genitourinary system and angiography. Chapter 9 explains how interventional radiology is used, including image-guided biopsy, vascular embolization and thermal ablation. Chapter 10 focuses on digital imaging systems and picture-archiving and communication systems (PACS), discussing network integration, data management, and cybersecurity. Chapter 11 looks at dental and maxillofacial imaging, including panoramic radiography and cone-beam CT. Chapter 12 explains how to use imaging in children by designing special protocols that help reduce radiation and consider their developing anatomy. Chapter 13 covers imaging of bones, joints and soft-tissue injuries using radiography, MRI and ultrasound. Chapter 14 covers the use of CT angiography, MRI and echocardiography in cardiovascular imaging. Chapter 15 finishes with a section on neuroimaging which explains CT and MRI of the brain, functional MRI and how these methods are applied to stroke and neurodegenerative conditions.

The book is written for medical students, radiology residents, technologists and practicing doctors who want a thorough but easy-to-understand guide. People in biomedical engineering, research and administration in healthcare will find the information about technology, workflow and safety useful.

INTRODUCTION TO DIAGNOSTIC IMAGING

1

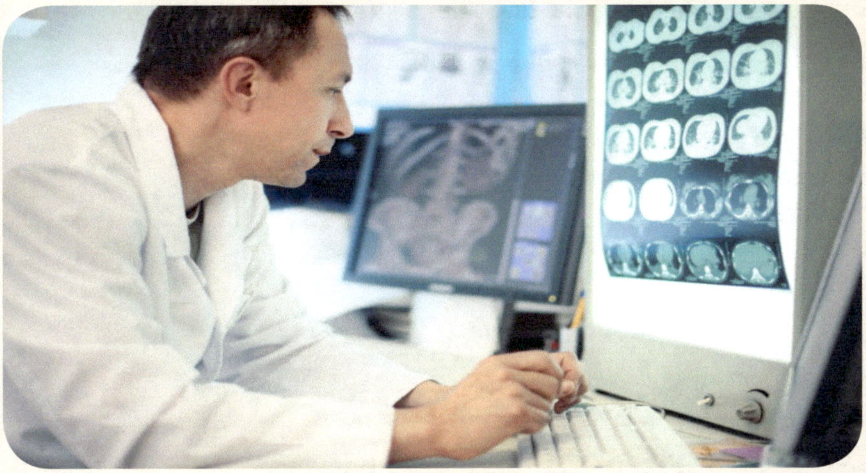

LEARNING OBJECTIVES

After studying this chapter, you will be able to:

1. Describe the history of diagnostic imaging.
2. Identify and differentiate between various types of diagnostic imaging.
3. Explain the fundamental principles of imaging techniques.
4. Analyze the clinical applications of diagnostic imaging.
5. Evaluate the safety and risks of diagnostic imaging.
6. Define future trends in diagnostic imaging.

Introduction

Medical technology has really changed how we do healthcare, especially in checking what's going on inside our bodies. Today, doctors use diagnostic imaging which includes X-rays, CT scans, MRIs and ultrasound, to detect problems early and know what is happening. Every type of scan is different; an X-ray can be done quickly, but an MRI often shows more about soft tissues. What really matters is choosing the right tool to address the clinical question, so that patients get the best results. If we look further, diagnostic imaging is not just about taking images inside the body. Usually, it forms a bigger process that helps doctors choose treatments and monitor the development of the disease. Because radiologists and specialists need to know anatomy, pathology and technology, their training is often tough and thorough. On top of that, they sometimes add contrast agents, like gadolinium-based ones, to make certain tissues pop, which really helps when looking at conditions linked to the liver or central nervous system (Haneder et al., 2015). As time has gone on, imaging has focused more on patient safety, introducing new tools and changing procedures to reduce risks. Generally speaking, it's not only about capturing clear images but also about using predictive models to estimate how various imaging choices might affect patient management (Leening et al., 2014). Safety is important and agencies watch for any side effects caused by contrast agents. As a result, in diagnostic imaging today, you notice a combination that covers both the technical process and the obligation to ensure patients are safe and well cared for.

Overview of Diagnostic Imaging

The fast advancement of technology has made diagnostic imaging very important in current healthcare. These days, you can use X-rays, CT scans, MRIs and ultrasounds to look inside the body and see different views. Early detection by medical staff means they can start treatment sooner. The latest addition is 3D imaging and AI which often help improve both accuracy and speed. As an illustration, AI algorithms are able to detect anything unusual in images with great accuracy which can reduce mistakes made by people. All in all, using these modern approaches in imaging appears to be the best way to improve care for patients and make work easier. Imaging has a key part in how healthcare providers look after patients. It is necessary to identify the issue in craniosynostosis before choosing surgery. Generally, the guidelines point out that the correct imaging is important to tell craniosynostosis apart from other similar issues. Sometimes, telling synostotic from non-synostotic cases can be confusing, but following set guidelines allows doctors to refer patients to the right specialists for treatment. This blend of imaging with overall treatment planning shows how these advances impact care in so many specialties (Mathijssen, 2020). We should not forget that having powerful imaging tools also means we have a strong responsibility to act ethically. Health professionals should review all the choices, making sure the patient's health is considered and the guidelines are followed—at times, it is not obvious which one to choose. They need to weigh the pros and cons of each imaging test, as choosing can sometimes be difficult. Groups like the European Society of Cardiology point out that combining solid clinical judgment with up-to-date evidence is key (Cosentino et al., 2019). Ultimately, it is not just about mastering the tech; it is also about understanding the deeper effects on patient safety and treatment success (Figure 1.1).

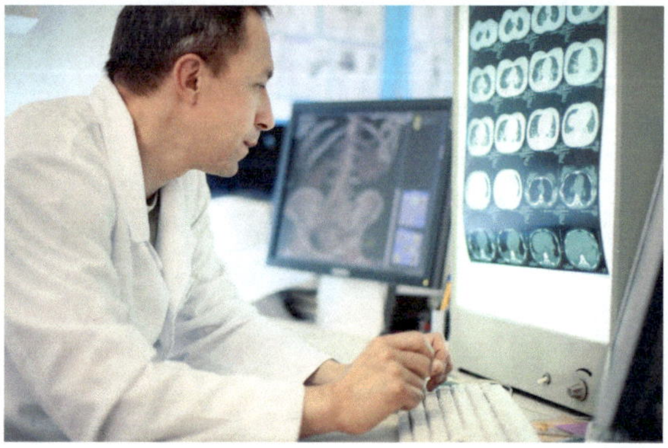

Figure 1.1. Diagnostic Imaging.

Source: https://www.healthimages.com/content/uploads/sites/2/2019/10/radiologist.jpg.

Importance in Modern Medicine

Modern diagnostic imaging has changed medicine today. Thanks to ultrasound, MRI and CT scans, doctors are able to see inside the body and detect problems earlier which helps them plan better treatments. For instance, prenatal ultrasound is important because it provides useful details that can help lower risks for both the mom and the baby and sometimes prevents invasive tests. In most cases, as healthcare evolves, imaging remains central to quick diagnosis and smart, preventative care, all while matching the wider goal of better treatment strategies (Malinger et al., 2020). Imaging doesn't stop at helping in the clinic, either. Today, researchers are using these approaches to explore details of diseases that were not possible before. Most of the time, researchers use this non-invasive approach to see how new treatments work which helps drive progress and supports decisions backed by strong evidence. Many studies point out that providing more access to these methods is crucial, since earlier inequalities delayed the progress of medicine. Discussions about raising imaging standards and guidelines are still ongoing, pushing the field steadily into a more progressive future (Buchbinder et al., 2020). Also, diagnostic imaging builds bridges between different specialists. Since patient care is so involved, radiologists, oncologists and various experts frequently join to review imaging results and plan treatments together. By reviewing cancer patient images as a team, experts can decide on the best treatment and also spot early signs of the cancer returning which supports better communication among team members. Over time, organizations like the International Society of Ultrasound in Obstetrics and Gynecology (ISUOG) have chipped in by sharing best practices and setting standards, which reinforces a culture of collaboration and continual learning in healthcare (Malinger et al., 2020).

Common Terminology Used in the Field

Precision in language matters in imaging tests in medicine. Doctors may say radiography, ultrasound or CT scans which are all methods for looking inside the body. Usually, the first step is radiography which uses X-rays to take pictures of bones and tissues to find any fractures. Ultrasound sends high-frequency sound waves into the body to reveal soft tissues and organs (you often see it used in pregnancy checks or abdominal exams). Another kind of scan is computed tomography or CT which divides the body into thin slices to find tumors or deep injuries. Properly using these terms allows all members of the medical team to understand the imaging reports together. In addition, contrast agents and artifacts are very important in all this. Contrast agents make internal details easier to see—usually helping with CT and MRI scans—by being given orally or injected which allows radiologists to distinguish between different tissue densities. Artifacts, by contrast, are strange errors in images that might hide actual problems or even seem to show problems that don't exist. People in this field need to know how these work to avoid misinterpreting images during both shooting and review. If these terms are noticed, the accuracy of the diagnosis goes up which means better care for patients and more efficient use of imaging. Imaging professionals are having to adapt their language because of the arrival of new technology. Recently, digital imaging and image fusion are terms you hear more frequently. Instead of film, digital imaging uses electronic files which makes it simpler to handle, access and edit pictures. When different scanning methods are combined, the results can give a clearer picture of a patient's health which supports more accurate diagnoses and makes treatment planning easier. As new technologies appear, the imaging field learns and adopts new words and practices to address today's needs. Knowing these new terms helps professionals use modern tools with confidence and also improves how specialists talk to each other about patients.

1.1. History of Diagnostic Imaging

Learning Outcome

1. Understand the early methods of diagnosis.
2. Explore the development of the X-ray technology.
3. Evolution of imaging techniques over the decades.

Diagnostic imaging has turned the whole idea of looking inside the body on its head. In 1895, Wilhelm Conrad Roentgen found X-rays by accident which allowed doctors to see inside the body without surgery. At that point, it became possible to see fractures, tumors and other strange things which altered the way things worked. In the 20th century, ultrasound and CT scans were introduced, giving doctors another safe way to find out about many conditions. Because of these methods, doctors could rely on better results and needed fewer risky surgeries, clearly showing that technology is vital in healthcare today. Advances in imaging have followed along with progress in science and changes in public health. In general, the introduction of MRI in the late 1970s made it possible to see soft tissues in detail, mainly benefiting diagnosis of brain and muscle problems. With time, digital technology has helped imaging techniques become both smarter and more efficient at analyzing pictures. In addition, people are using advanced computer methods to put together a lot of data and help guide decisions about diagnoses. Big data in healthcare, for example, shows how pooling imaging info can lead to better patient outcomes and firmly establish these techniques as a backbone of modern medicine (Dash et al., 2019). At the same time as new technologies, ethical matters and caring for patients have gained significance. The new rules now address consent, privacy and correct use of imaging tools, reflecting the growing importance of patient rights and autonomy. Since imaging is used more and more by healthcare providers to decide on treatments, ethical practices are becoming very obvious. Many times, this involves getting patients' opinions and letting their choices guide how imaging is carried out. In this way, diagnostic imaging keeps evolving—not just technologically, but also as it grapples with the sometimes messy, always vital realm of ethics and patient care (Schalock et al., 2021) (Figure 1.2).

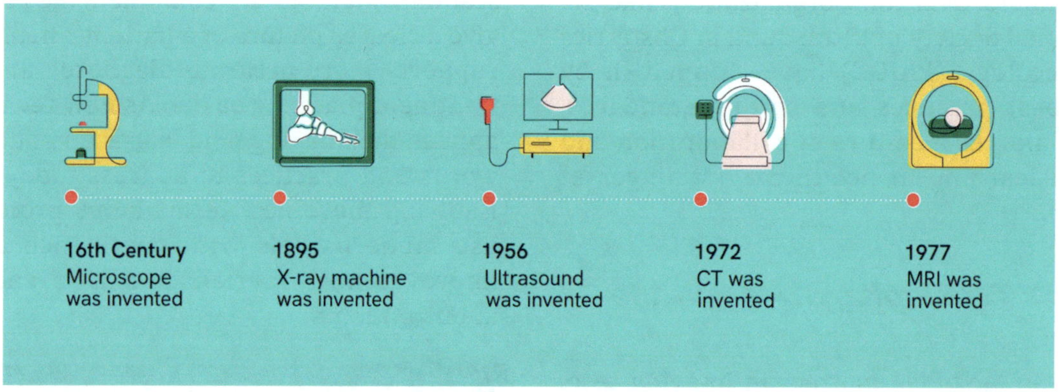

Figure 1.2. The invention of the microscope to using MRIs, major breakthroughs in imaging technology have helped scientific researchers and medical professionals all over the world see inside the human body in greater detail and with greater clarity.

Source: https://chanzuckerberg.com/blog/the-past-present-and-future-of-medical-imaging/.

1.1.1. Early Methods of Diagnosis

Diagnostic imaging's rise has reshaped how we spot and treat diseases—blood disorders in particular have felt the impact. Before, doctors would mostly look at symptoms and use simple methods; for example, they would examine peripheral blood smears to spot unusual cell shapes that might mean leukemia. Those approaches worked, but they were slow and highly dependent on the people working at the time. Today, machine learning is a major help, allowing clinicians to examine blood smear images with great accuracy. In most cases, studies even report detection accuracies above 97%, which kind of shows how much the old protocols in hematology are being upended (Ghaderzadeh et al., 2021). Turning to oncology, a similar story unfolds. Initially, radiographs and CT scans were the main tools, but these often did not reveal malignant problems, especially those affecting bones. Because of these boundaries, it wasn't unexpected that new, advanced approaches began appearing. SPECT/CT and PET/CT which are molecular and hybrid imaging techniques, are now being used, providing better and earlier detection of skeletal metastases.

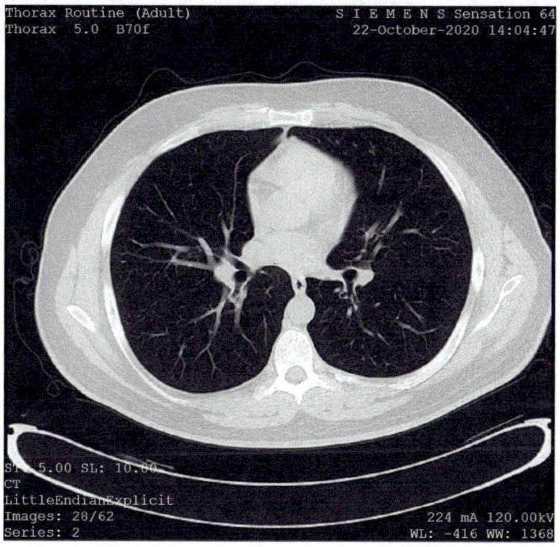

Figure 1.3. Evolution of medical imaging.

Source: By Ptrump16 - Own work, CC BY-SA 4.0, https://commons.wikimedia.org/w/index.php?curid=114999332.

Although adoption into everyday practice has been somewhat uneven, there's a growing body of evidence (Cook et al., 2020) suggesting that these innovations help refine diagnostic accuracy and shape treatment plans more effectively. In general, using advanced imaging in hematology and oncology is similar to the trend of precision medicine in healthcare. The previous approaches, useful as they were, stopped doctors from exploring certain aspects of medicine. Thanks to digital technology and AI, the way doctors diagnose has been improved and changed in some ways. As ML algorithms improve in handling blood data, they could make it much quicker and cheaper to find leukemia in routine diagnostics. Further, with hybrid imaging offering a fuller, multi-faceted look at disease progression, the future of diagnostic imaging looks poised to be not just more accurate and efficient, but also far more centered on patient care (Cook et al., 2020; Ghaderzadeh et al., 2021) (Figure 1.3).

1.1.2. Development of X-Ray Technology

X-ray technology burst onto the scene and changed how medicine looks at the human body. In 1895, Wilhelm Conrad Roentgen found a way to look inside the body without surgery which seemed almost like magic to people then. Soon, doctors started using X-rays to find broken bones, tumors and different conditions with a clarity that was usually unbeatable. With time, the use of radiography grew into digital imaging which is faster and provides clearer pictures. New techniques like computed tomography (CT) now give us 3D views that can sharpen treatment plans, generally speaking. Digital platforms are now changing the way X-ray imaging is done even more. Modern digital radiography uses less radiation and gives clearer images because of the combined efforts of smart sensors and software. Doctors can easily look at, change and share these images on the screen which makes it simpler to ask for a second opinion. Because of the digital shift, issues are now easier to notice and patients tend to receive treatment sooner which has led to better results overall. There are still new developments in diagnostic imaging technology. Photoacoustic imaging (PA), which blends optical tricks with ultrasound methods, is emerging as a promising alternative to traditional X-ray techniques, especially in identifying early signs of breast cancer. Some studies suggest that PA might even replace both

X-ray mammography and ultrasonography for early-stage diagnosis (Hilgerink et al., 2011). As research into these novel techniques moves forward, the overall field of medical imaging appears set to expand further—mixing a range of tools to enhance both diagnostic precision and patient comfort, all while working along with well-established methods like X-rays (Rakhmonovna et al., 2023).

1.1.3. Evolution of Imaging Techniques Over the Decades

Imaging has come a long way, and it is changed the game for how doctors work and how patients feel. In the early 1900s, radiography was introduced as the main method to see bones and the harder parts of the body. In the 1950s, ultrasound was able to show images of soft tissues as they moved which gave clinicians more useful information. In the '70s, CT came into use, allowing doctors to see inside the body in a way that was never possible before. As a result, doctors could make diagnoses more accurately and use fewer invasive tests which helped the field move towards a patient-focused approach. More recently, imaging moved on to some serious upgrades. MRI which became popular in the 1980s, provided clear images of the body and its functions, without introducing extra risks from ionizing radiation. Later on, editing and processing images became much better. Because of digital pathology and whole slide imaging, healthcare experts can now review and share digital images for remote check-ups and teamwork, regardless of their location. As noted in Jain et al. (2020), when you combine machine learning and AI, it feels like diagnostic imaging is stepping into a whole new realm that promises finer diagnosis and more personalized treatment plans. Although things are always evolving, it is obvious that imaging is shifting toward safer and more advanced ways to examine the body. Methods like multiphoton microscopy and molecular imaging are helping us observe what cells do and the biochemical reactions taking place inside them. The change is partly due to the desire for tests that are safer and more comfortable which is causing biopsies to become less common. With observations such as those in Schalock et al. (2021), it is evident that the future holds ever more refined tools—tools that should help boost diagnosis precision, track treatments better, and ultimately hand clinicians the power to care more effectively.

1.2. Types of Diagnostic Imaging

Learning Outcome

1. Identify and describe the early diagnostic methods used in medicine.
2. Explain the development and significance of X-ray technology in medical diagnostics.
3. Define computed tomography (CT) scans.

Diagnostic imaging has changed how medicine works over time. X-rays got things going by using radiation to create images of bones and some tissues and they are still helpful for finding broken bones or infections. The next advance was CT scans which usually generate cross-sectional images of the body. It becomes easier to handle problems like tumors or internal bleeding with this new method. For example, MRI is able to show soft tissues in great detail and it does not use ionizing radiation. Selecting the correct type of image is important, since it affects both the clinical questions and keeping patients safe. X-rays, CT scans and ultrasound are now all part of the mix. People like it a lot because it is easy to use and shows what's happening as events unfold. It uses sound waves that move very fast to form images and is most helpful in obstetrics, cardiology and examining the abdomen. It is very useful for observing a fetus grow and for performing biopsies, since seeing what is happening in real time matters a lot. Ultrasound is preferred over X-rays for pregnant women and kids since it does not use ionizing radiation. In some sense, using ultrasound demonstrates that modern medicine aims to be safer while maintaining excellent diagnostic results. Lately, nuclear medicine techniques like PET and SPECT scans have become more important. They depend on radioactive tracers to observe cell activity and they are most useful in oncology for finding tumors and checking the effectiveness of treatment. Seeing cellular activity allows doctors to notice things that might be missed by standard imaging tests. AI and machine learning are also getting involved, adding more information to what images can show us, although sometimes the details are surprising. At the same time, as imaging methods keep evolving, there's always that need to balance progress with ethics — guidelines remind healthcare professionals to use these advances carefully (Mach et al., 2019; Williams et al., 2018) (Figure 1.4).

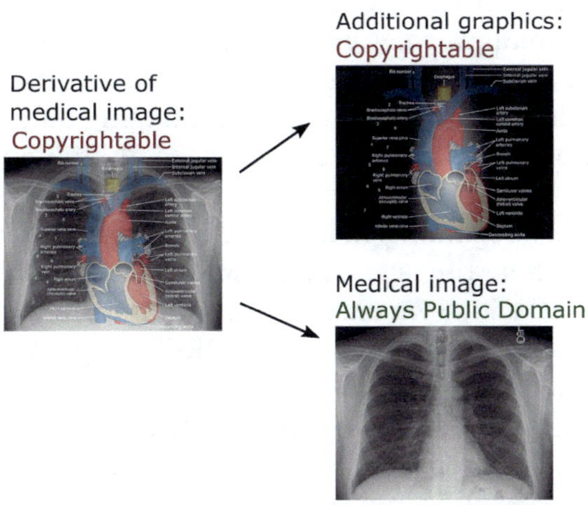

Figure 1.4. Components of different diagnostic imaging techniques.

Source: By Mikael Häggström, from source images by ZooFari, Stillwaterising and Gray's Anatomy creators - editFile: Heart diagram-en.svg by ZooFari (Attribution-Share Alike 3.0 Unported license).File:Trachea (transparent).png (From Gray's Anatomy, Public Domain)File:Chest_Xray_PA_3-8-2010.png by Stillwaterising (Public Domain)Further outline of venous system:(2011). "A pictorial essay: Radiology of lines and tubes in the intensive care unit." Indian Journal of Radiology and Imaging 21 (3): 182. DOI:10.4103/0971-3026.85365. ISSN 0971-3026.Synthesis by: Mikael Häggström, CC BY-SA 3.0, https://commons.wikimedia.org/w/index.php?curid=63226966.

1.2.1. X-Ray Imaging

Medical diagnostics has changed over time, and one major part of that shift is how we use different imaging tools. X-rays make it possible to detect broken bones and may reveal early signs of cancer. Being a radiologist is not always easy, as you must deal with different image quality and a wide variety of diseases, so you really need to understand the basics of imaging. This situation, generally speaking, is why many in the field are pushing for smarter tech and new methods—to boost both accuracy and speed in assessments, ultimately leading to better patient care (Islam et al., 2023). For example, the introduction of CT in the 1970s completely changed the way things worked. With CT scans, doctors could see clearer and more detailed images of the body and they didn't need to operate to examine certain complex structures. In general, better pictures allow clinicians to deal with difficult neurological or orthopedic problems. It is interesting how X-ray ideas have moved beyond the basics to power these advanced diagnostic tools, and there's a lot of optimism that upcoming techniques will keep redefining how we evaluate and manage diseases (Prichard et al., 1992). And the evolution hasn't stopped. New developments in X-ray imaging, especially with digital radiography and a bit of artificial intelligence (AI) thrown into the mix, are making it easier and quicker to read those images—even though the occasional hiccup with quality or resolution still lingers. Since many people prefer less invasive testing, the ongoing improvements in X-ray technology are very timely. As the healthcare system gradually adopts these fresh innovations, diagnostic imaging—with X-rays at its core—remains a crucial meeting point between cutting-edge technology and hands-on clinical know-how, all helping pave the way for more personalized patient care (Islam et al., 2023) (Figure 1.5).

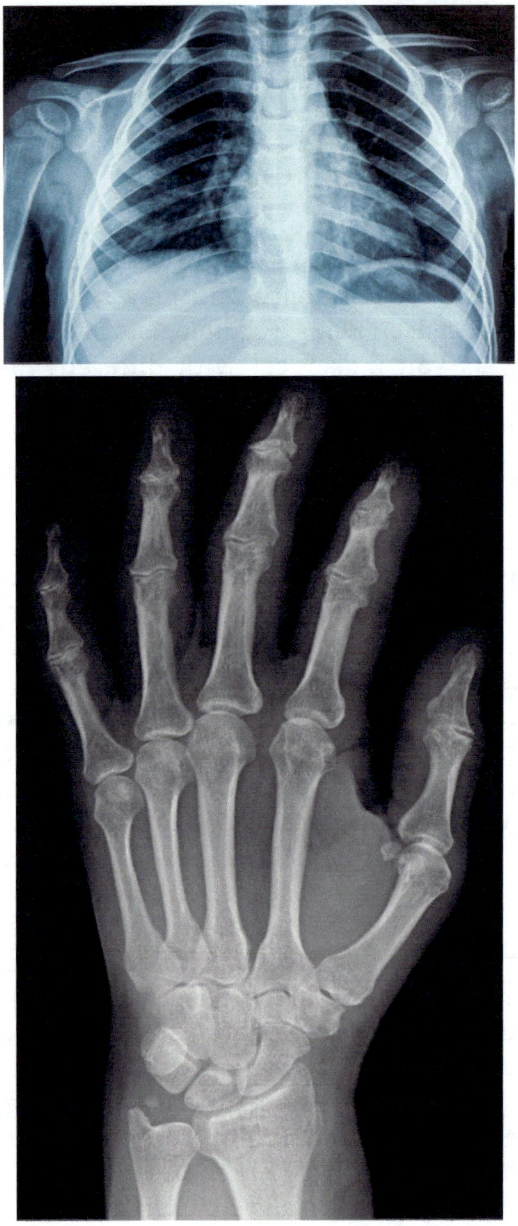

Figure 1.5. X-rays.

Source: By Ptrump16 - Own work, CC BY-SA 4.0, https://commons.wikimedia.org/w/index.php?curid=115012214.

1.2.2. Magnetic Resonance Imaging (MRI)

Advanced imaging has shifted how we look at diagnosing diseases. These days, we don't just see pictures—we get clues about what's going on inside the body. MRI is a favorite tool for doctors because it produces very clear images of soft tissue without exposing you to radiation. MRI scans use powerful magnets and radio waves to make a clear image of the organs which allows doctors to notice any irregularities with great accuracy. Nowadays, many doctors use MRI for both routine imaging and to assess brain function which helps identify problems. Because it is flexible and very accurate, it has become important in fields such as oncology and neurology. When you look closely at neurodegenerative conditions, MRI plays an even more important role. Multiparametric MRI—thanks to newer developments—has boosted our ability to assess diseases like amyotrophic lateral sclerosis (ALS), generally speaking. These MRI changes may also be used by doctors as signs that motor neuron problems are under consideration. When different imaging data are combined, clinicians can more easily tell apart ALS from disorders that could be confused with it at the beginning. In most cases, as this research unfolds, setting up standard MRI routines should fine-tune how we diagnose and monitor patients (Kassubek et al., 2020). MRI's importance doesn't stop at mere diagnosis either. It is a main tool in the effort to solve the mysteries of neurodegeneration. We have not found out the exact reason for these conditions, so we should study the biology further. Specific techniques that rely on transition metals and lanthanide ions have made it possible to catch certain neuropathological markers and these methods are useful along with PET and SPECT. Thanks to these new imaging approaches, researchers are now able to combine information about brain structure with information about brain function, gradually learning how several factors interact in neurodegenerative diseases. This evolving picture not only paves the way for better diagnosis but also might steer us toward more effective treatments (Sedgwick et al., 2020) (Figure 1.6).

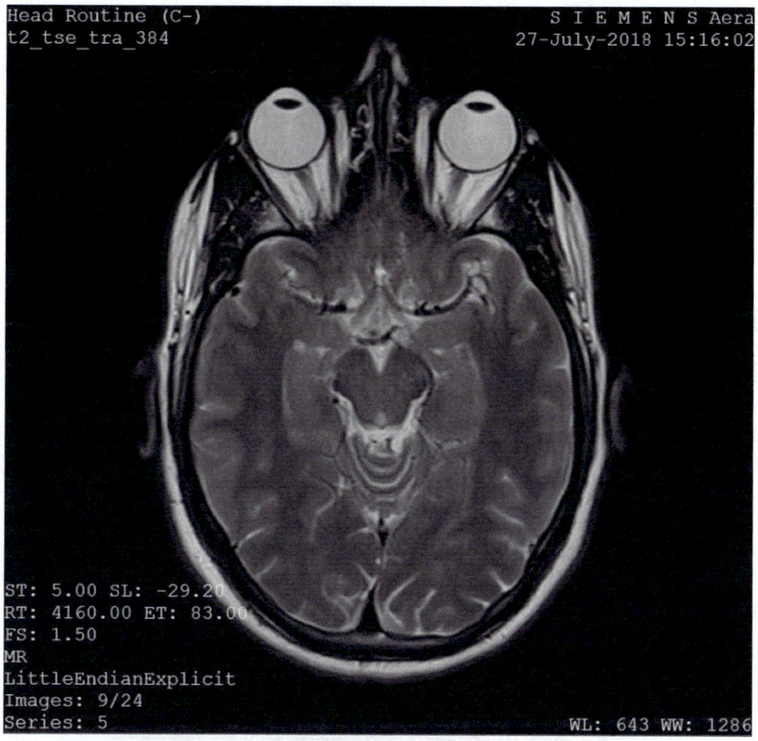

Figure 1.6. Magnetic resonance imaging (MRI).

Source: By Ptrump16 - Own work, CC BY-SA 4.0, https://commons.wikimedia.org/w/index.php?curid=115011738.

1.2.3. Computed Tomography (CT) Scans

Modern diagnostic tools have reshaped how we see the human body—CT scans, for instance, have become a major player. Ever since the early 1970s, CT technology has been developed and now covers a wide range of medical cases, mainly in examining the head. They help doctors see inside the body in detail, showing things that might be missed by other types of imaging. It is important to know how head CT requests are handled, since this guides daily work and influences future research in diagnostic imaging. A review of a retrospective study from a tertiary health center in north-central Nigeria shows some different aspects of head CT orders. The study sifted through 350 case files and generally found that men made up a large chunk of patients receiving head CT scans, largely because traumatic brain injuries (TBI) emerge more frequently among them. TBIs were involved in about 22% of the cases which proves the importance of reliable imaging, especially when every second matters in acute care. Oddly enough, a good number of these scans came out normal—hinting that sometimes, clinical suspicions don't completely line up with what appears on the images (Zhang et al., 2024). Having this insight really helps doctors decide when to order imaging tests. Recently, AI, especially advancements in natural language processing, has begun to change the way CT interpretation is done. A recent study used GPT-4 to look for cerebral hemorrhages in CT scans of the brain. While GPT-4 performed well in some cases, it had difficulties with certain types of hemorrhages which means that more detailed knowledge is still needed to handle these situations. AI can be very useful in radiology by helping to improve efficiency and accuracy, especially when there are not enough radiologists. As diagnostic imaging continues to evolve, blending these modern techniques with traditional methods may eventually lead to better patient outcomes in the future (Zhang et al., 2024) (Figure 1.7).

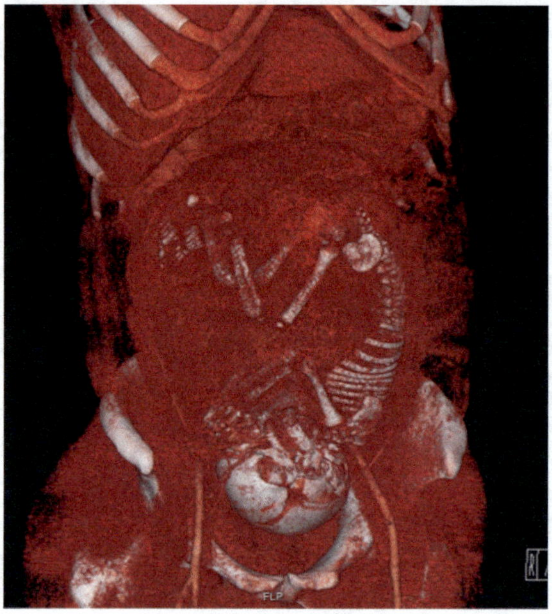

Figure 1.7. Computed tomography (CT) scan.

Source: By Mikael Häggström, M.D. Author info- Reusing images- Conflicts of interest: None Mikael Häggström, M.D. Consent note: Written informed consent was obtained from the individual, including online publication. - Own work, CC0, https://commons.wikimedia.org/w/index.php?curid=61722886.

Test Your Knowledge

1. How does MRI differ from CT scans in terms of the type of imaging technology they use and the kind of tissues they are most effective at visualizing?
2. What is the primary advantage of using a CT scan over an MRI when diagnosing trauma-related injuries, such as fractures?

1.3. Principles of Imaging Techniques

Learning Outcome

1. Explain the basic physics behind X-rays.
2. Discuss magnetic fields in MRI.
3. Define computation and reconstruction in CT.

Imaging has advanced a lot, making it much easier to see problems inside the body. With the help of ultrasound, CT and MRI, doctors are able to see inside us in great detail. High-resolution ultrasound, for example, has turned out to be a real game-changer when checking thyroid nodules—a point underscored by recent American Thyroid Association (ATA) guidelines that lean on using these imaging clues for deciding on fine-needle aspiration biopsies. These recommendations, built on heaps of research and everyday clinical insights, offer a more flexible plan for handling common thyroid issues (Haugen et al., 2015). Therefore, using these imaging techniques allows doctors to find problems early and clearly see what is happening which helps decide on the best treatment. Knowing how these imaging tricks work is very important for everyday medical diagnosis. CT uses radiation and MRI uses magnetic properties of hydrogen to produce important images. Many times, deciding between ultrasound and MRI for a soft tissue lesion depends on where the problem is located and how comfortable the patient can be during the scan. Also, using new computer techniques to analyze images often improves the accuracy of diagnoses by handling complex data in unexpected ways. Ongoing research and hands-on developments are steadily boosting clinicians' confidence in picking the best method for each patient (Ritchie et al., 2015). It is very important to read these images correctly to guide clinical decisions. Both radiologists and doctors should consider what the scans show, what the patient says and the lab results, even if some details do not match perfectly. Using standard imaging protocols, for example in thyroid nodules, helps avoid errors and makes it simpler to repeat the results. Another interesting area is molecular imaging which pairs regular scans with biological signals to see inside the body at the cellular level in real time. Because of this, treatments can be given earlier and are more likely to be tailored to each patient. Overall, knowing how these imaging methods work not only boosts diagnostic precision but also unlocks new directions in patient care (Haugen et al., 2015).

1.3.1. Basic Physics Behind X-Rays

The use of X-rays has made a big difference in medical imaging, uniting physics with ordinary healthcare in ways that are often surprising. They have a lot of energy and very short wavelengths which allow them to move through materials and tissues in ways that might seem unusual. Photons from an X-ray tube shoot through the body and depending on the tissue, some are absorbed while others pass through. Radiation is absorbed by bones more than by soft tissues which is why bones appear white and soft tissues appear dark on X-rays. Because of this uneven absorption, X-rays can highlight the inside of the body and help doctors identify different health problems which is why X-ray physics is important. X-rays are made by speeding up electrons and directing them toward a target which is usually tungsten. In the tube, electrons get accelerated by a high voltage and then smash into tungsten atoms; here, two major events go down: there's Bremsstrahlung (or "braking" radiation) and characteristic radiation. When electrons approach the tungsten nucleus, they slow down and release photons which is called Bremsstrahlung and when inner electrons are displaced and outer electrons take their place, X-rays are released, a process called characteristic radiation. Basically, how strong and penetrating the rays are depends on the energy of the photons and knowing how these processes work both improves the technology and helps set up proper safety measures in clinics. X-rays are important for therapy as well as for diagnosis in many medical areas. Now that digital technology is more advanced, X-rays are frequently used together with it to improve image quality and accuracy. For example, CT scans create detailed cross-sectional images using X-rays which show much more than what basic radiographs are able to display. Lately, machine learning has started to help analyze images which is streamlining the process of making diagnoses. It's quite interesting to watch how combining old physics with new technology can change how patients are cared for, even if there are some bumps along the way. As Lundervold et al. (2018) suggest these advances in machine learning applied to X-ray imaging are promising—a small but significant step towards smoothing out challenges and boosting efficiency in how we interpret and use these vital images (Figure 1.8).

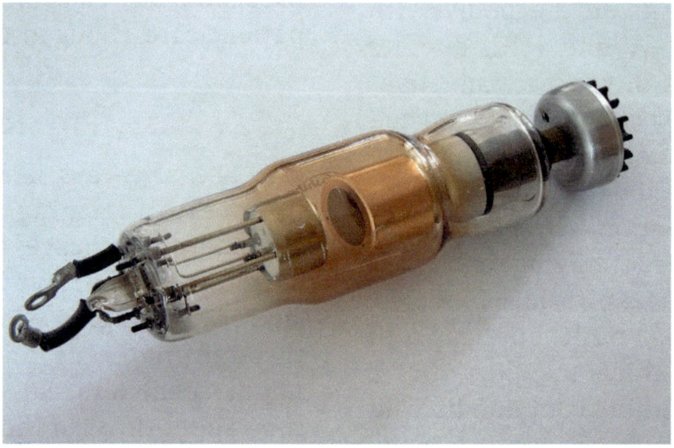

Figure 1.8. The X-ray tube.

Source: By Kyle Senior - Own work, CC BY-SA 4.0, https://commons.wikimedia.org/w/index.php?curid=118428178.

1.3.2. Magnetic Fields In Magnetic Resonance Imaging (MRI)

MRI demonstrates the unusual ways physics and medicine are connected. It applies strong magnetic fields to change the position of hydrogen nuclei in the body which helps create clear images of what is inside. Typically, these machines use a field strength between 1.5 and 3 Tesla (T), which usually works just fine for clinical needs. These days, systems that operate at lower fields, for example 0.1 to 0.55 T, are getting some attention. They tend to cut costs and even allow patients to be positioned with more freedom, which can be a boon in places with limited resources (Hei et al., 2021). The setup of radiofrequency pulses and gradient fields plays a big role in determining the final image, in addition to the magnets. Hydrogen atoms exposed to a strong magnetic field start to vibrate at a specific frequency which we call nuclear magnetic resonance. After that, when the atoms relax in response to radio pulses, the fine features of soft tissues are revealed. Many times, MRI is able to show anatomical features more clearly than other methods and it does not use ionizing radiation. Over time, thanks to advances in algorithms and imaging tweaks, the sensitivity of these machines has only gotten better, proving invaluable for diagnosing a wide range of conditions (Hei et al., 2021). People are starting to focus on how changing magnetic field strengths in MRI can influence the technical, social and economic parts of healthcare. More people can now benefit from MRI diagnostics because high-performance, low-field systems are more efficient and are being used in different places. It seems that this shift is meant to help more people receive important imaging services. Low-field MRI allows clinicians to provide these services to a larger group of patients and as affordable and accessible care is becoming more important, it could help fill gaps in medical imaging while still giving good results for different health problems.

1.3.3. Computation and Reconstruction in Computed Tomography (CT)

CT image making isn't a simple routine. The conversion of raw CT scan data into pictures is done by clever computer programs that reconstruct the images and this is a difficult process. Raw data goes through a series of steps that use unusual math along with finding the best balance between image quality and radiation. Since cutting down on radiation is very important, making sure that balance is right, even if it leads to a bit of extra noise or clutter, is necessary. Most of the time, as these methods advance, they gradually help us notice even the smallest changes, proving how important better computation is. Low-dose CT scans throw another wrench into the works. You reduce the amount of radiation and, in general, you could get more noise and extra artifacts in the images.

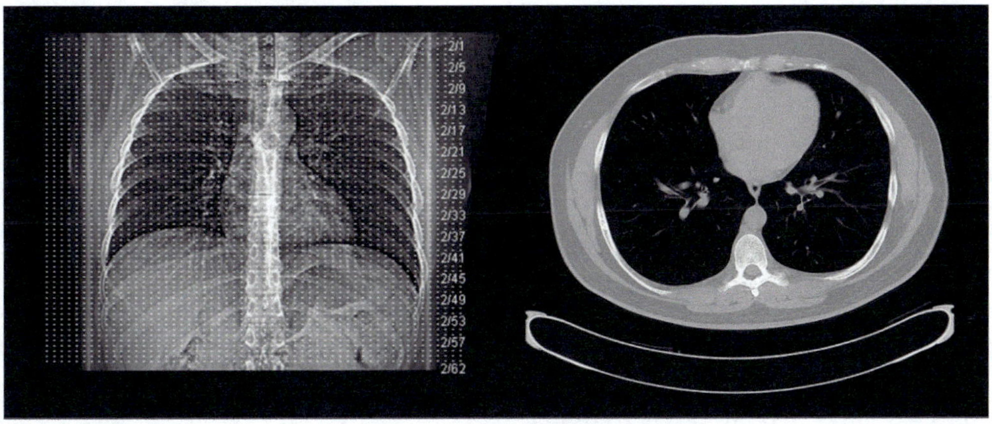

Figure 1.9. Comparison with iterative reconstruction algorithm for clinical CT images. (a1) and (a2) FBP reconstructed LDCT images. (b1) and (b2) ASIR reconstructed LDCT images. (c1) and (c2) ASDL processed result for the LDCT images in (a1) and (a2).

Source: By Ptrump16 - Own work, CC BY-SA 4.0, https://commons.wikimedia.org/w/index.php?curid=123692659.

Sometimes, radiologists have a hard time reading these less clear images which has encouraged many researchers to experiment in the labs. Many researchers are working on different ways to remove noise during the reconstruction phase, without losing essential details. One interesting way is to use deep learning which can reduce the noise in reduced-dose scans without making the images too blurry. Methods that stress similarity and Wasserstein techniques are applied to both boost the signal-to-noise ratio and maintain details needed for a proper evaluation. Another important development is generative adversarial networks or GANs which have made a big impact in low-dose imaging. By using concepts from optimal transport, GANs can reduce noise in images without affecting the important features which is necessary for reliable diagnoses. Their ability to judge the structure of images is so similar to human vision because of their loss function. To put it simply, radiologists can better understand the images even if they have some special characteristics. As advancements in these computer techniques keep unfolding, the overall promise for better patient outcomes appears significant, with imaging that's not only enhanced but also gentler in terms of radiation (Figure 1.9).

Test Your Knowledge

1. What is the role of high-energy electrons in the generation of X-rays within an X-ray tube?
2. How does the interaction of X-rays with matter lead to the formation of an image in diagnostic radiology?

1.4. Applications of Diagnostic Imaging

Learning Outcome

1. Understand the role of imaging techniques in detecting diseases.
2. Explain how imaging is utilized in planning effective treatment strategies.
3. Discuss the importance of monitoring patient progress.

Technological leaps have turned diagnostic imaging on its head. AI is now used in almost every type of imaging and images and how they are read by doctors seem more advanced and intelligent. Now, radiologists experience a streamlined process and the technology handles reducing radiation and speeding up image delivery. Often, the main focus is on patient safety and accurate results which is why this process is preferred. Whether it is chopping an image into sections or dipping into predictive bits that hint at a problem, AI is gradually reshaping care in ways that matter (Antonoli et al., 2023). As an example, in oncology, catching cancer early changes everything. Researchers have found that AI plays a role in handling difficult cases, for example lung cancer which is known to be dangerous. It helps to spot pulmonary nodules and suggests that some of them might be related to tumors. Such findings usually help doctors decide on treatment and predict outcomes which often results in fewer deaths. The combining of AI with imaging, overall, marks a big step forward in tackling cancer's many challenges (Qin et al., 2022).

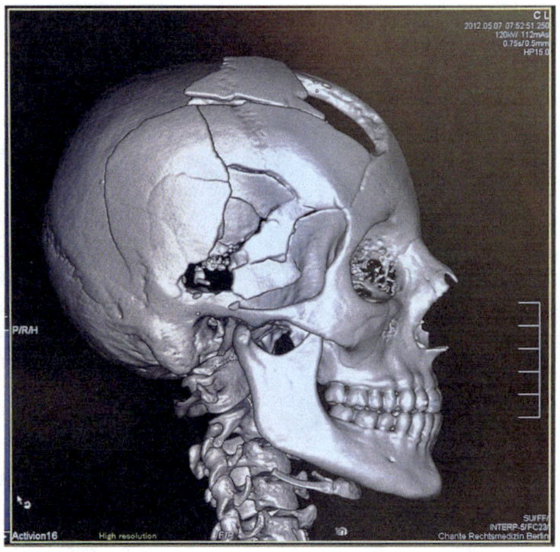

Figure 1.10. Key applications of medical imaging in diagnosis.

Source: By Prof. Dr. Michael Tsokos - Prof. Dr. Michael Tsokos, FAL, https://commons.wikimedia.org/w/index.php?curid=22886395.

Other than AI, the main tools for diagnostic imaging are still X-rays, MRI and CT scans. If you have a broken bone, an X-ray can quickly reveal the problem, but an MRI is better for looking into soft tissue concerns that might not be clear on X-ray images. There are also CT scans which are valued for taking cross-sectional pictures quickly in emergency situations. Combining these methods in daily work proves that a mixed imaging strategy is very important for understanding a patient's condition. In the end, blending the old with the new not only keeps healthcare on its toes but also paves the way for better patient management overall (Antonoli et al., 2023) (Figure 1.10).

1.4.1. Role in Disease Detection

Medical technology improvements have changed how we spot diseases these days. Using imaging, doctors can see inside the body and CT scans, MRI and ultrasound are able to detect small details that might go unnoticed. Take thyroid cancer in the U.S., for example; many experts now point to sharper imaging picking up tiny, local tumors (often leading to what some call overdiagnosis (Kitahara et al., 2022). It proves that these tools can help us notice problems early, but they can also warn us about issues that do not require treatment. It is not limited to detecting cancer early; imaging also lets doctors watch diseases develop and see if the treatment is working. In most cases, in conditions like Alzheimer's, doctors are now leaning on imaging biomarkers to follow the disease's inner workings rather than just its outward signs (Clifford et al., 2018).

By going from checking symptoms to studying the biology, doctors can often intervene earlier. Using several imaging approaches gives a fuller, sometimes confusing, view of a patient's health, so care can be tailored to each individual. Imaging is now used in preventive medicine and public health, as well as its main role. More screening programs are using tools like mammography to flag people at risk even before clear signs show up (Kitahara et al., 2022). As our understanding of illnesses such as Alzheimer's deepens, imaging biomarkers slip into research settings, hinting at a broader shift in detecting diseases in their earliest hints (Clifford et al., 2018). In general, this approach supports both early treatment and ongoing studies to find out why diseases happen which is useful for healthcare.

1.4.2. Use in Treatment Planning

Diagnostic imaging has flipped the script on how we plan treatments in healthcare today. Doctors now use MRI, CT and ultrasound to look inside the body and find out what is happening. Many times, these images are used to help doctors design the right treatment for a patient; for example, oncologists may use them to find the tumor's location and if it is spreading which can lead to surgery, radiation or chemotherapy. Because advanced imaging is so exact, the treatments are often more suitable for the patient which leads to better outcomes and sometimes saves money. AI has played a big role in how this process is carried out. AI algorithms are able to quickly find any tiny issues in images, making image analysis more precise. With AI in the imaging process, doctors can review images more quickly and design treatment plans that are right for each patient. Most of the time, these systems can handle large amounts of data quickly, so decisions are made more accurately and speedily, especially in cases with several conditions. This whole blend of AI and imaging is gradually proving itself vital in boosting diagnostic precision and overall healthcare quality, as several studies suggest (Luís Coelho, 2023). Linking imaging findings with electronic health records (EHRs) stands as another notable leap forward. By integrating in this way, communication between specialists and general practitioners is improved and all team members know what the images mean for the patient. Combining images with a patient's background, lab results and current care plans allows doctors to make plans that handle both urgent and future health concerns. Showing images in this manner helps treatments work better and makes patients feel more satisfied. As the landscape of healthcare continues to shift, the close relationship between imaging and treatment planning remains a key part of truly patient-centered care, playing its role in the ongoing push for better outcomes (Kuwaiti et al., 2023).

1.4.3. Importance in Monitoring Patient Progress

Modern healthcare is a real maze, especially in those high-pressure intensive care units. Imaging tests are important because they show doctors what is happening with a patient at the moment. Easy tests such as bedside ultrasound or CT scans, can detect dangerous problems quickly before they get worse. Many times, these tools go beyond helping with decisions and actually improve the quality of care and reduce the number of deaths. There's no arguing that keeping an eye on patient progress through imaging stands at the heart of effective treatment, even if it might sometimes be overlooked (Rajšić et al., 2021). Then, consider what the COVID-19 crisis taught us. In general, the pandemic revealed that having a timely and accurate diagnosis is very important and delays can completely alter a patient's situation. The crisis not only involved fighting the virus; it also made clear that groups who are marginalized struggled most with access to diagnostic services. Improving access to imaging, therefore, is essential because it helps decisions and treatments happen faster which can save lives. Recent reports even hint that broadening these diagnostic tools could cut down on preventable deaths (Fleming et al., 2021). It seems that technology will play a major role in the future of healthcare. These terms are more than just trends; they're providing new opportunities for patients who are far from medical centers. No matter if tests are simple or involve imaging, these advances can help both patients and providers in ways that were not expected. It is obvious that developing these areas is very important for establishing a strong healthcare system. The mix of cutting-edge imaging with constant patient monitoring helps systems adapt to new threats while working to ensure everyone gets the timely care they need (Fleming et al., 2021; Rajšić et al., 2021) (Figure 1.11).

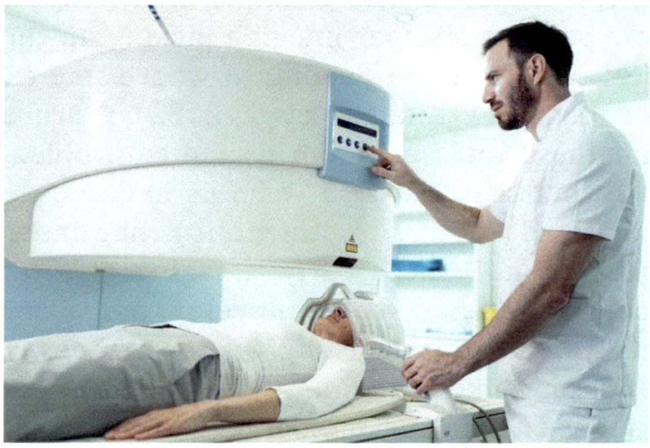

Figure 1.11. Importance in Monitoring Patient Progress.

Source: https://orthomiami.com/wp-content/uploads/2023/11/Can-Diagnostic-Imaging-Help-in-Monitoring-Treatment-Progress.jpg.

Test Your Knowledge

1. How do imaging techniques like X-rays and MRI contribute to the early detection of diseases such as cancer?
2. In what ways do imaging technologies, such as CT scans, assist in planning the precise delivery of radiation therapy for cancer patients?

1.5. Safety and Risks

Learning Outcome

1. Discuss radiation exposure concerns.
2. Define contrast agent reactions.
3. Explain the guidelines for safe imaging practices.

Doctors now use diagnostic imaging to understand many different conditions. It allows doctors to look inside the body in ways that were not possible before, but the use of advanced techniques can also cause some real safety issues, mainly from the ionizing radiation in CT scans and X-rays. When patients are in serious danger, the benefits are usually more important than the risks, but doctors still have to be careful about the possible harm from repeated treatment. Getting too many or too long scans with radiation could result in injuries and, in certain cases, raise the risk of cancer. Good, sensible protocols should be in place so that imaging is only performed when there's a real clinical reason (Wichmann et al., 2020). In general, managing risks well is important for using these technologies and ensuring patient safety. COVID-19 caused complications, proving that diagnostic imaging can sometimes be linked to patient safety concerns. Because of the virus, tests such as echocardiography were now considered ways for the virus to spread, putting both patients and healthcare workers at risk. Due to the increased risk for workers, using proper PPE and sorting imaging requests by risk level and the purpose of the test is very important. In most cases, sticking to infection control guidelines—like those suggested by the American Society of Echocardiography—ensures that imaging keeps going safely while cutting down on exposure risks (Kirkpatrick et al., 2020). By taking such an involved approach, everyone's welfare is supported, even as the world is dealing with a pandemic. Ethics is another major concern and it appears to be just as important as the technical parts. Doctors should balance their kindness with making sure they and their patients are not put in danger. When deciding on imaging tests, ethics helps us determine if the risks are greater than the benefits which was often true during the pandemic. Training staff on the newest safety rules and technology can help patients and manage risks. In general, focusing on ethical practices and patient safety—with a bit of informed decision-making thrown into the mix—plays a huge part in pushing diagnostic imaging forward in modern healthcare (Wichmann et al., 2020) (Figure 1.12).

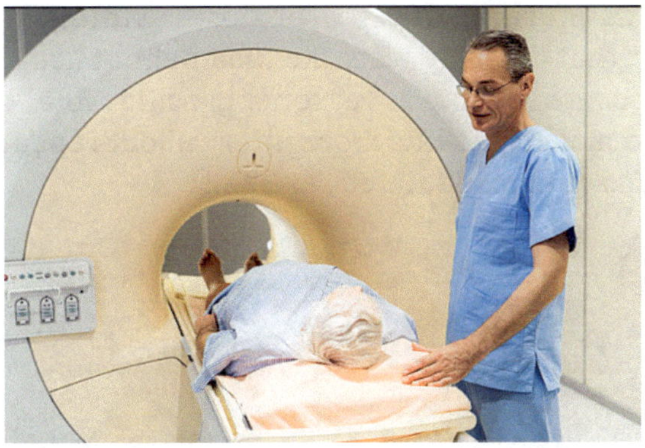

Figure 1.12. Managing risks well is important for using these technologies and ensuring patient safety.

Source: https://domf5oio6qrcr.cloudfront.net/medialibrary/2043/conversions/w1010c16207233089387-thumb.jpg.

1.5.1. Radiation Exposure Concerns

As more people lean on diagnostic scans to get answers about their health, a lively discussion has sprung up about the risks tied to radiation. Many people have to weigh the clear benefits of accurate diagnostics against the concern about exposure to ionizing radiation. Usually, standard radiographs, CT scans and CBCT have different levels of radiation—so it's good to know what the numbers mean. They play a vital role in getting the correct diagnosis, yet they also cause real safety issues. Sometimes, realizing that the radiation level isn't interestingly different from everyday exposure can ease those worries and help patients decide whether a scan is needed (Pereira et al., 2023). Using PET scans along with CT scans is now common in oncology for finding out the stage of a disease and planning treatments. Using these advanced methods requires us to pay attention to both accurate images and the safety of the patient. For hybrid PET/CT imaging, the benefits for diagnosis are clear, but it also adds to the concern about radiation exposure, mainly when contrast media is used. Research shows that using contrast can, in some cases, push radiation doses up by as much as 250% over doses without it, a fact that not only tests the idea behind keeping exposure "as low as reasonably achievable" but also makes patients more jittery about repeated scans (Shamsuddin et al., 2022).

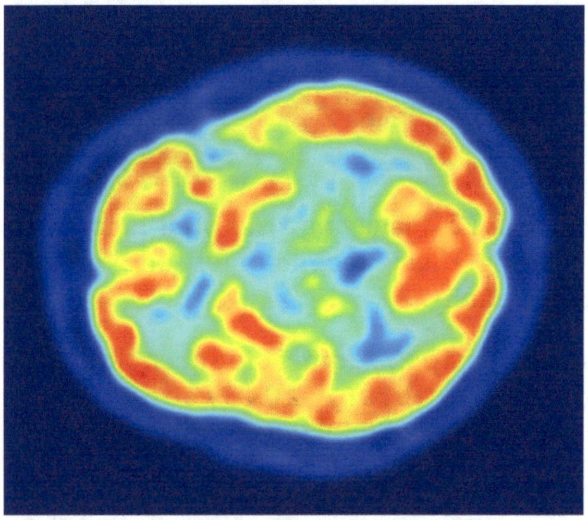

Figure 1.13. Radiation from PET CT scan.

Source: By Jens Maus (http://jens-maus.de/) - Own work, Public Domain, https://commons.wikimedia.org/w/index.php?curid=404690.

Resolving these radiation questions requires learning about the advantages and disadvantages of each imaging method. Doctors should be able to discuss these points in a simple, sometimes relaxed way that helps patients trust them. A major part of this talk focuses on radiation safety guidelines which help both clinicians and patients know what to do. If healthcare providers concentrate on lowering risks, for instance by improving scan settings and sticking to well-tested methods, patients can feel more confident about radiation. At the end of the day, keeping an open and honest dialogue about safety goes a long way in encouraging people to go ahead with these important diagnostic procedures, without letting worry get in the way (Pereira et al., 2023) (Figure 1.13).

1.5.2. Contrast Agent Reactions

Contrast agents improve imaging so that technicians can observe body details more easily on CT and MRI scans. They may cause different reactions in people—sometimes only a mild irritation, but sometimes more significant responses. It is important to know how chemicals and drugs interact with our bodies to prevent risks. Using iodinated media in CT scans has sometimes brought about allergy-like symptoms in a few people which is why doctors usually screen patients and may give them pre-medication if they have a history of sensitivity. Knowing how to handle and predict these reactions is very important for safer imaging which is a sign that imaging practices are always evolving. Nanotechnology has brought in small materials that help with better imaging and more precise treatments. Also, these nanomaterials may cause the immune system to react in unexpected ways. Recent reviews (Patra et al., 2018) show that these nano-sized carriers might sometimes provoke reactions that no one saw coming, which means thorough testing—and a watchful regulatory eye—are absolutely necessary. Researchers must continue to balance making these agents effective and safe which is still a major challenge. In real practice, medical staff should be alert to how patients respond to the contrast agents used. Guidelines and recent literature (Marrero et al., 2018) suggest that traditional checks, like a careful look at patient history, should be combined with the newest insights on contrast media options. Patients must be told about the risks involved so they can choose the right imaging tests. Thanks to advanced imaging and new materials, doctors can find health problems more accurately and prevent serious side effects. An environment that values ongoing awareness (and yes, a bit of unpredictability) not only boosts patient outcomes but also helps build trust—a real win for patient-focused care (Figure 1.14).

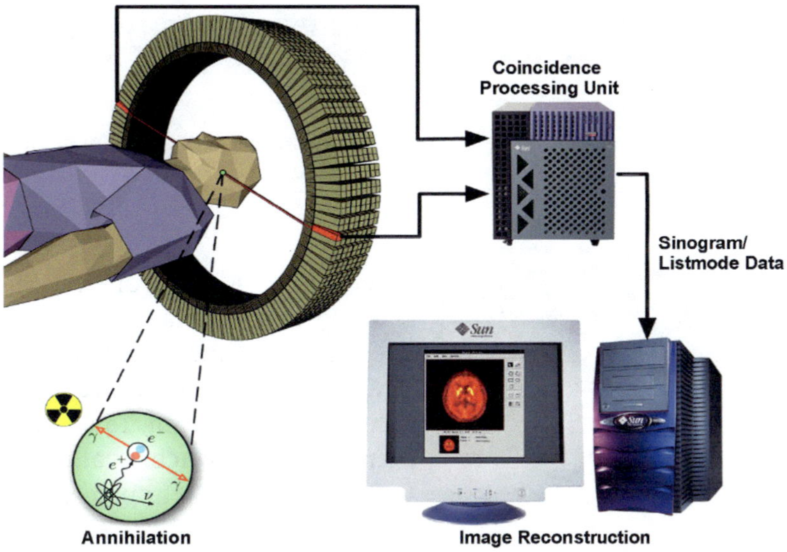

Figure 1.14. Contrast agent, a drug that enhances CT scans, is sometimes skipped because of concerns about side effects.

Source: By Jens Maus (https://jens-maus.de/) - own work - part of master thesishttps://jens-maus.de/ftp/langner_mscthesis.pdfhttps://jens-maus.de/ftp/langner_mscthesis.bib, Public Domain, https://commons.wikimedia.org/w/index.php?curid=401252.

1.5.3. Guidelines for Safe Imaging Practices

Safety is a top issue in diagnostic imaging—patients and care providers alike keep a keen eye on it. These guidelines aren't just rules; they actually protect against the risks that can happen during imaging tests. For example, it is very important to wear personal protective gear during an echocardiogram in situations where the risk is high such as during a pandemic. The American Society of Echocardiography even points out that triaging echo studies based on urgency and patient benefit is a smart move (Kirkpatrick et al., 2020). Such steps ensure that both the practitioner and the patient are safe, since the tests do not endanger public health. It is very important to know about the risks of each imaging method when making decisions. Think about transesophageal echocardiography (TEE)—this one is known for cranking up the risk of aerosol generation, which can be a real headache during infectious outbreaks. This means that, most of the time, deciding whether to use TEE or a transthoracic echo is an important choice. When proper use criteria are followed, the decision process is smoother and unwanted exposure for both patients and staff is kept to a minimum (Prayer et al., 2017). Regular updates and being flexible with new guidelines allow providers to stay aware, since safety is always a priority when public health changes. Every facility should have its own set of practical rules that are right for it. There should be clear rules in hospitals about cleaning imaging equipment to prevent cross-contamination. It matters more because the equipment and settings at each institution can be very different. For example, echo machines must be well-cleaned, especially when they're used on patients with infectious conditions (Kirkpatrick et al., 2020). In addition, having people from various fields join forces can help these safety measures work better, despite some differences in wording or punctuation.

Test Your Knowledge

1. What are the potential health risks associated with radiation exposure during medical imaging procedures?
- What are some common adverse reactions to contrast agents used in medical imaging, and how can they be managed?

1.6. Future Trends in Diagnostic Imaging

Learning Outcome

1. Understand the recent advancements in medical technology and their impact on healthcare.
2. Explore the integration of artificial intelligence in medical diagnostics and treatment.
3. Define Potential for personalized medicine.

There are new developments in diagnostic imaging and AI is playing a role that is already affecting how we look after patients. AI is being used in imaging devices to help find diseases by going through a lot of data and noticing patterns that are difficult for humans to spot. So, it gives us a better chance to find illnesses early, treat patients more individually and avoid mistakes caused by humans reading the data. As these new tools become more common, healthcare providers will need to deal with ethical matters, privacy issues and always ensure that humans are in charge. Addressing these matters is key not just for upgrading imaging practices but also for keeping AI as a helpful partner in clinical settings (Alowais et al., 2023). In the future, wireless technology will play a big role in diagnostic imaging. Many believe that 6th-generation (6G) systems, expected sometime between 2027 and 2030, will dramatically improve data transmission—higher bandwidth, lower latency, and a boost in overall service quality are on the horizon. Generally, these improvements may assist with using tele-radiology and remote diagnostics in the future. In reality, this would allow healthcare professionals to care for patients remotely which helps more people receive quality care. It is not just a tech upgrade; it signals a shift that could lessen the geographic limits that have long kept top-notch imaging out of reach for many (Chowdhury et al., 2020).

Combining AI with advanced wireless systems could change how diagnostic imaging is done. We are moving toward a model where cloud computing, big data analysis and learning algorithms are all used to keep improving our techniques. These directions could improve how work is done, encourage specialists to cooperate and help predict what healthcare will look like in the future. With time, these improvements should help imaging be more accurate and also encourage more preventive care. In most cases, keeping up with these evolving trends is crucial for professionals and institutions aiming to stay at the forefront of diagnostic excellence, ensuring that patient care grows right along with our technological strides (Alowais et al., 2023) (Figure 1.15).

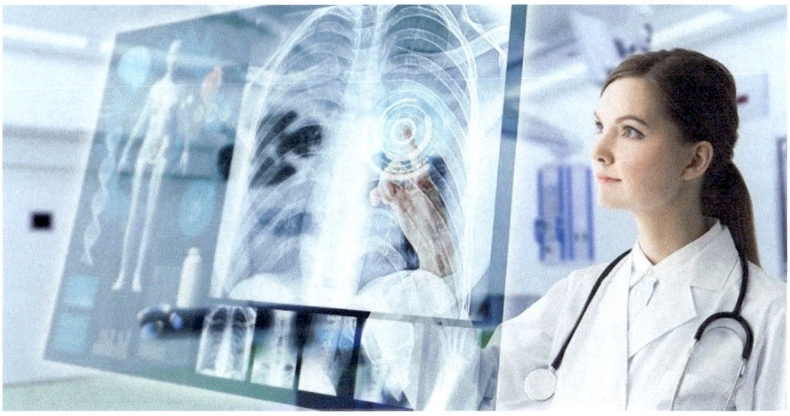

Figure 1.15. Future Trends in Diagnostic Imaging.

Source: https://www.astermedicalimaging.com/images/blog-images/emerging-techniques-inner.png.

1.6.1. Advancements in Technology

Diagnostic imaging has flipped the script over the past few years, shaking up our whole approach to diagnosing illnesses. Digital pathology has made cancer detection faster and more accurate. Using digital imaging and AI together is now common in histopathology and it allows pathologists to investigate difficult cases and improve precision medicine. Take, for example, automated whole slide imaging scanners. They manage to take very detailed pictures of whole glass slides and combine anatomy, medicine and molecular details into a single report. This big shift not only improves the diagnostic accuracy but also smoothens the day-to-day workflow in clinics (Shafi et al., 2023). At the same time, digital pathology was developing, other medical imaging methods were also changing, giving us more tools to address different health problems. Now, with CT scans, MRIs and PET scans, we can see inside the body in ways that were not possible before, even for problems like heart or brain disorders. New hybrid methods, like PET/CT—and don't forget the emerging three-dimensional ultrasound computed tomography (3D USCT)—serve up images with extra crispness and detail, sometimes in ways that even surprise us. Generally, clinicians believe these advances help them make more accurate diagnoses and move quickly to interventions and treatment planning. It is a clear sign that technology and patient care are moving closer together, one image at a time (Hussain et al., 2022).

There are so many exciting things ahead for diagnostic imaging. New technologies could bring about clearer images and also introduce new ways to handle complicated medical data. AI is now being used more often in medical imaging which could lead to faster detection of abnormalities by radiologists. As imaging tools advance and sometimes in unexpected ways, we might soon have real-time diagnostics that give immediate insights in busy clinics. Ultimately, all these innovations are set to rewrite the healthcare playbook, ensuring that diagnostic imaging stays at the heart of boosting patient outcomes while fueling deeper research into a variety of conditions (Hussain et al., 2022; Shafi et al., 2023) (Figure 1.16).

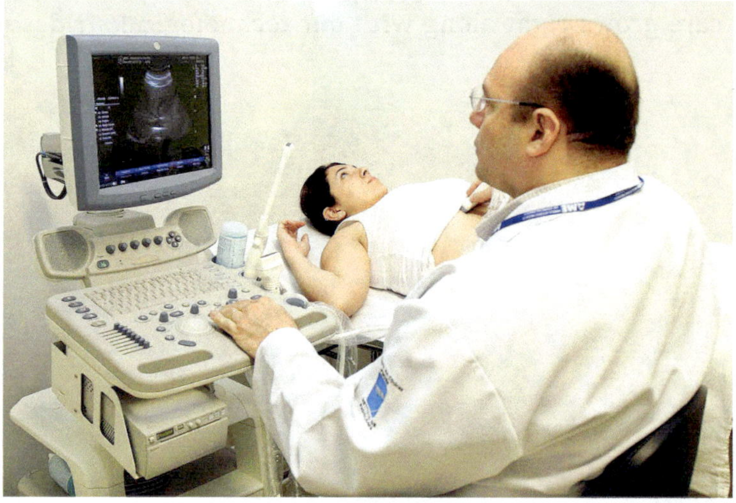

Figure 1.16. 3D Ultrasound tomography (UST) scanner.

Source: By Leval - Own work, Public Domain, https://commons.wikimedia.org/w/index.php?curid=3349818.

1.6.2. Integration of Artificial Intelligence (AI)

AI is shaking things up in diagnostic imaging—a real game changer for healthcare. Medical images are becoming more complex which means doctors need to make diagnoses more quickly and accurately. AI tools are now assisting radiologists and radiographers by finding important details in images which helps them work more efficiently and possibly achieve better outcomes for patients. (Rainey et al., 2021) reminds us that even though AI tech has come a long way, everyday use in clinics is still lagging. Most of the hesitation comes from people not wanting to disrupt their current work and deal with adding new systems to old ones. It is obvious that these issues must be solved so that AI can eventually perform well in healthcare, helping patients and making the system more efficient. For AI to help in these fields, healthcare professionals must be very familiar with it. Even if many agree that AI holds a lot of promise, a survey of UK radiographers, as noted in Rainey et al. (2021), showed a surprisingly big gap in the confidence and knowledge needed to use AI tools. Because these tools are unfamiliar, they might not be used effectively which could result in fewer chances to improve. In most cases, addressing these learning gaps seems essential. Special training programs can assist radiographers in gaining the skills required which leads to a more skilled and comfortable workforce using these new technologies. Teaching people about AI is important as we get closer to a future where AI will have a bigger role. Looking at the overall impact, AI is not only about making radiology work more efficient—it could lead to a new approach to diagnosing conditions. Seong Mun et al. (2021) point out that AI could eventually tie together info from radiology, pathology, and even genomics, which might just revolutionize patient management. This approach promises many benefits, but it also brings some problems. Radiology is still working on finding stable business approaches and proving that AI tools help doctors in their work. The main thing is for tech experts and healthcare providers to truly work together. Together, they can unlock what AI has to offer, positioning diagnostic imaging as a cornerstone of modern healthcare that can handle the many modifications and turns of patient needs (Figure 1.17).

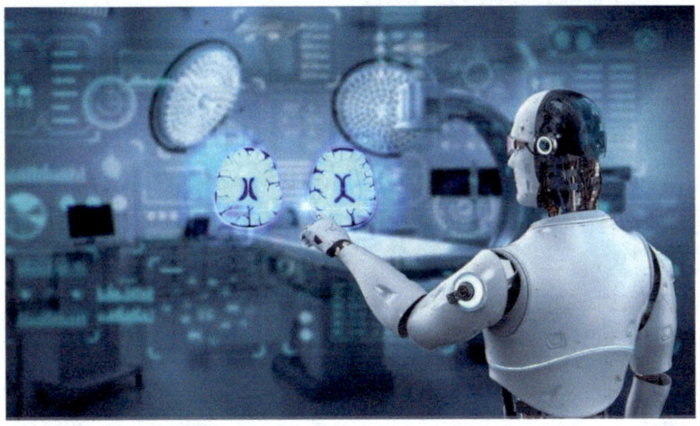

Figure 1.17. AI is shaking things up in diagnostic imaging—a real game changer for healthcare.

Source: https://media.licdn.com/dms/image/v2/D5612AQFUCMpOVsZt7A/article-cover_image-shrink_720_1280/article-cover_image-shrink_720_1280/0/1694956022027?e=2147483647&v=beta&t=-sWu6ixAXjnWgPWeOrwB8PMm5ykaDo2H2WU_yVbM1uA.

1.6.3. Potential for Personalized Medicine

Breakthroughs in imaging are changing how we think about personalized care. Modern machines are used for more than just making pretty pictures – they provide insights that are much deeper than what traditional tests offer. Many doctors are choosing to use advanced scans like MRI and PET which can detect details about tumors and other diseases that were not visible before. Most of the time, this new method both improves diagnosis and helps create individualized treatment plans for patients. With better imaging technology, more patient data is being used to guide decisions which helps patients receive better, more personalized care. AI is now being used to help interpret the huge amount of imaging data. AI can spot patterns that humans might not see right away which is like having a helpful assistant who quickly detects any unusual signs – this is especially useful for problems such as cancer or heart problems. Most of the time, AI is now combining lots of data and helping doctors design treatment plans that fit each patient. In general, this digital partner helps doctors gain better understanding of images and also promotes care based on solid evidence. Of course, challenges remain – ethical concerns, data safety, and the need for human oversight are still very much part of the mix (Alowais et al., 2023). Combining detailed pictures with tailored care gives patients new opportunities to be involved. Sharing easy-to-understand imaging results allows patients to understand their health more clearly which can improve their trust and increase their chances of sticking to treatment. And with new tools like ChatGPT coming into play, there's even more potential for improving health literacy and personal learning about medical care (Sallam, 2023). Often, being aware of the details of their diagnosis encourages people to be more involved in their care which can help them feel better. In general, using advanced imaging, personalized medicine and honest patient conversations is helping healthcare become more complete and modern—even if it sometimes causes a few problems.

Test Your Knowledge

1. How does prolonged radiation exposure during medical procedures potentially impact human health?
2. What are the key steps to take if a patient experiences an allergic reaction to a contrast agent during imaging?

Summary

Diagnostic imaging keeps changing as tech moves forward. MRI, CT scans and similar tools have brought about big changes in how we detect and treat health problems. Future healthcare workers should learn not only how the devices function, but also how they will be used and what ethical issues they bring. If people really grasp what imaging is capable of, they are in a stronger position to manage the real-world problems in modern medicine. AI makes the imaging process more unpredictable when it joins the team. Even though smarter machines can help with diagnosis, some people are not sure if we can always trust them or if we should always involve a human. It is generally necessary to understand these technology changes well. It is usually important for schools to teach students both practical skills and how to understand and work with the amazing results from AI, so that healthcare teams can handle both technology and its uniqueness. The future of diagnostic imaging looks bright if we handle things correctly. Normally, achieving those big technology advances involves being cautious and ethical. It is now thought that using blockchain for traceability could help ensure both improved quality and safety. Overall, investing in both new tech frameworks and smart teaching strategies is key to moving diagnostic imaging forward, leading to a healthcare system that's more nimble and patient-focused (Dasaklis et al., 2022; Holmes et al., 2023).

Adhering to established guidelines is key in diagnostic imaging—getting it right means better care for patients. Craniosynostosis is a good example; the guidelines keep shifting as more studies and clinical experiences appear. The Dutch Society for Plastic and Reconstructive Surgery kicked off a revision by pulling together a broad mix of evidence from medical literature and even weighing what patients think (Mathijssen, 2020). They used the latest research and better ways to detect problems during pregnancy to make diagnosis more accurate and referrals easier which benefited children with the condition. Keeping up with new imaging standards improves the quality of images and makes it easier to look after patients. People who read these images in healthcare must use both their technical knowledge and clinical understanding. Ultrasound, X-ray and 3D CT scans all have special strengths and weaknesses in finding craniosynostosis. Understanding these differences, even in subtle ways, helps nail an accurate diagnosis and shape treatment plans that tend to lead to better surgical results (Mach et al., 2019). Ultrasound is commonly used to check infants and 3D CT scans are used when more detail is needed for further evaluation. If issues are found quickly and patients are referred promptly, they will not have to wait for care. The values and preferences of patients must always be considered. Many parents prefer to get quick and accurate assessments at local healthcare centers which highlights the importance of good referral systems and teamwork among clinicians. The real challenge is balancing these patient desires with the more comprehensive checks that tricky cases might demand (Mathijssen, 2020). Usually, these guidelines are built on scientific proof, the newest imaging methods and focusing on what is best for the patient. This mix helps both guide care and help healthcare providers stay current with new guidelines, even when the process is sometimes messy.

KEY TERMS FROM THIS CHAPTER

- 3D imaging
- CT scan (computed tomography)
- Fluoroscopy
- Interventional radiology
- PET scan (positron emission tomography)
- Ultrasound
- Contrast media
- Digital imaging
- Image-guided surgery
- MRI (magnetic resonance imaging)
- Radiology
- X-ray

Critical Thinking Questions

1. **Who is credited with the discovery of X-rays, marking the beginning of diagnostic imaging?**
   a. Marie Curie
   b. Wilhelm Conrad Roentgen
   c. Thomas Edison
   d. Alexander Fleming
2. **In what year were X-rays discovered?**
   a. 1885
   b. 1895
   c. 1901
   d. 1915
3. **Which of the following imaging techniques uses ionizing radiation to create images of the body?**
   a. MRI
   b. Ultrasound
   c. CT Scan
   d. PET Scan
4. **What is the primary advantage of Magnetic Resonance Imaging (MRI) over X-rays?**
   a. Lower cost
   b. Faster imaging
   c. Better soft tissue contrast
   d. Use of ionizing radiation
5. **What substance is often used in diagnostic imaging to improve the visibility of internal structures?**
   a. Anesthetic
   b. Contrast agent
   c. Antibiotic
   d. Saline solution

Short Answer Questions

1. Who is known as a pioneer in the field of diagnostic imaging and what did they do that was especially important?
2. State what three types of diagnostic imaging are commonly used and what they are used for.
3. What basic idea does X-ray imaging use to form pictures of the body?
4. What is the usual role of MRI in medical diagnostics and what is better about it than a CT scan?
5. What are some risks that can happen if a person is exposed to diagnostic imaging such as X-rays and CT scans, many times?
6. Which new advancement or trend is coming to diagnostic imaging and how might it support better care for patients?

Answers to Critical Thinking Questions

1. (b); 2. (b); 3. (c); 4. (c); 5. (b)

References

1. Al Kuwaiti, A., Nazer, K., Alreedy, A. H., AlShehri, S. D., Almuhanna, A., Subbarayalu, A. V., Al Muhanna, D., et al. (2023). A review of the role of artificial intelligence in healthcare. *Journal of Personalized Medicine, 13*, 951. https://doi.org/10.3390/jpm13060951.
2. Alowais, S. A., Alghamdi, S. S., Alsuhebany, N., Alqahtani, T., Alshaya, A., Almohareb, S. N., Aldairem, A., et al. (2023). Revolutionizing healthcare: The role of artificial intelligence in clinical practice. *BMC Medical Education, 23*, Article 698. https://doi.org/10.1186/s12909-023-04698-z.
3. Ayo-Farai, O., Olaide, B. A., Maduka, C. P., & Okongwu, C. C. (2023). Engineering innovations in healthcare: A review of developments in the USA. *Engineering Science & Technology Journal, 4*(6), 381–400. https://doi.org/10.51594/estj.v4i6.638.
4. Bowlus, C. L., Arrivé, L., Bergquist, A., Deneau, M., Forman, L., Ilyas, S. I., Lunsford, K. E., et al. (2022). AASLD practice guidance on primary sclerosing cholangitis and cholangiocarcinoma. *Hepatology, 77*, 659–702. https://doi.org/10.1002/hep.32771.
5. Buchbinder, R., Underwood, M., Hartvigsen, J., & Maher, C. G. (2020). The Lancet Series call to action to reduce low value care for low back pain: An update. *Pain, 161*(Suppl 1), S57–S64. https://doi.org/10.1097/j.pain.0000000000001869.
6. Chia, D. M., Hameed, M., Ugande, A. A., & Wuave, R. B. (2023). Pattern of head computed tomography requests, common indications and findings at a tertiary health center in North-Central Nigeria. *EAS Journal of Radiology and Imaging Technology*. https://www.semanticscholar.org/paper/eb91214c009f2593b2e74dd52898f132d94bc256 (accessed on 23 May 2025).
7. Chowdhury, M. Z., Shahjalal, M., Ahmed, S., & Jang, Y. M. (2020). 6G wireless communication systems: Applications, requirements, technologies, challenges, and research directions. *IEEE Open Journal of the Communications Society, 1*, 957–975. https://doi.org/10.1109/ojcoms.2020.3010270.
8. Coelho, L. (2023). How artificial intelligence is shaping medical imaging technology: A survey of innovations and applications. *Bioengineering, 10*(12), Article 1435. https://doi.org/10.3390/bioengineering10121435.
9. Cook, G., & Goh, V. (2020). Molecular imaging of bone metastases and their response to therapy. *Journal of Nuclear Medicine, 61*(6), 799–806. https://doi.org/10.2967/jnumed.119.234260.
10. Cosentino, F., Grant, P. J., Aboyans, V., Bailey, C. J., Ceriello, A., Delgado, V., Federici, M., et al. (2019). 2019 ESC Guidelines on diabetes, pre-diabetes, and cardiovascular diseases developed in collaboration with the EASD. *European Heart Journal, 41*, 255–323. https://doi.org/10.1093/eurheartj/ehz486.
11. Cruz-Jentoft, A. J., Bahat, G., Bauer, J. M., Boirie, Y., Bruyère, O., Cederholm, T., Cooper, C., et al. (2018). Sarcopenia: Revised European consensus on definition and diagnosis. *Age and Ageing, 48*, 16–31. https://doi.org/10.1093/ageing/afy169.
12. D'Antonoli, T. A., Stanzione, A., Bluethgen, C., Vernuccio, F., Ugga, L., Klontzas, M. E., Cuocolo, R., et al. (2023). Large language models in radiology: Fundamentals, applications, ethical considerations, risks, and future directions. *Diagnostic and Interventional Radiology, 30*(1), 80–90. https://doi.org/10.4274/dir.2023.232417.
13. Dasaklis, T. K., Voutsinas, T. G., Tsoulfas, G. T., & Casino, F. (2022). A systematic literature

review of blockchain-enabled supply chain traceability implementations. *Sustainability, 14*(4), Article 2439. https://doi.org/10.3390/su14042439.

14. Dash, S., Shakyawar, S. K., Sharma, L., & Kaushik, S. (2019). Big data in healthcare: Management, analysis and future prospects. *Journal of Big Data, 6*, Article 54. https://doi.org/10.1186/s40537-019-0217-0.
15. Fleming, K. A., Horton, S., Wilson, M. L., Atun, R., DeStigter, K., Flanigan, J., Sayed, S., et al. (2021). The Lancet Commission on diagnostics: Transforming access to diagnostics. *The Lancet, 398*(10315), 1997–2050. https://doi.org/10.1016/s0140-6736(21)00673-5.
16. Ghaderzadeh, M., Asadi, F., Hosseini, A., Bashash, D., Abolghasemi, H., & Roshanpour, A. (2021). Machine learning in detection and classification of leukemia using smear blood images: A systematic review. *Scientific Programming, 2021*, Article 9933481. https://doi.org/10.1155/2021/9933481.
17. Haneder, S., Kucharczyk, W., Schönberg, S., & Michaely, H. (2015). Safety of magnetic resonance contrast media: A review with special focus on nephrogenic systemic fibrosis. *Topics in Magnetic Resonance Imaging, 24*(2), 57–65. https://www.semanticscholar.org/paper/8b75a762b255b10b1ad2727d00d5bcf0b29e09ae (accessed on 23 May 2025).
18. Harry, A. (2023). The future of medicine: Harnessing the power of AI for revolutionizing healthcare. *International Journal of Multidisciplinary Sciences and Arts, 2*(1), 36–47. https://doi.org/10.47709/ijmdsa.v2i1.2395.
19. Haugen, B. R., Alexander, E. K., Bible, K. C., Doherty, G. M., Mandel, S. J., Nikiforov, Y. E., Pacini, F., et al. (2015). 2015 American Thyroid Association management guidelines for adult patients with thyroid nodules and differentiated thyroid cancer. *Thyroid, 26*, 1–133. https://doi.org/10.1089/thy.2015.0020.
20. Heiß, R., Nagel, A. M., Laun, F. B., Uder, M., & Bickelhaupt, S. (2021). Low-field magnetic resonance imaging. *Investigative Radiology, 56*(11), 726–733. https://doi.org/10.1097/rli.0000000000000805.
21. Hilgerink, M. P., Hummel, J. M., IJzerman, M. J., & Manohar, S. (2011). Assessment of the added value of the Twente Photoacoustic Mammoscope in breast cancer diagnosis. https://core.ac.uk/download/pdf/11481011.pdf.
22. Holmes, W., Bialik, M., & Fadel, C. (2023). Artificial intelligence in education. In *Data Ethics: Building Trust: How Digital Technologies Can Serve Humanity* (pp. 621–653). Globethics Publications.
23. Hussain, S., Mubeen, I., Ullah, N., Shah, S. S. U. D., Khan, B. A., Zahoor, M., Ullah, R., et al. (2022). Modern diagnostic imaging technique applications and risk factors in the medical field: A review. *BioMed Research International, 2022*, Article 5164970. https://doi.org/10.1155/2022/5164970.
24. Islam, S., Al Nasim, M. A., Hossain, I., Ullah, M. A., Datta, K., Monjur, M., et al. (2023). Introduction of medical imaging modalities. https://www.semanticscholar.org/paper/e481bc94be41f9e10ce7b77f704b1eacfe7a66e2 (accessed on 23 May 2025).
25. Jack, C. R., Bennett, D. A., Blennow, K., Carrillo, M. C., Dunn, B., Budd Haeberlein, S., Holtzman, D. M., et al. (2018). NIA-AA research framework: Toward a biological definition of Alzheimer's disease. *Alzheimer's & Dementia, 14*, 535–562. https://doi.org/10.1016/j.jalz.2018.02.018.

26. Jain, D., Torres, R., Celli, R., Koelmel, J. P., Charkoftaki, G., & Vasiliou, V. (2020). Evolution of the liver biopsy and its future. *Translational Gastroenterology and Hepatology, 6*, 20. https://doi.org/10.21037/tgh.2020.04.01.

27. Kassubek, J., & Müller, H. P. (2020). Advanced neuroimaging approaches in amyotrophic lateral sclerosis: Refining the clinical diagnosis. *Expert Review of Neurotherapeutics, 20*(3), 237–249. https://doi.org/10.1080/14737175.2020.1715798.

28. Kirkpatrick, J. N., Mitchell, C., Taub, C., Kort, S., Hung, J., & Swaminathan, M. (2020). ASE statement on protection of patients and echocardiography service providers during the 2019 novel coronavirus outbreak: Endorsed by the American College of Cardiology. *Journal of the American Society of Echocardiography, 33*(6), 648–653. https://doi.org/10.1016/j.echo.2020.04.001.

29. Kitahara, C. M., & Schneider, A. B. (2022). Epidemiology of thyroid cancer. *Cancer Epidemiology, Biomarkers & Prevention, 31*, 1284–1297. https://doi.org/10.1158/1055-9965.EPI-21-1440.

30. Leening, M., Vedder, M., Witteman, J., Pencina, M., & Steyerberg, E. (2014). Net reclassification improvement: Computation, interpretation, and controversies. *Annals of Internal Medicine, 160*(2), 122–131. https://www.semanticscholar.org/paper/958c1d2bdfb450b8ca2150e953 63c3e06db6ed16 (accessed on 23 May 2025).

31. Liebschner, D., Afonine, P. V., Baker, M. L., Bunkóczi, G., Chen, V. B., Croll, T. I., Hintze, B. J., et al. (2019). Macromolecular structure determination using X-rays, neutrons and electrons: Recent developments in *Phenix*. *Acta Crystallographic Section D: Structural Biology, 75*, 861–877. https://doi.org/10.1107/S2059798319011471.

32. Lundervold, A. S., & Lundervold, A. (2018). An overview of deep learning in medical imaging focusing on MRI. *Zeitschrift für Medizinische Physik, 29*, 102–127. https://doi.org/10.1016/j.zemedi.2018.11.002.

33. Lyon, A. R., López-Fernández, T., Couch, L. S., Asteggiano, R., Aznar, M. C., Bergler-Klein, J., Boriani, G., et al. (2022). 2022 ESC Guidelines on cardio-oncology developed in collaboration with the European Hematology Association (EHA), the European Society for Therapeutic Radiology and Oncology (ESTRO), and the International Cardio-Oncology Society (IC-OS). *European Heart Journal, 43*, 4229–4361. https://doi.org/10.1093/eurheartj/ehac244.

34. Mach, F., Baigent, C., Catapano, A. L., Koskinas, K. C., Casula, M., Badimón, L., Chapman, M. J., et al. (2019). 2019 ESC/EAS Guidelines for the management of dyslipidemias: Lipid modification to reduce cardiovascular risk. *European Heart Journal, 41*, 111–188. https://doi.org/10.1093/eurheartj/ehz455.

35. Malinger, G., Paladini, D., Krajden Haratz, K., Monteagudo, A., Pilu, G., & Timor-Tritsch, I. E. (2020). ISUOG Practice Guidelines (updated): Sonographic examination of the fetal central nervous system. Part 1: Performance of screening examination and indications for targeted neurosonography. *Ultrasound in Obstetrics & Gynecology, 56*(3), 476–484. https://doi.org/10.1002/uog.22145.

36. Marrero, J. A., Kulik, L., Sirlin, C. B., Zhu, A. X., Finn, R. S., Abécassis, M., Roberts, L. R., et al. (2018). Diagnosis, staging, and management of hepatocellular carcinoma: 2018 practice guidance by the American Association for the Study of Liver Diseases. *Hepatology, 68*(2), 723–750. https://doi.org/10.1002/hep.29913.

37. Mathijssen, I. M. J. (2020). Updated guideline on treatment and management of craniosynostosis. *Journal of Craniofacial Surgery, 32*(2), 371–450. https://doi.org/10.1097/scs.0000000000007035.

38. Mun, S. K., Wong, K. H., Lo, S. C. B., Li, Y., & Bayarsaikhan, S. (2021). Artificial intelligence for the future radiology diagnostic service. *Frontiers in Molecular Biosciences, 7*, Article 614258. https://doi.org/10.3389/fmolb.2020.614258.

39. Patra, J. K., Das, G., Fraceto, L. F., Campos, E. V. R., Rodriguez-Torres, M. P., Acosta-Torres, L. S., Díaz-Torres, L. A., et al. (2018). Nano based drug delivery systems: Recent developments and future prospects. *Journal of Nanobiotechnology, 16*, Article 71. https://doi.org/10.1186/s12951-018-0392-8.

40. Pereira, R., Sabri, H., Pereira, P., & Wang, H. (2023). Associated risks with periodontal X-rays or CBCT scans, are there any? *Clinical Advances in Periodontics*. https://www.semanticscholar.org/paper/15b8d4dd606ca90fce9c546e49d8bc00c2f13a8d (accessed on 23 May 2025).

41. Perkins, R. B., Guido, R. S., Castle, P. E., Chelmow, D., Einstein, M. H., García, F., Huh, W. K., et al. (2020). 2019 ASCCP risk-based management consensus guidelines for abnormal cervical cancer screening tests and cancer precursors. *Journal of Lower Genital Tract Disease, 24*(2), 102–131. https://doi.org/10.1097/lgt.0000000000000525.

42. Prayer, D., Malinger, G., Brugger, P. C., Cassady, C. I., De Catte, L., De Keersmaecker, B., Fernandes, G. L., et al. (2017). ISUOG practice guidelines: Performance of fetal magnetic resonance imaging. *Ultrasound in Obstetrics and Gynecology, 49*, 671–680. https://doi.org/10.1002/uog.17412.

43. Prichard, J., & Brass, L. (1992). New anatomical and functional imaging methods. *Annals of Neurology, 32*. https://www.semanticscholar.org/paper/ea1dbeb74b7205f22372d9f1d5906f84f65e553d (accessed on 23 May 2025).

44. Qin, P., Luo, Y., Chen, Y., Li, J., Xie, D., & Ye, T. (2022). Artificial intelligence in clinical applications for lung cancer: Diagnosis, treatment and prognosis. *Clinical Chemistry and Laboratory Medicine (CCLM), 60*(12), 1974–1983. https://doi.org/10.1515/cclm-2022-0291.

45. Rainey, C., O'Regan, T., Matthew, J., Skelton, E., Woznitza, N., Chu, K. Y., Goodman, S., et al. (2021). Beauty is in the AI of the beholder: Are we ready for the clinical integration of artificial intelligence in radiography? *Frontiers in Digital Health, 3*, Article 739327. https://doi.org/10.3389/fdgth.2021.739327.

46. Rajšić, S., Breitkopf, R., Bachler, M., & Treml, B. (2021). Diagnostic modalities in critical care: Point-of-care approach. *Diagnostics, 11*(12), Article 2202. https://doi.org/10.3390/diagnostics11122202.

47. Ritchie, M. E., Phipson, B., Wu, D., Hu, Y., Law, C. W., Shi, W., & Smyth, G. K. (2015). lemma powers differential expression analyses for RNA-sequencing and microarray studies. *Nucleic Acids Research, 43*(7), e47. https://doi.org/10.1093/nar/gkv007.

48. Sallam, M. (2023). ChatGPT utility in healthcare education, research, and practice: Systematic review on the promising perspectives and valid concerns. *Healthcare, 11*(6), Article 887. https://doi.org/10.3390/healthcare11060887.

49. Schalock, R. L., Luckasson, R., & Tassé, M. J. (2021). An overview of *Intellectual Disability: Definition, Diagnosis, Classification, and Systems of Supports* (12th ed.). *American Journal on Intellectual and Developmental Disabilities, 126*(6), 439–442. https://doi.org/10.1352/1944-7558-126.6.439.

50. Sedgwick, A. C., Brewster, J. T., Harvey, P. K., Iovan, D. A., Smith, G., He, X. P., Tian, H., et al. (2020). Metal-based imaging agents: Progress towards interrogating neurodegenerative disease. *Chemical Society Reviews, 49*, 2886–2915. https://doi.org/10.1039/c8cs00986d.

51. Senapati, S., Mahanta, A. K., Kumar, S., & Maiti, P. (2018). Controlled drug delivery vehicles for cancer treatment and their performance. *Signal Transduction and Targeted Therapy, 3*, Article 7. https://doi.org/10.1038/s41392-017-0004-3.

52. Shafi, S., & Parwani, A. V. (2023). Artificial intelligence in diagnostic pathology. *Diagnostic Pathology, 18*, Article 61. https://doi.org/10.1186/s13000-023-01375-z.

53. Shamsuddin, N. S., Sudin, A. E. L. T., Mohamad, N. S., Abdul Razak, H. R., & Mansor, M. S. (2022). Comparing radiation dose between contrast-enhanced and non-contrast-enhanced CTAC acquisition in 18F-FDG-PET/CT examination. *Health and Wellness II*. https://www.semanticscholar.org/paper/77c97e55a79416c1c0f88b4664b481c216991e20 (accessed on 23 May 2025).

54. Soxibova, Z. R., & Nasriddinov, B. Z. (2023). Ultrasound examination as an important part of clinical diagnostics. https://core.ac.uk/download/612988262.pdf (accessed on 23 May 2025).

55. Wichmann, D., Sperhake, J. P., Lütgehetmann, M., Steurer, S., Edler, C., Heinemann, A., Heinrich, F., et al. (2020). Autopsy findings and venous thromboembolism in patients with COVID-19. *Annals of Internal Medicine, 173*, 268–277. https://doi.org/10.7326/M20-2003.

56. Williams, B., Mancia, G., Spiering, W., Rosei, E. A., Azizi, M., Burnier, M., Clement, D. L., et al. (2018). 2018 ESC/ESH Guidelines for the management of arterial hypertension. *European Heart Journal, 39*, 3021–3104. https://doi.org/10.1093/eurheartj/ehy339.

57. Yang, Q., Yan, P., Zhang, Y., Yu, H., Shi, Y., Mou, X., Kalra, M. K., et al. (2018). Low-dose CT image denoising using a generative adversarial network with Wasserstein distance and perceptual loss. *IEEE Transactions on Medical Imaging, 37*(6), 1348–1357. https://doi.org/10.1109/tmi.2018.2827462.

58. Zeppenfeld, K., Tfelt-Hansen, J., Riva, M., Winkel, B. G., Behr, E. R., Blom, N. A., Charron, P., et al. (2022). 2022 ESC guidelines for the management of patients with ventricular arrhythmias and the prevention of sudden cardiac death. *European Heart Journal, 43*(40), 3997–4126. https://doi.org/10.1093/eurheartj/ehac262.

59. Zhang, D., Ma, Z., Gong, R., Lian, L., Li, Y., He, Z., Han, Y., et al. (2024). Using natural language processing (GPT-4) for computed tomography image analysis of cerebral hemorrhages in radiology: Retrospective analysis. *Journal of Medical Internet Research, 26*. https://www.semanticscholar.org/paper/525929e9d10551438464f32ee4f6b70712e5830d (accessed on 23 May 2025).

RADIOGRAPHIC IMAGING (X-RAYS)

2

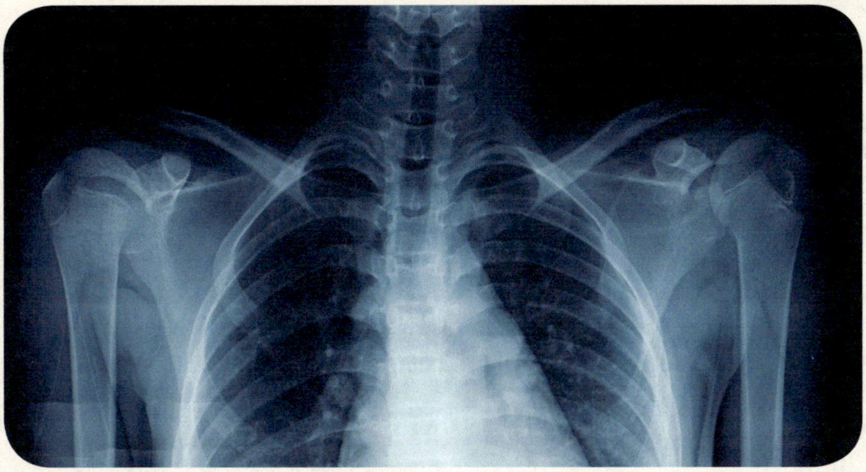

LEARNING OBJECTIVES

After studying this chapter, you will be able to:

1. Understand the fundamental principles of X-ray imaging.
2. Identify and describe the various types of X-ray imaging.
3. Explore the different medical applications of X-ray imaging.
4. Define the safety and risks of X-ray imaging.
5. Examine recent advancements in X-ray technology and their impact on diagnostics.
6. Understand the ethical considerations.

Introduction

Medical imaging has come a long way, changing how doctors see inside our bodies without the need for surgery. X-ray technology, for instance, uses the fact that different tissues soak up radiation at different rates to deliver pictures that show bone strength, soft tissue differences, and other health issues. In places like orthopedics, dentistry, and emergency settings—where a quick, reliable look inside is crucial—this non-invasive approach has become a real game changer. The shift to digital radiography has pushed things even further, making images crisper and helping patient care overall. Ultimately, knowing how X-rays work remains vital for both clinicians and patients, since it sits at the very core of modern medical practice. Striking the right balance between getting a high-quality image and keeping radiation doses low is key when using radiographic methods. Practitioners generally follow the "As Low As Reasonably Achievable" (ALARA) principle—a guideline that pushes for minimal radiation exposure while still securing useful diagnostic details. Interestingly, research shows that increasing the source-to-image distance (SID) can improve image detail and cut down the effective dose by about 19.2% to 23.9% (Bath et al., 2013). These findings, in most cases, urge those in the field to update their techniques and routines occasionally, so that practices stay both safe and effective. A mix of refined methods and clear guidelines on SID adjustments truly helps keep radiographic work balanced. The rapid strides in digital radiography have opened up a range of new possibilities that keep transforming diagnostic processes. Take, for example, studies on the equine foot—where the need for multiple views has been eased by advanced image processing techniques, reducing both study times and patient radiation exposure (Whitlock et al., 2016). The power to tweak images after they're taken not only improves diagnostic clarity but also minimizes extra radiation risks. This trend shows a clear shift from routine practices to more efficient, flexible approaches as technology and clinical needs evolve—often in surprising ways. In most cases, such changes highlight the importance of ongoing training and a fresh look at techniques, even if the updates sometimes come with small imperfections leading to a slightly uneven style in the way we describe these processes.

Definition of Radiographic Imaging

Seeing inside an object without breaking it open has changed the game in so many areas like medicine and industrial testing. X-rays, for example, serve as the backbone of what we now call radiographic imaging. Radiologists and technicians can snap pictures of a body's inner workings or the hidden layers of different materials, pulling out details that would otherwise be out of reach. The process is pretty straightforward: X-ray beams are fired at a subject, and the resulting image shows variations in density across different tissues or materials. This naturally helps in flagging issues—fractures, lesions, and other irregularities—while also checking material quality in non-destructive tests (Carpenter et al., 1976). Digital imaging, in most cases, has taken this a step further, sharpening these pictures and boosting overall diagnostic accuracy. At its core, radiographic imaging banks on how X-rays interact differently with diverse densities. As they travel through anything from bone to soft tissue, the rays get absorbed at levels tied to both density and atomic makeup. For instance, denser bone tends to show up as a lighter area, while regions with air or less solid material come off much darker.

These subtle, yet important contrasts give clinicians key insights into physical conditions or structural hiccups. Besides that, the overall picture quality also hinges on how you set things up—the distance from the X-ray source to the subject, and exactly where the detector sits, can seriously impact clarity and minimize distortions (Whitlock et al., 2016). Generally speaking, even slight tweaks in the setup can make all the difference. Radiographic imaging isn't just the domain of hospitals and clinics—it is found a home in many other sectors too. In medicine, besides mapping out the skeletal system and spotting diseases, it even lends a hand during interventions. On the flip side, industries rely on this technique for non-destructive testing, which is crucial when checking the soundness of infrastructure like aircraft or bridges. Both worlds lean on a solid background in X-ray physics and imaging know-how to pinpoint defects and anomalies effectively. With ongoing improvements in computer-aided image analysis, figuring out those complex images has become more refined, leading to better diagnoses and tighter quality controls. Overall, the wide-ranging use of radiographic imaging keeps it at the forefront across many diverse applications (Figure 2.1).

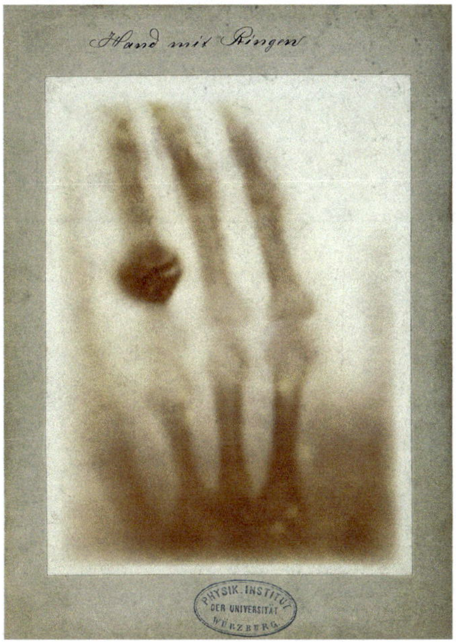

Figure 2.1. Radiographic Imaging.

Source: By Wilhelm Roentgen - Source 1: [1] Source 2: [2], Public Domain, https://commons.wikimedia.org/w/index.php?curid=12354709.

Historical Background of X-Ray Technology

Wilhelm Conrad Rontgen stumbled on X-rays back in 1895, and that single moment ended up shifting how we see inside the body. He was busy exploring cathode rays when, curiously enough, a fluorescent screen lit up even several feet away from an electrified cathode tube. It suddenly hit him that unseen rays could slip through solid objects—a discovery that opened the door to a noninvasive way for doctors to check internal structures. This unexpected tool gave physicians a fresh peek at the inner workings of the human form and sparked improvements in radiographic examinations that kept evolving over the years (Sakano et al., 2021). As the 20th century unfolded, this new imaging tool began to transform medical training almost as much as patient care. Radiological schools popped up, and training programs for radiologic technologists got underway—each step generally speaking aimed at building a workforce that could handle increasingly complex machines. In 1951, the Radiological X-ray Technologist Act was put in place to regulate the practice and set educational standards, underscoring the need for professionals who could guarantee patient safety while managing advanced imaging systems. In most cases, these changes not only cemented the importance of X-ray technology in healthcare but also highlighted that robust educational programs must keep pace with rapid technological progress (Sakano et al., 2021). Today's radiology still carries the legacy of those early experiments. Digital imaging, computed tomography (CT) and magnetic resonance imaging (MRI) have combined in surprising ways to push diagnostic capabilities to new levels. Radiologists now rely on advanced software to polish images and unravel complex data, while the call for skilled technologists remains as strong as ever. Colleges, for instance, have shifted to bachelor's degree programs that aim to equip future experts both with hands-on technical skills and creative problem-solving abilities. This ongoing evolution in education mirrors a global drive to let imaging technology and patient care grow together, step by step (Sakano et al., 2021).

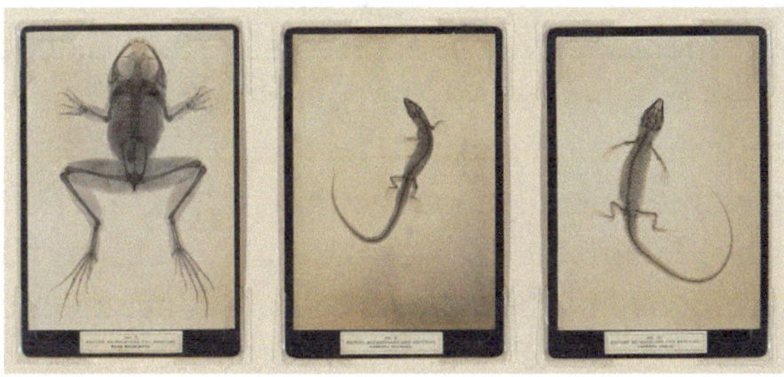

Figure 2.2. Timeline of X-ray imaging.

Source: By James Green / James H. Gardiner - https://collections.britishart.yale.edu/catalog/orbis:12428971, Public Domain, https://commons.wikimedia.org/w/index.php?curid=112773861.

Importance of X-Ray in Modern Medicine

X-ray imaging has changed how doctors approach patient care. Instead of following a strict textbook method, this tool lets clinicians take a quick, non-invasive peek inside the body—revealing everything from broken bones and dental troubles to more complex issues like tumors and infections. Over time, as diagnostic methods evolved, few techniques reshaped care quite like X-rays.

They give near-instant feedback—vital in emergencies—allowing for rapid treatment decisions. In most cases, new tech improvements have sharpened the image quality, nudging diagnostic accuracy even further. It is no wonder hospitals keep turning more to X-rays as an essential part of modern medicine. X-rays aren't just for spotting problems; they help guide treatments too. Take fluoroscopy, for example.

This real-time imaging method shows dynamic internal processes, which can be a real game-changer when doctors are placing a catheter or performing a gastrointestinal study. Being able to watch what's happening live means potentially fewer mistakes and safer procedures. Advances in digital X-ray technology have made these methods even more accessible and faster to use—and that helps when every second counts. Public health efforts also lean on X-ray tech in a big way, especially in screening programs. Chest X-rays, for instance, are commonly used to flag early signs of tuberculosis or lung cancer, which can lead to better survival rates once detected. Mammography works similarly for breast cancer, showing how X-rays can act as a preventive tool rather than just a diagnostic one.

These screening programs not only help catch issues early but also nudge people to keep up with regular check-ups. As research keeps uncovering new roles for X-rays, their preventive benefits become even clearer—improving individual outcomes and strengthening public health systems alike.

2.1. Principles of X-Ray Imaging

Learning Outcome

1. Understand the basic physics of X-ray production.
2. Define the interaction of X-rays with matter.
3. Discuss image formation and processing.

X-ray imaging works on the idea that different tissues in our body absorb X-rays in their own way. As the rays travel through, they bump into various materials that differ in density—each reacting a bit differently. Bones, being on the denser side, capture more of the X-rays and end up looking almost white on the film; softer tissues let more rays slip through, which makes them appear darker. This natural contrast, in many cases, helps doctors pick out problems like fractures or tumors. In short, knowing how X-rays interact with tissues is pretty much at the heart of getting good radiographic images (Nagel et al., 2010). Besides the body's natural traits, a host of technical settings plays a big role in the final image. For example, the kilovoltage (kV) generally decides how well the rays can push through denser tissue. And then there's the milliamperage (mA), which sets the number of photons produced – in other words, it influences how sharp the image turns out. Even the length of the exposure time matters; a tad too long can sometimes lead to unwanted motion blur. Balancing all these factors carefully is key to getting a clear picture while keeping radiation levels as low as reasonably possible. In recent years, there have been some cool upgrades in X-ray technology. Digital radiography, for instance, uses sensors that convert X-ray energy directly into digital images, so doctors can check the results almost immediately. In most cases, these new systems come with smart algorithms that naturally boost contrast and clarity. There's also growing interest in techniques like tomosynthesis, where multiple images from different angles are used to build a sort of three-dimensional view. Overall, these innovations are slowly nudging aside traditional methods, driven by a need for better efficiency and improved patient safety (Du et al., 2018; Nagel et al., 2010).

2.1.1. Basic Physics of X-Ray Production

When electrons are pushed by a high-voltage field and slam into a target—usually tungsten because it is tough and handles heat well—they slow down fast, turning their motion into bursts of electromagnetic energy. This deceleration, what individuals call bremsstrahlung radiation, ends up creating most of the X-rays you see in a tube. Sometimes, too, the speeding electrons knock out inner electrons from atoms; then, outer electrons drop in to fill the gap, and that switch releases photons of very specific energies based on the differences between energy levels. In a way, these little interactions pile up to power effective radiographic imaging, which is pretty crucial for making everything work just right. Mixing in the physics with how the X-ray tubes are run adds another layer to the story. You can tweak the image quality and the radiation dose just by adjusting the tube current (measured in milliampere), which changes how many electrons hit the target at once—even a slight shift can make a noticeable difference. Then there's the tube's voltage; bumping it up gives the X-rays a stronger kick, letting them cut through denser stuff like bones. But, of course, all these settings have to be managed carefully because too much exposure might inadvertently raise the chance of radiation damage—a concern that touches on both technical limits and ethical responsibilities, in most cases challenging us to strike just the right balance. Over time, advances in X-ray tech have been pushed not only by a need to understand these basics better but also by the drive for sharper, more precise imaging methods. Digital systems now play a big role in enhancing both the capture and processing of X-ray images, often providing improved contrast and better diagnostic clarity. Digital radiography, for example, lets professionals manipulate images in real-time, which can be a huge advantage when immediate assessment is needed. Techniques like computed radiography and direct digital radiography, using flat-panel detectors to turn X-ray photons into digital signals, have made evaluations much more reliable. Ongoing research, with its constant tweaks and tests, continues to open up new possibilities in radiographic imaging, paving the way for ever more effective medical diagnostics (Du et al., 2018) (Figure 2.3).

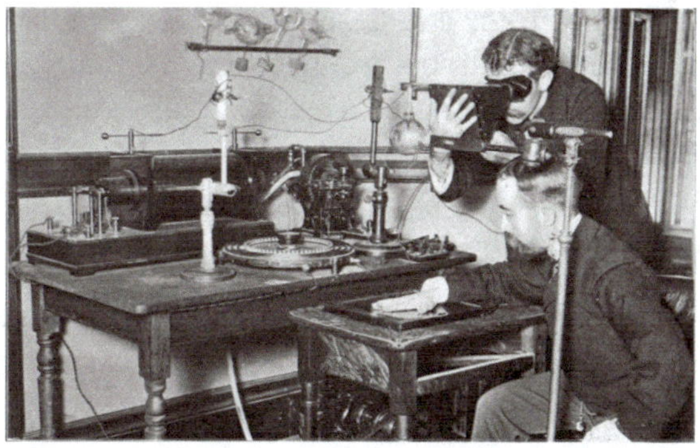

Figure 2.3. Production of X-rays.

Source: By William J. Morton - Downloaded 2007-12-23 from William J. Morton and Edwin W. Hammer (1896) The X-ray, or Photography of the Invisible and its value in Surgery, American Technical Book Co., New York, fig. 54 on Google Books, Public Domain, https://commons.wikimedia.org/w/index.php?curid=3272036.

2.1.2. Interaction of X-Rays with Matter

X-rays behave in ways that depend a lot on their energy and basic physical traits. They can interact with different stuff in unexpected ways – sometimes they get completely absorbed (often called the photoelectric effect), sometimes they bump into particles and scatter about (that's the Compton effect), and occasionally you even get Rayleigh scattering mixed in. In dense materials, photoelectric absorption tends to eat up the X-rays entirely, which in turn boosts the contrast needed to tell soft tissues apart from bone. When the X-rays are in an in-between energy range, though, Compton scattering takes hold and the rays end up going in various directions, which can make images a bit blurry. All of these interactions, repeatedly influencing clarity and diagnostic usefulness, remind us that choosing the right X-ray energy for each material is pretty important in both medical and industrial settings. The push for better radiographic imaging rides on how well we grasp these nuances. For example, sophisticated software now helps to control the X-ray sources and detectors, making imaging more precise than before. In fields like analyzing cultural artifacts, automated systems even steer the X-ray source and detector with surprising finesse – a move that trims down scanning time and lessens operator fatigue.

A recent study showed that a tomographic system with upgraded control software managed to capture clear images of valuable artworks, proving that technology and the uniqueness of X-ray interactions go hand in hand when reshaping radiographic methods (Tisbeni et al., 2017). Generally speaking, insights like these underscore how the merging of physical behavior and tech progress leads to better imaging techniques. More recently, new systems that blend neutron and X-ray CT have started showing promise in non-destructive testing. These setups, which harness the differing strengths of two radiation types, can pick up on details even when samples contain materials with nearly identical atomic numbers. The dual-technique approach seems to reveal subtle details that a single imaging method might easily miss. In most cases, using measures like modulation transfer function and detective quantum efficiency becomes key to assessing how well the system performs, thereby giving better insights into image quality. By embracing these cutting-edge tools, researchers are now uncovering a deeper understanding of material properties and complex structures, steadily pushing the envelope of what we consider conventional radiographic imaging (Sinha et al., 2013) (Figure 2.4).

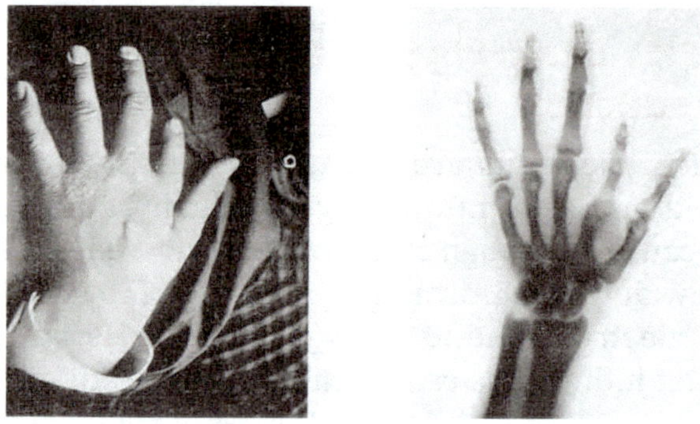

Figure 2.4. Interaction of X-rays with matter.

Source: By Albert Londe (1858-1917) - "Nouvelle iconographie de la Salpétrière" (Tome 9; plaque XXI) See here, Public Domain, https://commons.wikimedia.org/w/index.php?curid=12352684.

2.1.3. Image Formation and Processing

Radiographic imaging is all about nailing down the details that make a proper diagnosis tick, and it turns out that how we form and tweak those images matters more than ever. Digital methods have shaken things up, making image capture faster and crisper. When you mix in smart algorithms that work with X-ray data, radiologists can spot body structures with a clarity that wasn't possible before. It is almost like the way we see things gets a bit more intuitive—an extra nudge that makes abnormalities easier to catch while also offering a better sense of spatial relationships within the body. There's a growing push, in most cases, to keep refining these techniques so that the diagnosis remains spot-on and medical interventions can happen in good time. Artificial intelligence (AI) has now come into play, and honestly, it is a pretty big deal for image analysis. AI systems are getting good at picking up complicated patterns hidden in the imaging data, and that extra boost in accuracy means a lot. By leaning on these computational tricks, radiologists can turn a qualitative look at an image into something more quantitative—something studies have backed up (Kents et al., 2021). The speed and precision that come with AI-assisted diagnostics help not only in flagging issues but also in cutting down on missteps.

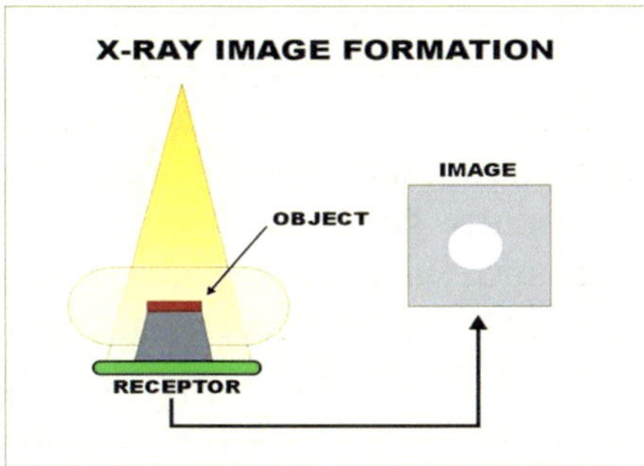

Figure 2.5. X-ray image formation.

Source: http://www.sprawls.org/resources/XRAYCON/module.htm.

This becomes especially important with respiratory ailments, where detecting problems early can make a real difference in treatment. Taking a closer look at newer imaging techniques, there's also been some cool progress with X-ray phase-contrast imaging, or X-PCI for short. This method makes it a whole lot easier to see low-density materials that usual X-rays might just blur over, which means soft tissues—like cartilage—get a clearer picture than ever before (Horng et al., 2021). It is almost as if you're getting a peek at tissue details nearly as fine as a microscope could offer, minus the hassle of complicated staining. With X-PCI, both researchers and clinicians get to explore tissues down at nearly the cellular level; this extra layer of insight helps in tracking how diseases develop and tissues slowly break down. Overall, it opens up fresh avenues for diagnosis and a deeper look into how our bodies work (Figure 2.5).

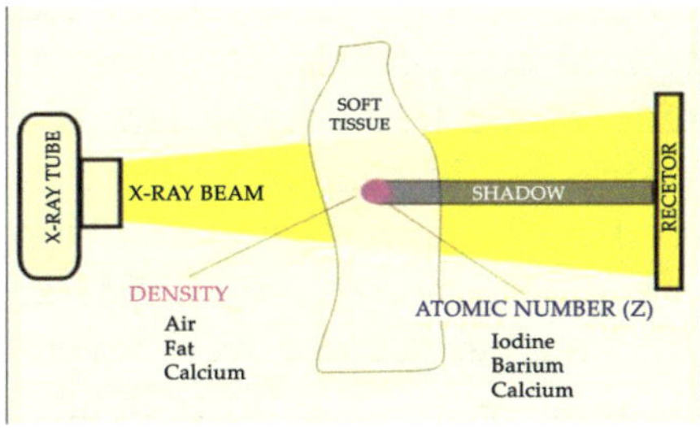

Figure 2.6. The image contrast produced by an object depends on its attenuation of the X-ray beam.

Source: https://lh6.googleusercontent.com /proxy/agkirtEDX1kZlxbSvqBkZ3GSQ8FMu5PaHJpEBGjDszvWxZjtWzTzb9NvOLqj1E87mlDGiqHb4OAai3_Nmznj9HojXF4EUQ.

Test Your Knowledge

1. What are the key physical processes involved in the production of X-rays?
2. How do X-rays interact with matter, and what are the main types of interactions that occur?

2.2. Types of X-Ray Imaging

Learning Outcome

1. Define conventional radiography and computed tomography (CT).
2. Discuss about fluoroscopy.

Medical technology has pushed X-ray imaging into all sorts of new directions - each type now finds its own role in diagnosing issues. Conventional radiography, which many doctors use first, gives a flat, two-dimensional view that's handy for spotting broken bones or assessing dense tissues. But traditional methods eventually hit their limits. That's why techniques like CT and fluoroscopy emerged. CT scans slice the body into cross-sectional images to show fine details, while fluoroscopy lets you watch bodily processes in real time - for example, seeing contrast material travel through the gut. This evolution shows how important clear, precise imaging has become. New developments keep expanding X-ray capabilities in unexpected ways. Digital X-ray technology has, in most cases, turned things on their head by not only boosting image quality but also streamlining the workflow—often even lowering radiation exposure for patients. Instead of relying on film, these devices turn X-rays into digital signals that radiologists tweak to make abnormalities pop out. Sharing images instantly with colleagues is now easier too, which helps when multiple opinions are needed. Some advanced algorithms in image processing have even started revealing conditions that older methods might have missed. Generally speaking, as this tech moves forward, the chance for faster, more accurate patient diagnoses is huge. There are also specialized forms of X-ray imaging that cater to unique fields like breast and dental health. Take mammography: it uses low-dose X-rays for early cancer screening and, thanks to digital systems, now offers clearer images that help catch tumors sooner. On the dental side, radiography is key in uncovering oral issues and planning treatment. High-resolution techniques have reached a point where even subtle problems can be detected, which ups patient care. As different branches of medicine keep picking up on these specialized methods, the overall world of diagnostic radiography grows more expansive—and that promises a deeper, more informed approach to medical practice.

2.2.1. Conventional Radiography

Conventional radiography works by taking advantage of how different tissues absorb X-rays in their own unique ways, which ends up giving us images with varied contrast. When a patient is exposed to X-rays, denser parts like bones tend to soak up more radiation than the softer, surrounding tissues—this results in a film that shows many grays. This basic idea helps radiologists spot what's normal and what isn't. Technique matters a lot here; even small things like how you position the patient or pick your imaging settings make a big difference. New methods, such as spatial frequency encoding that looks at data unique to each tissue type, boost the detail and aid in getting a more accurate diagnosis (Gielen et al., 2012). In many cases, these tweaks have reshaped the way radiographs are interpreted in clinical practice. In the clinic, the perks of conventional radiography are pretty clear—it's generally accessible and cost-effective. Unlike advanced scans like MRI or CT that call for pricier, high-tech gear, a routine X-ray is done in no time and with simpler equipment, which is crucial in emergencies where every second counts. Almost every healthcare facility has an X-ray machine, so doctors can quickly get real-time insights into a patient's condition, which helps steer treatment decisions promptly (Gielen et al., 2012). It is a reliable, fast tool that still holds a vital place in today's diagnostic arsenal. That said, there are also some drawbacks that practitioners need to keep in mind. Because the images produced are essentially two-dimensional, it can be tricky to evaluate complex anatomical structures or separate overlapping tissues—issues that sometimes complicate diagnosis. Also, there's always a lingering concern about too much radiation exposure, even if modern methods have cut that risk down, particularly for kids and pregnant women. Some of the advanced processing techniques—like the encoding strategies mentioned earlier—help sharpen the clarity and specificity of the images (Gielen et al., 2012). Overall, being mindful of both the strengths and weaknesses of conventional radiography is key when it is used alongside other imaging tools (Figure 2.7).

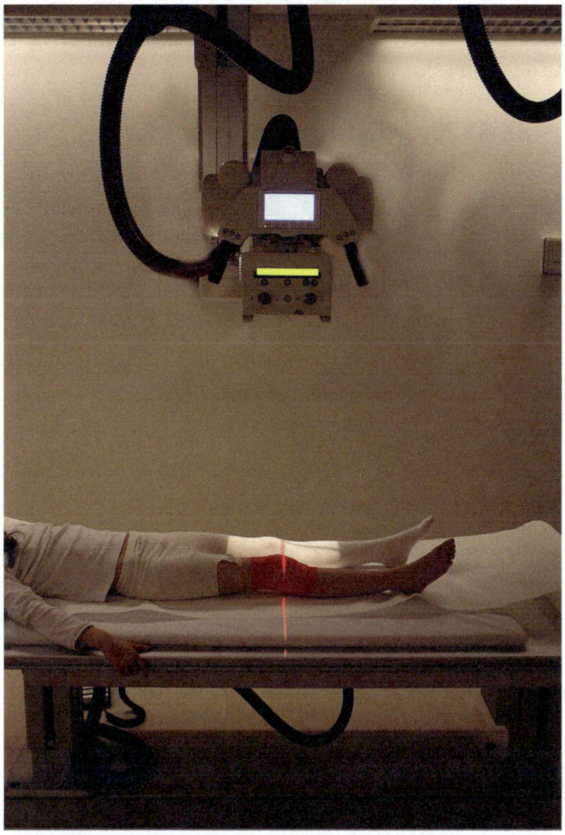

Figure 2.7. Conventional radiography.

Source: By Thomas Bjørkan - Own work, CC BY-SA 3.0, https://commons.wikimedia.org/w/index.php?curid=24676248.

2.2.2. Computed Tomography (CT)

Modern medicine now leans on advanced imaging in ways that clearly stand out. CT scans, or computed tomography, jump to the forefront by producing high-resolution cross-sectional images of the body—a step up from the flat, two-dimensional views you get with traditional X-rays. Instead of a simple picture, CT delivers a detailed, three-dimensional look that lets clinicians see internal structures with striking clarity. This kind of comprehensive view proves vital, especially in complex cases where a precise diagnosis is needed. You can see that many medical fields tap into these benefits, as the insights from CT images help guide treatment choices and surgical plans. In most cases, this extra image detail not only sharpens diagnostic accuracy but also improves overall patient outcomes, underlining CT's essential role in today's radiographic imaging practices. CT works using a clever blend of X-rays and computer processing to capture its detailed images. During a scan, X-ray beams spin around the patient—snagging multiple slices of data that later get pieced together into vivid cross-sectional pictures. Often, these reconstructions even pick up on subtle differences in tissue density, making it noticeably easier to spot abnormalities like tumors, fractures, or internal bleeding. This heightened sensitivity has made CT the go-to method in urgent care settings. Sometimes, adding contrast agents into the mix further boosts the detail, enhancing the view of blood vessels and internal organs; it is like giving the images an extra layer of depth. In effect, CT offers a nuanced understanding of different pathologies, firmly anchoring it amid the broader tools of radiographic imaging. As imaging technology continues to spread its wings across the medical field, CT's role is evolving with a steady flow of new innovations. Improvements in scanning speed, reductions in radiation dose, and leaps in image quality all come together to support diagnostic precision while keeping patient safety in mind—even if these enhancements sometimes appear in unexpected ways. Consider, for instance, the emerging dual-energy CT: by differentiating materials based on their atomic numbers, it provides a fresh approach to evaluating conditions like pulmonary emphysema. Research generally indicates that blending CT with other modalities can improve the diagnostic sensitivity; indeed, some studies have compared CT with inventive X-ray techniques in certain settings (Durand et al., 2016). Moreover, the gradual introduction of machine learning algorithms into CT data processing hints at a future where automated image analysis could simplify diagnostic steps and enrich patient care protocols (Achterhold et al., 2013). Overall, these developments keep CT firmly on track as an indispensable element of modern radiology (Figure 2.8).

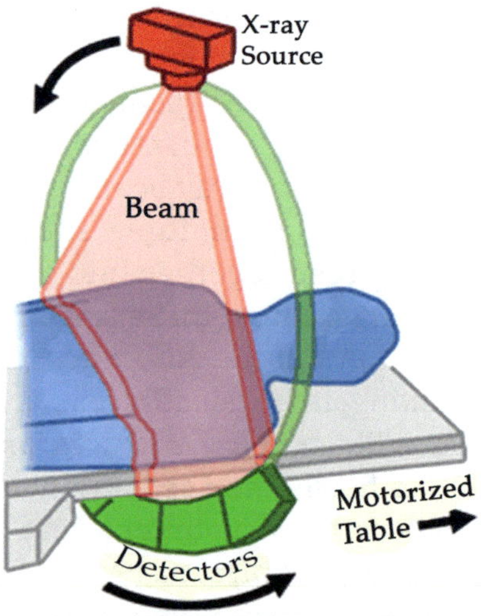

Figure 2.8. Computed tomography (CT).

Source: By FDA - https://www.fda.gov/radiation-emitting-products/medical-x-ray-imaging/computed-tomography-ct, Public Domain, https://commons.wikimedia.org/w/index.php?curid=99627315.

2.2.3. Fluoroscopy

Radiographic imaging brings together a mix of techniques that don't always follow a strict rulebook—each one doing its own thing. Take fluoroscopy, for instance; it is known for showing movement, which is a neat twist compared to your everyday X-ray that simply freezes a moment in time. In most cases, rather than capturing a single image, fluoroscopy uses a steady stream of X-rays to build a video-like sequence that lets you see internal structures working in real-time. You might see this used when doctors guide orthopedic procedures or check on how the gastrointestinal system is moving—it's all about identifying those little details that make a difference for both treatment plans and patient care. Put simply, this method blurs the line between standard imaging and live observation, carving out a unique place for itself in the world of radiography. Over the years, improvements in fluoroscopy have upped its game by not only making it work better but also by lowering the radiation risk.

Nowadays, digital fluoroscopy largely ditches the old film-based approach, giving sharper images while cutting down on exposure—a change that's as practical as it is innovative. Software tweaks now occur right on the spot to adjust exposure settings, ensuring that the images captured are top-notch, with both patients and providers benefiting from reduced risk. Generally speaking, the blend of AI and machine learning has taken image enhancement a step further, automating the process and easing concerns about radiation. In most cases, these technological shifts help ease worries, proving that when used correctly, fluoroscopy is both safe and effective. Fluoroscopy's role isn't limited to snapping moving pictures; it is also a key player in a range of therapeutic interventions. Think about minimally invasive procedures like catheter placements, biopsies, or even the administration of contrast agents—these all lean on fluoroscopy's real-time imaging to work smoothly. In the realm of interventional radiology, being able to see what's going on inside the body at the moment makes a huge difference in patient care, and even fields like gastroenterology get a boost when diagnosing issues with esophageal or gastric movement. There's even chatter about its potential in unexpected areas, such as space medicine, where advanced imaging like fluoroscopy could one day help with in-mission diagnostics (Pohlen, 2024). This emerging trend speaks volumes about the versatility and broad importance of the technique within the larger field of radiographic imaging (Chen et al., 2023) (Figure 2.9).

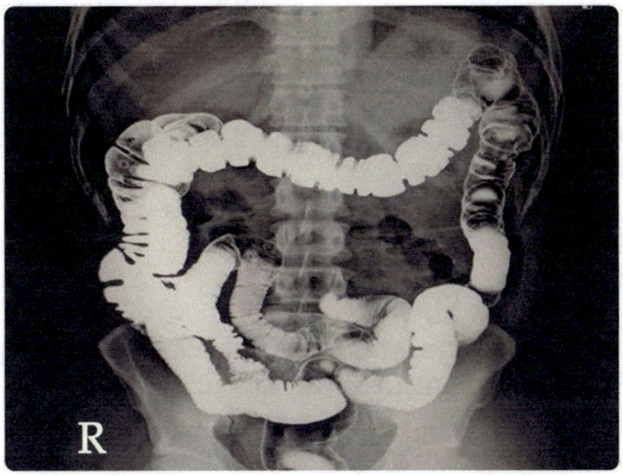

Figure 2.9. Fluoroscopy.

Source: https://d2jx2rerrg6sh3.cloudfront.net/image-handler/picture/2019/3/shutterstock_1098970352.jpg.

Test Your Knowledge

1. How does conventional radiography differ from computed tomography (CT) in terms of image acquisition and resolution?
2. What are some advantages and limitations of using conventional radiography compared to CT scans in medical diagnostics?

2.3. Applications of X-Ray Imaging

Learning Outcome

1. Understand the role of X-ray imaging in diagnosing conditions across different medical specialties.
2. Explore the application of X-ray technology in dental diagnostics.
3. Recognize the importance of X-ray imaging in emergency medicine.

New technology has shaken up how we do medical diagnostics—especially in X-rays. This method gives us a detailed look at our insides, which turns out to be super handy in countless clinical situations. In emergencies, for example, radiography is one of the first things we lean on to spot fractures or sudden injuries, letting teams jump into action quickly. At the same time, its use spills over into routine check-ups and even preventive care. It is key in identifying early signs of problems like tuberculosis or some cancers, showing just how crucial a quick intervention can be. With improvements like digital radiography, not only do the images get clearer, but patients also end up getting less radiation—addressing those ongoing worries about safety and effectiveness in diagnostics (Leo et al., 2023). X-rays aren't just about making an initial diagnosis either; they also guide important treatment steps. Think of procedures like biopsies or minimally invasive surgeries where having a clear picture helps doctors hit the mark. In radiation therapy, for instance, these images let clinicians see where a tumor is and how the surrounding tissue lines up. Now, with newer approaches like cone-beam computed tomography (CBCT) offering 3D views, planning treatments has become a lot more precise. This extra precision is especially vital in complex techniques such as stereotactic radiosurgery, where pinpointing the right spot can mean the difference between protecting healthy tissue and causing unnecessary damage. In other words, X-ray imaging stands at a crossroads between diagnosing and treating, showcasing its many roles in modern healthcare (Lee et al., 2015b). Lately, the mix of AI with X-ray imaging has been turning heads in the medical world. Deep learning algorithms are now busy going through radiographic images, boosting how well we can detect and classify diseases. For instance, some programs that interpret chest X-rays have shown they can pick up on pneumonia and other lung issues at rates that rival—even sometimes outperform—human radiologists. This progress is a real lifesaver in busy settings where every second counts. Generally speaking, ongoing research is also taking a close look at issues like data privacy and bias in these algorithms, trying to smooth out any kinks for ethical use. As these AI-driven applications keep evolving, the chances for better patient outcomes and more efficient healthcare systems become more and more apparent, underlining how important X-ray imaging is in today's medicine (Leo et al., 2023b) (Figure 2.10).

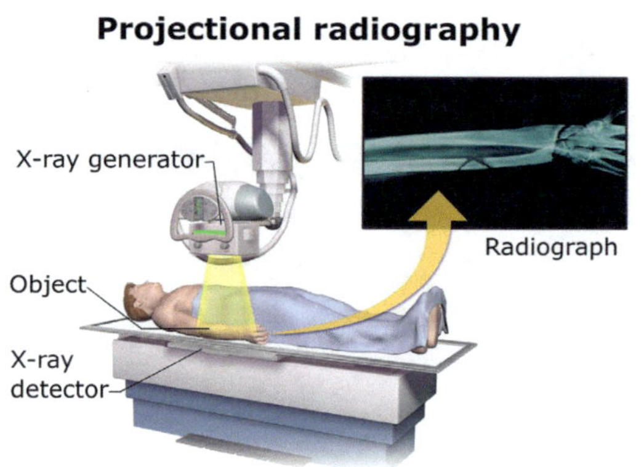

Figure 2.10. X-ray applications.

Source: By Blausen Medical Annotations by Mikael Häggström - By Blausen Medical., CC BY-SA 4.0, https://commons.wikimedia.org/w/index.php?curid=58054654.

2.3.1. Diagnostic Purposes in Various Medical Fields

Advanced imaging has shifted how we diagnose things in medicine. X-rays, for example, do more than just reveal bones—they help us check soft tissues, spot organ problems, and even track disease processes. Capturing high-res images has changed the game for noticing fractures, spotting tumors, and flagging infections. Digital systems thrown into the mix have smoothed out routine workflows in clinics and hospitals, so doctors can, in most cases, decide on treatments a bit faster and improve patient care overall. In hospitals it is not simply a matter of installing new gadgets; the whole use of radiographic imaging depends on what's going on inside the organization as well as on rules set by health ministries (Nor et al., 2010).

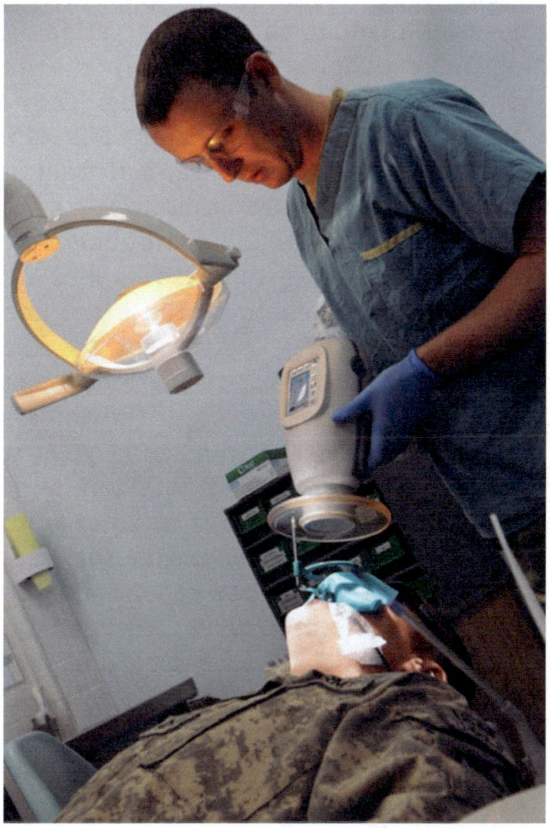

Figure 2.11. Providers can use X-rays to diagnose broken bones, arthritis, infections in your lungs, spine conditions and teeth issues.

Source: By US Army - http://www.army.mil/-news/2011/04/21/55379-deployed-dentists-test-lightweight-mobile-x-ray-system/, Public Domain, https://commons.wikimedia.org/w/index.php?curid=15026673.

Take Malaysia, say—the give-and-take between hospital managers and external regulators can mean that service quality and access end up varying a lot from one facility to the next. That kind of push-and-pull underscores why strategies have to mesh internal aims with public policies. Plus, the very act of rolling out X-ray tech often reshapes roles among the care team, encouraging radiologists, technicians, and other staff to work together more closely while keeping the patient's needs front and center. Even with all its perks, radiographic imaging isn't without its risks—radiation exposure being a big one. It is crucial to manage these dangers to protect both patients and healthcare workers. Over time, clinical guidelines have emerged to limit overexposure during both routine diagnostic and interventional procedures (Martin et al., 2017). Some hospitals rely on checklists and dose alerts to catch errors that might lead to unplanned exposure, and, frankly, keeping an eye on these details is key. A solid understanding of radiation's impacts, combined with proactive safety measures, makes all the difference in maintaining trustworthy imaging practices; ongoing training and sticking to safety protocols remain essential for top-notch diagnostic work and patient safety (Figure 2.11).

2.3.2. Use in Dental Imaging

Sometimes a simple X-ray is all it takes to reveal what a routine check-up might miss. In dentistry, radiographic imaging isn't just another tool—it is a vital way to catch hidden cavities, gum issues, or other problems that a casual exam wouldn't uncover. The detailed picture provided by these scans often lets dentists craft treatment plans that are better suited to each patient's needs and, in many cases, lead to improved outcomes. Nowadays, procedures like root canals increasingly lean on these images to check how extensive an infection might be and to gauge treatment success (Lee et al., 2015a). Overall, it is about making sure the diagnosis and follow-up care are closely matched to what the individual patient needs. Beyond just spotting issues, dental imaging plays a key role in keeping tabs on treatment progress. For example, after a root canal, it is pretty ordinary for dentists to order follow-up X-rays—not merely to tick a box, but to keep an eye out for things like reinfection or fillings that aren't quite right. These extra images help offer a deeper look at how treatments are holding up, sometimes even guiding tweaks in future care. Recent advances in digital imaging, as some studies note, seem to boost accuracy in identifying troubles like canal leakage or less-than-ideal obturation (Lee et al., 2015a).

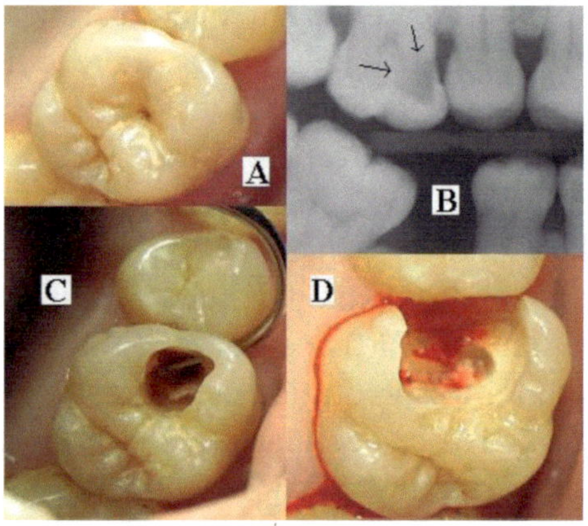

Figure 2.12. Dental X-rays.

Source: By Original uploaded by DRosenbach (Transferred by wikiLeon) - Original uploaded on en.wikipedia, CC BY 3.0, https://commons.wikimedia.org/w/index.php?curid=12339287.

In a way, the jump to digital not only sharpens diagnostic skills but also ends up educating practitioners about what works best day-to-day in modern dental practice. Of course, all this progress brings up the need to carefully weigh in on radiation exposure—especially in kids and other sensitive groups. It is not unusual for parents to feel a bit uneasy about the idea of their children being exposed to ionizing rays, mostly because the risks aren't always clearly explained right off the bat. Simple educational steps, like handing out brochures, can help ease those concerns by boosting understanding and making guardians more comfortable with necessary procedures. Ultimately, it is a balancing act: harnessing the benefits of radiographic imaging while also taking seriously the potential risks, ensuring that both patients and their families are well-informed throughout the process (Figure 2.12).

2.3.3. Role in Emergency Medicine

Emergency medicine thrives on quick, accurate diagnoses, which can change how patients do. Radiographic imaging - think X-rays - ends up being a lifesaver in this setting. They let doctors see inside the body almost instantly, which speeds up spotting trauma, fractures, and other sudden issues so that help can come fast. Getting this info on the fly not only boosts rapid decision-making but also shapes what comes next in treatment. In the often hectic chaos of an emergency department, the knack for reading an X-ray swiftly can seriously up the overall care, sometimes making all the difference in patient outcomes. X-ray imaging goes way beyond just telling doctors what's wrong; it is used in many different ways in emergencies. For example, portable X-ray machines in trauma bays allow for on-the-spot checks—no need to shuffle patients around, which cuts down on delays in critical moments. This proves especially handy when every second counts in life-threatening injuries. Sometimes, these images also help track the development of sudden conditions, proving over and over just how integral they are in emergency care. In most cases, having adaptable X-ray tech around shows its versatility and solidifies its stand as a cornerstone in emergency medicine. Beyond basic diagnostics and procedural support, X-rays also shape whole patient management and discharge plans. Often, what appears on an X-ray sets off a chain reaction—like spotting an internal hemorrhage that pushes for immediate surgery, instantly drawing up a rapid treatment plan. Sometimes, integrating these findings into electronic health records makes it easier for care teams to chat and coordinate their next moves. In essence, the many uses of radiographic imaging not only quicken the first assessments but also nurture a broader, more holistic approach to patient care, confirming just how critical it remains in modern medical practice (Du et al., 2018) (Figure 2.13).

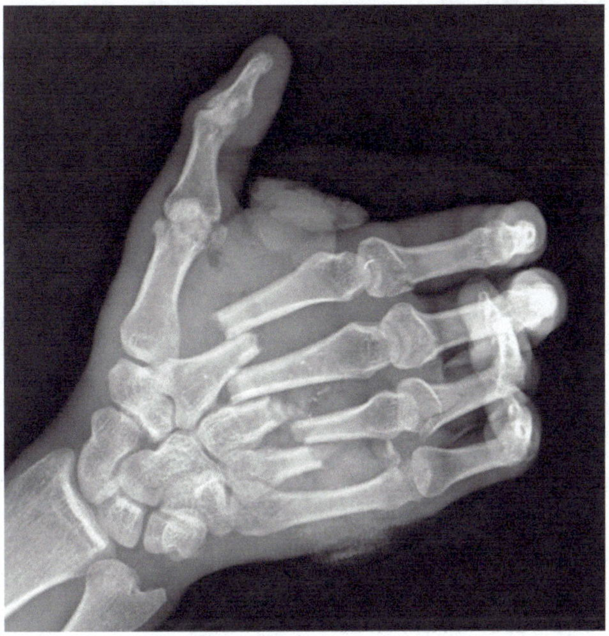

Figure 2.13. X-ray radiograph in the emergency room.

Source: https://www.researchgate.net/figure/ray-radiograph-in-the-emergency-room_fig1_343190209.

Test Your Knowledge

1. How is diagnostic imaging used in various medical fields to aid in patient diagnosis and treatment planning?
2. What role does X-ray imaging play in dental imaging, and what are its primary uses in dental diagnostics?

2.4. Safety and Risks

Learning Outcome

1. Understand the radiation exposure and its effects.
2. Identify key safety measures in X-ray procedures.
3. Define regulations and guidelines for X-ray use.

Safety in radiographic imaging isn't something you can overlook. Radiation risks are ever-present, especially during procedures where things can go awry unexpectedly. Sometimes, equipment uniqueness or simple human oversights lead to doses higher than intended. Solid training – focusing on getting the hang of operating every piece of equipment – makes a big difference in cutting down these mishaps. Simple steps, like using checklists and pausing briefly before a procedure, can lower the chance of extra exposure. Hospitals often lean on clear guidelines about handling overexposure, which in turn boosts overall patient care (Martin et al., 2017). Keeping up with new technology is another key part of managing these risks. It turns out that clinging to older methods, like relying on lead X-ray vest gear, isn't as safe as it once seemed. Generally speaking, recent research shows that modern digital devices can target the X-ray beam more precisely, hitting only what's needed. This focus makes a noticeable dent in unnecessary radiation. Further, if those old vests aren't cared for properly, they might even expose patients to lead themselves. So, letting both patients and providers in on what's new helps everyone make smarter, safer choices in medical and dental imaging (Deker et al., 2020). Even with all these improvements, concerns still linger. The idea of unpredictable, long-term effects from even small doses of radiation keeps both patients and health professionals on their toes. This worry is especially true for vulnerable individuals, like pregnant patients, where any stray exposure might bring extra risks. A practical system that learns from each incident and keeps the radiation safety conversation going can ease these fears. When hospitals foster a culture of accountability—with clear, though sometimes imperfect, reporting practices—it not only handles issues right away but also helps reduce the chances of repeat problems, which ultimately builds more trust among patients (Martin et al., 2017).

2.4.1. Radiation Exposure and Its Effects

Radiation exposure in medical imaging has always been a bit of a balancing act. Think about X-rays: we used to rely on lead aprons to shield patients, but nowadays, that old trick is mostly out of style. New gadgets like digital radiography and sharper collimation have pretty much taken over, honing in on just the spot where the beams are needed. Generally speaking, these advances mean we can lower doses substantially. It is a good idea for both patients and healthcare individuals to know that many of the traditional safety practices simply aren't as necessary as they once were (Deker et al., 2020). In veterinary work, the scene isn't all that different. Consider the imaging used for equine feet—that dual dorsoproximal–palmarodistal oblique shots that used to be the go-to method are getting a fresh look. Nowadays, digital radiography paired with better post-processing techniques lets practitioners snap one solid image instead of a bunch, which cuts down on radiation exposure for both the animals and the people treating them. Some recent work even suggests there's no major difference between those newer images and the older multiple shots approach, so sometimes one well-taken image does do the trick (Whitlock et al., 2016). All this talk about radiation isn't just technical banter—it is about keeping risks low. Even though diagnostic X-rays are generally safe, stacking up those little doses over time can, in most cases, raise the chance of cancer or other health issues. Sure, even low amounts of radiation shouldn't be taken lightly.

That's why sticking with the latest imaging tech and regularly tweaking safety guidelines is so important: it helps us protect patients while still getting the clear pictures we need (Deker et al., 2020) (Figure 2.14).

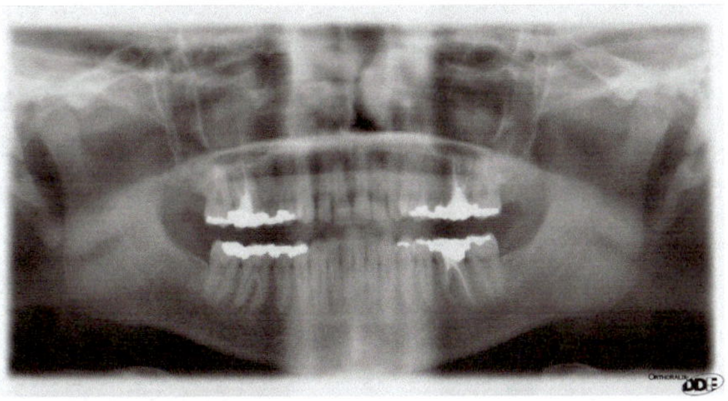

Figure 2.14. Radiation dose in X-rays.

Source: Public Domain, https://commons.wikimedia.org/w/index.php?curid=95297205.

2.4.2. Safety Measures in X-ray Procedures

Safety in radiographic imaging isn't just an afterthought—it is the cornerstone of every procedure. Strong protocols should be in place to keep radiation exposure low, especially when performing diagnostic or interventional tests. Many international guidelines generally suggest that training staff to operate imaging machines properly and adjust their settings on the fly is key. In most cases, this kind of training not only improves how well procedures work but also cuts down significantly on overexposure risks. For instance, introducing checklists and taking brief pauses before starting can act as important safety checkpoints. Dose alerts during procedures—providing near-real-time updates on exposure—often prove crucial in stopping accidents before they happen. All these measures, coupled with clear communication and practical safeguards, help build a robust safety framework in radiology departments, addressing many of the pressing radiation risks (Martin et al., 2017). When accidental overexposures occur, the radiology team must be ready with clearly defined policies and action plans. It helps if every team member knows exactly what their role is; this leads to a quick, organized response and faster identification of the root causes. Having a well-documented process for calculating doses and assessing the risks tied to any exposure incident often makes a world of difference. For example, if radiation unexpectedly affects organs, skin, or even a fetus, accurately estimating the dose—whether expressed in general terms rather than hard numbers—becomes essential for immediate and long-term care. This clearer way of communicating potential health effects aids decision-making and eventually paves the way for better safety measures, nurturing a culture that puts patient safety first in radiographic practices (Martin et al., 2017). Learning from past incidents is another vital element of safety in X-ray procedures.

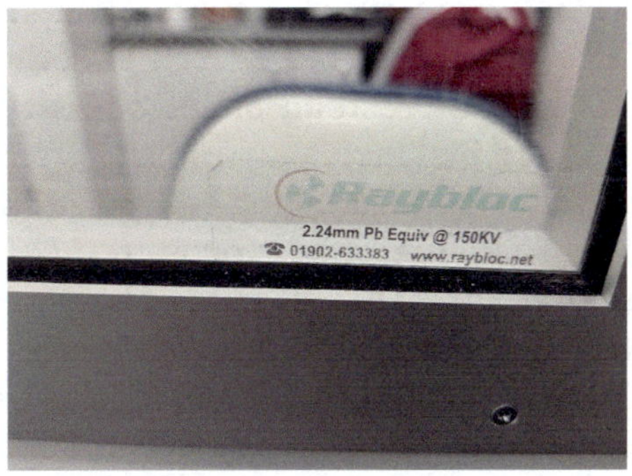

Figure 2.15. Safety precautions before an X-ray.

Source: By Andy Mabbett - Own work, CC BY-SA 4.0, https://commons.wikimedia.org/w/index.php?curid=138442771.

As healthcare providers navigate the complex landscape of imaging technology, they must accept that mistakes, like accidental exposures, can happen—and these events offer invaluable lessons. Often, digging deeper into such incidents reveals issues like equipment glitches or procedural missteps that need thorough addressing. Integrating these lessons into training programs and everyday practices can help staff avoid repeating errors. Besides, routine audits that check both machine performance and adherence to safety guidelines serve as proactive ways to spot and fix potential hazards. Ultimately, true safety in radiography comes from more than just following strict rules; it requires ongoing education, a bit of flexibility, and a constant readiness to tackle emerging challenges in patient care (Martin et al., 2017) (Figure 2.15).

2.4.3. Regulations and Guidelines for X-Ray Use

X-ray technology gives us great diagnostic benefits, but keeping patients safe isn't always straightforward. A strong set of rules is needed to strike that balance—lowering radiation exposure while still getting the clear images we depend on. Sometimes, when staff lack proper training in using the equipment or fine-tuning the procedures, dangerous overexposures can happen. For example, guidelines mention the importance of using checklists, taking a timeout before procedures, and setting up dose alerts to keep risks down (Martin et al., 2017). These steps, repeated over time, help everyone learn from past mistakes and show that regular training and sticking to policies matter. Guidelines also lay out clear responsibilities for each healthcare worker involved in radiographic imaging. In most cases, formal policies are set up to look into any unintended overexposures so that issues can be quickly investigated. When a patient accidentally gets too much radiation, it becomes critical to work out exactly how much dose hit each organ. This kind of estimation not only reveals potential problems but also points the way for practical improvements. As the current framework suggests, building accountability within hospitals helps boost the response to incidents and cut down on future errors (Martin et al., 2017). Overall, this approach protects patients while also improving the overall effectiveness of imaging practices. The day-to-day operations in healthcare do more than affect patient safety—they also leave their mark on the environment. Hospitals, for instance, play a part in environmental challenges through activities like generating medical waste and managing equipment sterilization, including during X-ray procedures. Guidelines are now broadening their focus to include these environmental issues, nudging facilities toward greener practices. This means not only careful disposal of outdated or damaged equipment but also smarter purchasing decisions that lessen upstream and downstream impacts. By combining patient safety with environmental care, the framework encourages a more rounded approach to radiologic practices—addressing all aspects in a way that's ethical and beneficial for the wider community.

Test Your Knowledge

1. What safety measures should be followed during X-ray procedures to protect both patients and healthcare workers?
2. What are the key regulations and guidelines that govern the safe use of X-rays in medical imaging?

2.5. Advances in X-ray Technology

Learning Outcome

1. Understand the key advancements in digital radiography advancements.
2. Explore recent innovations in imaging techniques.
3. Identify emerging trends and future trends in X-ray technology.

Radiographic imaging has taken an interesting turn lately, completely reshuffling how we spot problems in patients. Nowadays, you see digital systems, CT scanning, and even AI all churning out super detailed images that old film-based methods just couldn't match. Switching to digital has not only sped up how fast images are obtained and processed but also lets doctors jump on diagnoses much quicker – in most cases, this means treatments can start sooner. AI, for instance, picks up on small irregularities that might slip past the human eye, yet real experts say the breakthrough comes from X-ray technicians, nurses, and clinicians all pitching in together, which also helps keep radiation exposure low. All of this change signals a major, if sometimes messy, shake-up in radiographic imaging practices (Alsubhi et al., 2024). There's another twist to this story in lung cancer. Traditional chest X-rays can easily overlook tiny lung lesions, and by the time these are spotted, the disease might have already progressed to a tough stage to treat. Now, grating-based imaging has popped up as a fresh method that boosts how soft tissues look, using the unique interplay of X-rays and biological tissues to make even minute changes stand out. This technique, which leans on interferometric ideas, seems to highlight subtle structural details that standard methods miss. Some studies, especially in *in vivo* models, hint that this approach could outdo conventional radiography, offering a promising new avenue for early lung cancer detection (Bölükbas et al., 2019). At the same time, as radiographic tech races ahead, safety hasn't taken a backseat—not by a long shot. With all these innovations, it becomes crucial to fold solid safety protocols into every step so that patients and healthcare workers aren't put at unnecessary risk. Radiologists, technicians, and nurses often team up (sometimes a bit unpredictably) to make sure safety checks are in place, even if the exact methods shift here and there. These efforts boost awareness about potential radiation pitfalls and help everyone stick to best practices, even if some guidelines get a casual tweak along the way. In the end, combining fancy new imaging techniques with practical safety measures definitely paves the way for more effective diagnoses and better overall care (Alsubhi et al., 2024) (Figure 2.16).

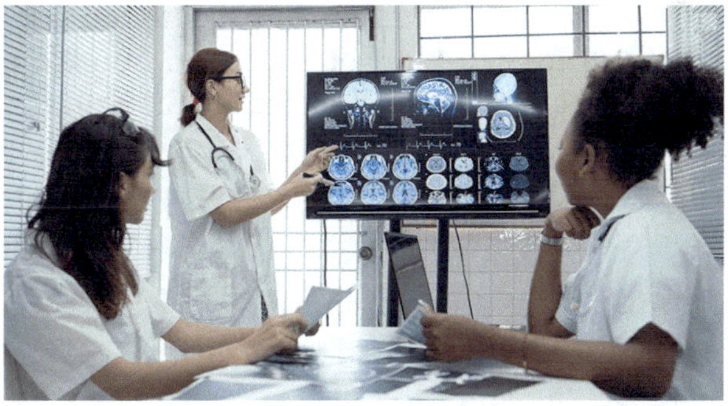

Figure 2.16. Advances in X-ray Technology.

Source: https://images.myacare.com/uploads/AdminBlogs/4deffc460d66459b961f42edad6b4656.webp.

2.5.1. Digital Radiography Advancements

Digital radiography has shaken up the whole imaging scene—it's not just about switching from film to digital detectors, but about capturing images faster and with better sharpness. Clinicians now obtain pictures that come out clear and immediate, which means patients get shorter exposure times and fewer issues like motion blur that could mess up a diagnosis. Studies, in most cases, show that even a little movement during an X-ray can throw off the detection of key anatomical points; so quick, smooth imaging is pretty important. With more clinics and hospitals leaning into digital methods, adding AI and clever motion-correction tools is seen as a must to keep image quality high (Martin et al., 2025). A side benefit of going digital is how it brings medical teams together in a more natural way. Images are now shared easily between different professionals, letting everyone from radiologists to technicians take a closer look when something doesn't seem right, thereby boosting overall patient care. Sometimes, the system even encourages a bit of back-and-forth chat among the team, which can help catch potential issues early and smooth out treatment plans. Plus, newer safety checks—like smarter ways to manage radiation doses—are getting their due as technology improves. In this kind of setting, when X-ray techs, nurses, and doctors combine their efforts, the end result is often better care with fewer risks from unnecessary exposure (Alsubhi et al., 2024).

And there's more—new digital advances keep reshaping how we approach radiographic imaging. Portable digital units and real-time processing, for example, let doctors act quickly when every second counts, like in emergencies. These developments not only boost diagnostic strength but also bring a kind of flexibility that fits well in varied places, from busy hospitals to smaller outpatient clinics. The ever-changing nature of digital imaging even sparks more research and pushes toward standardizing methods across different settings. As tech keeps evolving, sticking to safety protocols and nurturing teamwork among specialists remains key to reaping the full benefits of digital radiography, ensuring both top-notch care and patient safety (Alsubhi et al., 2024; Martin et al., 2025) (Figure 2.17).

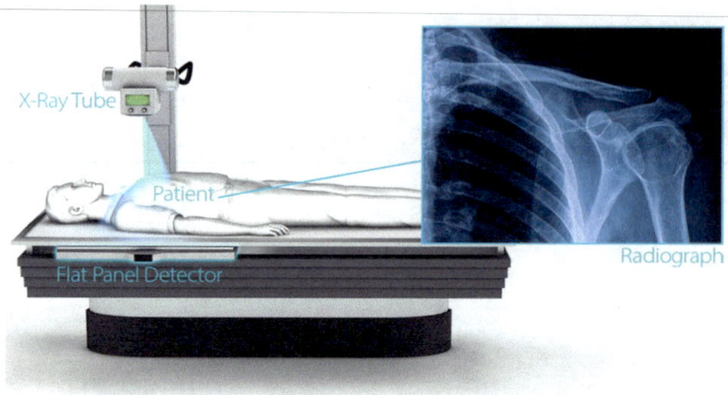

Figure 2.17. In digital X-rays, the X-ray machine uses a sensor to capture the image, and the resulting image is immediately available on a computer screen.

Source: https://www.mavenimaging.com/hs-fs/hubfs/Digital_X-ray_Systems_1390x956.jpg?width=1390&height=926&name=Digital_X-ray_Systems_1390x956.jpg.

2.5.2. Innovations in Imaging Techniques

Medical and dental imaging has changed a lot lately. We've moved on from the old film-based X-rays to digital methods that capture images almost immediately. Digital X-rays emerge on the screen with great detail, and doctors can tweak them—adjusting brightness, contrast, or even cropping—to better fit the case at hand. In many instances, these simple modifications help sharpen diagnoses and speed up treatment plans, leading to better care overall (Rayyani et al., 2024). Advanced techniques like CT scans and cone beam CT (CBCT) have recharged how we view the inside of the body. Now, doctors can see full 3-D pictures of intricate anatomical details, which is key when things get complex. In dentistry—say, for checking out cranio-facial irregularities or planning surgeries—CBCT has become nearly indispensable. Shifting toward volumetric imaging means that even those stubborn, deep-seated lesions are caught more reliably than with old 2-D images, which often just don't cut it anymore (Bansal et al., 2020). The move to digital isn't just a tech upgrade;

it also impacts budgets and day-to-day operations. Switching from analog to digital cuts down on storage hassles and slashes costs related to films and supplies. Further, the quick retrieval and sharing of images encourage a more collaborative, team-based approach to patient care. Generally speaking, as patient expectations and the complexity of conditions continue to rise, embracing new tech becomes more of a must than a luxury. Overall, these imaging innovations are paving the way for a more efficient, effective—and yes, more patient-centered—healthcare system (Rayyani et al., 2024).

2.5.3. Future Trends in X-Ray Technology

X-ray technology isn't the same as it used to be. Nowadays, digital tools are taking over from those old film-based methods. This change speeds up how images are captured and, in most cases, makes them crisper and more detailed. Using digital X-ray systems, doctors can sort out diagnoses and plan treatments a lot faster—which naturally helps patients feel better quicker. There's even been fresh progress with things like CT scans (especially the photon-counting kind), which shows that the field still cares a lot about getting things exactly right. Some current research (Rayyani et al., 2024) even hints that these tweaks are filling in the gaps left by older tech, keeping the practice of radiography on a solid, evolving track. Trends now suggest that the way we handle X-ray images is all set for a big change. Increasingly, AI tools are getting used to read these images—machine learning algorithms now help spot oddities with a surprising knack for accuracy. This kind of innovation lightens the load on busy healthcare teams, letting them focus on the trickier cases that need more attention.

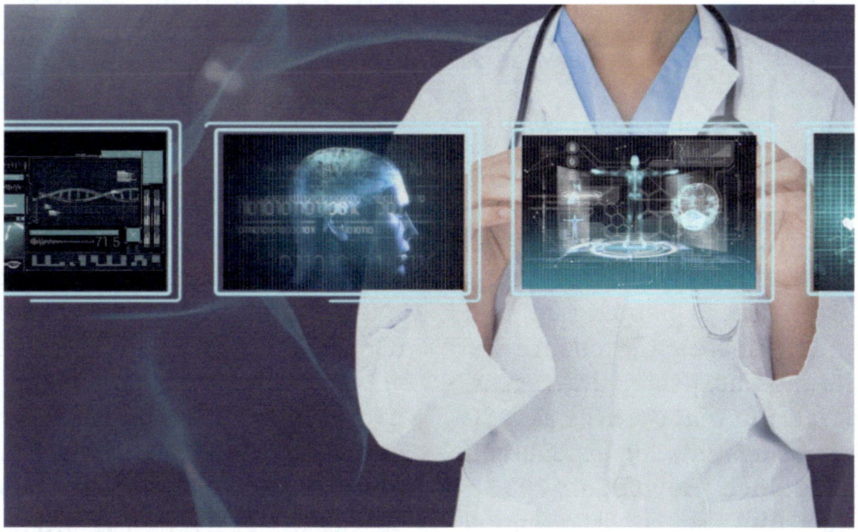

Figure 2.18. X-ray technology.

Source: https://www.verifiedmarketreports.com/images/blogs/01-24/Digital%20X-Ray%20Systems.png.

There's also been a growing buzz around tele-radiology, where experts can check out X-rays from far-away places. In a lot of studies (Rayyani et al., 2024), researchers note that these advancements are reshaping work routines and making it easier to get top-notch radiology insights wherever they're needed, which in turn ups the overall quality of patient care. People are also talking more about the environmental side of X-ray tech. It seems likely that soon both manufacturers and hospitals will lean toward greener materials and energy-smart systems when rolling out new equipment. Generally speaking, this move is a big deal since it fits with a broader push for cleaner practices in healthcare. New sensor technologies—designed to keep a watchful eye on equipment performance (and sometimes even with a few uniqueness)—promise to boost safety, ease maintenance, and cut down on waste. In short, this shift toward sustainability isn't just about caring for the planet; it also helps make X-ray imaging more reliable and efficient, pointing toward a more holistic future for healthcare (Figure 2.18).

Test Your Knowledge

1. What are some recent innovations in imaging techniques that have improved the accuracy and efficiency of X-ray technology?
2. What future trends in X-ray technology are expected to enhance diagnostic capabilities and reduce patient exposure to radiation?

2.6. Ethical Considerations

Learning Outcome

1. Define patient consent and autonomy.
2. Evaluate how to balance the diagnostic benefits of imaging with potential health risks.
3. Explain the addressing disparities in access to imaging.

Ethical issues in radiographic imaging matter—a lot—especially in patient safety and well-being. New digital equipment keeps popping up, and with every innovation, there's the chance for both major benefits and unexpected drawbacks. One report even points out that over the past 20 years, the average ionizing radiation exposure in the U.S. has nearly doubled (Boyd et al., 2013); naturally, that sends ripples of concern among health professionals. As technology marches on, radiologic technologists need a down-to-earth ethical guide to ensure that while they use these advances, patient care remains front and center. Clinical decisions and ethical responsibilities don't always dance in step; in fact, radiologists and technologists often end up juggling tough calls. It is not a neat balance—diagnostic goals sometimes clash with the need to cut down exposure risks. In many cases, digging into what drives a practitioner's choice (and examining subtle attitudes) reveals everyday ethical puzzles that the field faces (Boyd et al., 2013). Pressures from hospital rules or even social expectations can push professionals away from solid ethical ground, making it clear that more practical training and candid talks about best practices might help ease these dilemmas. Looking at the whole picture, addressing ethics in radiographic imaging means embracing both education and a supportive work culture. A safety culture within radiology departments, after all, boosts professionals' capacity to prioritize patient care and keep radiation risks low. Research generally shows that a technologist's approach to patient protection is often shaped by their education, work experiences, and even the vibe of their workplace (Boyd et al., 2013). Some institutions now roll out educational programs focused on real-world ethical decision-making, and these efforts seem to lift the quality of care considerably. In the end, a holistic take on ethics not only helps patients but also builds a profession rooted in integrity and responsibility—cornerstones for shaping the future of medical imaging (Figure 2.19).

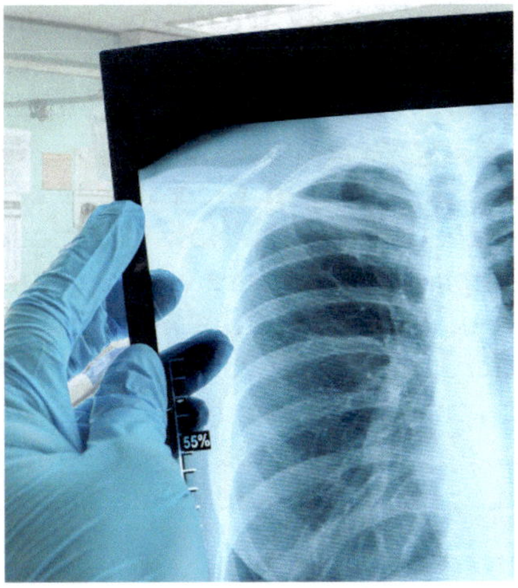

Figure 2.19. Ethical issues in radiographic imaging matter—a lot—especially in patient safety and well-being.

Source: https://cdn.who.int/media/images/default-source/imported/radiation/radiological-imaging.tmb-1200v.png?sfvrsn=2440411e_2.

2.6.1. Patient Consent and Autonomy

Patient consent and autonomy carry major weight, especially in radiographic imaging. It is not simply a matter of signing a form - it means making sure patients know what a procedure involves, including its risks and benefits. Often, when patients get clear explanations and feel listened to, they end up more confident in making decisions about their care. Studies generally suggest that better understanding is linked to higher satisfaction. In real-world settings, open and honest communication between radiographers and patients builds trust, which is key for both ethical practice and better health outcomes. Radiographers today aren't just behind the camera anymore; they're stepping into roles that require them to interpret imaging results too. Take, for example, the red dot system in the United Kingdom - a method that shows how expanding responsibilities makes clear, shared decision-making even more essential. When radiographers take the time to explain what they find collaboratively, patients tend to feel more involved in their own care. In many cases, this shift means that every professional on the team must be well-versed in both ethical and legal aspects of consent, offering information that is concise yet complete, even if it sometimes comes across as a bit unpolished. In areas with fewer resources - say, in parts of South Africa or other underserved regions - dealing with patient consent can get even more complicated. When there aren't enough radiologists, radiographers and other medical practitioners have to lean on each other, and while informal methods of reading images can speed up urgent treatments, they also bring along ethical and legal headaches. Establishing some clear guidelines about what radiographers should do might help balance these quick decisions with the need to protect patient rights. Overall, ensuring that patients understand their imaging not only fosters transparency and respect but also tends to boost patient care and satisfaction, even in settings that are far from ideal.

2.6.2. Balancing Benefits and Risks

Advanced imaging has taken a new turn with modern tech. Nowadays, radiography shows things we once missed, uncovering a range of conditions even before they fully develop. You see, when doctors use tools like X-rays and CT scans, they can catch issues—including something as serious as COVID-19—quite early, which often turns the tide for patients. At the same time, though, there's always that worry about ionizing radiation; it is not without its long-term baggage. In most cases, clinicians end up trying to strike a balance—getting the best diagnostic picture while not overexposing anyone to unnecessary risks. It is a bit of a juggling act. Mixing traditional imaging with newer approaches like AI and deep learning has also turned out to be a game changer. Research generally suggests that heavy-duty models—think ResNet152 or VGG16—can boost our ability to spot conditions like pneumonia and even COVID-19 from X-ray snaps, sometimes hitting accuracy levels near 99%. Still, these advances aren't all roses; data quality issues, biases in the training sets, and sometimes the very reasoning behind AI outputs can be pretty tricky. Addressing these glitches is key so that we don't let AI lead to misdiagnoses or an overdependence on technology, which means careful oversight remains essential. Even as X-ray techniques push forward, it is clear we need a solid ethical game plan, especially when dealing with more sensitive groups like children or pregnant women. For example, the repeated use of X-rays in these cases calls for a thoughtful weighing of radiation risks against immediate diagnostic benefits. New techniques—like the Dual Imaging and Diffraction (DIAD) method—offer a glimpse into a future where radiographic analysis might get better without ramping up the hazards of traditional methods. By blending different modalities, researchers can get a more rounded understanding of what's going on without bombarding patients with excessive radiation. Overall, this innovative trend highlights the need for ongoing research and a careful, sometimes even cautious, approach so that we keep improving patient outcomes while always putting safety first (Besnard et al., 2024; Xue et al., 2023).

2.6.3. Addressing Disparities in Access to Imaging

In many rural and resource-strapped areas, getting proper imaging services is a real struggle that hits patient care hard. Some places have tried new approaches—mobile diagnostic units (MDUs) for instance—and the results can be pretty encouraging. In western Kenya, one project pushed a generator-powered X-ray machine around several small health facilities. Since the project kicked off, over 4,500 chest X-rays have been done, with roughly 30% showing some form of abnormality. This kind of example shows that mobile units can work while also pointing out the pressing need for flexible, community-tailored solutions (Abuya et al., 2018). Still, even when MDUs make a positive mark, practical obstacles keep cropping up. Infrastructure challenges, like unreliable power supplies and the difficulties of moving heavy equipment around, tend to slow things down. Often, the issues go further—transmitting and reporting the X-rays in such remote settings is hit by tech shortfalls and not enough trained staff. Generally speaking, tackling these mixed-up hurdles—such as better training local healthcare workers and setting up sturdier communication channels for radiographic data—is essential to make these services as effective as they can be (Abuya et al., 2018). Not only do these problems haunt rural areas, but they also impact vulnerable groups like children in developing countries. Pediatric imaging has its own uniqueness, needing both special gear and a certain expertise to keep things safe. In many African nations where the number of kids is rising, there's an urgent call for better imaging support to deal with issues like tuberculosis and pneumonia.

Test Your Knowledge

1. How can healthcare providers balance the diagnostic benefits of X-ray imaging with the potential risks of radiation exposure?
2. What strategies can be implemented to address disparities in access to imaging services across different populations or regions?

Summary

Radiographic imaging has taken a fresh turn lately, with X-ray technology stepping up its game in the medical world. These days, AI is thrown into the mix, generally boosting both accuracy and speed. You might catch a study somewhere hinting that AI systems can nail the details in panoramic X-rays, which suggests they could be a handy sidekick to the old-school methods—especially since things can get pretty tricky in dental and medical checks. AI's impact goes beyond just sharper diagnostics. In many cases, its ability to flag issues like periapical lesions and dental cavities is sparking a real breakthrough in identifying early diseases. Some recent dental tech chats even point out that AI has shown notable precision when mapping out root canal details, which is an encouraging sign for endodontics. These improvements not only help fine-tune treatments but also build a bit of trust among doctors who rely on these AI insights for more confident decision-making. Still, adding AI to the mix isn't all smooth sailing. There's a fair bit to consider in patient privacy, data security, and the ever-present risk of algorithmic bias. Generally speaking, as we lean more on AI in healthcare, it is crucial to set up guidelines that keep ethical issues in check while making sure diagnostic precision stays top-notch. Balancing technological progress with a healthy dose of caution will be key in shaping future radiographic practices—something ongoing research and debate should help nail down, as shown in studies (Asgary et al., 2024; Katarzyna et al., 2022).

Radiographic imaging has come a long way with leaps in technology that now let us diagnose conditions much more clearly. Advanced scanning tools have blended into areas you might not expect, like checking the integrity of aircraft structures. Research on nondestructive testing — using radiography to inspect materials without causing any harm — shows just how efficient this approach can be (Andronikou et al., 2011). Generally speaking, these tech upgrades not only sharpen diagnostic precision but also lay the groundwork for improved treatment strategies. It is clear that for many in healthcare, staying current with these innovations is more than just a nice-to-have. Every healthcare setting seems to set up radiographic equipment differently, driven by behind-the-scenes policies as well as outside regulations. A study in Malaysian hospitals, for example, pointed out that the Ministry of Health played a big part in how imaging technologies were deployed and used, stressing that both internal policies and external rules can shape the process (Nor et al., 2010). In most cases, it turns out that success with radiography isn't just about having advanced tech—it is also about navigating the broader policies and conditions that affect a facility's readiness to adopt new methods. Recognizing these various layers is key to truly benefiting from radiographic imaging across institutions. Radiographic imaging isn't solely changing how diagnoses are made; it is also shifting the roles and interactions among healthcare professionals. Routine use of these advanced imaging techniques has helped to redefine what radiographers do, sparking new kinds of relationships between clinical staff and others working behind the scenes. Curiously enough, research noted that even though some job roles have evolved with the tech, the interaction between radiographers and radiologists has remained largely the same (Nor et al., 2010), this teaches us that while technology is a huge part of the picture, it is important to see how it influences everyday work dynamics. By paying attention to how advanced imaging, professional roles, and even the overall work culture come together, stakeholders can better handle the challenges of rolling out new imaging methods—ultimately leading to improved patient outcomes and smoother operations.

KEY TERMS FROM THIS CHAPTER

- Biopsies
- Chest x-rays
- Digital radiography (DR)
- Exposure time
- Gastrointestinal system
- Milliamperage (mA)
- Scatter radiation
- X-ray
- Catheter placements
- Computed radiography (CR)
- Dose optimization
- Gastric movement
- Grid (Anti-scatter grid)
- Radiograph
- Tube current (mA)

Critical Thinking Questions

1. **What is the primary component in the X-ray tube that produces X-rays?**
   a. Cathode
   b. Anode
   c. Rotor
   d. Filament
2. **Which type of radiation is primarily responsible for creating diagnostic X-ray images?**
   a. Beta radiation
   b. Alpha radiation
   c. Gamma rays
   d. Electromagnetic radiation
3. **In a chest X-ray, what color does air in the lungs typically appear on the image?**
   a. White
   b. Light gray
   c. Black
   d. Dark blue
4. **What is the purpose of using a grid in radiographic imaging?**
   a. To cool the X-ray machine
   b. To reduce scatter radiation
   c. To increase exposure time
   d. To magnify the image
5. **Which of the following factors does not directly affect the quality of a radiographic image?**
   a. kVp (kilovolt peak)
   b. mAs (milliampere-seconds)
   c. Patient positioning
   d. Patient's heart rate

Short Answer Questions

1. What are the fundamental principles behind X-ray imaging, and how does it work?
2. What are the different types of X-ray imaging techniques, and how do they differ?
3. How is X-ray imaging used in medical diagnostics and what are some common applications?
4. What safety precautions should be taken to minimize risks during X-ray procedures?
5. What are some recent advances in X-ray technology that have improved imaging quality and patient care?
6. What ethical considerations should be addressed when using X-ray imaging in medical practice?

Answers to Critical Thinking Questions

1. (b); 2. (d); 3. (c); 4. (b); 5. (d)

References

1. Abuya, J., Antani, S., Dhoot, R., et al. (2018). Implementing a mobile diagnostic unit to increase access to imaging and laboratory services in western Kenya. https://core.ac.uk/download/323075042.pdf.

2. Achterhold, K., Auweter, S., Bamberg, F., et al. (2013). Diagnosing and mapping pulmonary emphysema on X-ray projection images. https://core.ac.uk/download/12175665.pdf (accessed on 23 May 2025).

3. Alsubhi, S. K. M., Aloufi, M. A. T., Alharthi, A. K. Z., Alzhrani, H. A. T., Althagafi, M. A. A., Alharthi, F. R. A., Alshehri, M. M., et al. (2024). Comprehensive analysis of radiological innovations, safety protocols, and clinical applications in diagnostic imaging and collaboration between X-ray technicians, nurses, and clinicians. *Journal of Eco Humanism*. https://www.semanticscholar.org/paper/dbc6b4f0789339aff9846b26fb263cdbd0ee1d70 (accessed on 23 May 2025).

4. Andronikou, S., McHugh, K., Abdurahman, N., Khoury, B., Mngomezulu, V., Brant, W. E., Cowan, I., McCulloch, M., & Ford, N. (2011). Pediatric radiology seen from Africa. Part I: Providing diagnostic imaging to a young population. *Pediatric Radiology, 41*(7), 811–825. https://doi.org/10.1007/s00247-011-2081-8.

5. Asgary, S. (2024). Artificial intelligence in endodontics: A scoping review. https://core.ac.uk/download/618356561.pdf (accessed on 23 May 2025).

6. Bansal, R., Bawa, S. K. S., Chauhan, P., et al. (2020). A comprehensive review of new innovations in dental implant imaging techniques. https://core.ac.uk/download/327096886.pdf (accessed on 23 May 2025).

7. Bath, B., Bontrager, D., Brennan, B., Brennan, C., Brennan, D., Butler, D., et al. (2013). Reducing dose for digital cranial radiography: The increased source to the image-receptor distance approach. https://core.ac.uk/download/29844051.pdf (accessed on 23 May 2025).

8. Besnard, C., Marie, A., Sasidharan, S., Deyhle, H., James, A. M., Ahmed, S. I., Reinhard, C., et al. (2024). The DIAD approach to correlative synchrotron X-ray imaging and diffraction analysis of human enamel. *Chemical & Biomedical Imaging, 2*, 222–232. https://www.semanticscholar.org/paper/ac588b6088034144ab95cccd6793c646bbc127b2 (accessed on 23 May 2025).

9. Bölükbas, D. A., & Wagner, D. (2019). X-ray dark-field imaging of lung cancer in mice. *Lung Imaging and CADx*. https://www.semanticscholar.org/paper/54febadff3942a1d62567e1a9dd7b93a8388725c (accessed on 23 May 2025).

10. Boyd, B. L. (2013). Using the Theory of Planned Behavior as a predictor of radiologic technologists' use of patient radiation protection best practices: A regional study. https://core.ac.uk/download/232855648.pdf (accessed on 23 May 2025).

11. Brus-Sawczuk, K., Czajkowska, M., Ganz, S., Mijiritsky, E., Párkányi, L., Regulski, P., & Zadrozny, L. (2022). Artificial intelligence application in assessment of panoramic radiographs. https://core.ac.uk/download/528253028.pdf (accessed on 23 May 2025).

12. Bustos, A., de la Iglesia-Vayá, M., Pertusa, A., et al. (2019). PadChest: A large chest X-ray image dataset with multi-label annotated reports. https://core.ac.uk/download/328881801.pdf (accessed on 23 May 2025).

13. Carpenter, J. L., Jr., & Stuhrke, W. F. (1976). NDE: An effective approach to improved reliability and safety. A technology survey. https://core.ac.uk/download/pdf/42882888.pdf (accessed on 23 May 2025).

14. Chen, Y. L., & Chen, W. (2023). Radial planes in hip magnetic resonance imaging: Techniques, applications, and perspectives. *Journal of Magnetic Resonance Imaging, 60*. https://www.semanticscholar.org/paper/f96385e3d2ef59b6406ade4a0ab6da095ad4b41a (accessed on 23 May 2025).

15. Davies, J. C., & Lowe, A. (2025). Environmental implications of the healthcare service sector. https://core.ac.uk/download/pdf/9307987.pdf (accessed on 23 May 2025).

16. Deker, E., & Oakley, K. D. (2020). Lead X-ray vests: Pros and cons in dental radiography and patient education on radiographic technology. https://core.ac.uk/download/322936725.pdf (accessed on 23 May 2025).

17. Du, W., Zhao, Y., & Roy, R. (2018). A review of miniaturized non-destructive testing technologies for *in-situ* inspections. *Procedia Manufacturing, 16*, 16–23. https://doi.org/10.1016/j.promfg.2018.10.152.

18. Durand, A., Finck, M., Hammond, G., et al. (2016). Computed tomography and magnetic resonance diagnosis of variations in the anatomical location of the major salivary glands in 1680 dogs and 187 cats. https://core.ac.uk/download/42370872.pdf (accessed on 23 May 2025).

19. Gielen, I., et al. (2012). Diagnostic imaging of the canine stifle. In *Small Animal Arthroscopy, 30th International Workshop, Proceedings* (pp. 33–36). Ghent University. Faculty of Veterinary Medicine. Department of Medical Imaging and Small Animal Orthopedics.

20. Horng, A., Stroebel, J., Geith, T., et al. (2021). Multiscale X-ray phase contrast imaging of human cartilage for investigating osteoarthritis formation. *Journal of Biomedical Science, 28*, 42. https://doi.org/10.1186/s12929-021-00739-1.

21. Hwang, H. (2017). Knowledge, attitude and perception on radiation imaging among children's caregivers in the pediatric dental clinic. https://hdl.handle.net/2144/23797 (accessed on 23 May 2025).

22. Lee, D. K., Kim, S. V., Limansubroto, A. N., Yen, A., Soundia, A., Wang, C. Y., Shi, W., Hong, C., Tetradis, S., Kim, Y., Park, N. H., Kang, M. K., & Ho, D. (2015a). Nanodiamond–gutta percha composite biomaterials for root canal therapy. *ACS Nano, 9*(11), 11490–11501. https://doi.org/10.1021/acsnano.5b05718.

23. Lee, T. F., Yang, J., Wuu, C., Liu, A., Fang, F., & Yeh, S. (2015b). Radiation oncology and medical physics. *BioMed Research International, 2015*. https://www.semanticscholar.org/paper/201caa77d7fa1236624f58ab92dc56d38cbe713d (accessed on 23 May 2025).

24. Leo, L. M., Prabha, B., Gopinath, K. M., Tamilselvi, C., Mohanaprakash, T. A., & Naveen, P. (2023). Pioneering healthcare transformation: Deep learning and radiographic imaging for rapid COVID-19 diagnosis. *2023 3rd International Conference on Innovative Mechanisms for Industry Applications (ICIMIA)*. https://www.semanticscholar.org/paper/1c9783a9000789fe5784a1e88bf83d29f8d464ae (accessed on 23 May 2025).

25. Macovski, A. (2025). Radiographic applications of spatial frequency multiplexing. https://core.ac.uk/download/pdf/42858477.pdf (accessed on 23 May 2025).

26. Martin, C. J., Vassileva, J., Vano, E., Mahesh, M., Ebdon-Jackson, S., Ng, K. H., Frush, D. P., Loose, R., & Damilakis, J. (2017). Unintended and accidental medical radiation exposures in radiology: Guidelines on investigation and prevention. *Journal of Radiological Protection, 37*(4), 883–906. https://doi.org/10.1088/1361-6498/aa881e.

27. Martin, K., Katsaros, C., Brylka, R., Schwanecke, U., & Schulze, R. (2025). Influence of patient motion on definition of typical cephalometric reference points in digital horizontally scanning cephalometric radiography. *Head & Face Medicine, 21*(1), 18. https://doi.org/10.1186/s13005-025-00491-z.

28. Mohd Nor, R. (2010). The organizational implications of medical imaging in the context of Malaysian hospitals. https://core.ac.uk/download/1588563.pdf (accessed on 23 May 2025).

29. Olson, A. J. (2021). Visualizing research prototypes for a service dashboard and machine panel in radiographic workflow. https://core.ac.uk/download/646176561.pdf (accessed on 23 May 2025).

30. Pohlen, M. (2024). Space radiology: Emerging nonsonographic medical imaging techniques and the potential applications for human spaceflight. *Wilderness & Environmental Medicine.* https://doi.org/10.1177/10806032241283380.

31. Ramlaul, A. (2018). An exploration of the meaning and development of critical thinking in diagnostic radiography. https://core.ac.uk/download/287581658.pdf (accessed on 23 May 2025).

32. Rayyani, A. A., Shalalni, A. A., Radwan, A. H., et al. (2024). Digital X-ray imaging: Emphasis can be placed on developments in digital X-ray technologies and their applications in diagnosis and treatment. https://core.ac.uk/download/616775625.pdf (accessed on 23 May 2025).

33. Rossi Tisbeni, S. (2017). Development and optimization of the control software for a mobile computed tomography system for cultural heritage. https://core.ac.uk/download/129672738.pdf (accessed on 23 May 2025).

34. Sakano, Y., Muroi, K., Goto, M., Sakamoto, H., Morimoto, Y., Kyogoku, S., Sakai, T., et al. (2021). A contribution to the history of Japanese education systems for radiological technologists. *Juntendo Medical Journal, 68*, 44–51. https://www.semanticscholar.org/paper/69e2484f067e051d7098076053246b0836ef1389 (accessed on 23 May 2025).

35. Sinha, V. (2013). Design, development and characterization of a novel neutron and X-ray combined computed tomography system [Doctoral dissertation, Missouri University of Science and Technology]. https://scholarsmine.mst.edu/doctoral_dissertations/2094 (accessed on 23 May 2025).

36. Van der Venter, R. (2016). Reporting on radiographic images in after-hours trauma units: Experiences of radiographers and medical practitioners. https://core.ac.uk/download/188177818.pdf (accessed on 23 May 2025).

37. Vincent, C. R. (2024). Sensor analytics for subsea pipeline and cable inspection: A review (Master's thesis, Louisiana State University). https://repository.lsu.edu/gradschool_theses/5913 (accessed on 23 May 2025).

38. Whitlock, J., Dixon, J., Sherlock, C., Tucker, R., Bolt, D. M., & Weller, R. (2016). Technical innovation changes standard radiographic protocols in veterinary medicine: Is it necessary to obtain two dorsoproximal–palmar distal oblique views of the equine foot when using

computerized radiography systems? *Veterinary Record, 178*, 531. https://doi.org/10.1136/vr.103396.

39. Wonglee, S., Richards, C., Pornroongruengchok, W., Picha, P., Channuie, J., Khaweerat, S., & Liamsuwan, T. (2020). The 15th–18th terracotta doll investigation using a compact neutron tomography system at Thai Research Reactor. *Materials Research Proceedings, 15*, 239–243. https://www.semanticscholar.org/paper/b01dc582dba71f4ad1e8145dafc08bd8589c0127 (accessed on 23 May 2025).

40. Xue, X., Chinnaperumal, S., Abdulsahib, G. M., Manyam, R. R., Marappan, R., Raju, S. K., & Khalaf, O. I. (2023). Design and analysis of a deep learning ensemble framework model for the detection of COVID-19 and pneumonia using large-scale CT scan and X-ray image datasets. *Bioengineering, 10*(3), 363. https://doi.org/10.3390/bioengineering10030363.

COMPUTED TOMOGRAPHY (CT)

3

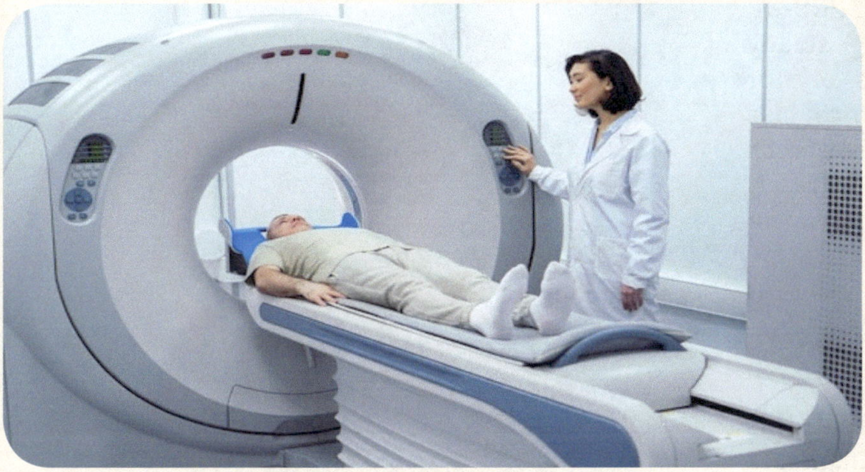

LEARNING OBJECTIVES

After studying this chapter, you will be able to:

1. Understand the basic principles of computed tomography.
2. Identify various types of CT scans.
3. Explore the clinical applications of CT in medicine.
4. Evaluate the advantages, limitations and risks of CT scanning.

Introduction

Medical imaging has come a long way. CT, for instance, now plays a major role in seeing what's happening inside the body—it lets doctors view anatomical details with a striking clarity. CT works by mixing smart algorithms with advanced detector systems to slice out images of the body, which, in most cases, makes diagnosing and planning treatments clearer. Sharper temporal and spatial resolution has made images better even as radiation doses drop, and adding modifications like dual- and multi-energy imaging has stretched CT's use into many different medical areas (Ákos et al., 2025). Precise diagnostics are more in demand than ever, so keeping radiation safe is a big deal. Diagnostic reference levels, or DRLs, act like a guide to ensure that radiation stays within safe bounds, especially for vulnerable groups like kids. Studies in different regions have looked at setting pediatric CT DRLs, and research—generally speaking—shows a lot of variation in DRL numbers across studies (Gyan et al., 2024). These efforts, really, not only make patients safer but also teach us more about how to use CT without extra ionizing radiation exposure. CT technology isn't standing still either. Advances in detector tech and image reconstruction keep pushing things forward, and photon-counting detector CT (PCD-CT) is one such breakthrough that's identifying attention. It promises even better image quality while keeping radiation levels low—a shift that underscores the imaging community's drive to fine-tune CT to meet both clinical and safety standards. Researchers are closely examining the ups and downs of PCD-CT, and it is becoming clear that ongoing, steady investment in this new technology is key for improved accuracy and broader clinical use (Ákos et al., 2025). Overall, blending these tech advancements with robust safety measures is what will shape the future of CT imaging in healthcare.

Definition of Computed Tomography (CT)

Imaging technology has come a long way—this shift has had a big impact on how diagnoses are made. CT, for example, uses X-rays to create detailed cross-sectional images that reveal layers of our internal anatomy. It is not simply a flat picture like traditional X-rays; instead, CT offers a sort of 3D view that helps doctors pick up on subtle abnormalities more clearly. Many times, clinicians find CT indispensable, especially when they're checking for trauma, tumors, or internal organ problems. Advancements in both the hardware and software sides have pushed CT even further, opening up multimodal imaging techniques that sharpen diagnostic details – and this is especially true in the fight against cancer (Wei et al., 2019). On top of that, CT is often combined with other imaging methods, like MRI or PET, to weave together both anatomical and functional data in one assessment. This mix isn't just a neat trick; it boosts diagnostic capabilities and even gives rise to the field of radiomics. Radiomics, generally speaking, uses algorithms to sift through the imaging data, extracting measurable features that shine a light on tumor characteristics and support stronger clinical decisions. Several studies have shown that fusing data from multiple modalities with machine learning can yield better prognostic outcomes than using just a single imaging approach, which reaffirms CT's role in personalizing medicine (Wei et al., 2019). Such progress has started to change the way professionals look at diagnostics, treatment planning, and patient care.

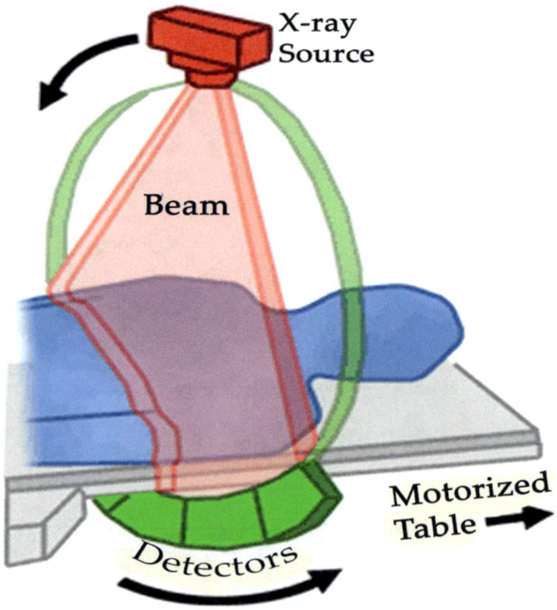

Figure 3.1. Drawing of CT fan beam (left) and patient in a CT imaging system.

Source: https://www.fda.gov/radiation-emitting-products/medical-x-ray-imaging/computed-tomography-ct.

Another point to note is how applying radiomics in CT isn't as simple as flipping a switch – the technical aspects count a lot. For instance, details like slice thickness and pixel size can sway image quality and the features that are picked up. Research often suggests that adjustments made during image acquisition and reconstruction do affect how reproducible radiomic features are, meaning that understanding these factors well is key to accurate interpretation. Detailed studies on texture and gray-level discretization have even shown methods to fine-tune CT scan analysis, making the images more clinically useful. In many cases, radiomics might just be the extra edge needed to increase diagnostic accuracy, refine treatment plans, and ultimately foster better outcomes for patients in this rapidly evolving field of medical imaging (Figure 3.1).

Historical Development of CT Technology

CT scanning changed the way we look inside the human body, and its rise wasn't a neat, step-by-step process. Back in the 1960s, breakthroughs in digital electronics and X-ray methods kind of collided and paved the way for this new tech. Godfrey Hounsfield, working at EMI Laboratories, rolled out the first CT scanner in 1971—a machine that could produce cross-sectional images of people. This whole development sparked a chain reaction; not only did it completely alter diagnostic routines, but it also pushed researchers to improve image resolution and speed. The jump from single-slice units to multi-slice scanners, for instance, slashed exam times and improved how finely doctors could see details in the images. As the machine got smarter and faster, the emphasis naturally moved toward making imaging safer and more efficient. Early on, worries about too much radiation from classic X-rays led to new safety checks and tech adjustments. Techniques like helical scanning and iterative reconstructions (IRs) emerged, aiming to keep the image quality high while cutting down the radiation dose. More recently, innovations such as photon-counting CT scanners have popped up, offering even better diagnostics while, in most cases, keeping radiation concerns in check. There's also a growing trend to weave artificial intelligence (AI) into how images are processed and analyzed, a move that seems to smooth out workflow and boost overall efficiency. Looking at CT's history today, it is clear that its evolution isn't just about technology—it also touches on broader social issues like healthcare access and the environment. The arrival of these advanced imaging methods naturally raised questions about who can afford such tools and whether these innovations widen the gap in healthcare availability, especially in underserved communities. Economic studies now suggest that we should balance neat technological wins with the need for affordability and fair access for all. Lately, there's even been discussion about using biodegradable contrast agents and energy-saving imaging processes to cut down on the environmental impact. All these layers show that, generally speaking, CT isn't just a scientific milestone; it has become a key player in discussions about sustainable and equitable healthcare practices (Kerna et al., 2024a) (Figure 3.2).

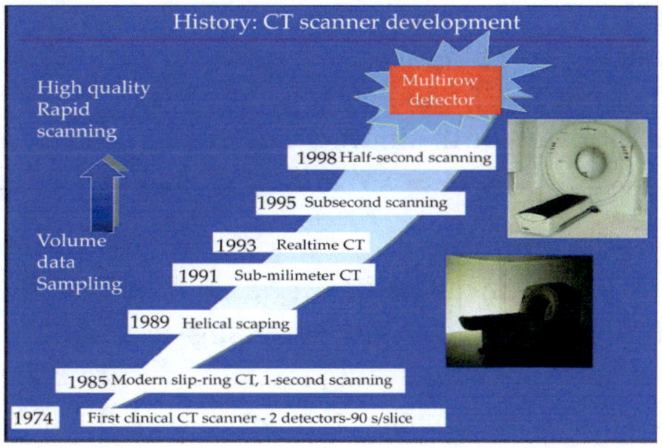

Figure 3.2. History: CT scanner development.

Source: https://thecommonvein.com/wp-content/uploads/2023/03/web-CT-018.jpg.

Importance of CT in Modern Medicine

A surge in new math techniques and faster computing has changed how we take a look at the body, especially with CT scans. Lately, tools like the TIGRE toolbox — a clever GPU-based solution — have managed to mix hard-to-grasp math with everyday CT work. This toolkit comes packed with smart number crunchers that sharpen image quality while keeping things simple for users. Its growing range means doctors now get more flexibility with shapes, and the calculations run quicker too, which opens up CT for use in lots of different medical situations. Its ongoing development, in most cases, keeps it at the cutting edge of diagnosis, tying new tech breakthroughs directly to what clinicians need, thereby cementing its pivotal role in modern healthcare (Biguri et al., 2024). In dealing with cancer and hormone disorders, CT has shown itself to be downright vital. It lets doctors see inside the body with such clarity that even small lesions, which are key in staging cancer, become obvious. When CT pairs up with PET scans, it almost becomes a double act — not only showing structure but also giving hints about a tumor's activity through metabolism. This mix often proves especially useful in endocrine cases, where identifying a tumor early on can change the treatment game. By casually blending what's functional with what's anatomical, CT and PET together provide a solid method for both finding cancers and tracking how treatments are working (Calderoni et al., 2024).

The non-invasive style is another big plus for patient care, offering a smoother, less uncomfortable diagnostic route. Its speed in capturing images can be a real lifesaver, particularly when emergencies arise and every second counts. In urgent cases, doctors can quickly check for issues like trauma, hidden bleeding, or sudden abdominal pain—oftentimes without needing any invasive goings-on. As technology steadily marches forward, CT's role in patient management is likely to grow even more, highlighting its central place in today's medicine. Generally speaking, this progress not only underlines its everyday importance in clinics but also points to why fresh research and tech upgrades are needed to keep improving diagnostic precision and treatment success.

3.1. Principles of Computed Tomography (CT)

Learning Outcome

1. Understand the basic mechanics of CT imaging.
2. Describe the role of X-rays in CT scans.
3. Define image reconstruction techniques.

This progress comes from some pretty basic physics ideas that aren't always obvious at first glance. At its heart, CT uses X-ray attenuation numbers – in plain terms, a way to gauge how different tissues soak up X-rays – to build slice-by-slice views of our inner body parts. This method gives us detailed images that go far beyond what standard X-rays can show. Innovations like helical scanning and multidetector setups started letting machines obtain continuously obtain data, which means images turned out sharper and scans happened much quicker. In most cases, having a strong grip on these physics basics turns out to be the secret sauce behind better diagnostic tools and improved patient care (Mński et al., 2024). Lately, new tech leaps have pushed CT imaging into exciting new territory. Take dual-energy CT (DECT), for example – it captures images at two different energy levels so that materials can be told apart based on how they react to X-rays; this is especially useful in vascular studies when figuring out the difference between iodine and calcium. At the same time, photon-counting computed tomography (PCCT) has begun making a splash by measuring the energy of every single photon, which may lower radiation doses while boosting both spatial and temporal detail. Generally speaking, DECT and PCCT represent a shift toward imaging methods that are not only more refined but also better at keeping patients safe without skimping on diagnostic accuracy (Mński et al., 2024). Understanding just how CT works isn't only about getting clearer pictures—

it also expands how we use it in clinics. As this technology keeps maturing, knowing its core elements lets radiologists tweak image settings and make smart acquisition choices. New approaches like volumetric rendering and advanced visualization have pushed CT into areas like radiation therapy planning and more precise localization. And when CT is mixed with other methods, say, PET scans, the result is an even richer peek into a patient's condition. Overall, this constant deepening of CT know-how sets the stage for better diagnostics and treatment planning, proving that weaving these principles into daily practice is absolutely essential (Alyami et al., 2023) (Figure 3.3).

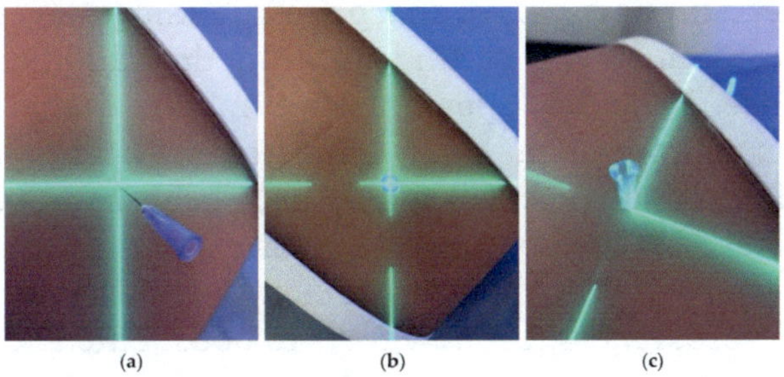

Figure 3.3. The green lines on the patient's body are light from a laser alignment system.

Source: Weigel K, Kubik-Huch RA, Baer-Beck M, Canstein C, Kostrzewa M. Evaluation of Accuracy and Performance of a Novel, Fully Gantry Integrated 3D Laser System for Computed Tomography Guided Needle Placement: A Phantom Study. *Diagnostics*. 2023; 13(2):282. https://doi.org/10.3390/diagnostics13020282.

3.1.1. Basic Mechanics of Computed Tomography (CT) Imaging

CT has changed the game in medical imaging, showing off a key physics idea in the way we diagnose illnesses. CT works by sending X-rays through the body and identifying them with detectors arranged around the patient. These X-rays get weakened differently by various tissues, which naturally builds up contrast and lets us piece together detailed cross-sectional views. In many cases, algorithms then take this messy raw data and turn it into images we can use. New developments—like photon-counting-detector CT (PCD-CT)—give these capabilities an extra boost. Generally speaking, PCD-CT offers sharper spatial resolution and a better contrast-to-noise ratio, which means diagnoses can be made more effectively. The way these systems operate illustrates how technology and medical practice are sort of combined together, changing not only how we diagnose but also how treatment plans are drawn up in everyday settings (Siegel et al., 2024). Even as detector technology keeps advancing, there's a real challenge in balancing the X-ray dose with the quality of the image. It a tricky situation where lowering radiation is important, yet doctors still need clear, useful images.

This balancing act—getting enough image detail without too much exposure—has driven ongoing tweaks in scanning methods and the algorithms that process the data. In earlier days, image processing mostly leaned on model-based approaches. Nowadays deep learning is opening up new frontiers, offering a significant jump in how well we can restore images. These new methods, which still build on some basic physics ideas, allow us to reconstruct high-resolution images from scans made at lower doses. As a result, clinicians get clearer pictures while keeping patient risk low, a sign of just how far imaging and computational advances have come (Dutta et al., 2024). Understanding CT imaging means also realizing that the way scans are done is adjusted for different clinical needs. Changes like tweaking slice thickness or adjusting how fast the X-ray tube rotates can notably impact image quality. Getting these parameters right is important not just for capturing the best possible images but also for meeting specific anatomical or disease-related requirements. With innovations like PCD-CT gaining ground, it has become even more essential to modify existing scanning protocols so their unique benefits are fully utilized. And, as data processing keeps evolving, the limits of what CT can do keep getting pushed further. This ongoing cycle of updates in both hardware and software highlights the ever-changing, dynamic role of CT in modern medical diagnostics (Siegel et al., 2024) (Figure 3.4).

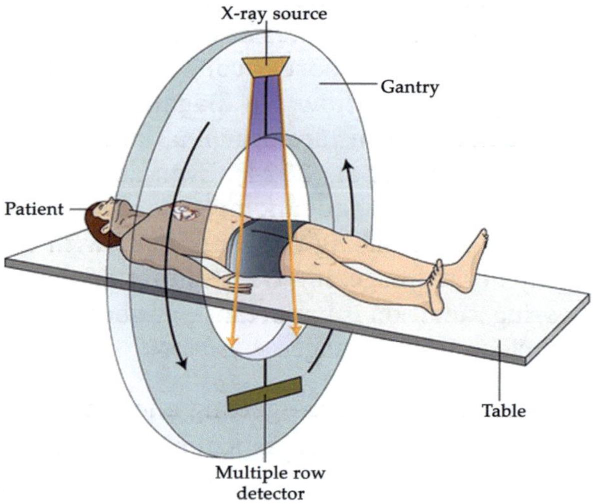

Figure 3.4. A cartoon depiction of a typical CT scanner.

Source: https://thoracickey.com/basic-principles-in-computed-tomography-ct/.

3.1.2. Role of X-Rays in Computed Tomography (CT) Scans

CT changed the game for looking inside the body in ways we hadn't seen before. It all started with X-rays, which essentially serve as the building blocks for CT imaging. Many X-ray images—taken here, there, and everywhere around the body—get mashed together to form a full-fledged 3D view. This jumble of images not only makes it easier for doctors to see what's going on (think tumors or even tiny fractures) but it also ups the accuracy big time. You can even fiddle with the X-ray data afterward to polish up the images for surgical planning and other interventions. In many cases, blending X-rays into CT scanning marked a turning point in how clinics run their imaging operations. Getting a feel for how X-rays and CT technology mesh together offers a peek into modern radiology's inner workings, when X-rays pass through the body, different tissues soak up the rays in varying amounts—dense bone hogs a lot of the exposure and pops up white, while muscles and organs show up in different gray tones. That natural contrast, repeated over and over, gives clinicians the edge they need to tell normal from abnormal tissues. Recent leaps in detector tech and image reconstruction algorithms (yes, sometimes they get a bit noisy) have sharpened CT images even more, all while cutting back on the radiation dose. Generally speaking, this means that CT scans rooted in X-ray data not only deliver sharper diagnoses but also help keep patients safer. The role of X-ray tech isn't standing still either—it is evolving right along with CT scans as researchers test new ways to boost efficiency and curb risks. For example, ongoing tweaks in X-ray settings, like dose modulation and IR (with a few slip-ups here and there), have made imaging both safer and more precise. Computer algorithms now help clean up the image noise, making sure that only the necessary amount of radiation is used. And there's the buzz about new applications, like dual-energy CT, where two different X-ray energy levels unravel more detailed tissue composition info. This kind of innovation not only broadens our diagnostic abilities but also helps in examining conditions that used to be tough to nail down. In most cases, as these advances continue chugging along, the influence of X-rays in CT imaging is bound to grow even further—paving the way for better patient care and smarter diagnostic strategies (Boonjindasup et al., 2024; Elkhadir et al., 2024) (Figure 3.5).

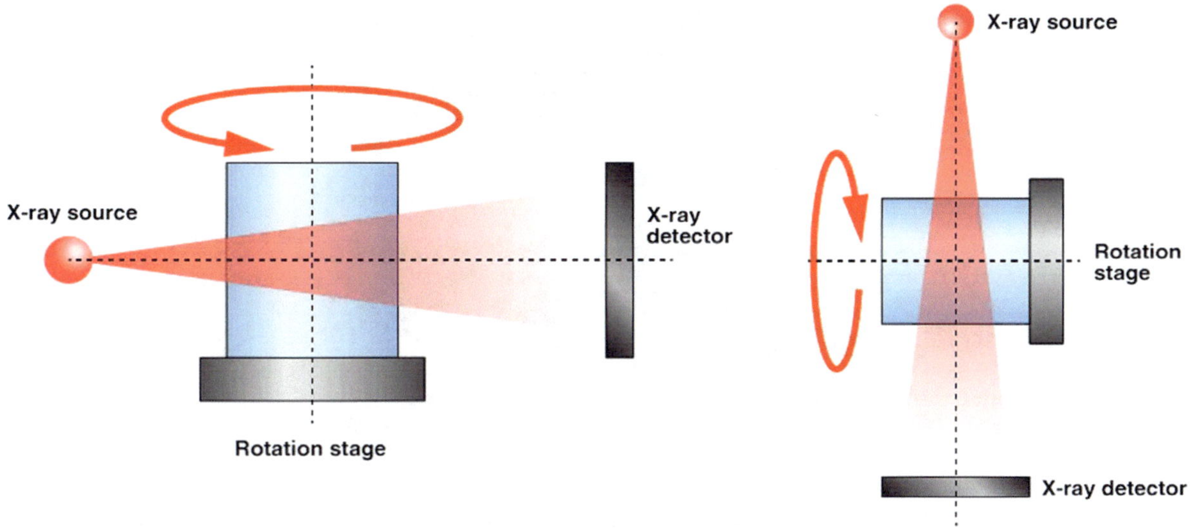

Figure 3.5. The X-ray CT structure.

Source: https://www.matsusada.com/column/words-ct.html.

3.1.3. Image Reconstruction Techniques

Technology has come a long way, and CT imaging now looks very different from the old days. What once worked—methods like filtered back projection (FBP) and iterative reconstruction (IR)—has started to run into trouble, especially when trying to keep radiation levels low. People are noticing that when you push for less radiation, the images don't always come out as clear or fast to reconstruct as before, so researchers have turned to ideas like AI and machine learning to see if they can do better. Recent work shows that convolutional neural networks (CNNs) and even their 3D cousins have become unexpected heroes in CT reconstruction. Many studies generally suggest that these deep learning approaches beat traditional methods by taking care of problems like noise and annoying artifacts.

It seems that using these more flexible algorithms gives you images that are easier to rely on for diagnostics, and in most cases, mixing deep learning techniques with CT scanning could boost both accuracy and efficiency in real clinical settings (Rahman et al., 2023). Applying deep learning to low-dose CT isn't just about solving old challenges—it also opens up many practical benefits for healthcare overall. Faster reconstruction times and better diagnostic accuracy mean that decisions can be made quicker when every second counts. Datasets such as the 2016 NIH-AAPM-Mayo collection have become key training grounds, helping these algorithms get robust and ready for real-world tests.

At the same time, we still face obstacles like high computational demands and the need for lots of training data. Overall, while the promise is huge, ongoing research and investment remain essential to fully tap into what deep learning can do for CT image reconstruction (Zhang et al., 2022) (Figure 3.6).

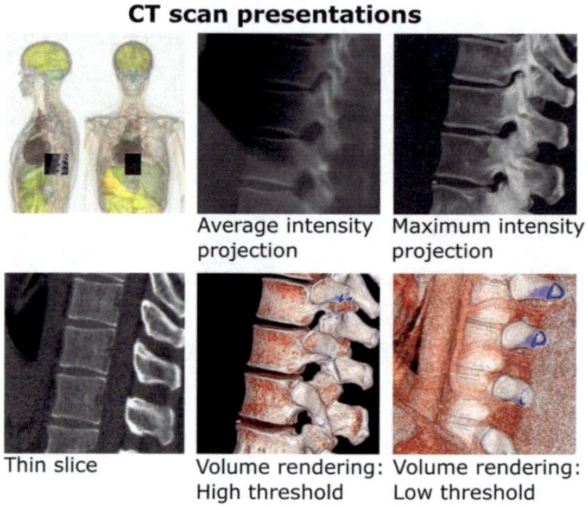

Figure 3.6. Types of presentations of CT scans: – Average intensity projection – Maximum intensity projection – Thin slice (median plane) – Volume rendering by high and low threshold for radiodensity.

Source: By Mikael Häggström & Anatomography, CC BY-SA 2.1 jp, https://commons.wikimedia.org/w/index.php?curid=60448994.

Test Your Knowledge

1. What are the basic mechanical components involved in CT imaging, and how do they work together to produce images?
2. How are X-rays utilized in CT scans to generate detailed cross-sectional images of the body?

3.2. Types of Computed Tomography (CT) Scans

Learning Outcome

1. Understand the basic principles of conventional CT scans.
2. Explore the features of spiral (Helical) CT scans.
3. Learn the principles and clinical uses of CT angiography.

CT has many different forms that suit various diagnostic needs. The standard CT scan takes several X-ray images from different angles and uses computer algorithms to stitch them into cross-sectional pictures – a method that's quite handy when examining the brain, chest, and abdomen. High-res CT and multi-slice CT have popped up recently, offering sharper images and quicker turnaround, which can help in emergencies or when tackling tricky anatomical details. Contrast-enhanced CT scans add another level of detail. By injecting a contrast dye, doctors can more easily pick out blood vessels and spot the odd tissue irregularity; in most cases, this means that differences in tissues stand out better. Generally speaking, these clearer images are key for accurate diagnoses and planning treatments – something especially important in oncology in evaluating tumors. Then there's dual-energy CT, which captures images at two energy levels. This approach helps differentiate materials based on their atomic makeup, proving useful for diagnosing issues like gout or urinary stone disease (Cynthia et al., 2020). New developments like dual-source and photon-counting CT keep pushing the boundaries. Dual-source CT employs two X-ray setups and detectors, obtaining images fast, which is particularly useful for capturing the beating heart. Photon-counting CT, by counting each photon passing through the body, produces exceptionally detailed images while cutting down on radiation exposure. All these innovations show that CT technology is constantly evolving, broadening its clinical applications—from untangling complex diseases to monitoring how treatments are working overtime (Zamhuri et al., 2021).

3.2.1. Conventional Computed Tomography (CT) Scans

Imaging technology has changed the game for medical diagnostics. CT scans, for instance, have become a real workhorse in clinics these days. They use X-rays to build detailed "slice-by-slice" pictures that help doctors see inside the body clearly. This makes it easier to spot issues like brain, lung, or abdominal problems—and often even catch tumors or internal injuries early. Of course, the flip side is that the radiation involved raises concerns about long-term effects. In most cases, ongoing upgrades in these machines aim to cut down on radiation without losing the detail needed for solid diagnosis. Digging into the tech side reveals that these scanners aren't just simple devices. They usually employ a rotating X-ray tube teamed up with many detectors that catch images from all sorts of angles. Then, sophisticated algorithms piece those shots together into high-resolution images—details that wouldn't be possible with older radiographic methods. Multi-slice scanning, for example, speeds things up, which proves handy in both emergency and routine outpatient care. Yet, sometimes the system shows its limitations: metal implants can cause odd artifacts, and a bit of image noise might lead to misinterpretations. In today's fast-paced clinical world, CT scans are taking on even more responsibility. Healthcare professionals lean on them heavily when rapid decisions are needed, sometimes in high-pressure emergencies. There's also a noticeable trend to mix conventional CT methods with emerging tools like photon-counting CT, which, generally speaking, helps boost image quality while lowering radiation doses. Ongoing studies are trying to sort out the best ways to use these scans across different patient groups and conditions. Overall, despite a few uniqueness here and there, CT scans remain a central player in medical imaging—constantly evolving to support better, more timely patient care (Figure 3.7).

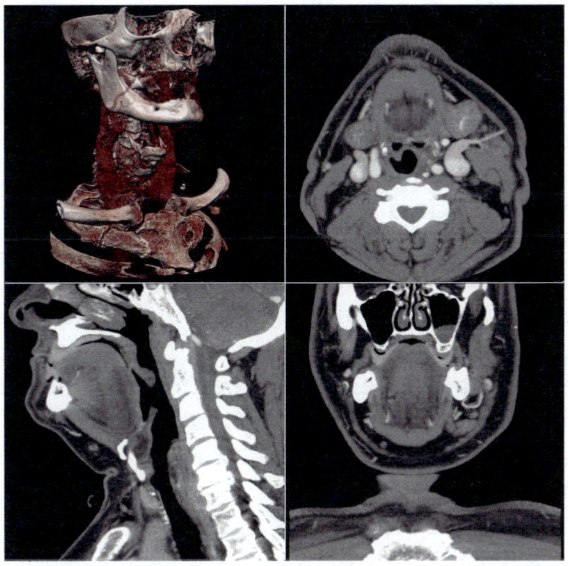

Figure 3.7. Typical screen layout for diagnostic software, showing one volume rendering (VR) and multiplanar view of three thin slices in the axial (upper right), sagittal (lower left), and coronal planes (lower right).

Source: By en: User: ChumpusRex - http://en.wikipedia.org/wiki/File:Ct-workstation-neck.jpg, CC BY-SA 3.0, https://commons.wikimedia.org/w/index.php?curid=6026473.

3.2.2. Spiral (Helical) Computed Tomography (CT) Scans

CT imaging has taken a interesting leap forward with new tech. Spiral CT scanning, for instance, now obtains data continuously while a patient moves through the machine—a real game changer compared to the old method of snapping one slice at a time. This continuous swirl of data collection not only speeds things up but also cuts down on those annoying motion artifacts, so the images show anatomy more truthfully. Doctors can twist and turn the resulting 3D dataset to get a full, flexible look at any area of concern, making it easier to spot details from different angles. In most cases, this shift brings faster, clearer scans that lead to better diagnosis. The buzz gets even richer when you throw dual-energy CT (DECT) protocols into the mix. Here, the scanner juggles two energy levels at once to tease apart different materials by their atomic traits. Generally speaking, low-energy monoenergetic decompositions from DECT boost soft tissue contrast noticeably – a handy trick, especially for tough cases like pancreatic cancer. It turns out that subtle, radiation-induced texture changes in the CT can be picked up more sharply with this approach, which means radiologists catch treatment responses with better precision. By tracking shifts in CT histogram features during therapy, clinicians—sometimes even noticing small shifts—can decide on patient care with more confidence (Noid et al., 2018). Then there's the emerging role of IR algorithms. These tools, built to reduce noise and keep radiation doses low, work in a step-by-step way that stands in stark contrast to the clunky traditional FBP methods. IR algorithms polish the images by gradually suppressing unwanted noise, resulting in sharper visuals even when you're not ramping up exposure. Sure, sometimes the old techniques left pesky artifacts in the mix, but these new computational tools sharpen the picture and boost diagnostic confidence. By tackling long-standing issues in CT imaging, IR algorithms are carving out a key role in everyday medical practice, making spiral CT just that much more useful for clinical decisions (Geyer et al., 2015) (Figure 3.8).

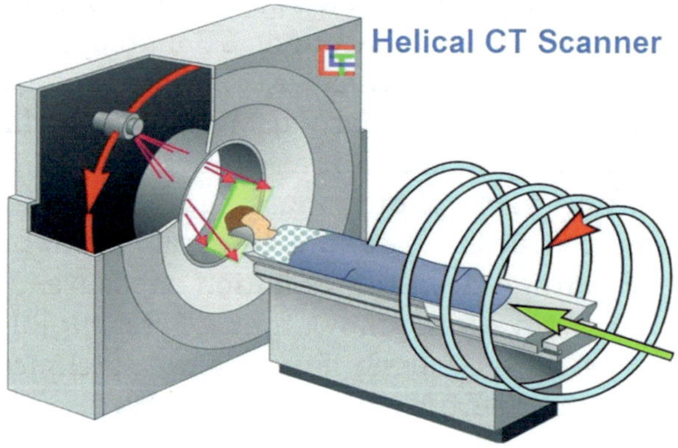

Figure 3.8. Spiral (Helical) CT scans.

Source: https://i.ytimg.com/vi/7Js5NwRPQ00/maxresdefault.jpg.

3.2.3. CT Angiography (CTA)

Imaging techniques have come a long way and changed how we check our blood vessels. CT angiography—often called CTA—now stands out by giving doctors a clear view of our vascular system without the need for invasive procedures. It works by using X-rays along with smart computer algorithms to produce detailed images of blood vessels. When a contrast dye is injected, doctors can tell tissues apart and spot blockages or unusual bulges. Generally speaking, advances like multi-detector CT systems have sped up scans, cutting down the time needed and often leading to better outcomes. Beyond its knack for producing high-resolution images, CT angiography (CTA) has found its way into many areas of medicine. For instance, it is widely used to look at cerebrovascular issues—helping diagnose things like ischemic strokes and irregular vessel formations where every minute counts. It is also now applied to study tumors, checking out how well they're supplied with blood, which shows just how adaptable the technique can be. This wide range of uses underlines why CTA is seen as a core tool in modern diagnostics. New advancements in radiology are continually pushing the limits of CTA. Researchers are mixing in methods like perfusion and even molecular imaging to get a better grasp on what's happening with blood vessels. These innovations not only improve diagnostic accuracy but also open the door to treatments that are tailored more closely to an individual's needs. Sure, challenges remain—like managing radiation exposure and ensuring top-notch quality in contrast agents—but the future does seem promising. As CTA evolves alongside leaps in AI and hybrid imaging techniques, its role in patient care keeps growing, paving the way for more targeted and effective therapies (Islam et al., 2025; Liu et al., 2024) (Figure 3.9).

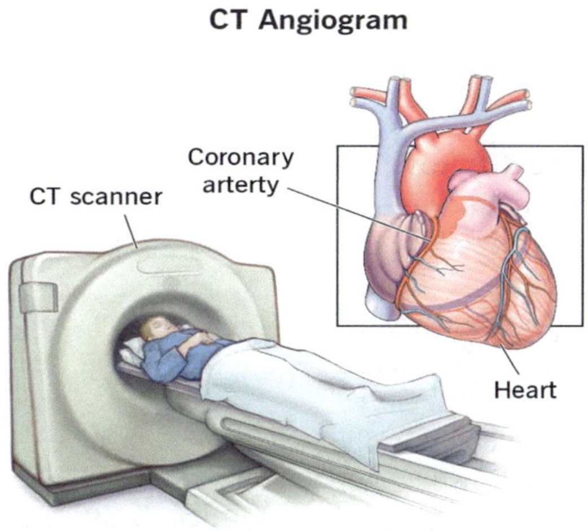

Figure 3.9. A CT angiogram allows your healthcare provider to see your blood vessels and tissues.

Source: https://my.clevelandclinic.org/health/diagnostics/16899-coronary-computed-tomography-angiogram.

Test Your Knowledge

1. How does a spiral (helical) CT scan differ from a conventional CT scan in terms of image acquisition?
2. What is the purpose of CT angiography, and how is it used to evaluate blood vessels in the body?

3.3. Applications of Computed Tomography (CT) in Medicine

Learning Outcome

1. Understand how CT imaging is used in diagnosing various diseases and medical conditions.
2. Explore the role of CT scans in preoperative planning and patient assessment.
3. Recognize how CT imaging helps in monitoring the effectiveness of medical treatments.

CT imaging has shifted how we do diagnoses in healthcare; it is not just fancy tech anymore—it's become a real game changer. High-res scans now let us spot everything from tumors and vascular issues to hidden injuries. With its ability to deliver clear cross-sectional views shot from different angles, CT helps doctors see all those complex details in our bodies. And generally speaking, when you mix in a bit of AI, it is even better at identifying those slight early signs of disease. Overall, these improvements smooth out the process and pave the way for treatments that feel much more tailored to the individual. Heart care is another area where CT flexes its muscles. Cardiac computed tomography angiography, or CTA, has become part of the regular routine to check on blood vessels and other odd changes. Recent upgrades have even managed to bring down radiation exposure—good news for anyone needing frequent scans. Sometimes 3D visuals and even virtual or augmented reality tools pop up, adding an extra layer of detail when doctors assess conditions like coronary artery disease. This mix of tech gives physicians a fresh, sometimes almost interactive, look at patient anatomy, which in turn leads to better, more informed clinical decisions. CT's role isn't limited to standard diagnostics either. Its applications have stepped outside the clinic, even showing promise in fields like agriculture where it aids in quality checks and precision management, and of course in advanced patient care. For example, using CT to guide needle biopsies is one clever trick that illustrates just how versatile it can be. Researchers are still digging into how these imaging breakthroughs can boost precision medicine and overall patient management. Sure, there are occasional bumps in fully rolling out these new approaches, but overall the evidence points to a future where CT transforms from a basic diagnostic tool into a key player across lots of healthcare areas (Sun, 2024; Wang et al., 2024) (Figure 3.10).

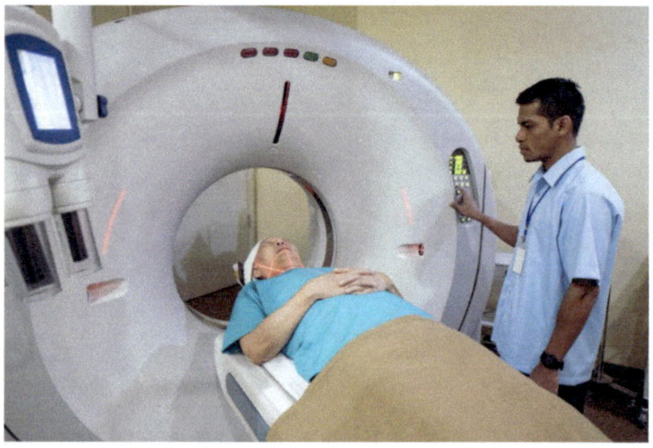

Figure 3.10. Computed Tomography (CT) in Medicine

Source: https://cdn-prod.medicalnewstoday.com/content/images/articles/153/153201/ct-scan.jpg.

3.3.1. Diagnosis of Diseases and Conditions

Medical imaging has come a long way and changed how we catch diseases. CT scans, for example, offer fast, clear images that help doctors notice even subtle problems. They're used for many things—from spotting cancers to checking injuries after accidents, and even for puzzling abdominal issues. Sometimes CT is paired with PET in a hybrid setup, which gives an extra look at how tissues work at a metabolic level. In most cases, this mix of methods means early detection and easier tracking of how a disease shifts over time, which boosts patient care overall (Hussain et al., 2022).

In inflammation, figuring out what's triggering it is super important. Chronic inflammatory conditions affect millions and often come with heavy costs in terms of suffering and even early death. Traditional scans like CT sometimes miss the finer details at the molecular level—details that are pretty key for planning treatment. New molecular imaging techniques seem promising, identifying tiny inflammatory markers with surprising sensitivity and clarity. This becomes especially relevant for conditions like rheumatoid arthritis or even certain heart diseases, where inflammation sits right at the center of the problem.

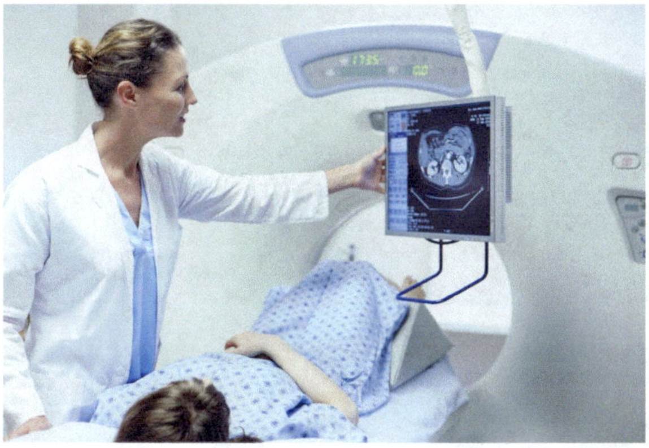

Figure 3.11. Diagnosis of Diseases and Conditions

Source: https://www.health.com/thmb/GNl2H9dmDbrPW6Q7gFrU3xr3XmE=/1500x0/filters:no_upscale():max_bytes(150000):strip_icc()/ctscan-GettyImages-493216325-63c244b9138f460f8529ecf076166864.jpg.

Researchers are, in most cases, working to sharpen these tools so that a deeper understanding of disease helps lead to more targeted care (MacRitchie et al., 2020). Diagnostic imaging is advancing, but it still faces a tricky trade-off. CT scans give us a level of anatomical detail that's hard to match, yet they expose patients to ionizing radiation, which isn't without its risks. Doctors often find themselves balancing the need for precise diagnosis with the potential harm from too much exposure. On top of that, new developments in CT—like dose-reduction strategies and improved ways of reconstructing images—are aiming to trim down that risk without sacrificing quality. It appears that as the technology improves, safety practices and ethical concerns will continue to evolve, ensuring that patient wellbeing stays in focus. Overall, ongoing research is promising not only a boost in image clarity but also a keen attention to keeping patients safe (Hussain et al., 2022) (Figure 3.11).

3.3.2. Preoperative Planning and Assessment

Preoperative planning matters a lot, especially when surgery demands a clear picture of the body's layout. Surgeons rely on CT scans to obtain high-definition images that reveal even the trickiest of anatomical details—images that help spot underlying issues and steer decisions on which technique to use. For example, in dogs with extrahepatic portosystemic shunt (EHPSS), CTA has proven useful by showing shunt shapes and even how intrahepatic portal veins branch, which in turn guides the surgical plan and helps predict the outcome (Takeuchi et al., 2025). In short, CT isn't just a tool for diagnosis; it weaves deep into the whole planning process. Modern advances, like blending CT with MRI and even 3-D imaging, add another layer to pre-surgery checks in many fields—take facial reconstructive procedures, for example. When scans lay out soft tissues and bones with such detail, surgical teams can get a better feel of the affected area and adjust their plans accordingly. Several studies, (Dave et al., 2024) in most cases, show that when doctors take a structured approach to assessing the area before surgery, precision goes up and patients tend to do better. CT imaging, then, becomes a bedrock component in shaping both diagnosis and the overall surgical strategy. Planning doesn't end when the surgery starts; it also plays a role in what happens afterward.

In that canine study mentioned earlier, CTA findings showed a link with intraoperative portal vein pressures—even though the grade of intrahepatic portal vein branching didn't majorly affect post-surgery complications, it still influenced the choice of surgical tactic (Takeuchi et al., 2025). This suggests that a thorough preoperative check can help anticipate complications and tweak surgical protocols. Overall, when surgeons take the time to plan carefully using tools like CT imaging, the result is smoother and better care for patients, whether we're talking about pets or people.

3.3.3. Monitoring Treatment Effectiveness

CT scanning has changed the way we check if a treatment is working. Doctors now lean on CT not just for planning but also to keep a live watch on how a tumor reacts—like when they use it to guide cryoablation on adrenal tumors. One study, for instance, showed a 91.7% success rate on the initial try with CT-guided cryo procedures, which kind of proves that having a good image can back up the treatment plan. The scans jump in early to set things up and then stick around during the procedure, letting clinicians tweak the approach in real-time, a shift that clearly bumps up patient survival rates (Pusceddu et al., 2024).

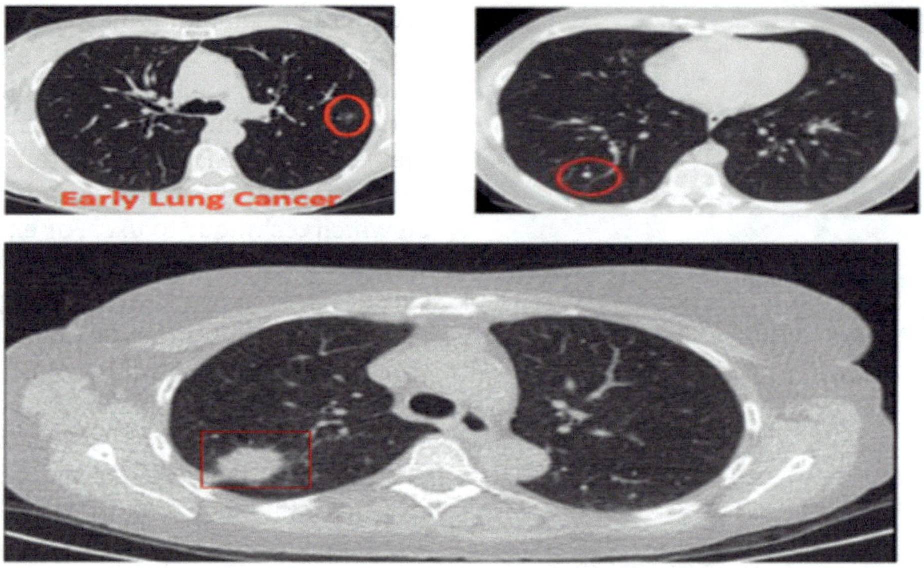

Figure 3.12. Uses of CT scan to predict and monitor cancer treatment.

Source: Shafi I, Din S, Khan A, Díez IDLT, Casanova RdJP, Pifarre KT, Ashraf I. An Effective Method for Lung Cancer Diagnosis from CT Scan Using Deep Learning-Based Support Vector Network. *Cancers*. 2022; 14(21):5457. https://doi.org/10.3390/cancers14215457.

Daily CT checks are now a big deal too, especially in cases like proton therapy for challenging cancers such as hepatocellular carcinoma (HCC). This technique locks in on the proton dose distribution details so closely that it gives a real sense of whether the treatment is hitting its mark. A retrospective review noted that keeping up with daily CT images helped maintain the intended dose limits for organs considered at risk, which shows that sticking to the plan is crucial—and sometimes even sparks a need for a quick re-plan when patient anatomy changes or positioning shifts unexpectedly. All of this regular monitoring ends up making the treatment safer and more effective for those in proton therapy (Maeda et al., 2023). Overall, using CT to keep tabs on treatments isn't just a side note in modern medicine—it is a full-on strategy. By providing detailed images, CT imaging lets healthcare teams make smarter decisions, which in most cases lifts both care quality and treatment outcomes. When you see high success with methods like CT-guided cryoablation alongside routine monitoring in proton therapy, it is clear that regular imaging checks aren't merely extras—they're a central part of how we treat patients today. As imaging continues evolving and new research comes into play, the door for even more personalized treatment plans is only likely to open wider, solidifying its key role in tracking treatment effects (Maeda et al., 2023; Pusceddu et al., 2024) (Figure 3.12).

Test Your Knowledge

1. How is CT imaging used in the diagnosis of traumatic injuries, such as fractures or internal bleeding?
2. What are some common medical conditions that can be assessed using CT scans, and how do they aid in treatment planning?

3.4. Advantages, Limitations and Risks of Computed Tomography (CT) Scanning

Learning Outcome

1. Understand the key benefits of CT scanning in medical diagnostics.
2. Identify the limitations and potential risks associated with CT scanning.

3.4.1. Advantages of Computed Tomography (CT) Scanning

Advancements in imaging have changed how we look at diagnoses in healthcare. CT scans, for example, give us surprisingly detailed cross-sectional views of the insides—slicing through tissues, organs, and even bones in ways that plain X-rays just can't match. It is quite something when you consider that these crisp images help doctors spot issues like tumors or fractures much more accurately. There's also this newer twist called photon-counting-detector computed tomography (PCD-CT) (Siegel et al., 2024) that ups the ante with better spatial resolution and improved contrast-to-noise ratios, generally leading to treatment plans that feel a lot more personalized. The speed of CT scanning goes hand in hand with its clarity, which, in most cases, is a real lifesaver. In emergency settings, every second counts; rapid scan times can make all the difference, allowing healthcare teams to assess critical conditions almost immediately. Modern CT systems often produce top-notch images in just seconds – a pace that's particularly impressive for trauma patients who need help fast. Moreover, PCD-CT manages to cut down radiation doses significantly while still keeping, or even boosting, image quality (Algın et al., 2024). This dose reduction is especially important for sensitive patients like children, where even a small extra exposure just isn't ideal. CT scanning doesn't stop at being clear and fast—it is also incredibly versatile. It finds a spot in everything from oncology to cardiology, helping not only with initial diagnoses but also with ongoing monitoring of disease progression. For instance, clear images are essential when tracking a tumor's response to therapy; the high specificity of PCD-CT lets clinicians differentiate between types of tissues in ways that are truly eye-opening (Algın et al., 2024). It even plays a part in interventional procedures, sometimes making minimally invasive techniques a safer bet. Overall, these varied strengths are setting new standards in medicine, showing how technology can blend detailed diagnostics with a strong focus on patient safety, even if the process isn't always perfectly polished (Figure 3.13).

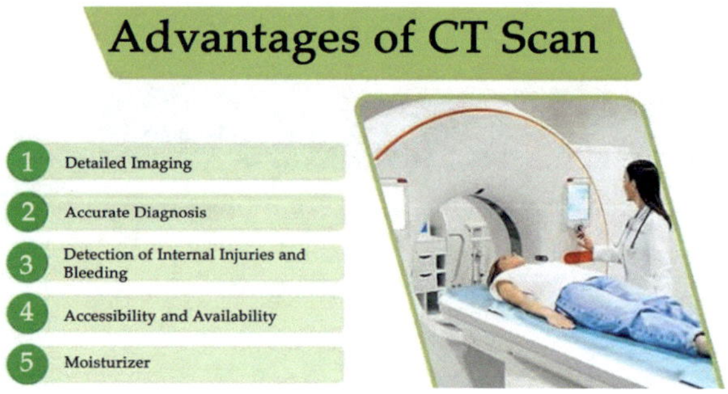

Figure 3.13. Advantages of (CT) Scanning

Source: https://www.instagram.com/sono.clinic/p/DBlK7yMO6Ef/.

3.4.1.1. Speed and Efficiency of Imaging

Imaging technology has come a long way, pushing us to rethink how speed and efficiency work in CT scans. With the pressure for fast diagnostic tests, obtaining images swiftly can improve patient outcomes. GPU-powered processing has turned into a kind of surprise hero here. For example, a Monte Carlo dose calculation tool called gCTD was built to check imaging doses during CT and cone beam CT (CBCT) scans. It not only cranks up computational efficiency—reportedly boosting speeds by around 400 times in some phantom tests—but also holds onto high accuracy (Briesmeister et al., 2011). Bringing in these newer computing techniques means that healthcare providers can offer diagnoses promptly while still keeping tight to radiation safety protocols. Figuring out how fast imaging blends with diagnostic accuracy is pretty crucial in CT technology. In emergencies, like trauma cases, every second counts, and quick image capture can make a big difference. Techniques that use graphics processing units can cut down image reconstruction time a lot without hurting quality. For instance, in photoacoustic CT with compressed sensing, a GPU-based setup speeds up reconstruction by roughly 24–31 times compared to old CPU methods. This gain not only makes it possible to act faster in critical moments, but it also produces better quality images that are key for solid diagnoses (Gao et al., 2020). In most cases, mixing speed with reliable imaging plays a central role in modern diagnostics.

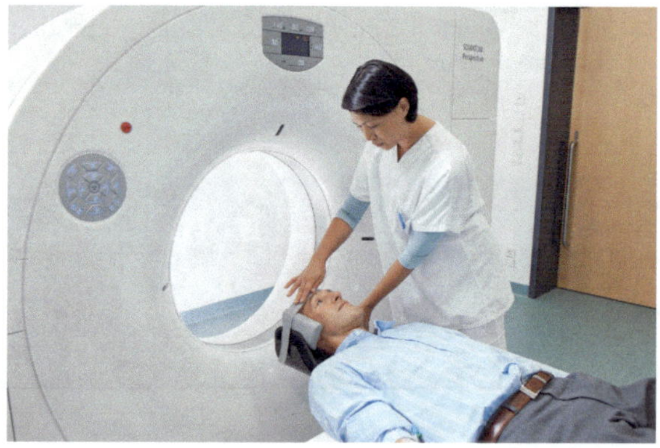

Figure 3.14. Imaging technology

Source: https://emerymed.com/wp-content/uploads/2018/06/CT-Scanner2.jpg.

There's a constant balancing act in imaging between moving fast and keeping high resolution. In CT scans, rushing things can sometimes cause unwanted artifacts or a drop in clarity if not handled right. Still, parallel computation methods seem to offer an encouraging fix. Enhanced algorithms now process huge amounts of data almost instantly—which is crucial as imaging demands increase. By tweaking these parallel systems, medical facilities can streamline their workflow and cut patient wait times, all while mostly keeping image data intact. The development behind tools like the gCTD system shows this isn't just about speeding things up; it also means keeping a careful eye on patient-specific dose management for better care outcomes (Briesmeister et al., 2011). Generally speaking, this mix of quick results and precise imaging sets the tone for today's evolving healthcare technology (Figure 3.14).

3.4.1.2. High-Resolution Images and Detail

High-resolution images play a key role in making CT scans work well, especially when doctors need to figure out what's going on inside. This method of imaging brings internal structures up close in a way that lower-resolution methods just can't, letting clinicians catch issues that might otherwise be missed. Getting these sharp images helps in making sure assessments are accurate and gives a closer look at tissue details and any problems present. Tools like photoacoustic computed tomography (PACT) mix different imaging styles to deliver crisp pictures of tissues. These advances show, quite clearly, that in image quality, sticking to proper spatial sampling is a must so that pesky artifacts don't mess up a diagnosis (Hu et al., 2020). Deep learning approaches are also shaking things up in CT image analysis, especially in breaking down complex structures. Researchers now use multi-resolution neural networks—technically speaking, networks that capture both minute details and broader context—to handle tricky datasets like 3D images of root structures, where every bit of precision counts. This balancing act helps tease apart fine features from the larger picture, and it ends up boosting segmentation accuracy. When you put these modern encoder-decoder networks side-by-side with older methods, the improvements are hard to miss, both qualitatively and quantitatively, proving that high-res imaging offers real clinical benefits (Soltaninejad et al., 2020). As imaging technologies keep evolving, they're opening up a whole new world of diagnostic precision in CT scans. Better imaging methods and smarter algorithms are teaming up to spark innovative ideas in various areas of medicine. For example, high-resolution CT is showing its worth in cancer care, where even the tiniest tumor details can steer treatment choices. The pursuit of ways to cut down aliasing artifacts—albeit sometimes with a few hiccups in the process—drives the academic community to keep refining these techniques. In most cases, as these high-res imaging methods and clever computational tools continue to merge, the scope for thorough patient evaluation and care climbs to new heights, setting a fresh standard in radiology and beyond (Hu et al., 2020) (Figure 3.15).

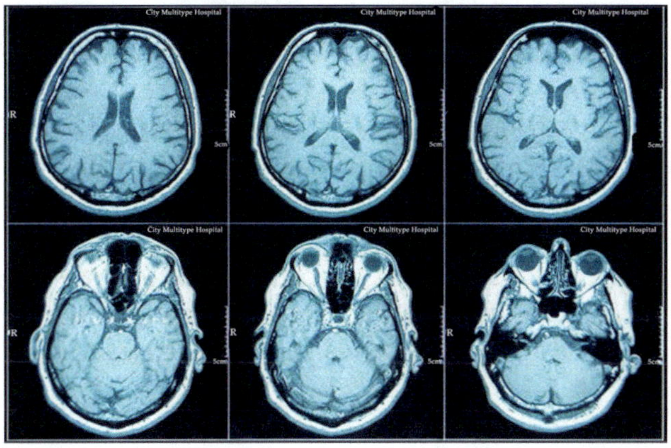

Figure 3.15. Brain CT scan high-resolution images.

Source: https://t3.ftcdn.net/jpg/02/59/88/92/360_F_259889262_ZSQKHFRbWlc9crqJVzHNo3VDKlyF7iKX.jpg.

3.4.1.3. Non-Invasive Nature of the Procedure

Medical imaging has come a long way from the old, cut-and-dry invasive methods, and today, CT stands out. CT gives doctors a clear look inside the body without having to make any incisions or perform biopsies—a fact that matters a lot when trying to minimize patient risk and discomfort. By harnessing the power of advanced imaging tools, clinicians can easily view intricate details of internal organs, which is especially useful in spotting issues like coronary artery disease or liver cirrhosis; identifying these early is key to planning good treatment. More people are turning to CT-based markers, such as fractional flow reserve, to help guide choices in care, thereby cutting back on the need for invasive coronary angiography, as noted in Becker et al. (2024). The appeal of CT isn't just about keeping patients comfortable; there's also a clear boost in diagnostic accuracy. Several studies suggest that mixing CT with other imaging techniques—MRI, for example—can improve how we spot complicated problems like liver cirrhosis. This blend of methods gives doctors a mix of detailed anatomical and functional data, reducing the dangers linked with older, more invasive tests. In many cases, these advances in sensitivity and specificity mean that early detection and steady monitoring of chronic conditions work hand in hand to prevent further complications, as reflected in the findings of Hassan et al. (2024). Non-invasive approaches in medical diagnostics mark a real shift towards care that puts patients first. As healthcare keeps evolving, the drive to cut down on invasiveness touches both the ethical and practical sides of medicine, always keeping patient welfare at its core. CT scans, when done non-invasively, offer a full picture of different conditions without overwhelming patients with uncomfortable tests. The ongoing tweaks to imaging algorithms and techniques not only boost the reliability of CT results but also broaden the scope of what we learn about a person's health, giving a more well-rounded view. Overall, our steady push to upgrade non-invasive diagnostic methods—backed by continuous research and fresh technological ideas—points to a promising future for CT as a central tool in effective medical assessment and disease management.

3.4.2. Limitations and Risks of Computed Tomography (CT)

CT imaging has changed how we look inside the body. It gives us amazingly clear, cross-sectional images, which is impressive on its own. But there's a flip side too—more and more studies point out some serious downsides. One big worry is the impact of radiation; when people get multiple scans, the cumulative exposure can raise the risk of radiation-related cancers. This issue has led many experts to wonder if every single scan is necessary. Traditional ways to gauge the dose, like using CTDI vol and ED, often fall short in showing the real amount of exposure patients get during scans (Bohanske et al., 2024). In most cases, this gap pushes clinics to keep reviewing their procedures so that the diagnostic advantages don't come at too high a long-term health cost. Figuring out CT results can also be trickier than it first appears, adding a whole new layer of concern. Different scanning techniques and choices in settings might change the quality of the images, and that's often largely because of how experienced the operator is or the choices they make. Even older methods, like biplanar radiographs, have their own issues such as observer bias and struggles with detecting subtle problems, which sometimes means a diagnosis gets missed or delayed. Lately, though, new techniques like CT-based Structural Rigidity Analysis (CTRA) are starting to show promise. Still, variations in how different observers score scans—and the differences between operators—remain a problem (Bohanske et al., 2024). Generally speaking, even with all the technological breakthroughs, the human side of things often muddies the waters, making standardized protocols and better training more urgent than ever. There's also the matter of how people feel when they get their CT results. The super-clear images can sometimes reveal incidental findings that weren't even the main focus, and these can stir up a lot of anxiety or even prompt unnecessary treatments. Patients might end up stressed out after hearing about these extra details, which can lead to more tests that carry their own risks without any obvious benefit. Doctors, too, have to be careful when sharing these findings to make sure everything is explained clearly—even if that means a few extra words here and there. In some cases, relying too much on CT scans might even kick off a runaway cycle of extra imaging, affecting both patient safety and healthcare costs. Overall, while CT technology gives us invaluable clues about what's going on inside, striking the right balance between its benefits and risks remains a tough challenge in today's medical world (Sabiniewicz-Ziajka et al., 2024) (Figure 3.16).

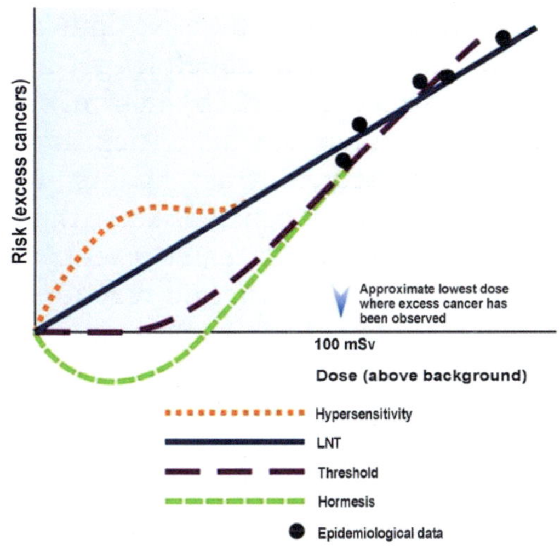

Figure 3.16. Different risks of CT scans.

Source: Garg M, Karami V, Moazen J, Kwee T, Bhalla AS, Shahbazi-Gahrouei D, Shao Y-HJ. Radiation Exposure and Lifetime Attributable Risk of Cancer Incidence and Mortality from Low- and Standard-Dose CT Chest: Implications for COVID-19 Pneumonia Subjects. *Diagnostics*. 2022; 12(12):3043. https://doi.org/10.3390/diagnostics12123043.

3.4.2.1. Exposure to Ionizing Radiation

CT—has changed how doctors figure out what's wrong, letting them see inside the body like never before. But it's not all smooth sailing; there's a downside with the ionizing radiation (IR) it uses, which can be a big deal, especially for kids and other sensitive groups. CT scans hit with a higher dose than your typical X-ray, so, generally speaking, the long-term risks—like the chance of developing cancer—shouldn't be ignored. Research shows that younger patients, still in full growth mode, might be extra vulnerable to these harmful effects. Because of these worries, experts have set up diagnostic reference levels (DRLs) to try and keep doses as low as possible during scans (Figure 3.17).

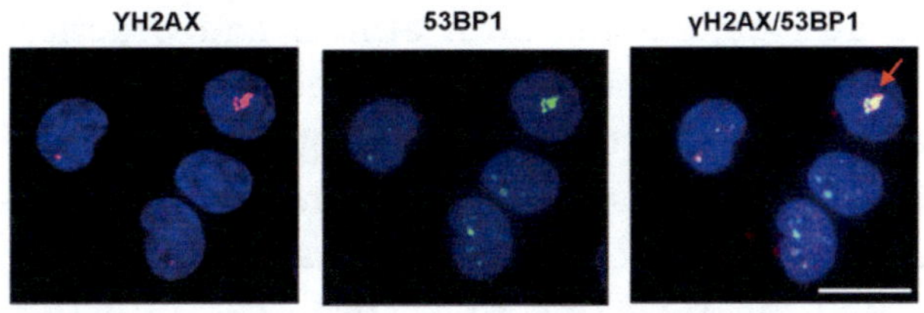

Figure 3.17. The figure shows representative images of γH2AX, 53BP1, and merging γH2AX/53BP1 foci in PBMCs from a healthy volunteer. Foci of different sizes including a giant focus (red arrow) are shown. The images were visualized by a fluorescence microscope using a 60x objective. Scale bar is 10 μm.

Source: Valente D, Gentileschi MP, Valenti A, Burgio M, Soddu S, Bruzzaniti V, Guerrisi A, Verdina A. Cumulative Dose from Recurrent CT Scans: Exploring the DNA Damage Response in Human Non-Transformed Cells. *International Journal of Molecular Sciences*. 2024; 25(13):7064. https://doi.org/10.3390/ijms25137064.

Safety comes first here; it is all about getting good images while still looking out for high-risk groups, particularly young ones (Tambe et al., 2024). In understanding how CT scans affect us with ionizing radiation, you've got to dive into the numbers behind the process. Every scan spits out data measured by things like the Dose Length Product (DLP)— a count of how much radiation the tissues soak up. And these figures are key when working out how much dose specific organs receive. New studies suggest that there's almost a straight-line link between DLP and a patient's age, which is pretty crucial for deciding on doses that fit different age brackets.

This insight lets healthcare providers tweak their scan methods, especially for kids who are far more sensitive to excess radiation; using set protocols (even if not perfect) helps them stick to safety guidelines (Kashcheev et al., 2023). Reducing exposure to ionizing radiation isn't just about one patient's care—it is a bigger public health issue. With CT scans being used more and more, the total radiation load on everyone starts to add up, raising both ethical and practical concerns. There's always a push to rework and refine the scanning techniques, continually checking the best ways to cut down unnecessary radiation without losing valuable diagnostic detail. By tweaking these processes, doctors and technicians help build a safety culture that spreads out to both healthcare providers and patients alike. Public awareness about radiation risks, combined with better, hands-on training for those doing the scans, is essential when handling CT imaging's tricky side. In the end, striking that balance between reducing exposure and getting accurate diagnostic results remains at the heart of radiology and patient care (Tambe et al., 2024) (Figure 3.18).

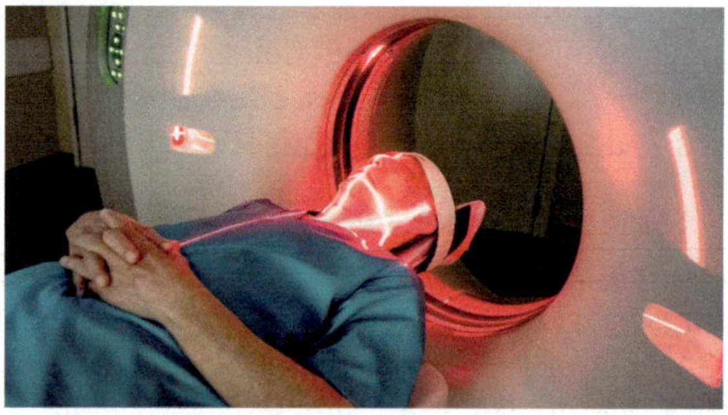

Figure 3.18. Exposure to Ionizing Radiation

Source: https://post.healthline.com/wp-content/uploads/2022/01/CT-scanner-body1.jpg.

3.4.2.2. Potential for Allergic Reactions to Contrast Agents

Imaging technology has flipped how we do diagnostics, but it is not all smooth sailing—there's a growing worry about the safety of contrast agents in CT scans. These agents play a big part in making images clearer, yet they can sometimes trigger allergic reactions. You might see cases where reactions range from a simple rash or some itching to severe, almost anaphylactic responses. A mix of things—not just patient history, but also the type of contrast used and individual sensitivity—often comes into play. That's why many clinics now screen patients ahead of time, so individuals with known allergies can hopefully get a safer alternative (Kerna et al., 2024b). Recently, some studies have pointed out an uptick in using non-ionic iodinated contrast agents, which most experts generally consider safer than the ionic ones. Still, even these "safer" agents aren't completely free of risk; allergic reactions can and do happen. Radiologists and medical staff need to be on their toes, identifying early signs of an allergic response so they can intervene quickly—after all, prompt action can lessen how bad things get. There's also been a move toward using things like predictive modeling and machine learning techniques to help gauge the risk of allergic reactions based on patient data (Xiong et al., 2022).

This more personalized approach not only improves diagnostic accuracy but also lowers the overall risks linked to contrast use. Diagnostic imaging is clearly shifting its focus toward both cutting risks and boosting the effectiveness of procedures. Efforts are underway to come up with new contrast agents that are less likely to spark an allergic response and to improve how patients are managed. For example, ongoing research into biodegradable and less allergenic agents holds some promise in reducing adverse outcomes in CT scans. Educating healthcare providers—and patients, too—about these risks goes a long way in making informed imaging choices. In most cases, as technology keeps evolving, the main aim remains steady: to deliver imaging that's safe, effective, and accessible while keeping a keen eye on the potential for contrast-related allergies (Kerna et al., 2024b) (Figure 3.19).

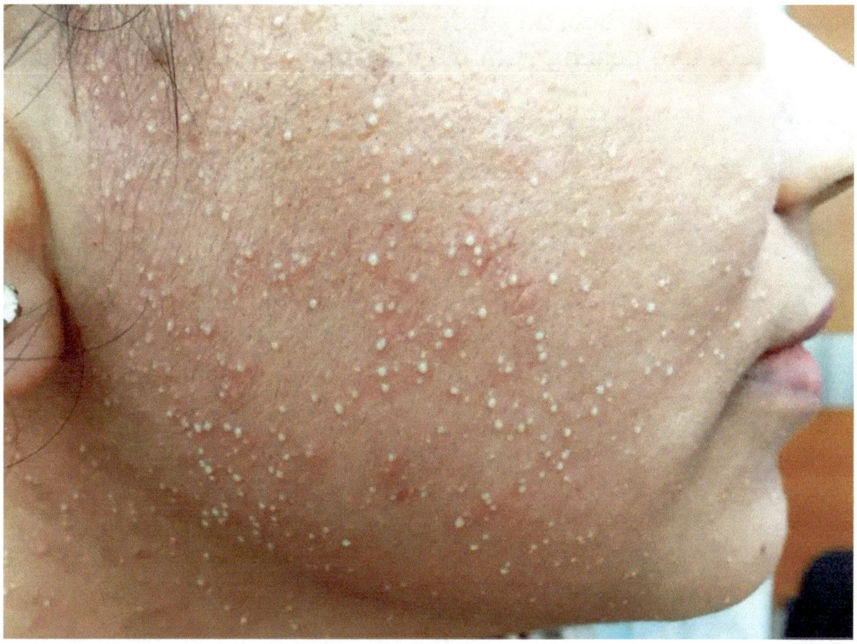

Figure 3.19. CT scan liquid gives woman rare allergy.

Source: https://punemirror.com/pune/civic/ct-scan-liquid-gives-woman-rare-allergy/cid5116481.htm.

3.4.2.3. Limitations in Soft Tissue Imaging

Modern imaging tools have boosted how we view different body parts, but soft tissue still proves tricky. Basic CT scans, for example, usually struggle a bit when trying to tell muscle, fat, and organs apart—mostly because water-filled tissues absorb X-rays almost the same way. Newer techniques, like photon counting detectors, are popping up to boost sensitivity, yet their knack for picking up those subtle differences is still being worked out. Also, the way X-rays pass through tissues of different thicknesses often means that, unless detectors are finely tuned, the images can vary a lot, putting limits on accurate diagnosis (Hameed et al., 2024). The usual CT approaches for soft tissue just don't cut it for every kind of situation, especially in complex fields like dental research. Recently, contrast-enhanced imaging—using special agents to brighten up the image—has been pushed forward in hopes of filling some gaps. For instance, some studies have shown that Lugol's iodine can help make soft tissues clearer, hinting at a promising way to ease traditional imaging issues. Still, these methods might not work equally well for every kind of soft tissue or medical scenario; in most cases, more tweaking and tests are needed to fully trust them. Overall, the need for thorough anatomical checks remains, since standard CT still sometimes misses the finer details of soft tissues (Hildebrand et al., 2024). In addition, even though there's a strong push to integrate these innovative methods into everyday CT imaging, practical problems still crop up. Extra training and adjustments in routine settings can make things less accessible—sometimes meaning that diagnostic results vary from one operator to another, or even from one piece of equipment to the next. As these imaging methods get more advanced, minor differences in how machines are calibrated or how they're used end up causing unexpected differences in the final images. This reality nudges us toward setting up clear guidelines and standards. Ultimately, while we continue to make progress in boosting soft tissue imaging, there's a constant balancing act between adopting new tech and dealing with ongoing practical limitations (Hameed et al., 2024).

Test Your Knowledge

1. What are the key advantages of CT scanning over other imaging techniques, such as X-ray or MRI?
2. What are the limitations and potential risks associated with CT scanning, particularly regarding radiation exposure?

Summary

CT imaging technology has come a long way and changed how we approach medical tests. Today, CT is seen as a must-have tool. Recent studies show that a method known as the Continuum Topological Derivative (CTD) can clean up images by cutting down noise—even handling tricky issues like quantum mottle noise in HRCT images. In some cases, adding this technique to every day diagnostics might help spot anatomical details with greater precision, marking a big step forward in both image clarity and patient care (Muthukrishnan et al., 2024). Deep learning also dives in to give CT a serious boost. These algorithms don't just speed up image reading; they help catch critical conditions (like COVID-19) early and offer valuable insights into lung nodules. After sifting through a wide range of studies on DL systems, it turns out that these tools are pretty essential for untangling the complex nature of CT image analysis. They not only lift diagnostic performance but also smooth over issues caused by data differences and heavy computational loads, underscoring deep learning's transformative role in modern radiology (Ahmad et al., 2024). Overall, these advances in CT techniques hint at a bright future for medical diagnostics. The CTD method and deep learning bring fresh angles that can lead to quicker, more accurate disease detection, which in turn improves patient outcomes. Generally speaking, more research and cross-field teamwork are needed to work through challenges like image interpretation and regulatory hurdles. The progress we're seeing now doesn't just raise the bar for imaging quality—it also lays the groundwork for future breakthroughs that might profoundly reshape healthcare policies and clinical practices (Ahmad et al., 2024; Muthukrishnan et al., 2024).

CT has changed the face of medical imaging. It gives us detailed three-dimensional views that help doctors figure out diagnoses and plan treatments more accurately. You can see this, especially in cases like cancers – non-small cell lung cancer (NSCLC) gets a lot of attention here. These days, some fresh ideas like radiomics are mixing things up; essentially, the process pulls many measurable data from CT scans that often link to how patients do. This extra detail lets clinicians adjust surveillance strategies to better cope with the many ways cancer can vary and come back, opening up new horizons for improved outcomes (Shi et al., 2018). In lung cancer treatment, CT has been a game changer in nailing down target volumes. The introduction of four-dimensional CT (4DCT) now provides a sharper look at the internal gross target volume (IGTV), which is pretty important for patients undergoing Stereotactic Body Radiation Therapy (SBRT). By leaning on deep learning methods, the precision of target delineation has shot up compared to old-school approaches. Research, in most cases, shows that patients getting SBRT benefit from these advances not just by having better treatment outcomes, but also by protecting the tissues around the tumor a bit more. The mix of CT and machine learning hints at a promising future in oncological care, steering treatment strategies onto a new path (Li et al., 2018). Bringing all these technical leaps together seems to signal a shift toward more personalized medicine, especially in cancer care using CT. When innovative imaging bumps up against predictive analytics, doctors can often predict how well a treatment will work and tweak care plans as needed. This blend of radiomic data and detailed imaging helps unwrap tumor behavior and even flags early signs of issues like metastasis or radiation-induced problems. As we keep polishing these techniques, there's a steady drive to boost patient survival rates by refining both diagnostic and treatment paths in our ongoing battle against cancer (Li et al., 2018; Shi et al., 2018).

KEY TERMS FROM THIS CHAPTER

- Convolutional neural networks (CNNs)
- CT reconstruction
- Dual-energy CT
- Image acquisition
- Multi-detector CT (MDCT)
- Radiation dose
- Radiomics
- Spiral CT (Helical CT)
- CT angiography
- CT scanner
- Filtered back projection (FBP)
- Image reconstruction
- Photon-counting detector CT (PCD-CT)
- Radiology
- Slice thickness
- Tomography

Critical Thinking Questions

1. **What does CT in medical imaging stand for?**
   a. Clinical Therapy
   b. Computed Tomography
   c. Contrast Technology
   d. Cranial Technique
2. **What is the primary advantage of CT over traditional X-ray imaging?**
   a. Lower radiation dose
   b. Faster image acquisition
   c. Ability to create cross-sectional images
   d. Better for imaging soft tissues
3. **Which component of the CT scanner rotates around the patient during the scan?**
   a. Patient table
   b. Detector array
   c. Gantry
   d. Contrast injector
4. **Why is contrast media sometimes used in CT imaging?**
   a. To reduce patient movement
   b. To decrease radiation exposure
   c. To enhance visualization of blood vessels and organs
   d. To improve bone clarity
5. **Which of the following conditions is not typically diagnosed using a CT scan?**
   a. Stroke
   b. Bone fracture
   c. Pneumonia
   d. Nearsightedness

Short Answer Questions

1. What are the basic principles behind how computed tomography (CT) creates cross-sectional images of the body?
2. What are the main types of CT scans, and how are they used in clinical practice?
3. In what ways is CT imaging applied across different areas of medicine for diagnosis and treatment planning?
4. What are the key advantages of CT scanning compared to other imaging methods?
5. What are the potential limitations and risks associated with CT scanning, especially regarding radiation exposure?

Answers to Critical Thinking Questions

1. (b); 2. (c); 3. (c); 4. (c); 5. (d)

References

1. Ahmad, I. S., Dai, J., Xie, Y., & Liang, X. (2024). Deep learning models for CT image classification: A comprehensive literature review. *Quantitative Imaging in Medicine and Surgery, 15*, 962–1011. https://www.semanticscholar.org/paper/605dd491037d04b2a8b0c866cfdb16f22b3760b0 (accessed on 23 May 2025).
2. Algın, O., Tokgoz, N., & Cademartiri, F. (2024). Photon-counting computed tomography in radiology. *Polish Journal of Radiology, 89*, e433–e442. https://www.semanticscholar.org/paper/4c5074cdc90d3c3d848bfbb83a1803d93b50fb39 (accessed on 23 May 2025).
3. Alyami, A. S. H., Lasloom, M. D., Lesloum, M. H. D., Al Mutarid, A. F. M., Alyami, S. H. H., Al Batnain, H. L. S., & Al Batnain, S. A. S. (2023). Simple physical principles and medical uses of computed tomography (CT) scan: A new assessment. *International Journal of Advanced Research*. https://www.semanticscholar.org/paper/78d1483124566598d0ce1ca3ef415b340671c8f5 (accessed on 23 May 2025).
4. Becker, L. M., Peper, J., van Nes, S. H., van Es, H. W., Sjauw, K. D., van de Hoef, T. P., Leiner, T., & Swaans, M. J. (2024). Non-invasive physiological assessment of coronary artery obstruction on coronary computed tomography angiography. *Netherlands Heart Journal, 32*(11), 397–404. https://doi.org/10.1007/s12471-024-01902-7.
5. Biguri, A., Sadakane, T., Lindroos, R., Liu, Y., Sabaté Landman, M., Du, Y., Lohvithee, M., et al. (2024). TIGRE v3: Efficient and easy to use iterative computed tomographic reconstruction toolbox for real datasets. *arXiv*. https://doi.org/10.48550/arXiv.2412.10129.
6. Bohanske, M., Momenzadeh, K., van der Zwaal, P., Hoogwater, F., Cory, E., Biggane, P., Snyder, B. D., et al. (2024). Computed tomography-based structural rigidity analysis can assess tumor- and treatment-induced changes in rat bones with metastatic lesions. *BMC Cancer, 24*. https://www.semanticscholar.org/paper/5494c092301e27167d09f3cf4e8af793d087400f (accessed on 23 May 2025).
7. Boonjindasup, W., Thomas, R. J., Yuen, W., & McElrea, M. (2024). Role of spirometry, radiology, and flexible bronchoscopy in assessing chronic cough in children. *Journal of Clinical Medicine, 13*. https://www.semanticscholar.org/paper/74b02a75c1300649ca884f1fd79e42b6aac3ad3a (accessed on 23 May 2025).
8. Briesmeister, J. F., DeMarco, J. J., Gu, X., et al. (2011). Fast Monte Carlo simulation for patient-specific CT/CBCT imaging dose calculation. *arXiv*. http://arxiv.org/abs/1109.3266 (accessed on 23 May 2025).
9. Calderoni, L., Giovanella, L., & Fanti, S. (2024). Endocrinology application of molecular imaging: Current role of PET/CT. *Journal of Endocrinological Investigation, 47*, 2383–2396. https://www.semanticscholar.org/paper/dc735ba8ff5f4af9f9763d13fd030b42131519ec (accessed on 23 May 2025).
10. Dave, B., Maniar, P., Kaur, N., Delapena, S. A., & Behnam, A. B. (2024). The role of advanced imaging in facial reconstructive surgery. *Journal of Surgery Care*. https://www.semanticscholar.org/paper/49d377029265e05b379c91e4f41ab1ce3c2bbc94 (accessed on 23 May 2025).
11. Dutta, S., Georgeot, B., Michetti, J., Basarab, A., & Kouamé, D. (2024). Unsupervised physics-inspired deep learning network with application to dental computed tomography image restoration. In *2024 IEEE International Symposium on Biomedical Imaging (ISBI)*. https://

www.semanticscholar.org/paper/3240a4177063215be640e1cf66a2e72a6f004bfd (accessed on 23 May 2025).

12. Elkhadir, A. M., & Yousef, R. M. B. (2024). Role of radiologic technologist specialist in plain image interpretation of adults in the Middle East: A radiologist's perspective. *Malaysian Journal of Medical Research, 8*(4), 1–8. https://doi.org/10.31674/mjmr.2024.v08i04.001.

13. Gao, M., Si, G., Bai, Y., Wang, L. V., Liu, C., & Meng, J. (2020). Graphics processing unit accelerating compressed sensing photoacoustic computed tomography with total variation. *Applied Optics, 59*, 712–719.

14. Geyer, L. L., Schoepf, U. J., Meinel, F. G., Nance, J. W., Jr, Bastarrika, G., Leipsic, J. A., Paul, N. S., Rengo, M., Laghi, A., & De Cecco, C. N. (2015). State of the art: Iterative CT reconstruction techniques. *Radiology, 276*(2), 339–357. https://doi.org/10.1148/radiol.2015132766.

15. Gyan, E., Subaar, C., Edusei, G., & Nyarko, L. A. (2024). Pediatric computed tomography diagnostic reference levels in Africa: A systematic review. *Journal of Medical Radiation Sciences, 72*, 139–147. https://www.semanticscholar.org/paper/e466106fe4549ca3057ee8b581ff840b3bdc4c57 (accessed on 23 May 2025).

16. Hameed, K., Zainon, R., & Tamal, M. (2024). Cadmium zinc telluride (CZT) photon counting detector characterization for soft tissue imaging. *ArXiv*. https://www.semanticscholar.org/paper/29b417f87b38066ffd250d68b99e7f96a618980b (accessed on 23 May 2025).

17. Hassan, M. S., Zhang, G., Latifi, K., Ullah, G., Hunt, D., Balagurunathan, Y., Abdalah, M. A., et al. (2017). Intrinsic dependencies of CT radiomic features on voxel size and number of gray levels. *Medical Physics, 44*, 1050–1062. https://doi.org/10.1002/mp.12123.

18. Hassan, S. H., Khan, F. M., Afridi, S., Younas, M., Khan, A., Ibrahim, M., et al. (2024). Diagnostic accuracy of MRI and CT scan in non-invasive evaluation of liver cirrhosis. *Pakistan Journal of Health Sciences*. https://www.semanticscholar.org/paper/954514cf002696d566ac0de2f374dc344c0f6beb (accessed on 23 May 2025).

19. Hildebrand, T., Humphris, Y., Haugen, H., & Nogueira, L. P. (2024). Contrast-enhanced micro-CT imaging of murine mandibles: A multi-method approach for simultaneous hard and soft tissue analysis. *Journal of Clinical Periodontology, 52*, 258–267. https://www.semanticscholar.org/paper/e6c504042913d117d0101de8d9e0741541bcb2d0 (accessed on 23 May 2025).

20. Hu, P., Li, L., Lin, L., & Wang, L. V. (2020). Spatiotemporal antialiasing in photoacoustic computed tomography. *IEEE Transactions on Medical Imaging, 39*(11), 3535–3547. https://doi.org/10.1109/TMI.2020.2998509.

21. Hussain, S., Mubeen, I., Ullah, N., Shah, S. S. U. D., Khan, B. A., Zahoor, M., Ullah, R., et al. (2022). Modern diagnostic imaging technique applications and risk factors in the medical field: A review. *BioMed Research International, 2022*, 1–19. https://doi.org/10.1155/2022/5164970.

22. Islam, M. R., Zohra, F. T., & Watabe, H. (2025). Current applications and advancements of state-of-the-art technology of PET-CT. *Bangladesh Journal of Nuclear Medicine, 28*(1), 149–155. https://doi.org/10.3329/bjnm.v28i1.79547.

23. Kashcheev, V. V., Pryakhin, E., & Menyailo, A. N. (2023). A method for assessing the radiation risk of medical exposure after computed tomography scan of children and adolescents based on data from scanning protocols. *Radiation and Risk: Bulletin of the National Radiation and*

Epidemiological Registry. https://www.semanticscholar.org/paper/402f1dca27f3f18e408c46f9175a394c26e33248 (accessed on 23 May 2025).

24. Kerna, N. A., Ngwu, D. C., Kadivi, K., Carsrud, N. V., Pruitt, K. D., Flores, J. V., Holets, H. M., et al. (2024a). Transformative advancements in diagnostic imaging: Reducing risks, enhancing accuracy, and promoting sustainability. *European Journal of Medical and Health Research, 2*(5), 153–172. https://doi.org/10.59324/ejmhr.2024.2(5).16.
25. Kerna, N. A., Ngwu, D. C., Kadivi, K., Carsrud, N. V., Pruitt, K. D., Flores, J. V., Holets, H. M., et al. (2024b). Transformative advancements in diagnostic imaging: Reducing risks, enhancing accuracy, and promoting sustainability. *European Journal of Medical and Health Research*. https://www.semanticscholar.org/paper/c618c1dac5672f139d256c1d31ebca23c449f0b9 (accessed on 23 May 2025).
26. Li, X., Deng, Z., Deng, Q., Zhang, L., Niu, T., & Kuang, Y. (2018). A novel deep learning framework for internal gross target volume definition from 4D computed tomography of lung cancer patients. *IEEE Access, 6*, 37775–37783. https://doi.org/10.1109/ACCESS.2018.2851027.
27. Liu, F., Yao, Y., Zhu, B., Yu, Y., Ren, R., & Hu, Y. (2024). The novel imaging methods in diagnosis and assessment of cerebrovascular diseases: An overview. *Frontiers in Medicine, 11*. https://www.semanticscholar.org/paper/9b5ad309eb30fed70f92d5ca2f92173a29382729 (accessed on 23 May 2025).
28. MacRitchie, N., Frleta-Gilchrist, M., Sugiyama, A., Lawton, T., McInnes, I. B., & Maffia, P. (2020). Molecular imaging of inflammation–Current and emerging technologies for diagnosis and treatment. *Pharmacology & Therapeutics, 211*, 107550. https://doi.org/10.1016/j.pharmthera.2020.107550.
29. Maeda, Y., Kobashi, K., Sato, Y., Tamamura, H., Yamamoto, K., Matsushita, K., Sasaki, M., et al. (2023). Effectiveness of CT-image guidance in proton therapy for liver cancer and the importance of daily dose monitoring for tumors and organs at risk. *Medical Physics, 50*(6), 3274–3288. https://doi.org/10.1002/mp.16433.
30. McCollough, C. H., Boedeker, K., Cody, D. D., Duan, X., Flohr, T., Halliburton, S. S., Hsieh, J., et al. (2020). Principles and applications of multienergy CT: Report of AAPM Task Group 291. *Medical Physics, 47*, e881–e912. https://doi.org/10.1002/mp.14157.
31. Muthukrishnan, V., Jaipurkar, S., & Damodaran, N. (2024). Continuum topological derivative–A novel application tool for denoising CT and MRI medical images. *BMC Medical Imaging, 24*. https://www.semanticscholar.org/paper/1566ff00bfbeddd512ca809a7bfd15bb535a98a9 (accessed on 23 May 2025).
32. Noid, G., Tai, A., Schott, D., Mistry, N., Liu, Y., Gilat-Schmidt, T., Robbins, J. R., & Li, X. A. (2018). Technical note: Enhancing soft tissue contrast and radiation-induced image changes with dual-energy CT for radiation therapy. *Medical Physics*. https://doi.org/10.1002/mp.13083.
33. Pusceddu, C., Faiella, E., Cau, C., Rinaldi, P., Melis, L., & Marsico, S. (2024). Computed tomography-guided cryoablation in treating adrenal metastases: A retrospective single-center study. *Diagnostic and Interventional Radiology (Ankara, Turkey)*. https://doi.org/10.4274/dir.2024.242956.
34. Rahman, H., Khan, A. R., Sadiq, T., Farooqi, A. H., Khan, I. U., & Lim, W. H. (2023). A systematic literature review of 3D deep learning techniques in computed tomography reconstruction.

Tomography, 9, 2158–2189. https://www.semanticscholar.org/paper/04dfe57859d2b669b9304bb199dd470479d59629 (accessed on 23 May 2025).

35. Sabiniewicz-Ziajka, D., Szarmach, A., Grzywińska, M., Gać, P., & Piskunowicz, M. (2024). Redefining radiation metrics: Evaluating actual doses in computed tomography scans. *Biomedicines, 12*(3), 600. https://doi.org/10.3390/biomedicines12030600.

36. Shi, L., He, Y., Yuan, Z., Benedict, S., Valicenti, R., Qiu, J., & Rong, Y. (2018). Radiomics for response and outcome assessment for non-small cell lung cancer. *Technology in Cancer Research & Treatment, 17*, 1533033818782788. https://doi.org/10.1177/1533033818782788.

37. Siegel, M. J., & Ramirez-Giraldo, J. C. (2024). Photon counting detector computed tomography in pediatric cardiothoracic CT imaging. *Radiology Advances*. https://www.semanticscholar.org/paper/f26a4ed2c7402adfe006aebef040dc125f861d21 (accessed on 23 May 2025).

38. Soltaninejad, M., Sturrock, C. J., Griffiths, M., Pridmore, T. P., & Pound, M. P. (2020). Three-dimensional root CT segmentation using multi-resolution encoder-decoder networks. *IEEE Transactions on Image Processing, 29*, 6667–6679. https://doi.org/10.1109/TIP.2020.2992893.

39. Stański, M., Michałowska, I., Lemanowicz, A., Karmelita-Katulska, K., Ratajczak, P., Sławińska, A., & Serafin, Z. (2024). Dual-energy and photon-counting computed tomography in vascular applications—Technical background and post-processing techniques. *Diagnostics, 14*. https://www.semanticscholar.org/paper/d1d253a652a1b4c8e4afac189fe91873fd7c5688 (accessed on 23 May 2025).

40. Sun, Z. (2024). Cardiovascular computed tomography in cardiovascular disease: An overview of its applications from diagnosis to prediction. *Journal of Geriatric Cardiology: JGC, 21*(5), 550–576. https://www.semanticscholar.org/paper/045ab8f2d03472d15d6bde146fedaaf57e808072 (accessed on 23 May 2025).

41. Takeuchi, R., Ishigaki, K., Iida, K., Ishikawa, C., Shiozawa, N., Yamaoka, S., Yamada, N., et al. (2025). Use of computed tomography angiography has potential in planning surgical treatment of an extrahepatic portosystemic shunt in dogs. *American Journal of Veterinary Research*. https://www.semanticscholar.org/paper/90dc936b3c3c9635a174c358b6daa8121784bce7 (accessed on 23 May 2025).

42. Tambe, J., Onana, Y., Dongmo, S., Chichom, A., Guegang, E., Ongolo-Zogo, P., Moifo, B., et al. (2024). Exposure to ionizing radiation from initial brain computed tomography for injuries in the South-West Region of Cameroon. *EAS Journal of Radiology and Imaging Technology*.

43. Varga-Szemes, Á., & Emrich, T. (2025). Photon-counting detector CT: A disrupting innovation in medical imaging. *European Radiology Experimental, 9*. https://www.semanticscholar.org/paper/3a29893e1a02682f2dbc96ad8be28389355c1732 (accessed on 23 May 2025).

44. Wang, Q., Xue, H., Martin, J. J. J., Hou, M., Cao, H., Dong, Z., Li, J., et al. (2024). Trends and applications of computed tomography in agricultural non-destructive testing. *Agriculture*. https://www.semanticscholar.org/paper/3121e83ac33263a12b8795a6fc8d53552a5d17ac (accessed on 23 May 2025).

45. Wei, L., Osman, S., Hatt, M., & El Naqa, I. (2019). Machine learning for radiomics-based multimodality and multiparametric modeling. *The Quarterly Journal of Nuclear Medicine and Molecular Imaging, 63*. https://doi.org/10.23736/s1824-4785.19.03213-8.

46. Xiong, X., Ding, Y., Sun, C., Zhang, Z., Guan, X., Zhang, T., Chen, H., et al. (2022). A cascaded

multi-task generative framework for detecting aortic dissection on 3-D non-contrast-enhanced computed tomography. *IEEE Journal of Biomedical and Health Informatics, 26*, 5177–5188. https://www.semanticscholar.org/paper/c9435e0bd96641235cb50f599d8735144c81bd40 (accessed on 23 May 2025).

47. Zamhuri, A., Lim, G. P., Ling, N., Tee, K. S., & Soon, C. F. (2021). MXene in the lens of biomedical engineering: Synthesis, applications and future outlook. *Biomedical Engineering Online, 20*, Article 87. https://doi.org/10.1186/s12938-021-00873-9.

48. Zanon, C., Pepe, A., Cademartiri, F., Bini, C., Maffei, E., Quaia, E., Stellini, E., et al. (2024). Potential benefits of photon-counting CT in dental imaging: A narrative review. *Journal of Clinical Medicine, 13*. https://www.semanticscholar.org/paper/f542934c65aa41def241d81841a87da9b3f94d6e (accessed on 23 May 2025).

49. Zhang, H., Li, S., Liu, Y., & Lu, H. (2023). [Application of deep learning in CT imaging]. *Journal of Biomedical Engineering (Shengwu Yixue Gongchengxue Zazhi), 40*(5), 1012–1018. https://doi.org/10.7507/1001-5515.202305015.

50. Zhang, M., Gu, S., & Shi, Y. (2022). The use of deep learning methods in low-dose computed tomography image reconstruction: A systematic review. *Complex & Intelligent Systems, 8*, 5545–5561. https://www.semanticscholar.org/paper/8182f5d3abfb9e0f831a9b23d7bdbd8078f1defb (accessed on 23 May 2025).

MAGNETIC RESONANCE IMAGING (MRI)

4

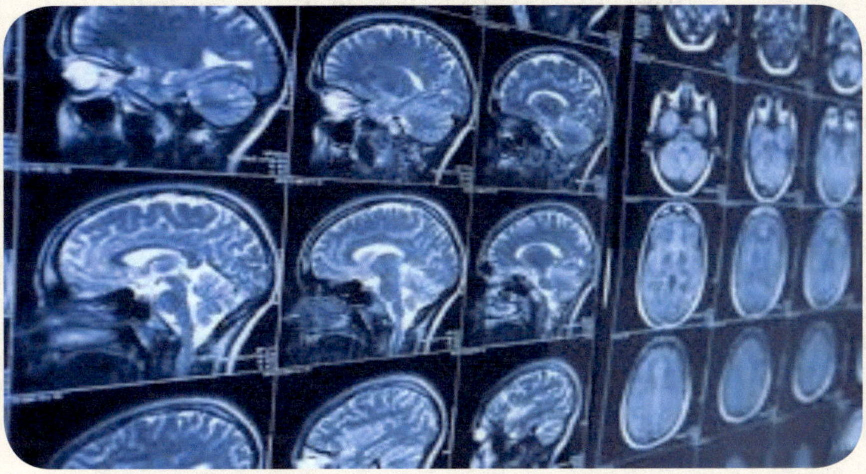

LEARNING OBJECTIVES

After studying this chapter, you will be able to:

1. Understand the basic principles of MRI.
2. Discuss the types of MRI Scans.
3. Explore the clinical applications of MRI in Medicine.
4. Explain the advantages, limitations and challenges of MRI.

Introduction

Medical imaging has come a long way, fundamentally changing how doctors look inside our bodies. MRI, for example, offers clear, sharp images without the risk of ionizing radiation. It works by tapping into the magnetic vibes of atoms—mostly hydrogen—in our tissues. This noninvasive method now plays a pivotal role not just in diagnosing brain and joint issues but also in the fight against cancer. Generally speaking, as MRI technology has improved, it has helped clinicians zero in on different types of tumors, which has led to treatments that are more targeted and, overall, better for patients. Switching gears a bit, MRIs have become increasingly important in assessing urological conditions. In bladder cancer, MRIs are now used to tell apart the more aggressive, muscle-invasive cases from the less serious, non-muscle-invasive ones—often by using the VI-RADS scoring system. This approach tends to outperform traditional methods like ultrasound and computed tomography (CT) urography, which have long been the standard for evaluating bladder cancer. In most cases, the enhanced detail from advanced MRI techniques not only refines cancer staging but also gives hints about how treatment might be working, marking a shift toward more personalized care in urological oncology (Masino et al., 2024). On the other hand, the reach of MRI isn't confined to oncology at all. Cardiac Magnetic Resonance Imaging (CMR) has earned a lot of praise for its impressive spatial details and the fact that it sidesteps ionizing radiation. Many clinicians rely on CMR for keeping an eye on heart conditions over time; it is often the chosen tool for long-term follow-ups and fine-tuning treatments (Jain, 2024). Its noninvasive, yet highly detailed imaging makes it a favorite among doctors, further cementing its role in routine checks and carving a path toward more individualized cardiac care.

Definition of Magnetic Resonance Imaging

MRI is one of today's standout imaging tools. It uses strong magnets and radio waves to snap detailed pictures of what's happening inside the body. This method avoids the ionizing radiation found in X-rays or CT scans, which in many cases can be a health worry. Instead, MRI offers a three-dimensional look at organs, tissues, and even hidden issues. It especially shines when checking soft tissues like the brain, muscles, and joints—places where more conventional scans can miss details. Ultimately, its clarity has made it a go-to choice for doctors looking to diagnose and monitor various diseases, helping to improve patient outcomes in real, measurable ways. New developments have pushed MRI far beyond basic imaging, extending its reach into different medical fields like radiotherapy.

Take multi-parametric MRI (mpMRI), for example. Blending several contrasting techniques, it has been shown to refine RT simulation processes and fine-tune treatment plans. In this light, mpMRI isn't just about diagnosis—it plays a significant part in planning treatments, especially for conditions such as cancer. Enhanced imaging helps spot the edges of tumors and assess nearby tissues, which is crucial for keeping unintended damage to a minimum. Overall, MRI is moving away from being solely a diagnostic gadget to a comprehensive tool that profoundly shapes clinical decisions, a trend that mirrors ongoing innovations in medical imaging. The mix of artificial intelligence (AI) with MRI is sparking a fresh wave of excitement. Recent studies generally suggest that applying AI algorithms can boost the efficiency of reading MRI outputs, easing the decision-making process for healthcare professionals.

For instance, deep learning techniques like Convolutional Neural Networks (CNN) might lead to faster, more accurate detection of abnormalities, ultimately lightening the workload for radiologists. This evolving blend of MRI and AI hints at a future where accuracy and productivity in imaging practice are taken to new heights. Researchers, in most cases, are exploring these synergies so that soon we might see even more advanced tools for clinical evaluation and treatment (Fıçıcı et al., 2023; Li et al., 2023) (Figure 4.1).

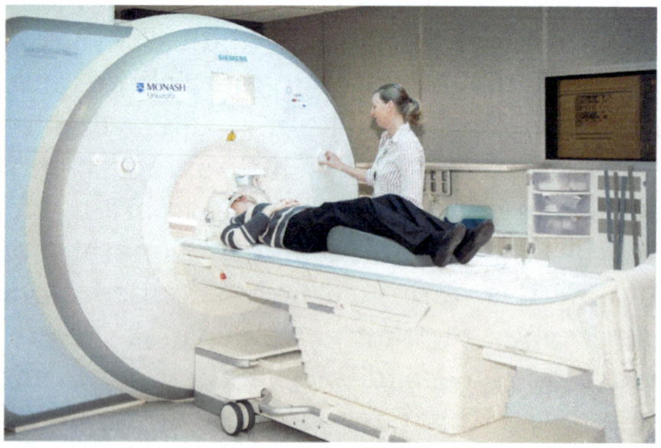

Figure 4.1. Magnetic Resonance Imaging

Source: http://contemplative-studies.org/wp/wp-content/uploads/2021/01/MRI-recording-effects2-Travis.jpg.

Historical Development of MRI Technology

MRI technology's journey is full of key moments that changed how we see the body through imaging. Back in the 1940s, experiments with nuclear magnetic resonance gave us the basic ideas behind MRI. Felix Bloch and Edward Purcell helped show what was happening at a physics level— their work even won them the Nobel Prize in Physics in 1952. Then, around the late 1970s, Raymond Damadian had the idea to use NMR for diagnosing health issues, making it possible to image soft tissues without the hazards of ionizing radiation. This break in thinking led to the first commercial MRI scanner by the 1980s, shaking up areas like oncology and neurology where seeing soft tissues clearly matters. The 1980s and 1990s saw MRI tech move at a fast pace, with improvements in imaging speed, clarity, and patient comfort coming all at once. Innovations like gradient coils and radiofrequency pulses ended up fine-tuning how images were captured, so that different tissues started to stand out in higher contrast.

Then came functional MRI (fMRI) in the early 1990s, which changed the game in studying the brain by noting shifts in blood flow—a sort of live map of brain function. As these advances piled up, MRI started to play a role in checking for a wider range of medical conditions and even helped guide procedures like vacuum-assisted breast biopsy (VABB). This growing flexibility shows that MRI isn't just for diagnosis but also plays a part in treatments. Today, the push in MRI tech is on ramping up magnetic field strengths and boosting the signal-to-noise ratio. Ultra-high field MRI machines—those working at 7 Tesla or more—offer a real breakthrough by capturing images with stunning fine detail, making it easier to spot tricky pathologies. While these systems are a powerful asset for clinical diagnosis, they also serve as a robust tool for research in areas like cognitive neuroscience and the life sciences. Of course, challenges like safety issues and wider accessibility still come up in discussion. Figuring out these obstacles while still pushing the boundaries of innovation will determine the future path of MRI technology, shaping better clinical results and fresh opportunities in research (Gupta, 2025; Qin et al., 2025) (Figure 4.2).

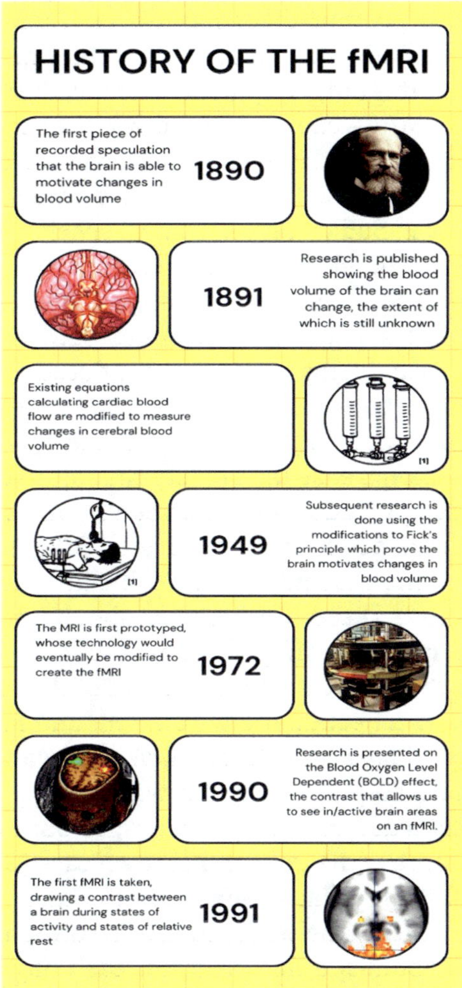

Figure 4.2. The history of fMRI.

Source: https://academic-med-surg.scholasticahq.com/article/123287-the-history-and-continued-evolution-of-functioning-magnetic-resonance-imaging-technology-fmri/attachment/244275.jpg.

Importance of MRI in Modern Medicine

Non-invasive imaging has reshaped how doctors care for patients today. Seeing inside the body without surgery isn't just cool—it has become a must-have in modern medicine. MRI, for example, is a standout tool in tackling complicated issues like a dissecting aortic aneurysm (DAA). DAA can be hard to pin down because its signs often look like those of other ailments, which makes getting a prompt diagnosis tricky. Traditional tests like ECGs and chest X-rays sometimes just don't cut it. That's why using advanced imaging such as MRI—capable of showing soft tissue with amazing clarity—is so important. Delayed diagnosis can lead to serious health problems, so regularly including MRI in clinical checks ups the chances of quick and effective treatment. These strengths don't end with making a diagnosis—it also plays a big part in keeping patients safe and at ease during scans. A recent study shows that when patients know more about the MRI process, it not only smooths out the workflow but also helps ease the anxiety that often comes with such procedures (Sumon et al., 2024). Many individuals get nervous before an MRI, mostly because the machine seems a bit intimidating or because there are worries about potential health risks. A simple, honest conversation before the scan can make a world of difference, setting up a friendlier environment and making the experience less stressful. When healthcare providers step in to explain what's happening, it builds trust and even encourages patients to take a more active role in their own care (Sumon et al., 2024). What's even more exciting is that MRI is shifting the whole idea of treatment. It is not just about spotting problems early any more; MRI is now crucial for fine-tuning treatments for each person's unique body. As medicine increasingly focuses on individual differences, real-time MRI lets doctors check if a treatment is working and adjust plans when necessary—a real boon in areas like oncology, where keeping an eye on tumor changes matters a lot. In this way, integrating MRI into everyday practice isn't just a technological upgrade; it marks a move toward smarter, more personalized care that values timely, evidence-based decisions (Sumon et al., 2024).

4.1. Principles of Magnetic Resonance Imaging (MRI)

Learning Outcome

1. Discuss the basic physics of magnetic fields and radio waves.
2. Describe the role of hydrogen atoms in imaging.
3 Define image formation and signal processing.

Magnetic Resonance Imaging (MRI) kicks into gear by playing with the way hydrogen nuclei – mostly the ones in water molecules – behave under a strong magnet. First off, a mighty magnetic field gets these little particles lined up, and then radiofrequency pulses give them a quick energy boost. As they relax (in their own time, really), they emit signals that get picked up and turned into images. Different tissues, thanks to factors like their water content and tiny molecular uniqueness, relax at varied speeds. In most cases, this means the scan picks up soft tissue details well, proving that MRI isn't just non-invasive but also a crucial part of modern diagnostics. Beyond the basics of snapping images, MRI is also stepping up its game by measuring specific conditions like iron overload syndromes. Generally speaking, techniques such as R2*/T2*-relaxometry let doctors figure out the level of iron buildup in organs like the liver and heart—without ever having to resort to a traditional biopsy. Since the paramagnetic nature of iron complexes distinctively changes the MR signal, clinicians can crunch numbers to get an idea of iron concentration. Methods like the signal intensity ratio (SIR) further tighten the accuracy of these readings, meaning that, in most cases, quantitative MRI helps fine-tune diagnoses, guide treatment choices, and even monitor how effective therapies are over time (Alibiev et al., 2024). Lately, fresh advances have pushed MRI even further—especially in slicing images into meaningful segments, a key step for spotting trouble areas. Innovations in deep learning have managed to automate part of the segmentation process to achieve clinical-level accuracy. Naturally, older supervised learning methods demanded huge piles of annotated data, which isn't always easy to come by. Now, emerging techniques that lean on self-supervised and few-shot learning are offering promising ways to work around these data issues. Overall, these new methods highlight its continuously evolving nature; its techniques keep adapting (despite some practical data constraints) to make diagnoses sharper and more reliable (Liu et al., 2024) (Figure 4.3).

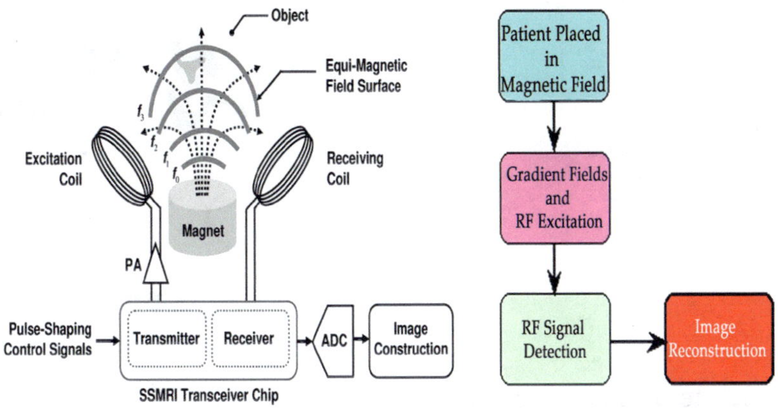

Figure 4.3. The basic principles of MRI.

Source: https://slideplayer.com/slide/5664295/.

4.1.1. Basic Physics of Magnetic Fields and Radio Waves

Magnetic imaging starts with plain physics. A strong magnet gets the hydrogen atoms in your body to line up—imagine those protons standing in neat rows. Then, quick radio pulses come along and ruffle that order for just a moment. As the protons settle back to normal, they fire off little bursts of radio energy that get picked up and turned into detailed views of the body's inner layout. This back-and-forth between magnets and radio waves isn't just clever science—it is what lets doctors tell different tissues apart, a big deal in making the right call. MRI shows its flexibility by playing with both magnetic fields and radio frequencies. In most cases, different tissues react in their own unique ways. Take fat versus water, for example their signals differ enough that the contrasts in an image can be a real lifesaver for clinical decisions. By tweaking the magnet's strength and adjusting pulse patterns, you can boost the image quality and trim down on unwanted distortions. It is this kind of adaptability that puts MRI in high demand across specialties like neurology and cardiology (Huo, 2025). Beyond just checking for problems, MRI has carved a niche in research too. Generally speaking, it is a go-to tool in projects from drug discovery to even veterinary studies. Compact, small-bore MRI systems have been key in deepening our grasp of various diseases, and linking lab discoveries with actual treatments. The basic idea of using magnets and radio waves goes further than imaging—it drives innovation and helps push modern healthcare into new territory (Saito et al., 2024) (Figure 4.4).

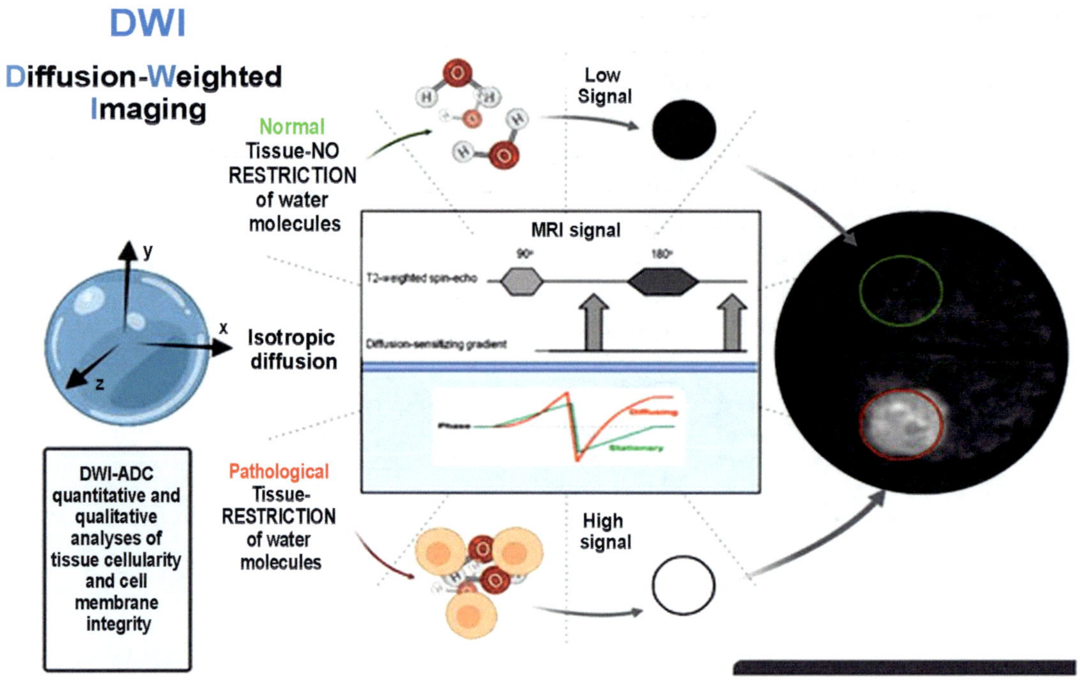

Figure 4.4. Basic principle of magnetic resonance imaging (MRI).

Source: Bruno F, Granata V, Cobianchi Bellisari F, Sgalambro F, Tommasino E, Palumbo P, Arrigoni F, Cozzi D, Grassi F, Brunese MC, et al. Advanced Magnetic Resonance Imaging (MRI) Techniques: Technical Principles and Applications in Nanomedicine. *Cancers*. 2022; 14(7):1626. https://doi.org/10.3390/cancers14071626.

4.1.2. Role of Hydrogen Atoms in Imaging

Magnetic fields and atoms have this oddly intimate dance that makes many imaging tricks possible—MRI being a standout. Hydrogen atoms, super common in body tissues, steal the show. In a strong magnet, these little nuclei line up; then, a burst of radio waves gives them a shove. They soon settle back, releasing energy as signals that get turned into pretty detailed images of our insides. This knack for tuning into hydrogen means you get top-notch photos without the worry of ionizing radiation exposure, which is generally why doctors lean on MRI for diagnostics and monitoring. Hydrogen's role isn't just about showing anatomy either. Take fMRI, for instance—here, tiny shifts in hydrogen signals hint at brain activity by tracking blood flow and oxygen usage in real-time (Figure 4.5).

In most cases, this helps untangle neurological uniqueness. And then there's diffusion-weighted imaging (DWI), where the movement of water molecules (full of hydrogen, naturally) is used to judge how healthy tissues are and flag any subtle changes. These methods, mixing everyday atomic behavior with clever tech, often provide insights that guide more personalized treatment strategies (Honnorat et al., 2024). Still, pinning imaging all on hydrogen isn't without its headaches. Challenges crop up, especially with picking the right solvents and imaging conditions. Recent work has even toyed with the idea of using proton-free liquids in *ex vivo* scans—a nod to growing concerns about traditional agents and their environmental footprint, the quest for alternatives that don't mess up hydrogen's signal while keeping safety and eco-friendliness in check is ongoing (Honnorat et al., 2024).

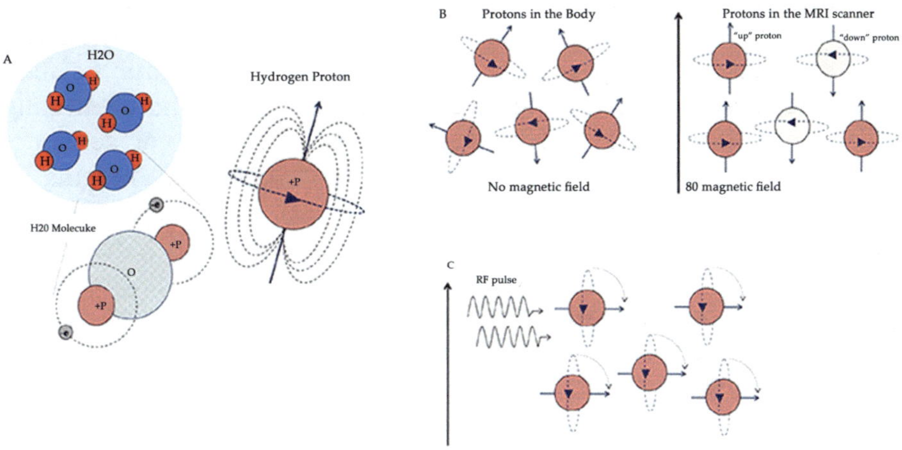

Figure 4.5. Hydrogen protons and how they behave in a magnetic field. (A) Water is made up of two hydrogen atoms and one oxygen atom. The hydrogen nucleus (shown in red as P+) contains one positive charge—a proton spinning around on its axis, which acts like a tiny magnet. (B) In the MRI scanner, the protons align with the B0 magnetic field, some "up" (red), and slightly less "down" (white). The total magnet field generated from all the hydrogen protons almost cancel each other out, leaving only the magnetic field from the small proportion of extra "up" protons, and it is this small magnetic field that we can measure using MRI. (C) When an RF wave/pulse with the same frequency as the proton's precessional frequency is turned on, the "up" protons flip away from the B0 field, as they absorb the RF energy.

Source: https://kids.frontiersin.org/articles/10.3389/frym.2019.00023.

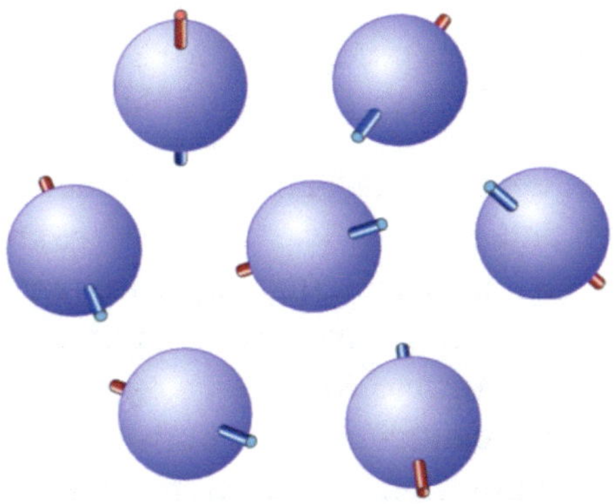

Figure 4.6. Without an external magnetic field, protons (hydrogen nuclei) are randomly oriented.

Source: https://www.analogictips.com/magnetic-resonance-imaging-part-1-how-it-works-faq/.

New solvent ideas could sharpen MRI's precision and also hit some broader sustainability marks. Overall, watching these evolving approaches reminds you just how complex—and a bit unpredictable—the field of medical imaging can be (Figure 4.6).

4.1.3. Image Formation and Signal Processing

Image formation with MRI isn't as mysterious as it might seem—it comes down to mixing the basics of nuclear magnetic resonance with how we fiddle with magnetization vectors. When the MRI machine fires off radiofrequency pulses, hydrogen nuclei inside our tissues start vibrating at rates that match the local magnetic field strength. Those vibrations eventually create signals that get captured over several rounds of image acquisition. You've got sequences like T2 Fast Spin Echo Fat Saturation (T2 FSE FAT SAT) and T2 Multiple Echo Data Imaging Combination (T2 MEDIC) that each tweak the contrast and clarity in unexpected ways. Varying the sequence settings adjusts the balance between the signal-to-noise ratio (SNR) and contrast-to-noise ratio (CNR) – a balance that's crucial for clear images, especially when imaging parts like ankles (Muzamil et al., 2023). Signal processing also gets a major boost from modern methods that polish up MRI images. Instead of letting noise and fuzzy details get in the way, clever algorithms work hard to lower that interference while sharpening up the resolution. In most cases, both the SNR and CNR are the key numbers used to judge how diagnostic an image is.

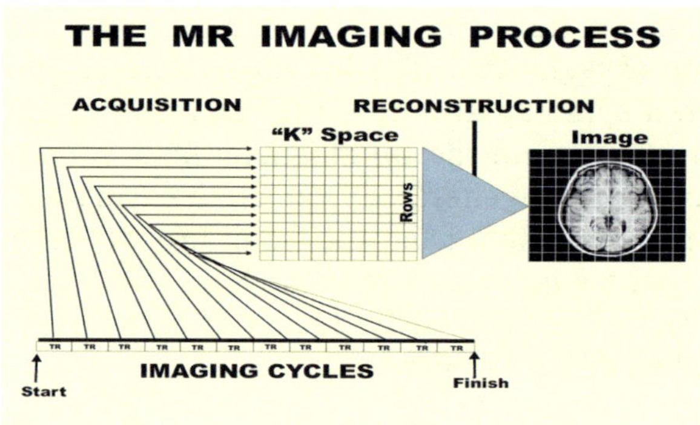

Figure 4.7. The MRI image processing.

Source: https://lh5.googleusercontent.com/proxy/MNMGP3ellRM7m3LjkWEoCXZo8oAOmLYh-nfgphLRpt2ZMnMICvHx67Cb7MoABfz8m25k2dYwO4nekjWkaMKseLOZHQc.

Some studies have generally shown that the T2 MEDIC sequence scores higher in these aspects, leading to images that are clearer and marred less by background interference (Muzamil et al., 2023). It almost seems like these signal processing improvements help doctors better tell apart abnormal tissues from healthy ones, which in turn boosts their ability to diagnose musculoskeletal disorders quickly and with better accuracy. New developments in MRI technology have also cracked the code on imaging hard tissues like cortical bone—a real headache in the past because low proton density gives off only a faint signal. Traditional methods just weren't up to the task. Lately, though, innovative acquisition techniques (including a few gradient-echo-based approaches) have been used to optimize how bones are visualized. This change is especially important, given that MRI is increasingly viewed as a radiation-free alternative to CT scans for musculoskeletal assessments. With the added use of post-processing steps—like generating synthetic CT images and even 3D modeling—MRI not only brings hard tissues into sharper focus, but it also plays a big role in treatment planning and diagnostics across various parts of the body; all of which shows how far we've come in both image formation and signal processing within this field (Figure 4.7).

Test Your Knowledge

1. How do magnetic fields and radio waves interact in MRI to produce detailed images of the body?
2. What is the role of hydrogen atoms in MRI imaging, and why are they crucial for generating high-quality images?

4.2. Types of Magnetic Resonance Imaging (MRI) Scans

Learning Outcome

1. Understand the basis of standard MRI Scans.
2. Describe the functional MRI (fMRI).
3. Learn the role of contrast-enhanced MRI.

MRI comes into its own in healthcare with an assortment of scan types that meet different medical needs. T1-weighted images, for instance, excel at showing off the details of our anatomy—they clearly separate fat from water, which makes it easier to check normal structures and even spot issues like tumors. T2-weighted scans, by contrast, are great at highlighting spots with extra fluid or swelling, as these areas usually stand out brightly; this can guide doctors when they're looking into strokes or signs of multiple sclerosis. Picking which scan to use can steer clinical choices in a big way, proving how MRI's subtle capabilities boost diagnostic accuracy across many scenarios. fMRI—that is, fMRI—adds another twist by tracking changes in blood flow to gauge brain activity. It is not about static pictures; rather, fMRI maps which parts of the brain are firing during specific tasks or in response to certain stimuli. This approach has, generally speaking, opened up exciting new paths in neuroscience, letting researchers probe into cognitive functions and conditions like depression and schizophrenia. Being able to see active brain regions in real-time enriches both clinical diagnoses and research studies, effectively bridging the gap between theory and practice. Plus, ongoing improvements keep fMRI evolving, steadily supporting better therapy plans and, in most cases, improved patient outcomes. Then there's the extra flavor of MRI with methods such as DWI and magnetic resonance angiography (MRA). DWI, for example, shines in spotting acute ischemic strokes by tracking how water molecules shift in tissues—a small clue that can prompt urgent intervention. MRA, on the other hand, zeroes in on blood vessels, delivering detailed images that are crucial for finding vascular problems or planning surgeries. Combining these specialized techniques shows just how flexible and resourceful MRI can be in a clinical setting. With further innovations on the horizon, MRI's role in patient care and clinical decision-making is only set to grow (Kirkpatrick et al., 2020; Zamhuri et al., 2021).

4.2.1. Standard Magnetic Resonance Imaging (MRI) Scans

Standard MRI scans have taken on a bigger role in clinical practice thanks to the infusion of new tech in MRI. Techniques like parallel imaging and compressed sensing now make these scans not only run faster but also deliver images with much sharper detail than before. The quicker capture times cut down on how long patients wait for diagnoses, all while keeping the image clarity intact. In musculoskeletal MRI, where nailing down joint and soft-tissue details is super important, these quicker methods make a difference. We often see that getting a handle on—and using—these tactics helps smooth out MRI workflows and supercharge the diagnostic boost (Yoon et al., 2023). In effect, coming up with new imaging strategies tackles older limits head-on, increasing the overall usefulness of standard MRI in many medical settings. Lately, there's been a surge of interest in sodium MRI, which might serve as a clever sidekick to the usual hydrogen scans. Since sodium (23Na) gives off the second strongest NMR signal in tissues, it offers an unexpected way to check on cell health and overall tissue vitality. This trick is especially handy when diseases are just starting out and anatomical changes aren't clear enough for a standard MRI to pick up. Still, sodium MRI faces its own hurdles—a rather low signal-to-noise ratio and longer scan times keep it from being a go-to in most clinics. That said, recent improvements in compressed sensing show promise in boosting the image quality and slicing down those long waits (Chen et al., 2021). Merging sodium imaging with traditional methods lets clinicians see a more complete picture of what's going on inside, underlining how standard MRI is constantly evolving. Mixing fresh coil designs and synthetic MRI sequences with conventional protocols can boost diagnostic accuracy and streamline workflow. These innovative ideas are all about sharpening signal pickup while leaning on AI to make imaging less of a hassle. For example, synthetic MRI can churn out several contrasts from a single acquisition, which means less overall scan time for a full assessment. New coil setups, on the other hand, aim to up both sensitivity and specificity, identifying small abnormalities that might slip by with traditional methods. Together, this blend of strategies not only speeds up the exam process but also raises the quality of images, proving that standard MRI continues to be an essential tool in modern diagnostics (Yoon et al., 2023). As these techniques keep evolving, they seem poised—if not ready—to redefine its role in healthcare (Figure 4.8).

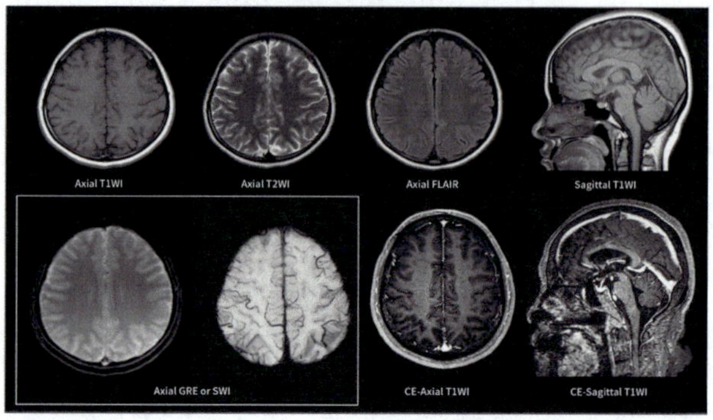

Figure 4.8. An example of a standard imaging technique of brain MRI. Brain MRI includes axial T1WI, axial T2WI, axial T2 FLAIR image, and sagittal T1WI.

Source: https://www.researchgate.net/publication/345962669/figure/fig1/AS:958747388149761@1605594598981/An-example-of-standard-imaging-technique-of-brain-MRI-Brain-MRI-includes-axial-T1WI.png.

4.2.2. Functional MRI (fMRI)

Neuroimaging tech has flipped the script on how we see brain issues—it became a must-have in clinics nowadays. fMRI, pops up as one standout method that checks out brain activity by watching blood flow changes. It relies on what we call the hemodynamic response—when neurons fire more, extra oxygen shows up in those brain spots. Research keeps pointing out that fMRI is used a lot in spotting epilepsy and planning surgeries, letting doctors map out brain networks and zero in on spots that need attention. Its steady integration into everyday clinical routines shows just how much promise advanced imaging has for crafting treatments that are truly personalized (Desale et al., 2024). Fancy software tools for fMRI analysis are coming along steadily—and generally speaking, they're changing the game in both labs and hospitals. Complex programs now help make sense of tangled brain connectivity patterns, sometimes in ways you wouldn't expect. These tools not only speed up studies but also hand over critical insights into what's going on inside the brain. Yet, every tool has its uniqueness and limits, so researchers must pick them carefully to get reliable results. Contemporary reviews even stress that digging into these methods boosts Fmri as a go-to approach in neuroscience research (Hussain Jaber et al., 2024). Understanding and using these evolving techniques remains a key, albeit sometimes messy, part of unlocking fMRI's full potential in both research settings and clinical trials. As the fMRI world keeps expanding, fresh opportunities—and challenges—continue to crop up. Machine learning and other cutting-edge computational tools are now being combined to fMRI analysis, helping us decode complex data sets for a deeper look at how the brain functions (and sometimes misfires). However, even though these innovations open up new paths in research, they still need strict validation to prove their worth. Plus, getting fMRI into everyday clinical use isn't without hiccups—issues like cracking standardized protocols and making sure imaging gear is available everywhere still need tackling. Ongoing discussions highlight how crucial teamwork and shared best practices are for guiding fMRI's future in personalized medicine (Desale et al., 2024). Overall, the steady evolution of fMRI looks set to push neuroimaging into new realms, aiming to offer better, more effective care for patients with neurological conditions (Figure 4.9).

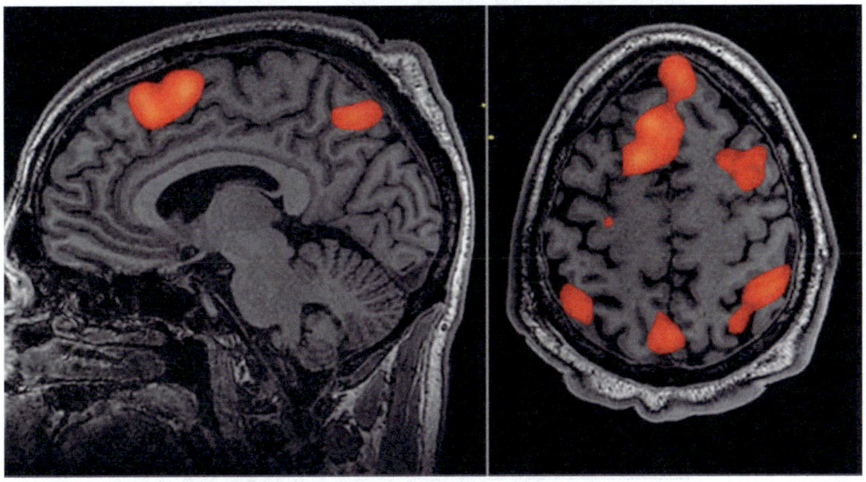

Figure 4.9. Functional magnetic resonance imaging (fMRI).

Source: https://media.post.rvohealth.io/wp-content/uploads/sites/4/2021/12/FMRI-brain-scan-1296x728-header-1024x575.jpg.

4.2.3. Contrast-Enhanced Magnetic Resonance Imaging (MRI)

Diagnostic imaging in cancer care has been taking some unexpected turns lately, especially in bladder cancer. Doctors used to rely almost solely on standard CT scans, but now there's a shift toward an MRI approach that uses contrast. This new method isn't just about snapping a picture; it digs into how tumors show up. It tells clinicians whether a tumor is invading the muscle or not—a detail that can change how treatment is planned. Using the VI-RADS scoring system along with this kind of MRI helps tailor treatments to the patient's specific needs (Masino et al., 2024). It is interesting how adding contrast agents to MRI ups the overall diagnostic game. Traditional gadolinium-based agents are still common since they boost the contrast between cancerous and normal tissue, making the images clearer. At the same time, emerging research is peaking at alternatives like nanodiamonds—tiny particles that seem to offer some cool advantages. They work by tweaking longitudinal relaxation times to improve signal-to-noise ratios and even assist in labeling cells for tracking inside the body. This fresh approach might offer a deeper glimpse into how tumors develop, all while cutting down on some of the risks linked with older gadolinium methods (Lazovic et al., 2023). Mixing advanced imaging with these newer contrast agents opens up a lot of clinical possibilities. Clinicians can now catch complex anatomical details—like the precise edges of a tumor or slight vascular involvement—with a clarity that wasn't always attainable before. This level of detail is important for planning operations and fine-tuning treatment strategies aimed at better outcomes. In most cases, such advancements signal a slow but steady evolution in MRI tech, nudging researchers to explore non-invasive methods even further. Overall, as contrast-enhanced MRI finds its footing in the medical field, it not only boosts diagnostics but also hints at a future where personalized medicine in oncology becomes a standard part of care (Masino et al., 2024) (Figure 4.10).

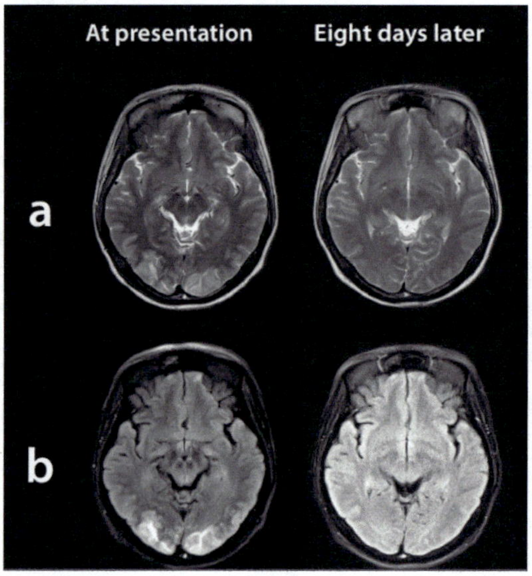

Figure 4.10. Contrast-enhanced MRI brain imaging: a. T2-weighted; b. T2-FLAIR of a patient with metastatic colorectal cancer who developed PRES following treatment with an anti-VEGF antibody and chemotherapy.

Source: https://www.researchgate.net/figure/Contrast-enhanced-MRI-brain-imaging-a-T2-weighted-b-T2-FLAIR-of-patient-with_fig1_281668337.

Test Your Knowledge

1. What is the basic procedure for performing a standard MRI scan, and what types of images does it produce?
2. How does functional MRI (fMRI) differ from standard MRI, and what is its role in measuring brain activity?

4.3. Applications of Magnetic Resonance Imaging (MRI) in Medicine

Learning Outcome

1. Understand the techniques of neurological imaging.
2. Define musculoskeletal imaging and cardiovascular imaging.

MRI changes the game in non-invasive diagnostics—it is one of those tools that generally surprises you with how clearly it shows soft tissues. It does more than just produce sharp images; in neurology, for example, it helps doctors check out the brain in ways that reveal things like tumors, multiple sclerosis, or even tiny blood vessel problems. fMRI, which kind of tracks shifts in blood flow, gives researchers a peek into brain activity; this aspect has opened up new questions about neurodegenerative and even psychiatric conditions. Overall, the technique plays a huge part in guiding treatment decisions and, in many cases, improving patient outcomes, making MRI a real cornerstone of today's medical imaging (Rabah et al., 2024). In oncology, MRI's knack for distinguishing diverse tissue types is absolutely vital for figuring out tumor details and staging them correctly. Lately, contrast-enhanced MRI has stepped in to spotlight aggressive cancer varieties—say, something like macrotrabecular-massive hepatocellular carcinoma (MTM-HCC). By tapping into advanced radiomics, oncologists can pull out measurable data right off the images, which then helps shape personalized treatments. This fresh approach, bolstered sometimes by machine learning models that refine preoperative predictions and ultimately prognosis, shows just how MRI can up the diagnostic game while nudging precision medicine forward (Zhang et al., 2023). MRI isn't just about the brain or cancer; it is also making waves in other specialties such as musculoskeletal imaging, cardiology, and pediatrics. In joints and soft tissue injuries, MRI gives detailed looks that often steer both diagnoses and treatment paths. In the cardiovascular world, it checks things like myocardial viability and heart wall motion abnormalities—pretty essential for thorough cardiac evaluations. And since it doesn't use ionizing radiation, it has become a go-to choice even for imaging young patients. As technology evolves—with newer tricks like DWI and spectroscopy popping up—MRI continues to adapt, bridging the gap between innovative techniques and everyday clinical practice, all while remaining an irreplaceable tool in the diagnostic toolkit (Rabah et al., 2024) (Figure 4.11).

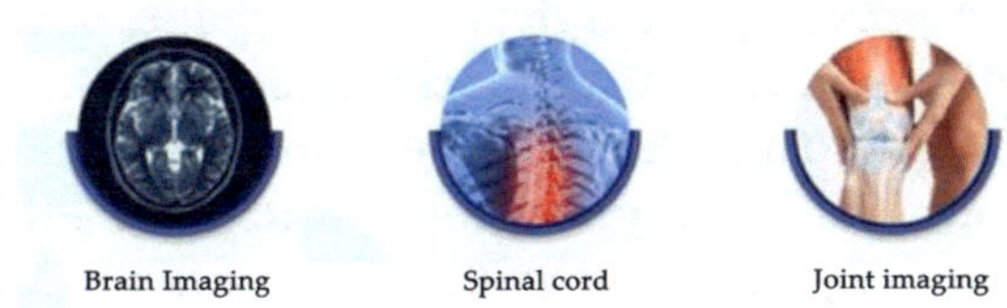

Figure 4.11. Key applications of MRI.

Source: https://external-content.duckduckgo.com/iu/?u=https%3A%2F%2Ftse1.mm.bing.net%2Fth%3Fid%3DOIP.gwMvZ_Ak-lNy2r743g2XjQHaDQ%26pid%3DApi&f=1&ipt=bc0b9ef34dbf1b126d1f0f0900a24ca2d35a0f590e069424bc707eef4b4cf560.

4.3.1. Neurological Imaging

Neurological imaging has taken a leap in recent years—advanced MRI techniques are now front and center. These new tools let us see not only the brain's structure but also how it works, and that's pretty key in spotting different disorders. Take fMRI as an example; it is almost like watching the brain in live action by capturing real-time shifts during neural tasks. Then there's diffusion tensor imaging (DTI), which unexpectedly gives us hints about white matter quality, a detail that's crucial for understanding conditions like multiple sclerosis and Alzheimer's. When you mix these methods together, they boost diagnostic accuracy and open up fresh avenues for research into how the brain's structure and function interact—paving the way for treatment options that are a lot more on target in clinical settings (Mahmoud et al., 2024). Another important piece is magnetic resonance spectroscopy (MRS); unlike your standard MRI which mostly shows anatomy, MRS zooms in on the brain's chemistry and metabolic changes at the cellular level. In many cases, this extra layer of detail proves especially handy for conditions such as epilepsy, where knowing the metabolic profile can shape treatment decisions. For instance, adding MRS into epilepsy care has helped experts better grasp both the physical and functional sides of the disorder, which in turn improves pre-surgical planning and post-op follow-up. And, with machine learning now stepping in to handle the heavy lifting of complex data analysis, the promise of MRS and MRI working together to decode brain pathologies and tailor patient care is becoming even more exciting (Desale et al., 2024). Neurological imaging isn't all smooth sailing, though—it is facing its own set of challenges alongside the opportunities. Sure, we're seeing sharper images and deeper insights thanks to modern tech, but fitting these innovations into everyday clinical practice can still be a real headache. Factors like cost, limited accessibility and the requirement for specialized training sometimes hold things back. Generally speaking, while ongoing MRI improvements and the allure of new imaging biomarkers point toward a future of more personalized medicine, much more research is needed to bridge the gaps—especially when trying to pin down how imaging results match up with clinical outcomes. In the end, pushing forward with these cutting-edge neuroimaging techniques might just revolutionize treatment approaches, helping us fine-tune interventions and improve patient results (Mahmoud et al., 2024) (Figure 4.12).

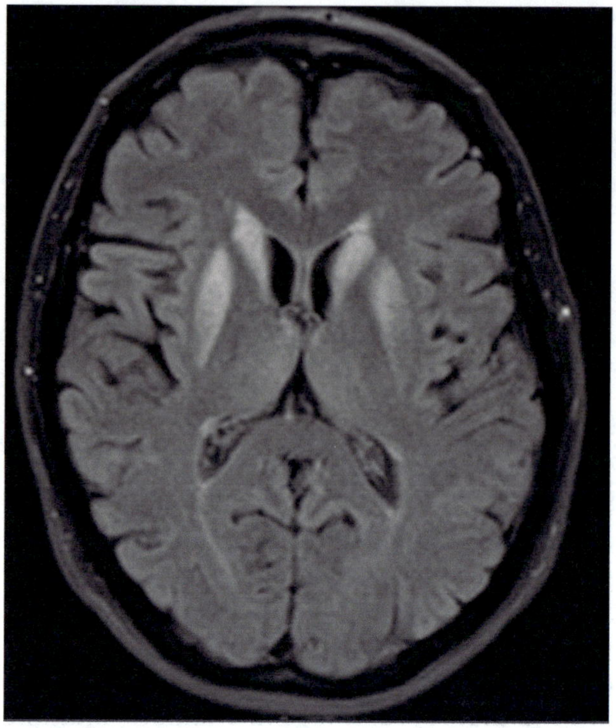

Figure 4.12. Neurological imaging.

Source: https://about.cmrad.com/hubfs/Neurology%20image.png.

4.3.2. Musculoskeletal Imaging

MRI has come a long way recently—doctors now have new ways to see problems in muscles and bones. Special sequences like zero echo time (ZTE) let them view those elusive short-T2 tissues that regular scans often miss. Using super-fast readouts, these ZTE methods pick up details in ligaments and tendons without the radiation worries linked to CT scans. It is a quicker process, and it cuts costs for both patients and healthcare systems, which is why this approach is identifying on (Fujisaki et al., 2023). UTE MRI, or ultrashort echo time imaging, has also shaken up traditional methods. This technique ramps up the usual scans by showing high-contrast images of tissues with short-T2 relaxation times—think of the osteochondral junction or the menisci. It mixes in different contrast tricks that help experts see not just the structure, but also how these tissues function. All this extra insight lets healthcare professionals shape treatment plans a bit more specifically, generally boosting patient outcomes (Afsahi et al., 2021). Quantitative UTE mapping is yet another new frontier that might change musculoskeletal imaging even more. Researchers are dabbling in methods like T1, T2*, and magnetization transfer ratio mapping. These techniques reveal the biochemical scene of tissues—details that would usually stay hidden. Measuring things like the macromolecular proton fraction and water content not only refines diagnosis but also makes it easier to track treatment results over time. Grasping these complex interactions could very well spur fresh ideas for therapies, further cementing MRI's role as a must-have tool in modern medicine (Afsahi et al., 2021) (Figure 4.13).

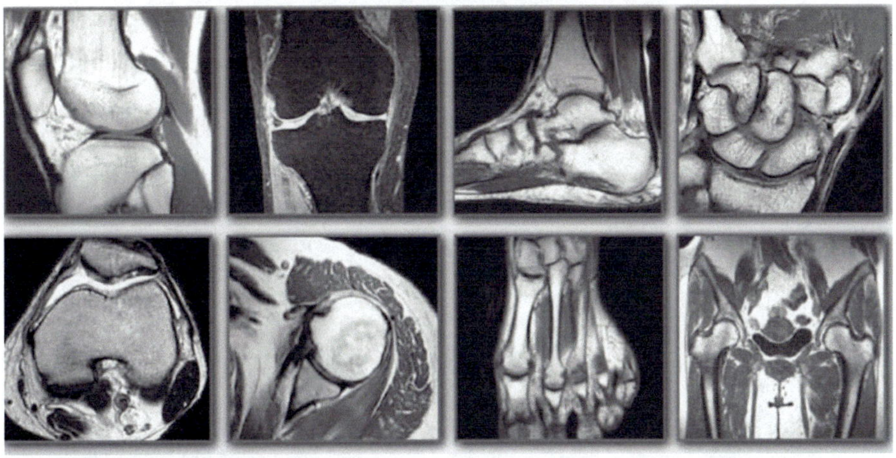

Figure 4.13. Musculoskeletal Imaging

Source: https://www.standupmriofbensonhurst.com/images/musculoskeletal-imaging.jpg.

4.3.3. Cardiovascular Imaging

Cardiovascular imaging has changed the game for heart diagnostics in ways we hadn't imagined—especially with the leaps in MRI technology. MRI, a non-invasive method, gives us detailed looks at the heart and blood vessels, all without exposing patients to ionizing radiation. New imaging sequences have come in handy for people with things like pacemakers by cutting down on image artifacts and yielding much clearer shots. It is pretty remarkable that wideband late gadolinium enhancement imaging has become such a go-to for checking myocardial viability, offering insights that help shape clinical choices. MRI keeps moving forward, proving again and again its key role in modern heart imaging, and ultimately boosting the reliability of patient care (Gut et al., 2024). There's also been a notable shift with AI stepping into cardiovascular imaging, opening up a new space for diagnostic precision. Machine learning algorithms, when applied to MRI, let clinicians tap into improved image processing that not only ups accuracy but also smooths out the bumps in older techniques. Deep learning, for example, has been used to rework image reconstruction, which means faster scans without losing essential details—this is especially crucial in cardiac MRI, where steps like under sampling can ease the patient's load while keeping quality intact. As these AI tools get smarter, they're getting better at spotting coronary artery disease and evaluating myocardial conditions, hinting at a future that leans to personalized medicine (Marey et al., 2024). Looking ahead, cardiovascular MRI seems set to break new ground and possibly redefine what we consider standard practice. Research into generative adversarial networks and similar AI-driven methods is expanding the horizon of what imaging can do, both in terms of precision and overall capability. That said, these advances bring along ethical challenges, like ensuring that AI outputs make sense and don't come with hidden biases in image assessment. In most cases, as AI becomes more woven into cardiovascular imaging, it is essential for doctors and researchers to keep an eye on these issues—balancing shiny innovation with the need for fairness and transparency. Striking that balance will be key to making sure these breakthroughs translate into genuinely better and more equitable patient care (Marey et al., 2024) (Figure 4.14).

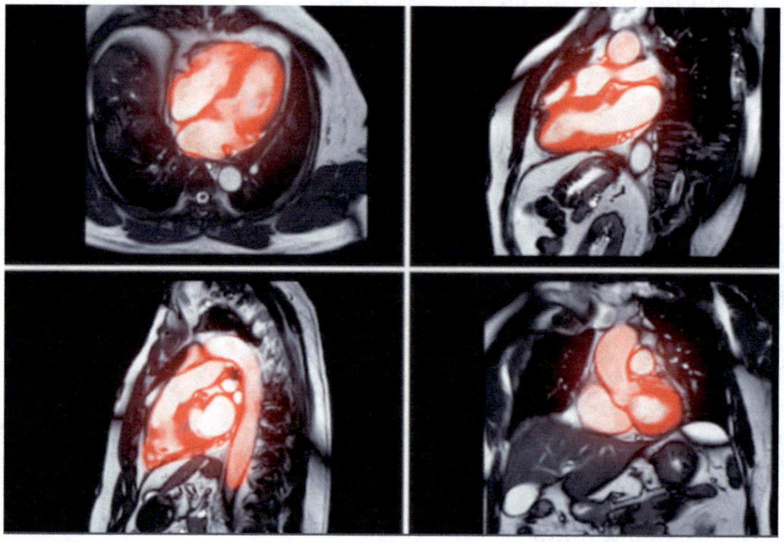

Figure 4.14. Cardiac MRI.

Source: https://s3-us-west-2.amazonaws.com/utsw-patientcare-web-production/original_images/Cardiac_MRI_hero_600x380.jpg.

Test Your Knowledge

1. How is neurological imaging used to diagnose conditions affecting the brain and nervous system?
2. What imaging techniques are commonly used in musculoskeletal imaging, and how do they help in diagnosing bone and joint disorders?

4.4. Advantages, Limitations and Challenges of Magnetic Resonance Imaging (MRI)

Learning Outcome

1. Discuss the advantages of MRI.
2. Define the limitations and challenges of MRI.

4.4.1. Advantages of Magnetic Resonance Imaging (MRI)

MRI stands out for its knack at revealing soft tissue detail in a way that few other imaging tools can match. It doesn't follow the old-school path of X-rays or CT scans. Instead, it uses a magnetic field teamed up with radio waves to generate crisp, detailed pictures – and all without ionizing radiation, which is a definite plus for patient safety. In many cases, when doctors suspect issues like anterior disc displacement in musculoskeletal problems, this method has shown its worth, especially when deep learning models help boost diagnostic accuracy (Lee et al., 2022). Overall, it ends up identifying soft tissue injuries that regular scans might easily overlook. The tool isn't just a one-trick pony, either. MRI pops up in several areas – neurology, cardiology, oncology, you name it. Take shoulder problems: it often takes the lead in sorting out rotator cuff tears, those common yet sometimes muddled diagnoses. Research generally points out that, while ultrasound can sometimes match MRI in spotting full-thickness rotator cuff tears, MRI tends to give a broader view, checking out nearby soft tissues and even subtle shifts in bone marrow (Elmorsy et al., 2017). This extra bit of detail often makes all the difference when mapping out treatment strategies and ultimately helps steer clinical decision-making. There's also the advantage of capturing images in several planes—a feature that helps doctors see how anatomical structures fit together in three dimensions. For example, if a patient has a joint disorder or a suspicious tumor, being able to view the area from different angles means that the diagnosis can become more refined, which in most cases, leads to better treatment planning. Advances like functional imaging and DWI have added layers to its capabilities, revealing insights into both tissue function and structure. MRI, by consistently disclosing key clues about what's going on inside, keeps reshaping medical imaging and, quite frankly, is a game changer for patient outcomes (Figure 4.15).

Imaging Techniques	Novel Finding	Clinical Advantages	Disadvantages
DIR, PSIR, MP2RAGE	CLs	Marker of disability and cognitive impairment	Acquisition time, availability of 3T and 7T MRI for better resolution
SWI, T2*, QSM	CVS, PRLs	Differential diagnosis (CVS); disability and disease progression (PRLs)	Availability of 3T and 7T MRI for better resolution, acquisition time
DTI	Pre-lesion alteration in NAWM	Early detection of new lesions	Lack of specificity
fMRI	Functional changes, plasticity, functional reserve	Study of fatigue and functional reserve	Lack of standardized protocol with high inter-subject variability

MT imaging	Pre-lesion alteration	Predicting long term disability accumulation	Lack of specificity and lack of standardized protocol
MRS	Neural integrity and functionality	Differential diagnosis	Lack of reproducibility and lack of standardized protocol
PET	Quantification of neuroinflammation	Quantification of demyelination and remyelination	Radiations

DIR: double inversion recovery; PSIR: phase-sensitive inversion recovery; MP2RAGE: rapid acquisition with gradient echo; SWI: susceptibility weighted imaging; T2*: gradient echo (GRE) derived R2/T2* maps; QSM: quantitative susceptibility mapping; DTI: diffusion tensor imaging; fMRI: functional MRI; MT imaging: magnetization transfer imaging; MRS: proton magnetic resonance spectroscopy; PET: positron emission tomography; CLs: cortical lesions; CVS: central vein sign; PRLs: paramagnetic rim lesions; NAWM: normal appearing white matter.

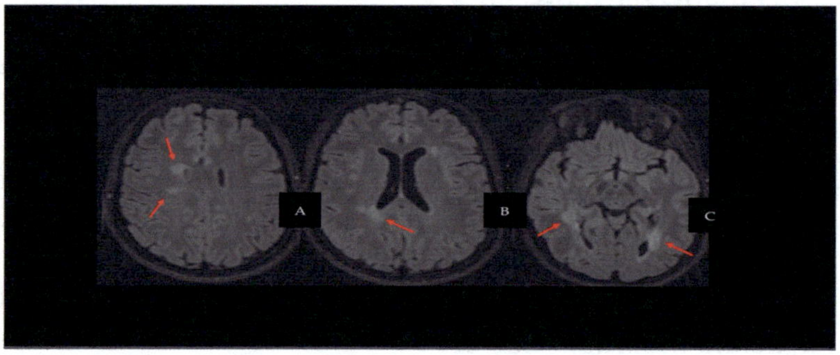

Figure 4.15. MRI advantages and disadvantages.

Source: Nistri R, Ianniello A, Pozzilli V, Giannì C, Pozzilli C. Advanced MRI Techniques: Diagnosis and Follow-Up of Multiple Sclerosis. *Diagnostics*. 2024; 14(11):1120. https://doi.org/10.3390/diagnostics14111120.

4.4.1.1. Non-Invasive Nature of the Procedure

MRI changed how we check things out inside the body—without any cuts or surgery. It pulls off detailed images using strong magnets and radio waves instead of relying on harmful radiation. This means doctors can inspect a mix of internal structures with ease, which often leads to spot-on diagnoses and better treatment plans. It is a safer option that cuts down on the stress and discomfort some invasive tests bring along. In most cases, this approach fits right in with today's focus on balancing accuracy and patient comfort. MRI's non-invasive design also lends itself well to many areas of medicine, like heart and brain care. Take cardiac imaging, for example; cardiac MRI often shines because it delivers crisp, time-sensitive details about the heart. Generally speaking, it lets clinicians follow the progress of heart conditions over time without exposing patients to radiation—something you don't usually get with other methods like echocardiography. This advantage proves handy when tracking disease progression or checking off treatment milestones, setting up a practical game plan for long-term care (Jain, 2024). Beyond the safety perks, MRI's gentle way of capturing images plays a big part in modern medical data processing. Sure, getting high-quality images isn't always easy; issues like background noise and movement can blur results. That's why new techniques—like some advanced filtering methods—are stepping in to help. For example, trilateral filtering has been showing promise, boosting the clarity of scans while keeping the non-invasive benefits intact. This blend of fresh image processing and MRI's inherent strengths not only refines the overall picture but also helps with detailed tissue classification, which is key for accurate diagnoses. In effect, MRI stands as both a non-invasive imaging tool and a beneficiary of continuous technological tweaks that sharpen its clinical role (Sriram et al., 2025) (Figure 4.16).

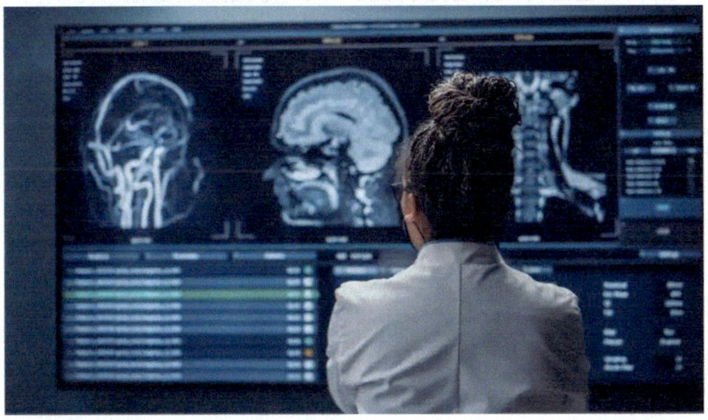

Figure 4.16. MRI changed how we check things out inside the body

Source: https://storage.googleapis.com/treatspace-prod-media/pracimg/u-2740/blogwebp_0_lHECByU.webp.

4.4.1.2. High-Resolution Images

Imaging technology has come a long way and, quite frankly, it reshaped how we diagnose diseases. MRIs, For example, now offer image clarity that makes precise treatment planning possible—when doctors see things in high resolution, lesion detection improves and interventions can happen sooner. Diffusion probabilistic deep learning techniques, for example, have lately become a game changer. Researchers now use these somewhat sophisticated models to transform low-quality scans into high-res images, sidestepping old problems like long scan times and limited equipment (Chang et al., 2024). This approach not only boosts MRI's diagnostic power but also streamlines clinical workflows, making high-resolution imaging more accessible while keeping patient safety and comfort in mind. The leap from low- to high-resolution imaging isn't just a small step forward; it might revolutionize neuroimaging. Take SynthSR—a clever method where AI helps convert routine MRI scans into high-resolution ones. It is especially useful in studies of brain structure in patients with neurological issues since the results often match those of true high-res scans (Iglesias et al., 2023). By effectively increasing the data set, this tool lets researchers delve into areas of brain morphology and pathology that were hard to explore before. In most cases, the extra detail not only enhances analytical insights but also helps tackle the age-old problem of small sample sizes in clinical research, ultimately leading to richer, more comprehensive findings. AI joining hands with MRI is just one sign of a broader move towards computationally enhanced imaging methods. Clear, sharp images reveal anatomical details that pave the way for earlier and more accurate diagnoses of complex conditions. Often, traditional methods can fall short, especially when every minute matters in a clinical setting. The new diffusion probabilistic framework, for lack of a better term, offers a boost—yielding high-quality images with noticeably improved signal-to-noise ratios compared to older interpolation methods (Chang et al., 2024). As the field continues to evolve, the benefits of high-resolution MRI stretch beyond mere diagnosis; they influence patient management and treatment outcomes, ultimately cementing their role in both today's medical practice and tomorrow's research initiatives (Figure 4.17).

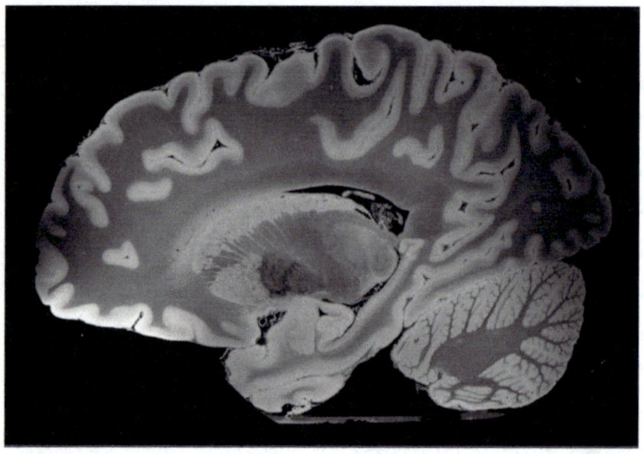

Figure 4.17. The highest resolution MRI scan of a human brain.

Source: https://kottke.org/plus/misc/images/brain-high-res-mri.jpg.

4.4.1.3. No Ionizing Radiation Exposure

Imaging techniques have come a long way and, these days, keeping patients safe is a big deal. MRI gives us detailed pictures of what's happening inside without using ionizing radiation. Instead of relying on X-rays or CT scans—which do expose you to radiation—MRI uses strong magnetic fields and radio waves, so you get the information you need with a lot less risk. Generally speaking, this means you can perform scans over time without worrying about the dangers of repeated exposure, making it a favorite for both doctors and researchers who need to keep patients safe. New MRI methods have started popping up that broaden their application in unexpected areas like cancer treatment and heart care. There are techniques like magnetic resonance spectroscopy and chemical exchange saturation transfer that let you peek into metabolic processes without any radioactive tracers. In fact, noninvasive metabolic MRI approaches have been used to map activities such as brown adipose tissue function in both animals and people—with Cr-CEST MRI showing promise in avoiding harmful radiation (Cai et al., 2024). Such breakthroughs show that MRI isn't just a workhorse for diagnosing conditions; it also offers a safer route for repeated examinations, helping us piece together how the body functions over time. It is also important to note that skipping the ionizing radiation makes MRI more widely acceptable—especially for groups like children and pregnant women, who are more vulnerable to radiation's effects. The noninvasive nature of MRI lets doctors monitor health conditions or treatment responses without adding extra risk for these sensitive populations. Ongoing research is constantly nudging MRI technology forward, expanding its capabilities while keeping patient safety front and center. Recent studies, for example, have urged a closer look at how we manage exposure to magnetic fields in the workplace, reinforcing that MRI can be both effective and safe (Comelli et al., 2024). Overall, this shift toward safer imaging practices is a real win—balancing the need for detailed diagnostics with a genuine concern for well-being.

4.4.2. Limitations and Challenges of Magnetic Resonance Imaging (MRI)

MRI technology brings impressive anatomical and functional insights, yet its complexity kicks up a host of challenges. For example thing, the upfront price isn't the only cost—it spills over into installation, maintenance, training, and day-to-day operations. This expensive upkeep can restrict access, especially in resource-strapped or underserved settings. Even when the machine is available, reading its sometimes subtle imagery demands deep expertise; a slight misinterpretation might easily snowball into a misdiagnosis, affecting treatment pathways. In most cases, radiologists do their best, but the inherent financial and human hurdles persist. Patients, too, add another layer to the conundrum. Not everyone fits neatly into the MRI protocol; staying perfectly still isn't simple for those grappling with claustrophobia, anxiety, or other conditions. Some individuals even come with metal implants or other contraindications that prevent safe scanning. Plus, any involuntary movement—or a lapse in maintaining stillness—can generate motion artifacts that muddy image quality. These issues, repeated again and again, underscore the pressing need for continuous improvements in imaging methods, ensuring that the technology serves all patients effectively. New tech like deep learning steps in with both promise and potential pitfalls for MRI enhancement. On one hand, innovative algorithms can improve how images are reconstructed and sharpen diagnostic accuracy; on the other, they spark concerns about data integrity and whether models are reliable enough. Typically, training such models demands enormous, well-labeled datasets—a resource-heavy requirement that isn't always easy to meet. Furthermore, the intricate process of model training sometimes falls prey to overfitting, which can yield less-than-accurate outcomes in real clinical settings. Generally speaking, striking a balance between harnessing these advanced tools and addressing their built-in limitations is critical. Ongoing collaboration among researchers, clinicians, and technologies (yes, that's how sometimes it goes) will be key to tipping the scales in favor of better patient care (Figure 4.18).

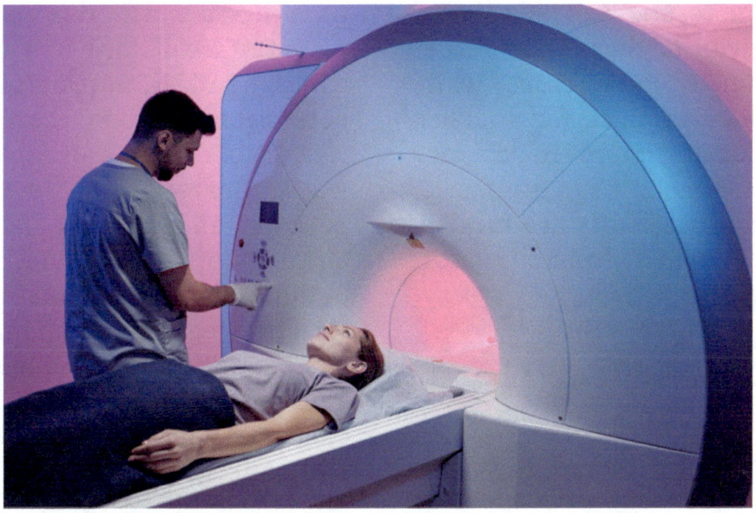

Figure 4.18. MRI technology brings impressive anatomical and functional insights

Source: https://cdn.prod.website-files.com/63bf3f41c3bc69578d823f01/6697b9b94e908c24f13d2b05_iStock-1337470128.jpg.

4.4.2.1. Cost and Accessibility Issues

MRI comes with a hefty price tag that affects both hospitals and patients. MRI gives excellent views of soft tissues, yet its steep costs mean that not every area can afford to update to the latest machines. Budgets are often too tight, so hospitals sometimes stick with older equipment, which can lead to longer waits for scans and delays in diagnosis and treatment. Plus, the need for specially trained operators only piles on extra expenses. In most cases, these money hurdles make it hard to roll out modern MRI technology widely—especially in under-resourced places. Cost isn't the only issue, though. Getting to an MRI scanner can be a challenge in itself. People with mobility issues or those living in remote regions often find that the few facilities available are clustered in big cities, leaving them at a disadvantage. This urban concentration tends to worsen the problem for individuals needing repeated exams or ongoing checks for conditions like cancer;

after all, staying on top of regular imaging is vital for early detection. Some studies also show that quick, timely scans are key in spotting diseases like HCC early on (Lee, 2025). Generally speaking, improving local infrastructure and transport options might be the only way to bridge this accessibility gap. Then there's the push to bring in new technology like computer-aided detection (CADe) systems, which can boost MRI's ability to pick up early signs of problems—especially for breast cancer screening. However, the high cost of these systems often puts them out of reach for smaller clinics (Jannatdoust et al., 2025). Even when a facility manages to invest, interpreting the results demands skilled professionals, which can further strain places already short on staff. In many cases, while these innovations offer promise for sharper, earlier diagnoses, balancing improved accuracy with affordability remains an ongoing puzzle; unless both cost and accessibility are tackled, not every patient will benefit from the latest advances in MRI imaging.

4.4.2.2. Patient Discomfort and Claustrophobia

Patients often face major hurdles when getting an MRI. Feeling uncomfortable or trapped is a real concern. The cramped space inside an MRI machine can trigger a burst of anxiety—especially for individuals who are already a bit claustrophobic. In fact, nearly 40% of patients who skip optional scans point to this very issue as the main reason for backing out. Besides, the overall experience isn't just about the tight space; the scanner's noise, odd positioning, and long procedure all add up. In most cases, tackling these everyday discomforts is key to keeping patients on board and ensuring the scans turn out well. The effects of feeling confined aren't limited to just making someone uneasy. They reach further, messing with mental well-being and even wrecking image quality. Patients who feel overwhelmed by anxiety often find it hard to stay still, which can blur images and throw diagnostic accuracy off course. Worse yet, the mental strain might push some people to forgo essential scans, delaying a diagnosis and subsequent treatment. Generally speaking, healthcare teams need to take the time to explain the process in plain language and build a more supportive vibe. Techniques like guided imagery or simple relaxation methods might help ease these nerves, making the ordeal a bit less taxing overall. New ideas are popping up to ease these MRI-related woes. Recent work has introduced something called the MRI-related distress scale (MRI-DS), designed specifically to measure anxiety during breast MRI. This tool gives doctors a better read on how stressed patients are before and during the scan. By using the MRI-DS, providers can set up more personalized interventions that not only ease claustrophobia but also boost comfort in other ways. Clearer, more relaxed chats between patients and doctors also seem to lead to better support measures aimed at reducing both physical and mental strain. Overall, these fresh strategies mark an important step toward making the MRI experience smoother and more effective, ultimately leading to more accurate diagnoses while keeping patient well-being front and center (Kang et al., 2024; Manuweera et al., 2024) (Figure 4.19).

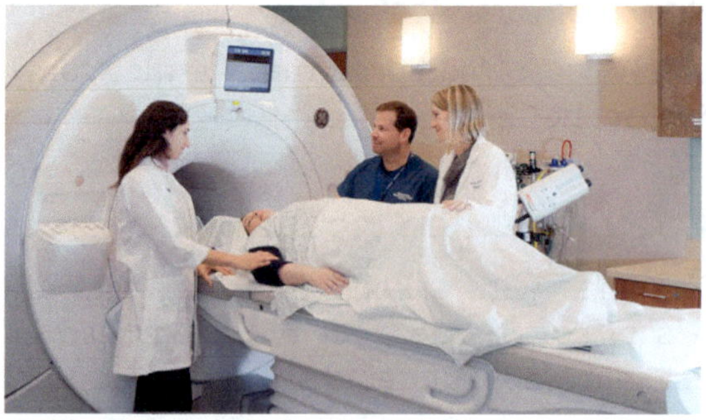

Figure 4.19. Patient Discomfort and Claustrophobia

Source: https://radiology.ucsf.edu/sites/radiology.ucsf.edu/files/fields/image/og/RadAbd-86.jpg.

4.4.2.3. Limitations in Imaging Certain Body Parts

MRI has come a long way in helping doctors see inside the body, yet some spots still give us headaches. Take the pelvic floor, for instance—it's a mess of overlapping structures and movements that show just how tricky imaging can be. Dynamic MRI works well to show the overall layout, but in identifying real-time motion—like the shifts seen in pelvic organ prolapse—it often falls short. The mix of detailed tissues and constant organ shifts makes it hard to get clear and useful images. Researchers have been trying, experimenting with contrast agents to brighten things up, but, frankly, finding that perfect contrast is still a major challenge in a lot of cases (Lv et al., 2023). Then there's the issue of movement. Patients moving, even the slightest breaths, plus the particular uniqueness of magnetic field strength, can mess with the final image quality. This problem pops up most clearly in busy parts of the body like the abdomen or chest where everything is always in motion. These little motion artifacts can sometimes blur the picture so much that important details might be misread. Even when doctors mix MRI with other imaging techniques to get a better look, the resolution and contrast needed to capture certain organs properly still remain elusive (Lv et al., 2023). When it comes down to looking at pelvic organs, the obstacles multiply. Sure, dynamic MRI does a decent job nailing the structure, but it bumbles when trying to capture how these parts work in real time. The pelvic region, with its jumble of overlapping features, tends to hide key diagnostic details—details that are usually vital for making the right call. So, while the technique does open some doors for functional analysis, it just isn't quite comprehensive enough for solid diagnosis and treatment planning, especially in tricky cases like pelvic organ prolapse where those subtle, dynamic changes matter.

Test Your Knowledge

1. What are the main advantages of MRI compared to other imaging techniques like CT or X-ray?
2. What are some common limitations and challenges associated with MRI, including patient-related and technical factors?

Summary

MRI has become a real game-changer in how we handle tough neurological disorders. It lets us see fine details of the brain's inner workings—details that shed light on conditions like epilepsy and gliomas. High-field MRI mixed in with machine learning tweaks, generally speaking, bumps up diagnostic precision, meaning treatments can be more closely tailored to each patient's needs. Recent studies even suggest that neuroimaging goes beyond just spotting issues; it plays a part in planning treatments and tracking how diseases evolve, ultimately boosting clinical outcomes and improving patient quality of life (Desale et al., 2024). That said, while MRI brings huge benefits, there are some hurdles to clear. For example, standardized reporting systems aren't always in place and weaving complex imaging data into everyday workflows can be tricky. Variations in radiologist expertise sometimes lead to results being misinterpreted, which complicates decision-making. In most cases, more interdisciplinary teamwork and fresh technological ideas are needed. Efforts focusing on aligning MRI protocols and upping data-sharing practices could help unlock the full potential of MRI as a reliable diagnostic tool, ensuring outcomes stay accurate (Koska et al., 2023). To wrap it up, the promise MRI holds for changing patient care in neurology is impressive—but it depends on persistent research and ongoing improvements. Incorporating radiomics along with machine learning not only sharpens diagnostic precision but also peels back layers to reveal the underlying biological processes, deepening our understanding of these disorders. Sure, getting to that point demands a joint effort among researchers, clinicians and technologists. Plus, emphasizing proper education and training for healthcare professionals could bridge the gap between cutting-edge tech and everyday practice, leading to better overall care. Ultimately, the future of MRI is a collaborative journey, one that's set to redefine modern medical imaging (Desale et al., 2024; Koska et al., 2023). MRI progress has pushed the boundaries in how we diagnose illnesses across many medical areas, not just one. Take breast imaging, for example; now, CADe systems have found their way into everyday practice. These tools, which mix classical machine learning with newer deep learning twists, are looking at lesions and trying to figure out their significance. Radiologists, in turn, get extra clues that help focus their judgment.

KEY TERMS FROM THIS CHAPTER

- Contrast agents
- Functional MRI (fMRI)
- Magnetic field
- MRI scanner
- Radio waves
- Relaxation time
- T1-weighted image
- Dissecting aortic aneurysm (DAA)
- Gradient coils
- Magnetic resonance
- Neuroimaging
- Radiofrequency pulses
- Signal intensity
- Vacuum-assisted breast biopsy (VABB)

Critical Thinking Questions

1. **Which of the following is the primary principle behind MRI?**
   a. Ionizing radiation
   b. Magnetic fields and radio waves
   c. Sound waves
   d. Electrical impulses
2. **In an MRI scan, what does the strong magnetic field primarily do?**
   a. It enhances the contrast of bone structures
   b. It aligns the hydrogen atoms in the body
   c. It increases the radiation dose
   d. It creates X-rays
3. **Which of the following is a major advantage of MRI over X-ray and CT scans?**
   a. It uses ionizing radiation
   b. It provides better soft tissue contrast
   c. It is faster than CT scanning
   d. It is less expensive
4. **What is typically used as a contrast agent in MRI to improve image clarity?**
   a. Iodine-based solution
   b. Gadolinium-based solution
   c. Barium sulfate
   d. Carbon dioxide
5. **Which of the following conditions is commonly evaluated using an MRI scan?**
   a. Bone fractures
   b. Pneumonia
   c. Soft tissue injuries (e.g., ligament tears)
   d. Dental cavities

Short Answer Questions

1. What are the fundamental principles behind how MRI imaging works, and how does it differ from X-ray or CT imaging?
2. What are the different types of MRI scans, and how are they used in clinical practice?
3. How is MRI applied in medicine to diagnose conditions related to the brain, spine, and joints?
4. What are the primary advantages of MRI over other imaging methods, such as CT or X-rays?
5. What are some limitations and challenges associated with MRI, including patient factors and imaging constraints?

Answers to Critical Thinking Questions

1. (b); 2. (b); 3. (b); 4. (b); 5. (c)

References

1. Afsahi, A., Ma, Y., Jang, H., Jerban, S., Chung, C., Chang, E., & Du, J. (2021). Ultrashort echo time magnetic resonance imaging techniques: Met and unmet needs in musculoskeletal imaging. *Journal of Magnetic Resonance Imaging, 55*. https://www.semanticscholar.org/paper/bfaf5fe3c18610744bc4ca1af7b24549310b26d1 (accessed on 23 May 2025).
2. AL Rabah, A. A. A., Binmhusien, M. A., Alotaibi, M. H., & Almalki, B. A. (2024). Magnetic resonance imaging (MRI): Principles, applications, and clinical utility. *Journal of Advances and Scholarly Researches in Allied Education, 21*(2, Special Issue). ISSN 2230-7540.
3. Alibiev, D., Zavadovskaya, V., Saprina, T., Musina, N., Murdinov, R., Zorkaltsev, M., & Kilina, O. (2024). Iron overload syndrome. Etiopathogenesis. Magnetic resonance imaging techniques for quantitative assessment of iron overload status: A review. *Diagnostic Radiology and Radiotherapy, 15*(1), 7–14. https://doi.org/10.22328/2079-5343-2024-15-1-7-14.
4. Cai, Z., Zhong, Q., Feng, Y., Wang, Q., Zhang, Z., Wei, C., Yin, Z., et al. (2024). Non-invasive mapping of brown adipose tissue activity with magnetic resonance imaging. *Nature Metabolism, 6*, 1367–1379. https://www.semanticscholar.org/paper/372e9e299946afb375a083db0064780f058c2b54 (accessed on 23 May 2025).
5. Chang, C. W., Peng, J., Safari, M., Salari, E., Pan, S., Roper, J., Qiu, R. L. J., et al. (2024). High-resolution MRI synthesis using a data-driven framework with denoising diffusion probabilistic modeling. *Physics in Medicine and Biology, 69*. https://www.semanticscholar.org/paper/9598320b46c043e90f6d476553b06db9cdf4781f (accessed on 23 May 2025).
6. Chen, Q., Shah, N. J., & Worthoff, W. (2021). Compressed sensing in sodium magnetic resonance imaging: Techniques, applications, and future prospects. *Journal of Magnetic Resonance Imaging, 55*. https://www.semanticscholar.org/paper/aa57dc89ad153d6c559ba8e0046a8702d5762f80 (accessed on 23 May 2025).
7. Comelli, M., Zoppetti, N., Burriesci, G., D'Agostino, S., Bogi, A., & Di Liberto, R. (2024). Technological developments in protection from non-ionizing radiation: Instrumental procedures and software to support operators. In *2024 4th URSI Atlantic Radio Science Meeting (AT-RASC)*. https://www.semanticscholar.org/paper/429abbaf91c330177d6e33fea01b0ae2c7728489 (accessed on 23 May 2025).
8. Desale, P., Dhande, R., Parihar, P., Nimodia, D., Bhangale, P. N., & Shinde, D. (2024). Navigating neural landscapes: A comprehensive review of magnetic resonance imaging (MRI) and magnetic resonance spectroscopy (MRS) applications in epilepsy. *Cureus, 16*. https://www.semanticscholar.org/paper/af7e40d432fb8f49784f39b492f7a27b0cdf5a65 (accessed on 23 May 2025).
9. Elmorsy, A., Keightley, A., & Flannery, M. (2017). Accuracy of ultrasonography (US) and magnetic resonance imaging (MRI) in detection of rotator cuff tears in district general hospital. *Polish Journal of Radiology, 82*, 634–637. https://www.semanticscholar.org/paper/a0d7d8a9f8675fc0869c7b06cb108b94253e2d53 (accessed on 23 May 2025).
10. Fıçıcı, C., Koçak, O., & Telatar, Z. (2023). Definition and classification of heart diseases from data obtained with echocardiography Doppler. In *2023 Medical Technologies Congress (TIPTEKNO)*. https://www.semanticscholar.org/paper/e656d554f393408c60c6771f9ab360f65f7c8fac (accessed on 23 May 2025).

11. Florkow, M., Willemsen, K., Mascarenhas, V., Oei, E., van Stralen, M., & Seevinck, P. (2022). Magnetic resonance imaging versus computed tomography for three-dimensional bone imaging of musculoskeletal pathologies: A review. *Journal of Magnetic Resonance Imaging, 56*, 11–34. https://www.semanticscholar.org/paper/85f3234b2c37e24723c2f7d83bf0a575b88c2a6d (accessed on 23 May 2025).

12. Fujisaki, A., Tsukamoto, J., Narimatsu, H., Hayashida, Y., Todoroki, Y., Hirano, N., Takeda, K., et al. (2023). Zero echo time magnetic resonance imaging; Techniques and clinical utility in musculoskeletal system. *Journal of Magnetic Resonance Imaging, 59*. https://www.semanticscholar.org/paper/c17fe198e6a6a571d10d854e53acdf5272fdd145 (accessed on 23 May 2025).

13. Gilyadova, A., Ishchenko, A., Puchkova, E., Mershina, E., Petrovichev, V., & Reshetov, I. (2023). Diagnostic value of dynamic magnetic resonance imaging (dMRI) of the pelvic floor in genital prolapses. *Biomedicines, 11*. https://www.semanticscholar.org/paper/b98298f26e320ed4d0dd91510c3628f210b90dba (accessed on 23 May 2025).

14. Gupta, A. (2025). *Vacuum-Assisted Breast Biopsy: A Comprehensive Overview*. https://www.semanticscholar.org/paper/a2519c45245096ffbd61aa0d56c3e8e2ef511678 (accessed on 23 May 2025).

15. Gut, P., Cochet, H., Stuber, M., & Bustin, A. (2024). Magnetic resonance myocardial imaging in patients with implantable cardiac devices: Challenges, techniques, and clinical applications. *Echocardiography, 41*(11), e70012. https://www.semanticscholar.org/paper/b2729a2d93b43817c4936e7fbc14b34e46112987 (accessed on 23 May 2025).

16. Honnorat, N., Mojtabai, M., Li, J., Smith, M., Seshadri, S., Bieniek, K. F., & Habes, M. (2024). A new halogenated solvent for *ex vivo* magnetic resonance imaging. *bioRxiv*. https://doi.org/10.1101/2024.06.05.597589.

17. Hossain, M., Shinde, R., Oh, S., Kwon, K. C., & Kim, N. (2024). A systematic review and identification of the challenges of deep learning techniques for under sampled magnetic resonance image reconstruction. *Sensors, 24*. https://www.semanticscholar.org/paper/8d131c88ceb066fba7dff0c68051a8a71d679353 (accessed on 23 May 2025).

18. Huo, Y. (2025). Magnetic resonance imaging applications and optimization analysis. *Theoretical and Natural Science, 80*, 101–106.

19. Iglesias, J. E., Billot, B., Balbastre, Y., Magdamo, C., Arnold, S., Das, S., Edlow, B., et al. (2023). SynthSR: A public AI tool to turn heterogeneous clinical brain scans into high-resolution T1-weighted images for 3D morphometry. *Science Advances, 9*. https://www.semanticscholar.org/paper/2a6d745158109c49204bef5c4c1aff4bce0ab108 (accessed on 23 May 2025).

20. Jaber, H. A., Al-Ghali, B. A., Kareem, M. M., Çankaya, I., & Algın, O. (2024). Exploratory data analysis methods for functional magnetic resonance imaging (fMRI): A comprehensive review of software programs used in research. *Al-Nahrain Journal for Engineering Sciences*. https://www.semanticscholar.org/paper/e999ba871c626685fe29679271e29114f070d18d (accessed on 23 May 2025).

21. Jain, P. (2024). An introduction and emerging techniques in cardiac MRI. *Central India Journal of Medical Research*. https://www.semanticscholar.org/paper/8c69bf02a28d9e6d103385cef13b609d36d22c0b (accessed on 23 May 2025).

22. Jannatdoust, P., Valizadeh, P., Saeedi, N., Valizadeh, G., Salari, H. M., Rad, H. S., & Gity, M. (2025). Computer-aided detection (CADe) and segmentation methods for breast cancer using magnetic resonance imaging (MRI). *Journal of Magnetic Resonance Imaging*. https://doi.org/10.1002/jmri.29687.

23. Kalekar, T., Gupta, A., & Kumar, M. (2024). 3-Tesla cardiac magnetic resonance imaging in primary dilated cardiomyopathy. *African Journal of Thoracic and Critical Care Medicine, 30*. https://www.semanticscholar.org/paper/2046f9142dc3f3232babdbb6c85913aac5fcdaed (accessed on 23 May 2025).

24. Kang, D., Kim, S., Han, J., Kim, Y., Cho, J., Lee, J. E., & Ko, E. S. (2024). Measuring patient-reported distress from breast magnetic resonance imaging: Development and validation of the MRI-related distress scale (MRI-DS). *Cancer Medicine, 13*. https://www.semanticscholar.org/paper/8448165acc13f5ed3a4f22b5de3aeeb4dcb1f187 (accessed on 23 May 2025).

25. Kirkpatrick, J. N., Mitchell, C., Taub, C., Kort, S., Hung, J., & Swaminathan, M. (2020). ASE statement on protection of patients and echocardiography service providers during the 2019 novel coronavirus outbreak: Endorsed by the American College of Cardiology. *Journal of the American Society of Echocardiography, 33*, 648–653. https://doi.org/10.1016/j.echo.2020.04.001.

26. Koska, I. O., Koska, Ç., & Fernandes, A. (2023). Automatic prediction of IDH mutation status of low-grade gliomas using radiomics and domain knowledge inspired features in magnetic resonance imaging. *Anadolu Kliniği Tıp Bilimleri Dergisi, 29*(2). https://doi.org/10.21673/anadoluklin.1378673 (accessed on 23 May 2025).

27. Kotadia, I., O'dowling, R., Aboagye, A., Crawley, R., Plein, S., Sztriha, L., Scott, P., et al. (2024). Predicting atrial fibrillation risk following embolic stroke of unknown source using cardiac magnetic resonance imaging. *Europace, 26*. https://www.semanticscholar.org/paper/39c00a56c2ed410e4c7843fd5a1fb328722c4b82 (accessed on 23 May 2025).

28. Lazovic, J., Goering, E., Wild, A. M., Schützendübe, P., Shiva, A., Löffler, J., Winter, G., et al. (2023). Nanodiamond-enhanced magnetic resonance imaging. *Advanced Materials, 36*. https://www.semanticscholar.org/paper/7b4e3b7868fd233390b99d7c3b1456a873810f21 (accessed on 23 May 2025).

29. Lee, D. H. (2025). Recent advances and issues in imaging modalities for hepatocellular carcinoma surveillance. *Journal of Liver Cancer*. https://www.semanticscholar.org/paper/8186ab61545a4644ac410c2968902e4d88ef2284 (accessed on 23 May 2025).

30. Lee, Y. H., Won, J., Kim, S., Auh, Q. S., & Noh, Y. K. (2022). Advantages of deep learning with convolutional neural network in detecting disc displacement of the temporomandibular joint in magnetic resonance imaging. *Scientific Reports, 12*. https://www.semanticscholar.org/paper/96aadcb01b14cf0908627270089bc6a75dd91c97 (accessed on 23 May 2025).

31. Li, T., Wang, J., Yang, Y., Glide-Hurst, C., Wen, N., & Cai, J. (2023). Multi-parametric MRI for radiotherapy simulation. *Medical Physics*. https://www.semanticscholar.org/paper/08e3b127c59783f69e36a17e6b33697bb5ea092f (accessed on 23 May 2025).

32. Liu, Z., Kainth, K., Zhou, A., Deyer, T. W., Fayad, Z. A., Greenspan, H., & Mei, X. (2024). A review of self-supervised, generative, and few-shot deep learning methods for data-limited magnetic resonance imaging segmentation. *NMR in Biomedicine, 37*(8), e5143. https://doi.org/10.1002/nbm.5143.

33. Lv, J., Roy, S., Xie, M., Yang, X., & Guo, B. (2023). Contrast agents of magnetic resonance imaging and future perspective. *Nanomaterials, 13*. https://www.semanticscholar.org/paper/5fd83d66c035b1d9b25f666106cfa969a28853a1 (accessed on 23 May 2025).

34. Mahmoud, A. A. Y., Ahmed, M. K. I., Mohammed, T. H. J., Hani, A. M. M., & Mahmoud, H. M. (2024). Development of magnetic resonance imaging (MRI) techniques for studying neurological changes associated with brain diseases. *European Journal of Medical Genetics and Clinical Biology*. https://www.semanticscholar.org/paper/1ee07ff84f66364da01eacab42e84a71e4aaf697 (accessed on 23 May 2025).

35. Manuweera, T., Karunakaran, K., Baechler, C., Rosales, J., Kleckner, A. S., Rosenblatt, P., Ciner, A., & Kleckner, I. R. (2024). Barriers and facilitators for participation in brain magnetic resonance imaging (MRI) scans in cancer research: A feasibility and acceptability analysis. *Research Square*. https://doi.org/10.21203/rs.3.rs-4595719/v1.

36. Marey, A., Serdysnki, K. C., Killeen, B., Unberath, M., & Umair, M. (2024). Applications and implementation of generative artificial intelligence in cardiovascular imaging with a focus on ethical and legal considerations: What cardiovascular imagers need to know! *BJR|Artificial Intelligence*. https://www.semanticscholar.org/paper/0e8e3b2828235f4372d65a7e840d88b8162c62c7 (accessed on 23 May 2025).

37. Masino, F., Eusebi, L., Muscatella, G., Montatore, M., Sortino, G., Giannubilo, W., & Guglielmi, G. (2024). Conventional and innovative imaging modalities in bladder cancer: Techniques and applications. *Digital Diagnostics*. https://www.semanticscholar.org/paper/6d2008a88d42df0af748955cdba6bf335a5bcb3a (accessed on 23 May 2025).

38. Moumaris, M. (2024). Advancements in magnetic resonance imaging: Transforming non-invasive diagnosis and treatment monitoring in radiology. *Journal of Life Sciences Research and Reviews*. https://www.semanticscholar.org/paper/7aae40b782edf35319696a6b7a45a88b0ca53928 (accessed on 23 May 2025).

39. Muzamil, A., Wandani, C., Hariyani, D., Rulaningtyas, R., Ain, K., Permatasari, P., & Astuti, S. (2023). Combination T2 multiple echo data imaging and fast spin echo fat saturation technique to improve image quality on ankle magnetic resonance imaging. *Rawal Medical Journal*. https://www.semanticscholar.org/paper/f1af6999e7433fec47236aaa18533157cf02e5f6 (accessed on 23 May 2025).

40. Qin, B., & Gao, J. (2025). Current status and perspectives of ultrahigh-field magnetic resonance imaging. *Acta Physica Sinica, 74*(7), 078701. https://doi.org/10.7498/aps.74.20241759.

41. Saito, S., & Ueda, J. (2024). Preclinical magnetic resonance imaging and spectroscopy in the fields of radiological technology, medical physics, and radiology. *Radiological Physics and Technology, 17*, 47–59. https://www.semanticscholar.org/paper/6fd029088fa0ef8963098cc046744af326e3226e (accessed on 23 May 2025).

42. Sriram, S., Vijayaraj, N., Srilekha, T., Praveena, M., & Murugan, T. (2025). GPU accelerated trilateral filter for MR image restoration. *IEEE Access, 13*, 63013–63028. https://www.semanticscholar.org/paper/7c6e5daecf8fec182856ae4d1b98244f2033561d (accessed on 23 May 2025).

43. Sumon, S., Rahman, M., Ahamed, M., Sikder, M., Abedin, M., & Akanda, A. (2024). Knowledge, attitude and practice (KAP) and health impacts of MRI among the patients attending MRI

in Dhaka city. *International Journal of Medical Imaging*. https://www.semanticscholar.org/paper/f18067ca88944652ef8f542c71bd73e4860f46f0 (accessed on 23 May 2025).

44. Yang, D., Liu, C., & Hu, Q. (2024). Diagnostic value of a magnetic resonance imaging (MRI)-based vertebral bone quality score for bone mineral density assessment: An updated systematic review and meta-analysis. *Quantitative Imaging in Medicine and Surgery, 14*, 7561–7575. https://www.semanticscholar.org/paper/ec0b513593eaa384e999fb1e129afb201da96d47 (accessed on 23 May 2025).

45. Yoon, M. A., Gold, G. E., & Chaudhari, A. S. (2024). Accelerated musculoskeletal magnetic resonance imaging. *Journal of Magnetic Resonance Imaging, 60*(5), 1806–1822. https://doi.org/10.1002/jmri.29205.

46. Zamhuri, A., Lim, G. P., Ma, N. L., et al. (2021). MXene in the lens of biomedical engineering: Synthesis, applications and future outlook. *Biomedical Engineering Online, 20*, 33. https://doi.org/10.1186/s12938-021-00873-9.

47. Zhang, Y., He, D., Liu, J., Wei, Y., & Shi, L. L. (2023). Preoperative prediction of macro trabecular-massive hepatocellular carcinoma through dynamic contrast-enhanced magnetic resonance imaging-based radiomics. *World Journal of Gastroenterology, 29*, 2001–2014. https://www.semanticscholar.org/paper/8f47181b8d617e26e69691ab76a4c9c224f863f9 (accessed on 23 May 2025).

ULTRASOUND IMAGING

5

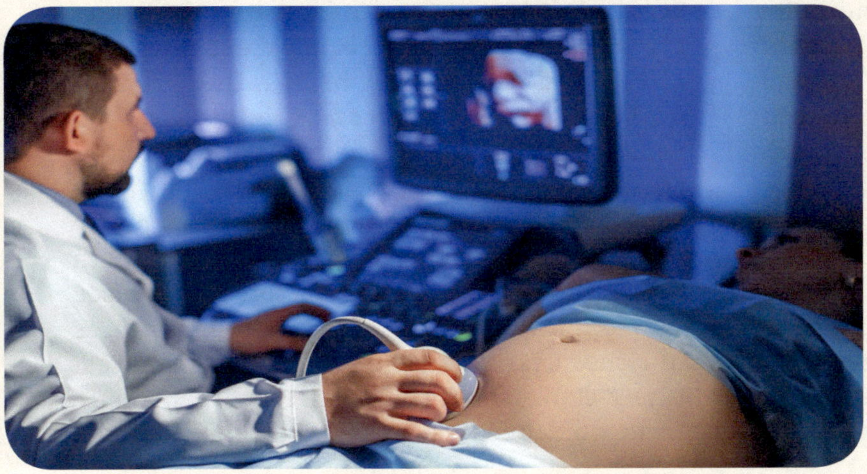

LEARNING OBJECTIVES

After studying this chapter, you will be able to:

1. Understand the principles of ultrasound technology.
2. Discuss the types of ultrasound imaging.
3. Explain the applications of ultrasound imaging in medicine.
4. Evaluate the advantages and limitations of ultrasound imaging.
5. Define future developments in ultrasound technology.

Introduction

Medical imaging has come a long way—ultrasound now plays a huge role in how we spot issues inside the body. This method, which simply uses high-frequency sound pulses to create images of internal structures, isn't invasive at all. It began as a basic tool and gradually morphed into something far more advanced, used in all sorts of medical areas. For example, breakthroughs in piezoelectric tech have combined old ideas with new, building ultrasound systems that shine in soft tissue imaging and overall diagnostic clarity. These changes make it clear that ultrasound isn't just for big hospitals—its impact on personal healthcare is getting noticed, as recent studies have shown (Zhang et al., 2023). Ultrasound's reach stretches to many parts of our anatomy, even into areas like the eyes that often slip under the radar. Even though the core physics behind it has pretty much stayed the same for over 50 years, the technology has taken off. What started as basic A-scan and B-scan methods has now given way to more refined Doppler imaging; meanwhile, fresh transducer designs and multielement arrays allow for dynamic, flexible imaging that fits the needs of various specialties. These tweaks not only promise better accuracy but also keep pushing the envelope, as noted in expert insights on today's and tomorrow's ultrasound tech (Silverman, 2023). Improving ultrasound systems remains a major focus as the field keeps evolving. New approaches—like flexible, conformable devices—show how the drive to boost both performance and access is ongoing. The blend between engineering know-how and medical insight opens up a lot of exciting possibilities, even if challenges such as choosing the right materials or perfecting manufacturing methods still pop up. Researchers are digging deeper into these issues, and the potential for ultrasound to further revolutionize diagnostics and personal healthcare looks truly expansive. Recent research roadmaps underline a steady commitment to breakthroughs that could define the next wave in biomedicine and health monitoring, ensuring ultrasound stays right at the center (Zhang et al., 2023).

Definition of Ultrasound Imaging

Ultrasound imaging changed the game in medicine. It doesn't need to break the skin or expose you to radiation - it just works in real time, giving us a peek inside the body. High-frequency sound waves are used to create pictures of soft tissues and organs, so doctors can check out internal details without making a cut. When a transducer sends out these sound waves, they bounce off various tissues and come back as images - kind of like natural echo-location, you might say. Over time, ultrasound methods have improved a lot, generally speaking, making diagnostic checks even clearer and useful in more areas. For example, in prenatal care, these scans give early insights into fetal development that help guide care for both mothers and infants. Then there's Color Doppler ultrasound, or CDUS as it is known, which now let's medical professionals watch blood flow in real time. In the past, bulky equipment and steep costs pretty much kept it on the sidelines in specialties like plastic and reconstructive surgery. But newer, smaller devices that still deliver high-definition images have eased those hurdles. With CDUS, surgeons can more precisely map out blood vessels and even pick out the best donor sites for flaps during reconstructive procedures. Studies hint that this technology also uncovers extra details about anatomical differences, adding more depth to surgical planning and execution (Miller et al., 2018). Overall, embracing these advanced ultrasound techniques brings the promise of better patient outcomes and increased satisfaction with surgical care. And then there's the rise of three-dimensional (3D) and four-dimensional (4D) ultrasound, which has pretty much revolutionized prenatal diagnostics. With breakthroughs like HD live, doctors can now see developmental stages in embryos and fetuses in richer detail than the old 2D scans allowed. It lets clinicians notice nuances—organ edges, little fluid pockets—that traditional imaging might have missed entirely.

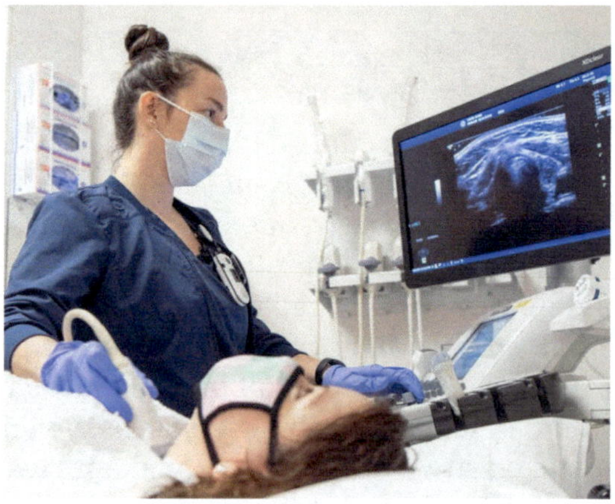

Figure 5.1. Ultrasound Imaging.

Source: https://my.clevelandclinic.org/-/scassets/images/org/health/articles/4995-ultrasound-imaging.

Spotting structural abnormalities early on is crucial for planning timely interventions and ensuring well-rounded perinatal care (Pooh, 2016). With ongoing tweaks in imaging algorithms and visualization techniques, ultrasound not only remains the top non-invasive option for prenatal checks but also continues to be a key player in keeping both maternal and fetal health on track (Figure 5.1).

Historical Development of Ultrasound Technology

Sound waves caught researchers' interest back in the early 1900s, when individuals were just beginning to figure out how they move. At first, rather than thinking about medicine, these studies mainly helped in spotting sneaky submarines during World War I – a step that led to the early use of sonar.

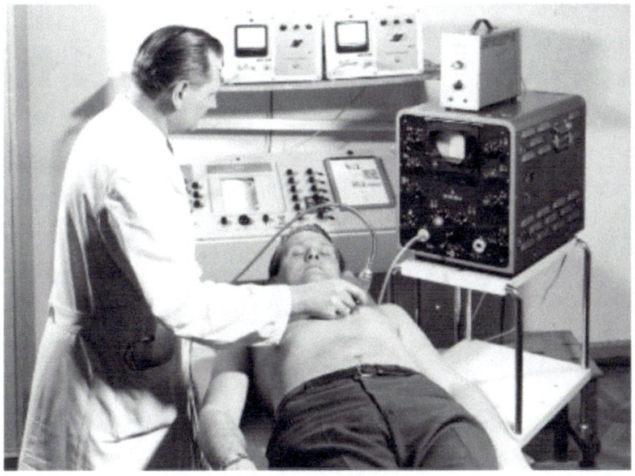

Figure 5.2. Ultrasound imaging grew into a reliable tool for patient care and diagnosis.

Source: https://www.siemens-healthineers.com/en-us/ultrasound/news-stories/history.

That maritime experiment, in many cases, eventually opened the door to looking inside the human body. By the 1950s, scientists had shifted gears and started using high-frequency sound pulses to create images of internal organs and tissues, paving the way for the first ultrasound machines. These early devices, though simple, allowed for a noninvasive peek inside our bodies, and through years of steady, sometimes uneven improvements, ultrasound imaging grew into a reliable tool for patient care and diagnosis (Figure 5.2).

Over time, as healthcare itself kept changing, ultrasound technology had to adapt to meet emerging needs. Portable ultrasound devices started appearing in the later decades of the 20th century, which meant doctors and radiographers could perform exams right at the patient's bed side or even in remote areas. This change not only improved diagnostic possibilities but also allowed professionals who weren't traditionally specialized in imaging to take on more responsibilities. In places like Zimbabwe, for instance, training radiographers to use ultrasound has been an important move toward easing the shortage of radiologists while making quality imaging more accessible. With a growing number of people able to both perform and interpret these exams, ultrasound has indeed cemented its role in many areas of medicine.

Lately, new modifications like contrast-enhanced ultrasound (CEUS) and super-resolution ultrasound (SRUS) have pushed the technology in exciting directions. CEUS now let's practitioners check tissue perfusion and blood flow with a clarity that is pretty crucial in more complex cases, while SRUS has stretched the usual boundaries, revealing microvascular details that go beyond the traditional diffraction limit. By combining both flat, two-dimensional views and more layered 3-dimensional perspectives, healthcare providers can now piece together images with an unprecedented level of detail. These breakthroughs, despite their occasional overlapping features, stir promise for better disease management and improved patient outcomes in clinical settings (Chinene et al., 2024; Ghosh et al., 2025) (Figures 5.3 and 5.4).

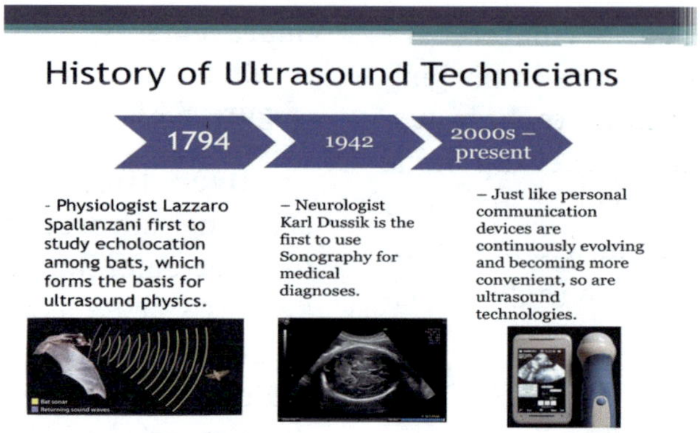

Figure 5.3. History of ultrasound technicians.

Source: https://image1.slideserve.com/2334334/history-of-ultrasound-technicians-l.jpg.

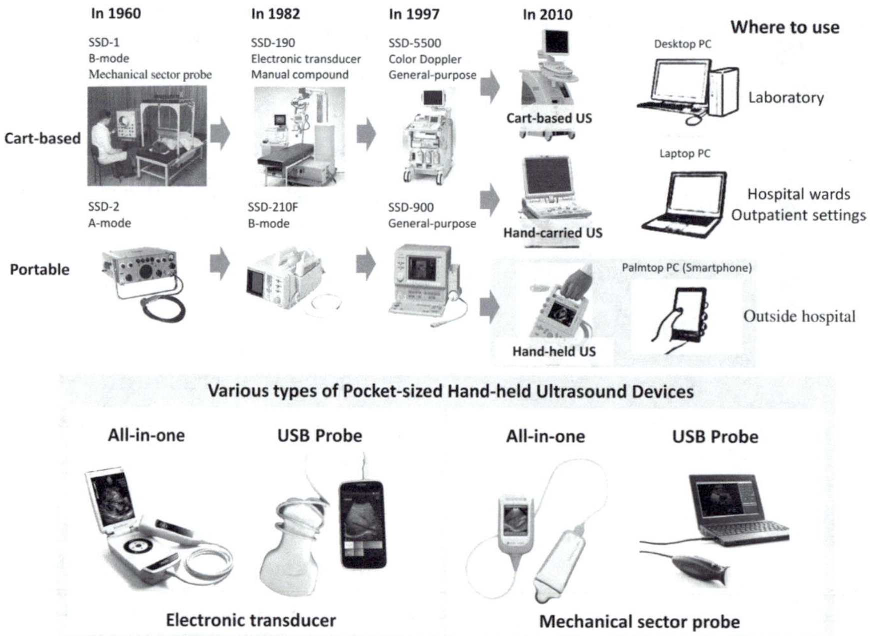

Figure 5.4. History of diagnostic ultrasound devices.

Source: https://www.researchgate.net/figure/History-of-diagnostic-ultrasound-devices_fig1_312247825.

Importance of Ultrasound in Modern Medicine

Ultrasound has become a fixture in everyday medical practice, shaking up how diagnoses are made and care is delivered. Its knack for showing images in real time means doctors can jump right into action, especially in keeping an eye on a growing baby—a task that can't wait. In many cases, spotting problems early during pregnancy isn't just useful; it is downright necessary. Newer developments—think portable units and improved imaging—have thrown a wider net, making these tools available even in settings that might not have all the bells and whistles. All together, these tweaks help clinicians reach more patients, proving that ultrasound is a real cornerstone in current healthcare. It is not only about diagnosing either. Ultrasound often lends a helping hand during treatments too. Consider procedures like biopsies or guided injections, where being able to view the target area on the fly boosts a doctor's confidence—thus keeping complications to a minimum. And nowadays, artificial intelligence (AI) is stepping in to lend a hand by picking out and separating important anatomical details, which in most cases fine-tunes clinical decisions (Gusev, 2025). These smart integrations have gradually transformed the way we not only detect issues but also how we go about fixing them. On top of that, ultrasound's influence stretches into medical physics, where safety standards and tech checks matter a lot. Diagnostic medical physicists work hard to keep ultrasound devices running just right, ensuring everything sticks to safety protocols while still delivering clear images (Gambo et al., 2024). These hands-on checks help ward off risks that could arise from a slip in quality control. As technology keeps evolving, a steady partnership between physicists and healthcare providers becomes even more important. In short, ultrasound isn't merely about better diagnostics—it is also about the teamwork and rigor needed to maintain high standards in patient care.

5.1. Principles of Ultrasound Technology

Learning Outcome

1. Understand the sound wave generation and propagation.
2. Describe the interaction of sound waves with tissues.
3. Describe the process of ultrasound image formation and interpretation.

Ultrasound tech grew out of some pretty basic ideas that shape how it works. Transducers sit right in the middle—they flip electrical signals into sound and then do the reverse, sometimes in ways that might seem almost magical. Lately, bulky piezoelectric transducer arrays—using thickness mode vibrations—have been obtaining attention in medical imaging, while newer types like piezoelectric micromachined ultrasound transducers (PMUT) and capacitive micromachined ultrasound transducers (CMUT) are making their mark. These newer devices use a flexural, thin-film approach that gives them a surprising boost in sensitivity and frequency response. Flexible ultrasound transducers built on these ideas are opening up fresh biomedical opportunities—they're not just improving images but are also lending a hand in sensing and even patient stimulation, all meeting a broad range clinical needs (Joshi et al., 2025). Getting to grips with ultrasound imaging means taking a good look at how sound travels through our tissues. Sound waves get tangled up with different tissues in ways that aren't always straightforward. For instance, acoustic impedance—which is a mix of tissue density and the speed of sound in that tissue—influences how much of the sound bounces back at different boundaries. Frequency also jumps in here, often forcing a tricky game of balancing clearer images against how deep the sound can go. In most cases, this interplay of reflection, attenuation, and overall wave behavior quietly sets the stage for creating reliable pictures of what's inside our bodies (Zhang et al., 2024b). Different fields coming together—like physics, engineering, and even materials science—have played a huge part in pushing ultrasound imaging forward. It is kind of a mixed bag where all these ideas merge to let us see more clearly and in innovative ways. As the flexibility in micromachined ultrasound transducers keeps getting better, suddenly there are new ideas for monitoring patients or doing non-invasive diagnostics. Generally speaking, with healthcare leaning more on automation and smarter systems for diagnostics, this blend of know-how is becoming heavier with meaning. Overall, this rough-and-ready mix not only reinforces the basics of ultrasound but also nudges it right to the cutting edge of medical imaging, paving the way for new types of diagnostic breakthroughs (Zhang et al., 2024b) (Figure 5.5).

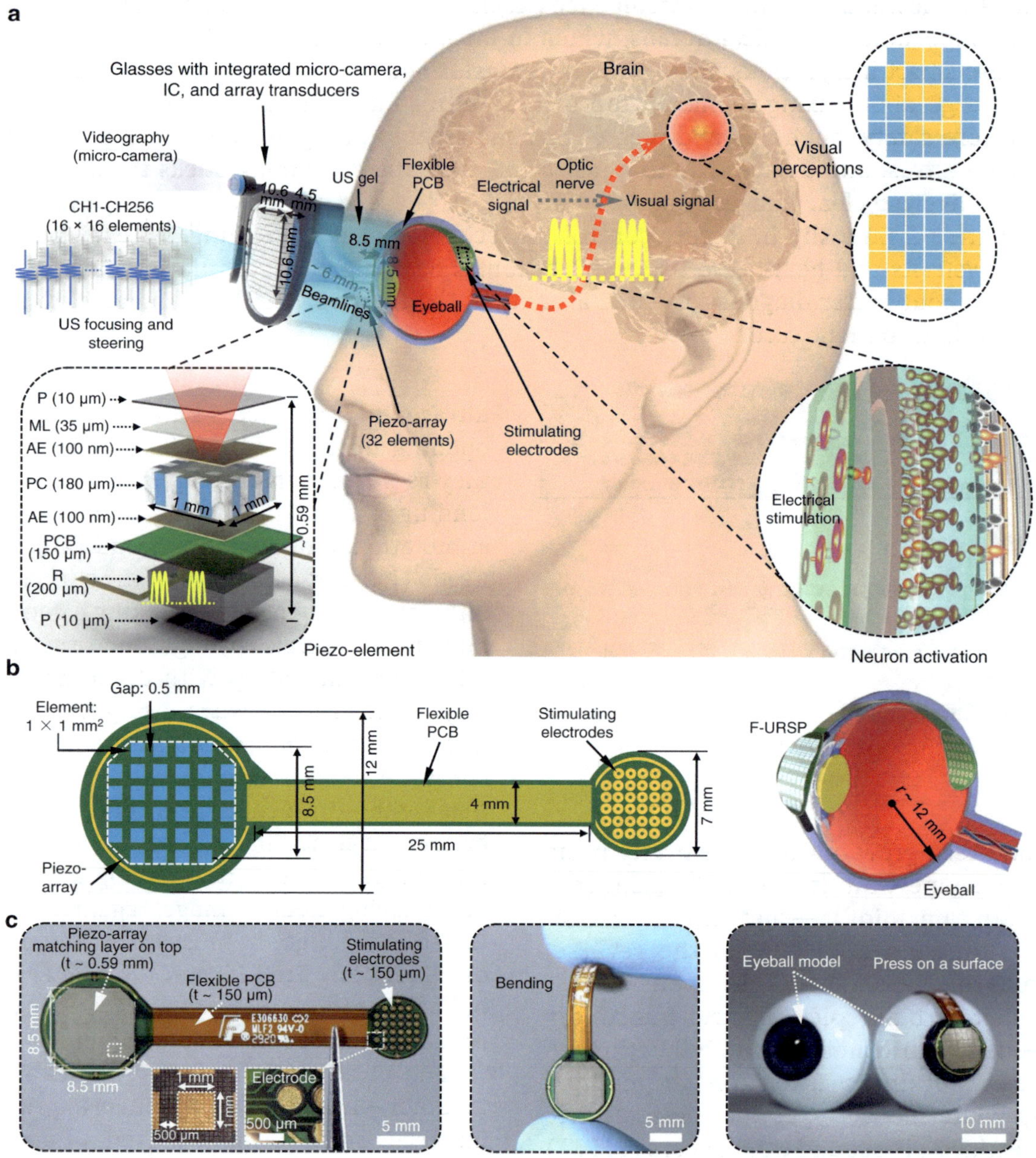

Figure 5.5. Piezoelectric effect and ultrasound.

Source: Jiang, L., Lu, G., Zeng, Y. *et al.* Flexible ultrasound-induced retinal stimulating piezo-arrays for biomimetic visual prostheses. *Nat Commun* **13**, 3853 (2022). https://doi.org/10.1038/s41467-022-31599-4.

5.1.1. Sound Wave Generation and Propagation

Ultrasound imaging kicks off with a neat play of sound waves. It starts when tiny vibrating crystals in the transducer turn electrical signals into mini bursts of mechanical energy. These little bursts shoot high-pitched pulses into the body, where they meet all kinds of tissues. As they travel, the pulses bounce, bend, or sometimes fade away, forming a kind of jumbled trail of echoes. Different tissues—thanks to how dense or stretchy they are—give back distinct echo patterns that help doctors figure out what's going on inside. In most cases, grasping how these sound pulses work is key to tweaking ultrasound tech and getting a crisper image for diagnosis. Refinements in imaging have also shown that taming the path of these sound waves isn't always straightforward—especially in high-intensity focused ultrasound (HIFU) surgery. Generally speaking, the unpredictable nature of sound makes it tough to nail down where all that energy converges, and that can throw off treatments. Add to that the pesky artifacts from shear waves, and things can get messy. Lately, new methods like Acoustic Radiation Force Impulse (ARFI) imaging have popped up. This approach delivers real-time visuals at rapid frame rates right before those shear waves start their unpredictable dance. Careful tests suggest that ARFI might just be the answer to honing in on the focus with better accuracy in surgeries, showing how a fresh take on imaging can change clinical outcomes. Chasing even better ultrasound images, researchers keep exploring how generative models can mix with the well-known physics of ultrasound. In most cases, boosting datasets with these models points to a clear need for a deeper look at sound wave behavior. Traditional methods often fall short because they simply don't capture all the nuances of how ultrasound pulses move through tissue—sometimes making the images less believable. By teaming up with a physics-based diffusion model crafted specifically for ultrasound, scientists are chasing after sharper, more lifelike images that truly mirror tissue details. This new strategy reminds us that getting into the nitty-gritty of sound dynamics is crucial for better imaging and ultimately more accurate diagnoses. In its own way, these advances not only push ultrasound tech forward but also deepen our hands-on understanding of how sound moves through the body's complex terrain (Figure 5.6).

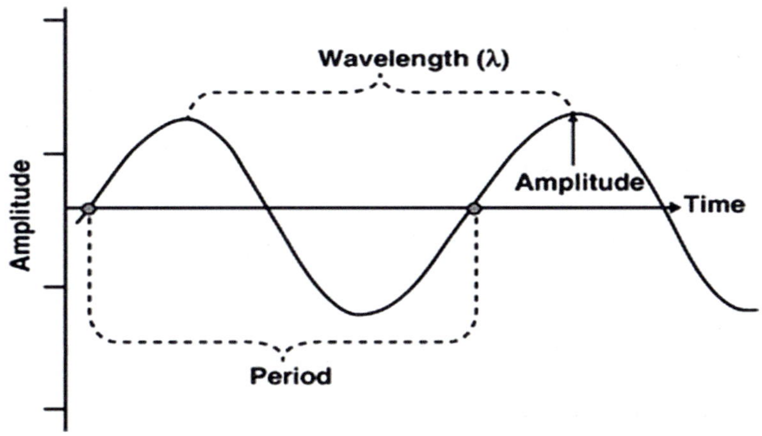

Figure 5.6. Characteristics of a sound wave: the amplitude of the wave is a function of the acoustical power used to generate the mechanical compression wave and the medium through which it is transmitted.

Source: https://radiologykey.com/physical-principles-of-ultrasound/.

5.1.2. Interaction of Sound Waves with Tissues

Sound waves behave in ways that matter when they pass through living tissue—a fact that underpins ultrasound imaging. As the waves move through areas in our bodies, they bounce back, bend off course, and lose energy; how they do this depends on the tissue's own traits like density and texture. The makeup of the tissue—its density and how its acoustic features are spread out—largely sets the stage for these effects. For example, how fast sound travels and how much of it gets absorbed are key details that need to be pinned down for clear, high-res images. There are clever algorithms that draw on data from multiple angles and juggle several scattering effects at once, which helps capture these acoustic nuances in the final image (Zotov et al., 2024). Even minor differences in tissue sound behavior can mean big changes in what the ultrasound shows. Sound's journey through tissue and the tissue's unique profile go hand in hand in pushing forward new imaging techniques. Ultrasound leans on the fact that biological tissues don't scatter sound too much, which leaves you with surprisingly sharp internal views. By keeping an eye on how sound waves spread and scatter as they hit areas with varying density and elasticity, experts can more easily sort out different kinds of tissue. Take tumors, for instance—they generally carry an altered acoustic signature compared to their healthier surroundings, offering vital clues for diagnosis. Newer methods, like tackling the inverse problems in image creation, help fine-tune how these sound signals are turned into visual details (Deán-Ben, 2023). This mix of sound behavior and imaging tech generally opens up the route to more precise diagnoses and better monitoring. To get the most out of ultrasound, you need a deep feel for the interplay between sound and tissue—covering not just the mechanical side but also the biochemical mix that changes acoustic behavior. Innovations such as blending optoacoustic with ultrasound methods remind us just how central these sound interactions are. Such hybrid techniques mix different contrast tools to deliver richer, more layered views of vascular features and tissue details. Research into how fast sound travels and how its energy drops off at different frequencies reveals clues about disease, pointing out specific problem spots (Deán-Ben, 2023). Overall, the ongoing push to sharpen these imaging ideas will keep boosting our knack for exploring complex tissues, eventually leading to better results in real-world clinical settings (Figure 5.7).

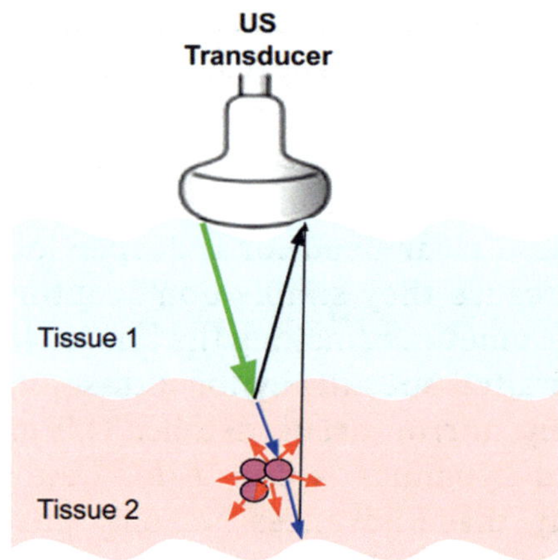

Figure 5.7. Ultrasound interaction with tissues. The green, black, red, blue arrows represent the incident wave, the specular reflection, the non-specular reflection, and the refracted wave, respectively.

Source: https://www.researchgate.net/figure/Ultrasound-interaction-with-tissues-The-green-black-red-blue-arrows-represent-the_fig1_367244137.

5.1.3. Image Formation and Interpretation

Ultrasound imaging isn't just about fancy equipment – it all starts when sound waves hit tissues and bounce around in unpredictable ways. When these waves are sent into the body they hit different structures, which in turn reflect and scatter signals that get turned into plain, two-dimensional pictures. This process helps doctors peek inside, making it easier to diagnose problems – think kidney stones, for example, where spotting them is absolutely crucial. Generally speaking, improvements in algorithms have gotten the picture clearer by fine-tuning how those signals are read, and new machine learning techniques have pushed detection even further, hinting at an exciting future for ultrasound in medicine. One snag with ultrasound imaging, however, is that artifacts and noise often mess up the true appearance of tissues. Speckle noise – a usual culprit in coherent imaging systems – can muddy things up, leaving clinicians to struggle with interpretation. In most cases, researchers have been busy tackling this problem, with various filters proposed that either keep most of the image intact or boost edge details. For example, some filters work particularly well in separating tumor regions, which directly affects how images are read. Enhancing image quality through these robust filtering methods not only helps achieve clearer visuals but also improves diagnostic accuracy, leading to better overall patient outcomes (Kapoor et al., 2017). Machine learning has also stepped into the spotlight, revolutionizing the whole ultrasound game. Recent studies have even used datasets with thousands of images to train models aimed at spotting things like kidney stones. The preprocessing and segmentation stages are key here, cutting down on noise and shining a light on the details that count. In many cases, pairing techniques like the Local Binary Pattern (LBP) with tools such as support vector machines (SVM) shows just how creative and effective these advances can be. Such developments not only speed up diagnoses but also act as early warning systems, potentially reducing risks associated with delayed treatment in conditions like nephrolithiasis (Hama et al., 2025) (Figure 5.8).

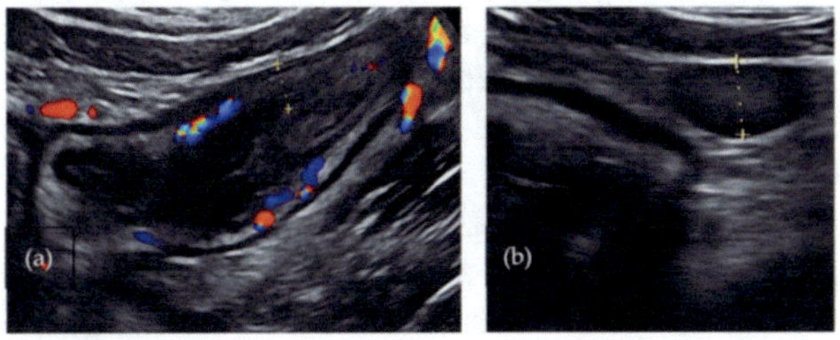

Figure 5.8. Schematic depiction of the sequence of image production by an ultrasound device.

Source: Aprile F, Vangeli M, Allocca M, Zilli A, Argollo MC, D'amico F, Parigi TL, Danese S, Furfaro F. Gastrointestinal Ultrasound in Infectious Diseases: A Comprehensive Review. *Medicina*. 2024; 60(9):1402. https://doi.org/10.3390/medicina60091402.

Test Your Knowledge

1. How are sound waves generated and propagated in ultrasound imaging?
2. How do sound waves interact with different body tissues to produce ultrasound images?

5.2. Types of Ultrasound Imaging

Learning Outcome

1. Explore the principles and applications of diagnostic ultrasound.
2. Understand the uses and techniques of therapeutic ultrasound in medical treatments.
3. Examine specialized ultrasound techniques (e.g., Doppler, 3D ultrasound).

Ultrasound imaging is remarkably adaptable; many types of scans have been created to meet specific clinical needs. The basic ultrasound, for instance, is used to track a baby's growth during pregnancy or simply check on organs in the abdomen. High-frequency sound waves produce live images that let doctors see inside the body, spot abnormal areas, and even guide certain procedures. It is a safe and accessible option that remains a go-to for early tests. Still, speckle noise often muddies the picture, hiding details and making interpretations tougher. Lately, researchers have been working on ways to cut back on this interference and boost image quality (Monika et al., 2025). Doppler ultrasound, on the other hand, dives into how blood flows within vessels. It uses the Doppler effect to measure movement, showing results in both colorful displays and spectral data – in most cases helping clinicians catch things like narrow passages or even clots. This non-invasive technique provides both a feel for the flow and solid numbers, which proves especially useful when looking at cardiovascular issues. Given that vascular problems are increasingly common, its real-time insights and evolving integration of deep learning techniques are making it an even more valuable tool for diagnosing and managing patient care (Nanthini et al., 2024). Then there are the 3D and 4D ultrasound methods that offer an even deeper glimpse into the body. These scans capture images in three dimensions – and with 4D, you get a live sequence that adds time into the picture. They give doctors a fuller view of fetal anatomy and can help spot potential issues earlier than usual, especially in obstetrics and gynecology. Although this advanced imaging can sometimes come with artifacts and varying interpretations, ongoing improvements remain key to keeping these techniques clear and reliable for daily use (Monika et al., 2025).

5.2.1. Diagnostic Ultrasound

Ultrasound technology has come a long way, reshaping how doctors diagnose problems across medicine. It wasn't too long ago that ultrasound was mainly tied to imaging expecting mothers, but now its use spills over into areas like heart care, stomach issues, and even cancer treatment. Its non-invasive approach and knack for giving real-time images let clinicians quickly zero in on problems—a real game changer when every minute counts. Digital image tweaks and smarter signal handling have also, in most cases, sharpened image clarity, which helps boost diagnostic accuracy. AI and machine learning are gradually joining the mix, nudging image analysis toward greater automation; this, in turn, can cut down on human mistakes and speed things along in busy clinical settings. Research these days leans heavily on deep learning to polish ultrasound's diagnostic chops even more. For example, one study put the EfficientNet-B7 model to work, boosting it with fresh image augmentation ideas to sort breast ultrasound scans. Techniques like Random Horizontal Flip and Color Jitter were thrown into the mix to balance out tricky class imbalances in the data, resulting in an impressive 99% accuracy on several performance metrics). Generally speaking, these innovations don't just dial up precision—they also ease the mental load on healthcare professionals who often operate under high-pressure conditions. Some projects even stretch beyond the borders of medical imaging. One notable effort blended methods from both medicine and agriculture to work on diagnosing pancreatic steatosis and checking crop health simultaneously (Gnanaraj et al., 2024). By tapping into tools like transfer learning and domain adaptation, this interdisciplinary model hit solid accuracy and specificity marks despite changing imaging conditions. Overall, this kind of cross-field experiment not only widens the scope of diagnostic ultrasound but also hints at a future where diverse areas of research come together in unexpected ways to improve imaging solutions (Figure 5.9).

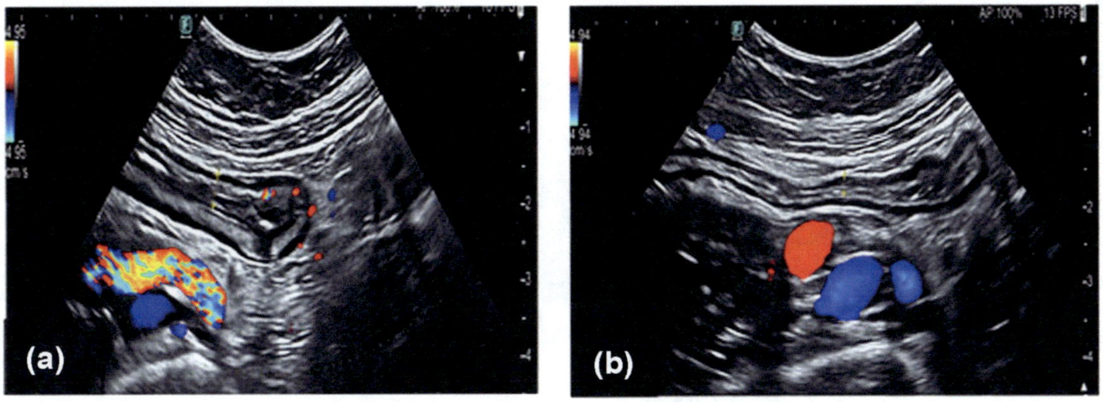

Figure 5.9. Diagnostic ultrasound.

Source: Aprile F, Vangeli M, Allocca M, Zilli A, Argollo MC, D'amico F, Parigi TL, Danese S, Furfaro F. Gastrointestinal Ultrasound in Infectious Diseases: A Comprehensive Review. *Medicina*. 2024; 60(9):1402. https://doi.org/10.3390/medicina60091402.

5.2.2. Therapeutic Ultrasound

Therapeutic ultrasound has come in and shifted how treatments get done—helping patients bounce back in unexpected ways. High-frequency sound waves, once used just for imaging, now step up to help repair tissue and ease pain. Studies keep pointing out that this method works with issues like musculoskeletal troubles and soft tissue healing, sometimes in ways that break the old surgery mold. A focused beam can zero in on a specific spot so that nearby areas aren't unnecessarily harmed. For example, it can break down stubborn scar tissue and spark collagen buildup, which in turn speeds up the healing process. It might even mean shorter recoveries and fewer risks overall. As more practitioners experiment with this approach, its role seems to be expanding, pushing us to look closer at the details of how it works. A neat trick of this method is how it changes tissue characteristics using controlled bursts of mechanical force. Sometimes, you get a continuous sound wave; other times, a pulsed beam—each nudging cells in its own unique way to boost repair at the microscopic level. In some cases, low-intensity pulsed ultrasound (LIPUS) is used, and research generally shows that it can kick osteoblast activity into gear, which may lead to faster fracture healing and even thicker bones. In a similar vein, when ultrasound elastography is thrown into the mix, as noted in Oglat et al. (2024), it can reveal just how stiff a tissue might be, giving therapists extra clues for fine-tuning treatments. This mix of imaging and healing tricks not only lifts treatment outcomes but also hints at the wider regenerative potential of ultrasound across many care settings—it makes a case for being a cornerstone in modern medicine. There's also a growing buzz that ultrasound's therapeutic uses pave the way for more personalized care.

Doctors can now use real-time imaging to watch how tissues react, adjusting treatment on the fly—something that's especially handy when managing stubborn conditions like heart failure, where no two patients are exactly alike. One set of ideas, outlined in Gamarra et al. (2025) for checking congestion through ultrasound, even shows how one tool can serve two roles: diagnosing and treating at the same time. This blend of functions kind of weaves a more holistic approach into patient care, making it both effective and a bit more flexible. As more research rolls in, it looks like the role of therapeutic ultrasound will only grow, promising better outcomes and, ultimately, happier patients (Figure 5.10).

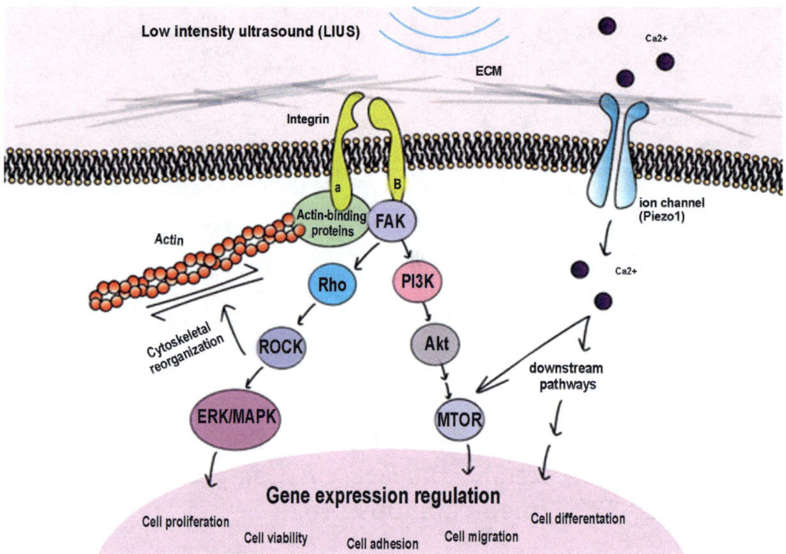

Figure 5.10. Therapeutic ultrasound.

Source: de Lucas B, Pérez LM, Bernal A, Gálvez BG. Ultrasound Therapy: Experiences and Perspectives for Regenerative Medicine. *Genes*. 2020; 11(9):1086. https://doi.org/10.3390/genes11091086.

5.2.3. Specialized Ultrasound Techniques (e.g., Doppler, 3D Ultrasound)

Ultrasound technology has come a long way. Doppler ultrasound and 3D imaging now let doctors see things that flat, two-dimensional scans just can't capture. Ultrafast Doppler, for example, now shows blood flow in incredible detail—even revealing the twists and turns of vessels in the brain or tumors. Using freehand scans tied to optical tracking, clinicians can build volumetric images that highlight tiny vessels, sometimes only a few hundred micrometers wide. This kind of clarity can help with planning surgeries and making decisions in the operating room (Verhoef et al., 2025). 3D ultrasound, on the other hand, gives us a fresh look at complex body regions. New freehand machines capture spatial data and reconstruct full 3D images using advanced optical calibration techniques. It is not just about spotting lesions; this method supports diagnosing everything from musculoskeletal issues to tricky vascular problems. Combining 3D B-mode images with Doppler and elasticity readings pushes ultrasound into new territory, broadening its diagnostic reach (Shen et al., 2024). Ultrasound imaging is rapidly evolving, and these techniques now offer unmatched precision and practical benefits in the clinic. Doppler provides a real-time look at blood flow, while 3D imaging lays out an all-encompassing view of anatomy—a boon for fields like cardiology, obstetrics, and oncology. This mix of approaches not only shows off ultrasound's versatility but also smooths out every day clinical routines. With ongoing research and technology leaps, the future promises even more detailed and flexible imaging, ultimately raising patient care standards and improving outcomes (Shen et al., 2024; Verhoef et al., 2025) (Figure 5.11).

Clinical studies carried out for tissue healing with different LIPUS therapies. (LIPUS parameters 30–100 mW/cm^2, frequency 1.5 MHz, 1 kHz, duty cycle of 20%).

NCT Number	Conditions	Interventions	Outcome
NCT00423956	Root resorption	LIPUS	Induced inflammatory root resorption
NCT00744861	Lumbar degenerative disc disease	LIPUS	Posterolateral fusion success
NCT00931749	Knee osteoarthritis	LIPUS	Knee cartilage thickness and volume
NCT01623804	Knee osteoarthritis	LIPUS	Pain and physical function
NCT02253212	Glioblastoma	LIPUS + Drug	Blood–brain barrier opening
NCT02034409	Osteoarthritis	LIPUS	Symptoms reduction
NCT02383160	Fractures	LIPUS	Time to union of scaphoid non-unions
NCT00667849	Tibial fractures	LIPUS	Healing of tibial fractures
NCT02872922	Diabetes mellitus	LIPUS	Changes arterial endothelial function
NCT03251807	Malocclusion	LIPUS	Dentoskeletal changes
NCT03119961	Brain diseases	LIPUS	Blood–brain barrier opening
NCT03347084	Brain diseases	LIFUP	Improvements in cognitive functioning
NCT03329482	Low back pain	LIPUS	Pain intensity of patients
NCT03744026	Glioblastoma	LIPUS + Drug	Blood–brain barrier opening
NCT03679507	Osteoarthritis in the knee	LIPUS	Pain intensity measure
NCT03657056	Temporal lobe epilepsy	LIFUP	Changes of the blood-oxygenation level
NCT03717922	Brain diseases	LIFUP	Auditory verbal learning
NCT04021420	Metastatic melanoma	LIPUS + Drug	Blood–brain barrier opening

NCT Number	Conditions	Interventions	Outcome
NCT04131387	Female stress urinary incontinence	LIPUS	Urinary incontinence questionnaire
NCT03868293	Drug resistant epilepsy	FOCCUS LIPUS	Reducing seizure frequency
NCT04406337	Osteoarthritis	LIPUS	Visual analog scale (Pain)
NCT04339972	Healthy adults	LIFUP	Analgesia

LIFUP: Low-Intensity Focus Ultrasound Pulsation.

Figure 5.11. 3D ultrasound.

Source: de Lucas B, Pérez LM, Bernal A, Gálvez BG. Ultrasound Therapy: Experiences and Perspectives for Regenerative Medicine. *Genes*. 2020; 11(9):1086. https://doi.org/10.3390/genes11091086.

Test Your Knowledge

1. How is therapeutic ultrasound used in medical treatments, and what conditions can it help manage?
2. What are some specialized ultrasound techniques, such as elastography or contrast-enhanced ultrasound, and how do they improve diagnostic accuracy?

5.3. Applications in Medicine

Learning Outcome

1. Define obstetrics and gynecology.
2. Explore using ultrasound in cardiology for diagnosing.
3. Examine the application of musculoskeletal imaging.

Ultrasound imaging has grown into an essential tool in modern medicine, thanks to leaps in technology that have reshaped both how we diagnose and treat patients. AI's arrival in this field, especially for prenatal imaging, has turned things on their head—a shift that cuts down on human error and lessens the need for skilled operators. The European Union's recommendations for ethical AI use give extra weight to these changes, generally speaking, since strict oversight helps both clinicians and patients feel secure about the results. With this blend, ultrasound paired with AI now seems ready to set new standards in medical imaging, providing a solid trust in the diagnostic process (Tonni et al., 2024). The role of ultrasound hasn't stayed put either. In recent years, it has made headway into musculoskeletal medicine, proving its versatility in quite unexpected ways. You see more and more ultrasound-guided procedures, particularly in minimally invasive settings like sports medicine and orthopedics, even if image quality and reliance on operator expertise still pose some challenges. In most cases, deep learning now steps in to clear up images and pinpoint details in tricky conditions, such as carpal tunnel syndrome or even osteochondritis dissecans. By breaking images down into manageable parts and isolating key structures, DL gives doctors the confidence to push forward with improved outcomes—a combining of traditional imaging with fresh, innovative techniques (Hattori et al., 2024). Looking forward, the future of ultrasound imaging in medicine is bright, largely because new ideas keep popping up when you mix real-time imaging with AI and DL capabilities. This combo not only sharpens diagnostic accuracy but also makes procedural guidance and therapeutic tasks easier to handle. As practitioners get access to these advanced tools, the potential to predict conditions more effectively becomes a real possibility. For example, timely screenings for issues like hip dysplasia or knee osteoarthritis may soon spur earlier and more effective interventions. Plus, investing in user-friendly, robust AI-assisted ultrasound systems is a must for broader acceptance in everyday clinical settings. In an era where medicine increasingly embraces multidisciplinary approaches, the partnership between ultrasound tech and AI is set to play a pivotal role in reshaping diagnostics and treatment methods (Hattori et al., 2024; Tonni et al., 2024).

5.3.1. Obstetrics and Gynecology

Integrating ultrasound imaging into obstetrics and gynecology has changed how prenatal care happens. High-frequency sound waves create live images that give doctors a peek into both fetal growth and the mother's overall condition. This method spots troubles early, which means potential issues get caught before they become serious. Techniques like 3D and 4D imaging add extra details that weren't there before, so practitioners can check for oddities more thoroughly. In most cases, these advances help ease worries for parents and support clinicians in managing high-risk or unusual pregnancies (Recker et al., 2024).

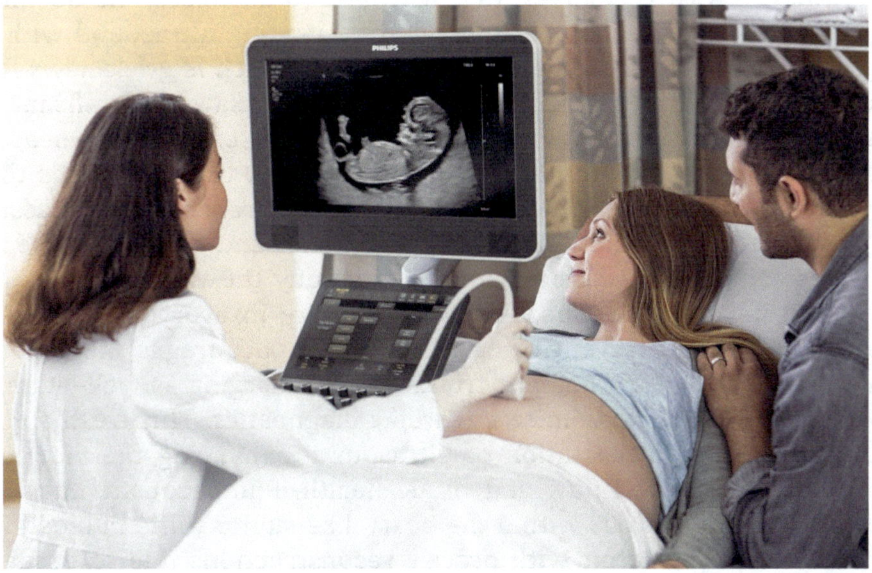

Figure 5.12. Obstetrics and gynecologic ultrasound.

Source: https://news.europawire.eu/wp-content/uploads/2017/09/Philips-will-showcase-its-wide-portfolio-of-OBGYN-ultrasound-tools-at-27th-World-Congress-on-Ultrasound-in-Obstetrics-and-Gynecology-ISUOG.jpg.

Look at cases of congenital issues—the value of ultrasound shines through here. Birth defects, especially those affecting the gut, emerge in only about 6 in every 10,000 births and sometimes show up later than expected. That delay makes those scans all the more vital. New imaging tools, like HDlive, let doctors see obstructions or modifications in the duodenum and intestines that standard scans might miss. Recent case studies, generally speaking, suggest that identifying these issues early leads to faster interventions, which can improve neonatal outcomes; indeed, these findings help tailor care plans to fit each situation (Wolder et al., 2024). Ultrasound's role isn't limited to just diagnosis—it also helps guide treatments. Continuous fetal monitoring during labor lets healthcare providers keep a close eye on the baby, so they can jump in if signs of distress appear. It also gives clues about the baby's position, which is essential when choosing a delivery plan. Occasionally, when checking nutritional status for both mom and baby, ultrasound is used to evaluate amniotic fluid and assess placental health. Overall, this more holistic approach means that different specialists end up working together, with ultrasound imaging forming a kind of backbone for making decisions that aim for the best possible outcomes for both mother and child (Recker et al., 2024) (Figure 5.12).

5.3.2. Cardiology

Ultrasound imaging has come a long way, offering doctors a closer look at the heart in ways that weren't possible before. You can now assess the heart's structure and function with surprising detail. Techniques like Doppler and echocardiography help reveal how the cardiac muscles are doing, check on the flow of blood, and even spot tiny structural uniqueness. It is an approach that avoids the risks of more invasive tests—always a win—and advances like 3D imaging mean the numbers are getting even more reliable. In most cases, blending ultrasound with smart tech like AI is opening up possibilities for more tailored treatments, which is great news for those dealing with heart issues. Ultrasound doesn't just capture images; it plays a significant role in gauging cardiovascular risk too. Take pulse wave velocity (PWV), for example—a neat biomarker that sheds light on artery stiffness, a key indicator of heart health. Using methods that include both Doppler ultrasound and Oscillo metric techniques, PWV measurements help classify patients who might face complications from conditions like hypertension and diabetes. Sure, methodological differences and other confounding factors sometimes muddy the waters, but generally speaking, standardizing these protocols could boost PWV's reliability in everyday practice. This, in turn, reinforces ultrasound's role in preventive cardiology and encourages more proactive care for those at risk (Pilz et al., 2024). New imaging frontiers are emerging as well—think photoacoustic imaging, which is starting to show promise in cardiac diagnostics. This fresh approach combines optical absorption with the fine resolution of ultrasound, enhancing the view of heart tissues, especially when checking on blood flow and tissue health. Photoacoustic imaging gives layered insights into the complex interactions within the heart, like subtle shifts in blood flow and oxygen levels, although it still struggles a bit with precise reconstructions due to tissue variability and limited view angles. Researchers are already working on overcoming these hiccups, and as these techniques mature and join forces with established ultrasound methods, we could soon see even more comprehensive heart evaluations that drive better patient outcomes (Zhang et al., 2024c) (Figure 5.13).

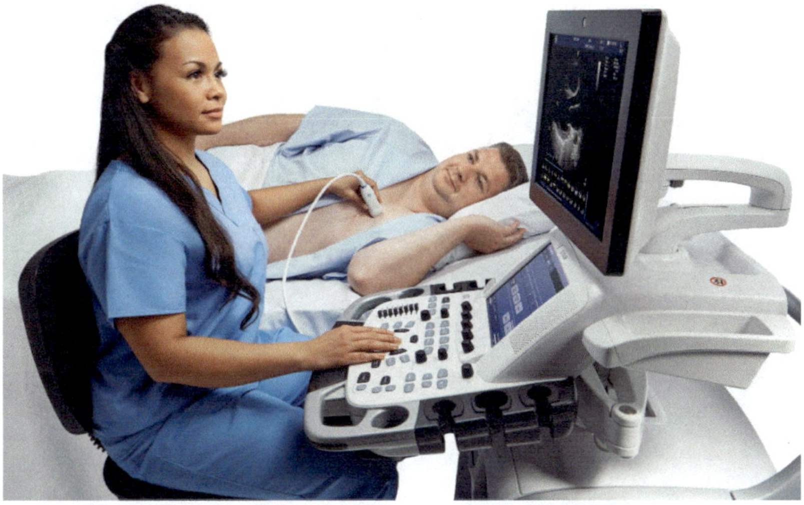

Figure 5.13. Cardiac ultrasound.

Source: https://www.itnonline.com/sites/default/files/field/image/X0000_GE_Vivid%20E9%20with%20XDclear%20Adult%20Echo.jpg.

5.3.3. Musculoskeletal Imaging

Real-time imaging of muscles and bones has changed the game for seeing injuries, especially around the shoulder and knee. The rotator cuff – which includes important players like the infraspinatus – is more than just a group of muscles; it helps keep the joint steady. When this area gets injured, the resulting issues can be crippling and call for quick checks. Using musculoskeletal ultrasound (MSK-US) is huge because it lets doctors see what's happening with that muscle and its tendon as it unfolds. Clear images of possible tears or ruptures often guide treatment choices and fine-tune rehab plans. Overall, these advanced scanning techniques give clinicians useful insights that shape their care plans and ultimately lead to better outcomes for shoulder problems (Manske et al., 2024). Looking at lower extremity evaluations, the posterior lateral knee can be pretty tricky to diagnose. Traditional imaging methods sometimes miss key details, leaving conditions like posterior knee pain without a complete explanation. Ultrasound imaging has stepped up as a vital tool by shedding light on those less-discussed ligaments and tendons. With systematic scanning – done in a way that feels almost intuitive – practitioners can spot issues like ligament sprains or even tears. Plus, adding ultrasound guidance helps boost diagnostic accuracy while cutting down on the risks during procedures. In a nutshell, this technique proves invaluable in both spotting and managing knee-related disorders, reinforcing its role in modern musculoskeletal assessments (Wu et al., 2024). Ultrasound imaging isn't just about making diagnoses; it deeply influences the treatment side of musculoskeletal disorders. Its real-time view lets care providers watch dynamic movements and treatment responses as they happen, which deepens the overall understanding of injury mechanics and recovery. In most cases, the non-invasive nature of ultrasound – along with its cost-effectiveness – makes it a top pick in many clinical settings. Generally speaking, as healthcare continues to evolve, weaving advanced ultrasound methods into everyday practice lifts clinical decision-making and helps patients stick to rehab protocols a bit better. By refining scanning techniques and pushing for improved operator training, ultrasound ends up being an essential tool that sharpens both diagnostic precision and the effectiveness of subsequent management plans (Manske et al., 2024; Wu et al., 2024) (Figure 5.14).

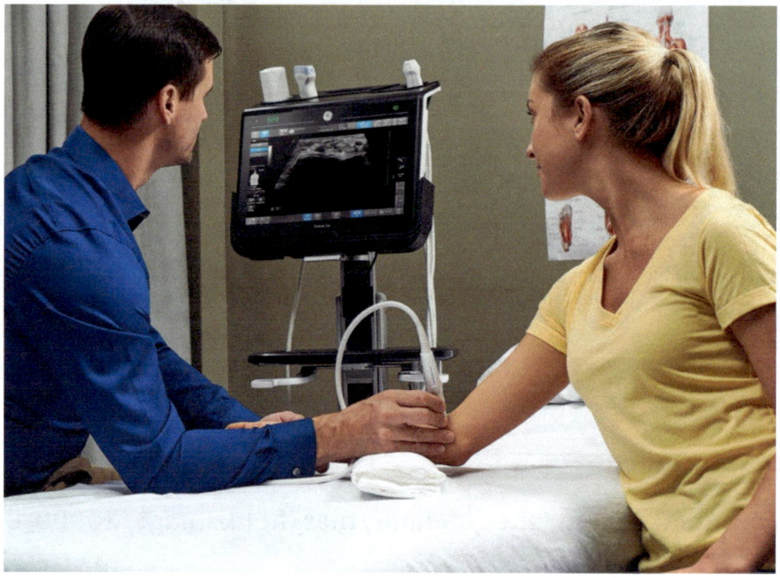

Figure 5.14. Musculoskeletal ultrasound.

Source: https://images-cdn.welcomesoftware.com/Zz04ZTc4YTBjOGNjNDcxMWVkODBmZDEyNmQxYmFmOWI1OQ==/venue-muskuloskeletal.webp.

t

Test Your Knowledge

1. How is ultrasound imaging used in obstetrics and gynecology to monitor fetal development and diagnose conditions?
2. What imaging techniques are commonly used in musculoskeletal imaging to diagnose bone, joint, and soft tissue disorders?

5.4. Advantages and Limitations of Ultrasound Imaging

Learning Outcome

1. Identify and evaluate the advantages of ultrasound imaging in medical diagnostics.
2. Analyze the limitations of ultrasound imaging.

5.4.1. Advantages of Ultrasound Imaging

Ultrasound imaging has become a go-to method in medicine thanks to its noninvasive way of revealing what's inside the body. It uses sound waves instead of the ionizing radiation seen in X-rays or MRIs—a shift that generally means safer exams. This safety boost matters for groups like pregnant women, where reducing radiation exposure is a top concern. Real-time images emerge during exams, giving doctors quick insights that often help them decide on the best next steps. In many practices, this easy-to-use technology speeds up diagnosis while keeping patient comfort and access at the forefront (Kamel et al., 2024). It is not all about safety—the cost factor is a big win, too. In most cases, ultrasound tends to be cheaper compared to pricier options like MRI and CT scans, easing the financial strain on healthcare systems. This affordability makes it popular in many settings, especially in emergency rooms or clinics where every minute counts. The fact that these machines are portable means that, quite often, they can be wheeled right to a patient's bedside for immediate checks, boosting convenience in acute situations. Mobile ultrasound tools are even transforming care in areas with fewer resources by literally bringing diagnostics to the patient (Gupta et al., 2024). Beyond simple diagnosis, ultrasound is branching into therapeutic uses as well. Its real-time feedback lends a hand in procedures like guided biopsies or fluid aspirations; these applications can help cut down recovery times and generally improve outcomes. The technique's knack for visualizing soft tissues and detecting blood flow makes it indispensable for assessing heart conditions, monitoring pregnancies, and examining musculoskeletal injuries. With ongoing enhancements—think 3D and 4D imaging—doctors are getting even more detailed views into body structures and functions. All these advances help secure ultrasound's role as a key player in modern medicine, one that meets a wide range of clinical needs while keeping the patient at the center (Kamel et al., 2024) (Figure 5.15).

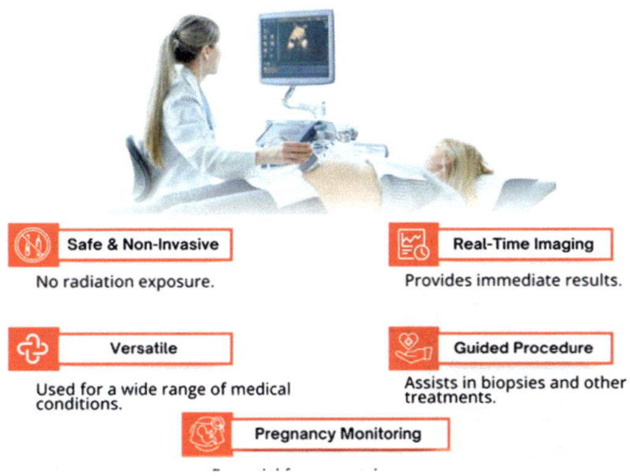

Figure 5.15. Benefits of ultrasound imaging.

Source: https://www.instagram.com/jabalpur_hospital/p/DFOn9FFtpEZ/.

5.4.1.1. Non-Invasive Nature

Medical imaging has come a long way, shifting focus toward techniques that skip the need for incisions. Ultrasound—one of the standouts—gives live, dynamic views inside the body, so doctors can peek at organs and tissues without any cutting involved. This method, which uses sound waves to form images, tends to lower both patient discomfort and the risks linked to more invasive tactics. In most cases, as ultrasound technology keeps evolving, it opens up new chances for sharper diagnosis while keeping safety front and center. Innovations like these remind us that non-invasive approaches play a key role in today's healthcare scene, ultimately nudging patient outcomes and satisfaction upward. Non-invasive imaging holds some serious promise in specialized areas, boosting how we diagnose while keeping risks at bay. Take its role in spotting issues like non-alcoholic fatty liver disease (NAFLD) for example—it shows off its versatility. Recently, research blending deep learning with ultrasound analysis reached some almost hard-to-believe numbers—precision hitting 99.8% and an AUC of 0.997, in most cases. These numbers suggest that sometimes these gentler techniques can match or even outdo their invasive counterparts.

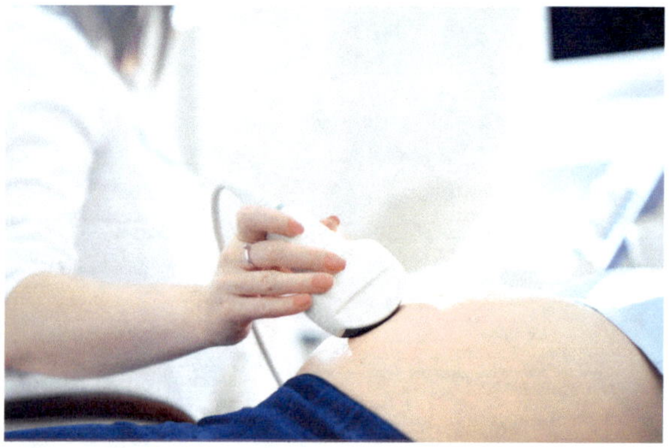

Source: https://arundelmedgroup.com/wp-content/uploads/2023/12/doctor-performing-ultrasound-scanning-her-pregnant-patient-1.jpg.

As more clinics start to adopt these advances, there's a good chance that leaning on non-invasive methods will only grow, gradually reshaping the overall healthcare picture. In dermatology, imaging without incisions is turning the tide on managing skin cancers such as basal cell carcinoma (BCC). High-frequency ultrasound (HFUS) and optical coherence tomography (OCT) have popped up as handy tools for checking tumor margins before surgery—even though they don't remove any tissue while mapping out the tumor's boundaries. This not only smooths out the process but also gives patients a clearer picture of what to expect, boosting their confidence. With these techniques finding more of a foothold in everyday medical practice — and even addressing worries about cost and recovery times—there's every reason to believe that non-invasive methods will keep shifting how we diagnose and treat conditions like BCC, paving the way for better overall care and satisfaction.

5.4.1.2. Real-Time Imaging Capabilities

Ultrasound imaging has come a long way, completely changing how doctors spot and handle conditions in real time. Cutting-edge tech—think AI and sleek electronics—has boosted these abilities in ways we didn't expect just a few years back. You can now watch blood flow or fetal movements live, which is key for getting assessments right and stepping in quickly. Newer devices pack more processing punch, making them work well even in places where resources or high-tech labs are scarce. These advances help smooth out workflows and bring diagnostics closer to patients, which in turn lifts the quality of care, faster, smarter tech means today's imaging isn't just about pretty pictures—it is become a core part of modern medical care, underscoring how tech and healthcare are getting more and more intertwined. You might also notice some neat breakthroughs in portable and wearable ultrasound systems. These aren't your run-of-the-mill machines; they employ advanced beamforming tactics to keep the imaging real-time and reliable. Plus, many of these gadgets come with wireless data sharing, letting caregivers monitor seriously ill patients around the clock, whether they're in a hospital or out in the field. By cutting down the traditional limits of imaging tools, these portable devices help doctors act fast—sometimes with life-saving results. New ultrasound probes, sporting fresh transducer technology, boost image quality without bogging down efficiency. In practice, merging real-time imaging with everyday medical routines means not just more accurate diagnoses but also a shift toward acting early on patient issues. That said, there are still hurdles to jump over—optimizing data transfer, especially in wireless real-time systems, remains tricky. In most cases, researchers have been tinkering with ideas like the vector quantized variational autoencoder model, which squeezes ultrasound radio frequency signals into smaller sizes. This method slashes the data by about 92% yet keeps the speedy real-time imaging flow over wireless links. By easing those bandwidth restrictions, such tweaks are nudging ultrasound imaging to spread wider in various clinical settings. Overall, as tech continues its upward march, mixing real-time imaging with AI and big data is set to further refine diagnostic tools and, eventually, reshape patient care in ways we're only beginning to imagine (Figure 5.16).

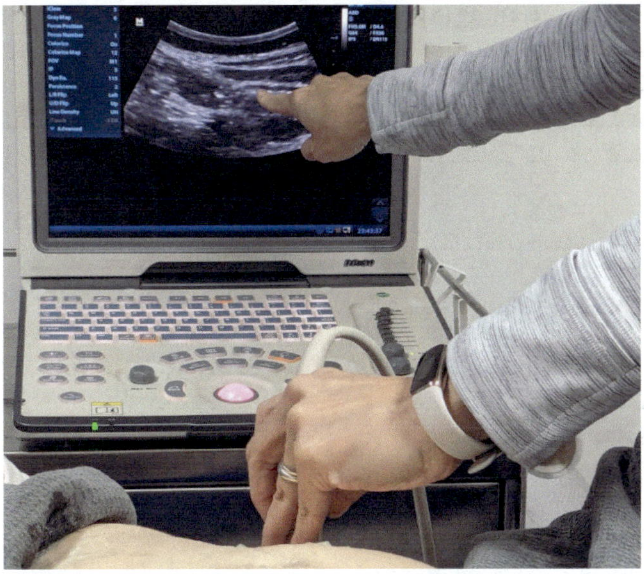

Figure 5.16. Ultrasound imaging has come a long way, completely changing how doctors spot and handle conditions in real time

Source: https://physio-central.com/cdn/shop/articles/real_time_ultrasound_for_men.png?v=1717131476&width=1000.

5.4.1.3. Safety and Lack of Ionizing Radiation

Medical imaging these days has made us rethink the balance between risk and reward. Ultrasound, for example, is getting a lot of attention because it doesn't hit patients with ionizing radiation—something especially critical in neonatology, where even small doses can be a real issue for little ones. Doctors can run scans over and over without worrying too much about radiation-related problems, which, in most cases, helps monitor patients effectively and even cuts down on overall healthcare costs related to radiation mishaps (Carnazzo et al., 2024). It is a handy tool that's proving its value time and again. On top of that, the ease with which ultrasound can be put to use makes it appealing across a range of settings. Point-of-care devices are popping up in places from busy emergency rooms to remote rural clinics. Unlike MRI or CT scans, which tend to be bulky and not so portable, these devices are light, quick to set up, and let physicians check things out in real time without long delays. It is kind of neat how the absence of ionizing risks not only boosts patient safety but also makes imaging more accessible in everyday practice (Abhimanyu et al., 2024). There's also been a steady stream of improvements pushing ultrasound technology even further. As clinicians dig into more complex procedures—like using it to guide needle insertions—the tech has been tweaked and refined, sometimes even getting a bit of robotic help to steer clear of vital structures. Generally speaking, these iterative breakthroughs help make the method both safer and sharper. Real-time imaging still plays a big part in its appeal, ensuring that as the challenges in modern medicine evolve, ultrasound is right there delivering timely, effective insights (Carnazzo et al., 2024).

5.4.2. Limitations of Ultrasound Imaging

Ultrasound isn't a simple tool—it comes with its own set of challenges that can sometimes hold back its overall accuracy. A lot of the time, the clarity of the images you see depends on how well the operator handles the equipment. Small differences in technique or even the way a transducer is held can change everything. Patient features, such as being overweight or having too much bowel gas, may also mess with the acoustic window, making images fuzzy. In most cases, this all points to a need for extra training and a heap of hands-on experience so that technicians can get reliable results. Recognizing these everyday variations is pretty essential for stepping up how ultrasound imaging is used in clinical settings. Another tricky part of ultrasound work lies in dealing with how clearly it can capture detail at different depths. Generally speaking, conventional ultrasound doesn't hit the spatial resolution mark set by alternatives like MRI or CT scans. That shortfall can make it hard to pick up on subtle changes or to tell similar-looking structures apart. Sure, ultrasound nails it when looking at superficial organs, but as you go deeper, sound waves tend to lose their oomph because of attenuation. Some studies even mention that this drop in image quality becomes a real headache for abdominal evaluations, where thicker tissue or overlying gas can hide important details. This means that for some patients or conditions, doctors might lean on a mix of imaging methods to get the complete picture. Finally, there's the whole issue of artifacts, which add another twist to the process by muddling up what's there. These odd distortions can emerge due to limits in equipment, settings tweaked by operators, and even natural differences in a patient's anatomy. You often see things like shadowing, enhancement, or reverberation creating confusing images that might mislead—even experts sometimes misread them, occasionally leading to misdiagnoses or oversights. Experts generally agree that tackling these artifacts is key if we're to up the game of ultrasound imaging accuracy. It seems that better processing techniques and smarter algorithms could play a big role in minimizing these hiccups, boosting the modality's clinical value (Oglat et al., 2024; Yang et al., 2024) (Figure 5.17).

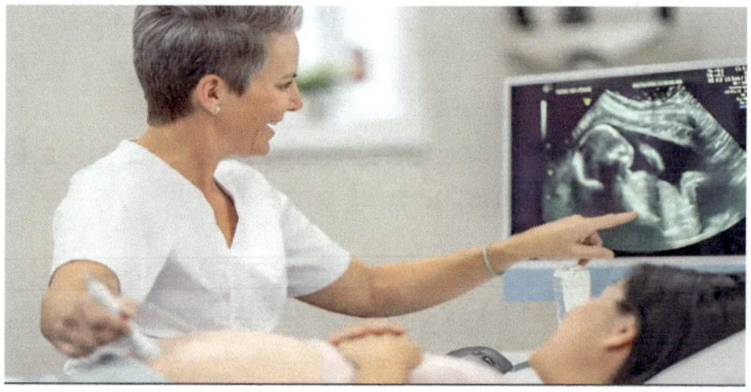

Figure 5.17. Limitations of Ultrasound Imaging.

Source: https://ehealthcommunity.org/wp-content/uploads/2025/03/limitations-of-ultrasound-in-diagnosing-certain-conditions-832x468.webp.

5.4.2.1. Operator Dependency

Ultrasound imaging is fraught with challenges because it leans so heavily on skilled operators.

This dependence often muddies diagnostic accuracy and consistency — something you see most clearly in those tricky cases where the operator's know-how counts. Recent studies, generally speaking, hint that deep learning might ease this load; for example, CNN-based models like SDFNet and U-Net have shown notable improvements when detecting subtle kidney issues (Chitra et al., 2025). Instead of strictly relying on human interpretation, these methods offer a fresh way to tackle the problem. Machine learning's promise isn't just about handing off tasks to computers; it also means making sure that the images from various devices come out clearly. The operator's experience, along with specific machine settings, can seriously impact image quality and, by extension, diagnostic outcomes. A new method in liver ultrasound diagnostics uses an augmentation process—one that simulates the natural variations in image quality among different devices. The findings indicate that when technicians employ these boosted models, the performance gaps tied to different machine setups shrink significantly. In most cases, older techniques like Histogram Equalization and CLAHE just don't hold a candle to this new two-step image tone augmentation (Cho et al., 2025). It isn't all about high-tech solutions, though; improving operator skills is equally key. Keeping ultrasound technicians in step with evolving technology through ongoing training proves essential—even if it is not always a one-stop fix. With advances in image processing and analysis unfolding rapidly, future work should concentrate on simulation-based training options, using tools like virtual or augmented reality to enhance skills. As diagnostic tools grow more sophisticated, the expectation that operators maintain top-notch image quality while interpreting complex scans becomes even more pressing. Ultimately, striking a better balance between human talent and modern technology appears to be the surest way to drive improved outcomes in ultrasound diagnostics.

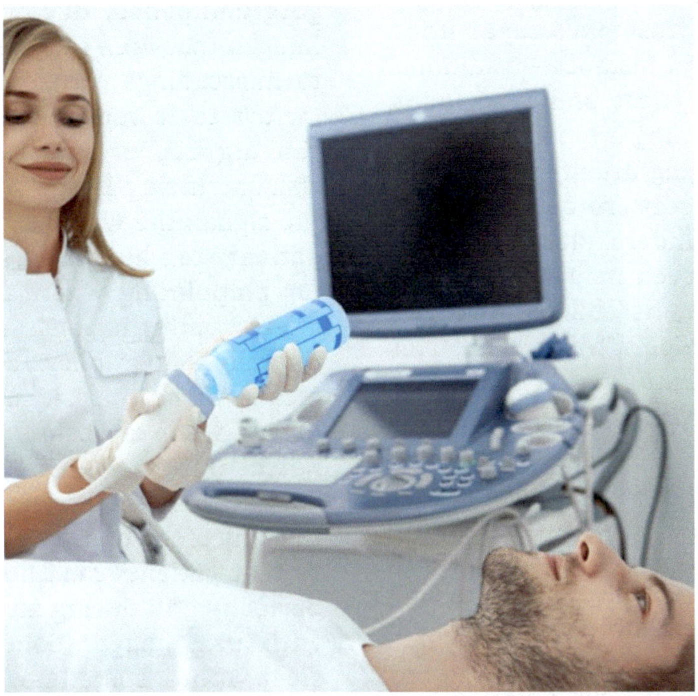

Source: https://www.southgatephysio.co.uk/wp-content/uploads/bfi_thumb/portrait-man-nurse-working-with-patient-scaled-3kam07munfenparz73ipe2.jpg.

5.4.2.2. Limited Penetration in Certain Tissues

Ultrasound imaging plays a big role in shaping diagnostic outcomes by how it interacts with different tissues. It is prized for being non-invasive and delivering live images, but when it meets tissues with unique acoustic traits, things can go sideways. For instance, when sound waves hit stubborn barriers like bones or air-filled pockets, they don't travel as they should – leading to murkier views and lower resolution that can throw off a diagnosis. Low signal-to-noise ratios just add to the confusion, making it hard to tell apart healthy from problematic tissue. Computer-aided needle segmentation, for example, helps in procedures like needle biopsies by easing these issues (Zhang et al., 2025). Generally speaking, tackling these obstacles is pretty crucial if ultrasound is going to live up to its potential in the clinic. Technical challenges aren't the only downside here, though; the way our bodies and certain diseases behave puts extra strain on ultrasound's capabilities. Take colorectal cancer, for instance—traditional methods often mix optical and ultrasound imaging, with each running into its own set of problems. Optical imaging usually stops at the surface because light scatters quickly, which leaves deeper tissues underexplored (Jia-Xi et al., 2024). Meanwhile, even though ultrasound can look further inside, its ability to capture molecular details just doesn't match up. This kind of split focus creates a diagnostic gap that might delay treatment when time is of the essence. Innovations like miniaturized handheld photoacoustic/ultrasound dual-modality probes are stepping in, blending deeper penetration with better molecular imaging to up the accuracy in tricky anatomical spots. Looking ahead, ongoing research might just break through the barriers of limited ultrasound penetration. Scientists are tweaking ultrasound frequencies and boosting the sensitivity of imaging systems to better capture complex tissue details. Plus, combining ultrasound with complementary techniques such as photoacoustic imaging seems promising—it can reduce that pesky interference from varied tissue types and improve both specificity and resolution. In most cases, these improvements could pave the way for earlier detection and more reliable monitoring of diseases in areas that have always been hard to image (Jia-Xi et al., 2024). Overall, these advances aren't merely technical upgrades; they hint at a whole new approach to using ultrasound in modern healthcare (Zhang et al., 2025).

5.4.2.3. Challenges in Imaging Obese Patients

Obesity is on the rise, and that throws a wrench into using ultrasound in medical imaging. Fat tends to sit deep under the skin, and the extra tissue can sap the strength of the ultrasound beam—generally speaking, this leads to weaker echoes that make it harder to see what's underneath. When the signal gets dampened, doctors might end up with images that aren't as clear, potentially leading to misreadings or oversights. Clinicians often switch to lower frequency transducers that can dig deeper into tissues—but then they risk sacrificing image resolution. It is not just the signal; the way the body's shaped in obese patients can hide the usual landmarks needed for pinpointing where to look, which in turn affects both diagnosis and therapy planning. Overall, sonographers and physicians have to pick up on how obesity muddles imaging results if they want to ensure patient care stays top-notch. Things get even more complicated when you factor in the patient's own body functions. In many cases, obesity worsens breathing issues so that patients can't hold their breath or stay perfectly still during an exam—this ending up with fuzzy images. Conditions like obstructive sleep apnea sometimes add another layer of difficulty; before a scan, additional checks or subtle adjustments might be necessary to cope with these challenges. This isn't just a technical glitch—it's a combination of physiological hurdles that mean the whole imaging process has to be more flexible, relying on teamwork among the healthcare staff to maneuver around the extra complications that come with increased body mass. The challenges of obesity don't stop at the imaging itself; they ripple out into broader patient management too. Health professionals increasingly recognize that changes in how the body processes drugs may force shifts in sedation choices during ultrasound-guided procedures. In critical settings—say, when rapid exams are needed for septic patients—the obesity-induced limitations can slow things down, even if technically the ultrasound is still in play. For instance, getting a clear picture quickly is key, even when the usual landmarks are obscured or the image is less crisp. Innovations like point-of-care ultrasound offer some hope, but practitioners must stay on their toes. In most cases, it means adapting continuously—mixing new technology with old-school technique—to manage both the technical and physiological challenges that obesity presents.

Test Your Knowledge

1. What are the main advantages of ultrasound imaging compared to other diagnostic imaging techniques?
2. What are some of the limitations of ultrasound imaging, particularly in terms of image quality and patient factors?

5.5. Future Developments in Ultrasound Technology

Learning Outcome

1. Explore recent advancements in imaging resolution.
2. Understand the integration with artificial intelligence with ultrasound imaging.
3. Examine the potential for portable ultrasound devices.

Ultrasound technology has changed the game in clinical practice. Once it was just a basic tool, but now 3D and even 4D imaging have turned it into a way to see details that were once hidden. Doctors get a clearer look at body structures, which means assessments are more on point. Meanwhile, AI—an ever-growing part of the mix—steps in to help analyze images automatically. This shift not only makes diagnoses more reliable but also widens ultrasound's use in areas ranging from obstetrics to oncology, giving a fresh push to personalized care (Doreen, 2025). There's also been a big buzz around CEUS, especially in cancer care. Traditionally introduced in the late 1960s, this technique has been refined over time with improved contrast agents that make images surprisingly crisp. In most cases, this means that medical pros are now better equipped to judge tumor features and decide on treatments that are just right for each patient. Put simply, as ultrasound starts to reveal tiny biological markers linked to disease, it opens an exciting door for precision medicine in oncology, fundamentally shaking up cancer diagnosis and treatment (Shi et al., 2025). Even the portability of these devices is changing how we think about accessing care. Compact ultrasound machines are popping up in settings you wouldn't have expected—ranging from remote clinics to emergency rooms—helping shorten the time it takes to get a quality check-up. Innovations such as microbubble technology are also beginning to play a role in imaging and therapy, hinting at a future where advanced diagnostics are available almost anywhere healthcare is needed (Doreen, 2025) (Figure 5.18).

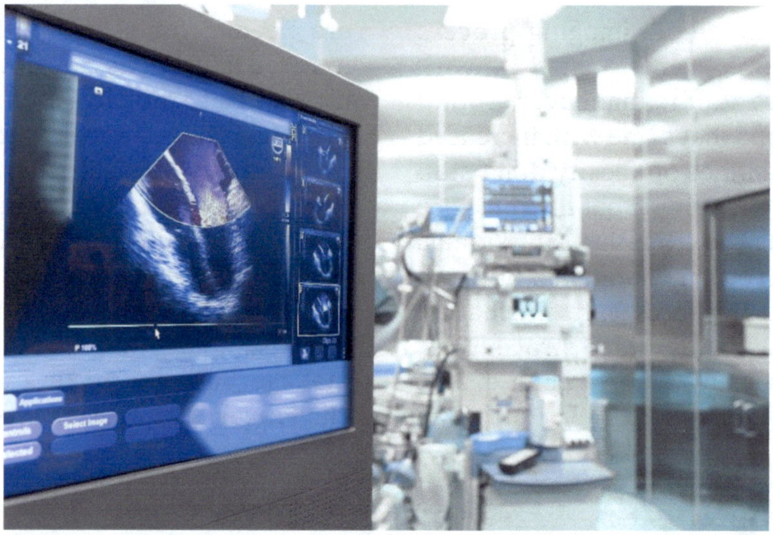

Figure 5.18. Ultrasound technology has changed the game in clinical practice.

Source: https://www.pbmchealth.org/application/files/cache/thumbnails/f370ad23cb0ece01c71bb9df85b37d09.jpg.

5.5.1. Advancements in Imaging Resolution

Ultrasound imaging has come a long way—its development keeps shaking up how we diagnose illnesses. Clearer picture details now let doctors spot things they used to miss. CEUS, which made its debut in 1968, kind of opened the door to newer imaging ideas. This method brings unique benefits in many clinical cases, especially when checking for hepatocellular carcinoma (HCC). In most cases, the sharper images not only boost diagnostic accuracy, but they also help us grasp the underlying biology of HCC, which in turn supports more personalized treatment strategies (Shi et al., 2025). Meanwhile, breakthroughs in acoustic sensors have pushed ultrasound imaging into new territories beyond the usual medical settings. Using high-frequency acoustic waves—sometimes reaching nearly 1 GHz—has amazed many by boosting spatial detail. This happens when acoustic and optical technologies are teamed up to convert signals more efficiently, allowing the detection of tiny details in the tissue microenvironment that were once overlooked. For instance, switching from traditional SiO2 fibers to more advanced As2Se3 tapered fibers shows just how far high-frequency and high-sensitivity detection have come (Bao et al., 2025). It is a striking step forward that keeps ultrasound imaging at the cutting edge of diagnostics. These advances don't stop at delivering better visuals; they also have a real impact on patient care and treatment decisions. Enhanced image resolution gives clinicians insights that shape both diagnosis and therapy. Often, picking up on subtle tissue changes early on can lead to swifter treatments that help improve outcomes. Generally speaking, as personalized medicine gets more popular, the detailed information from modern ultrasound techniques becomes even more important. So instead of just providing data, these methods deliver actionable clues that are changing how medicine is practiced—a transformation that goes way beyond mere technical upgrades (Figure 5.21).

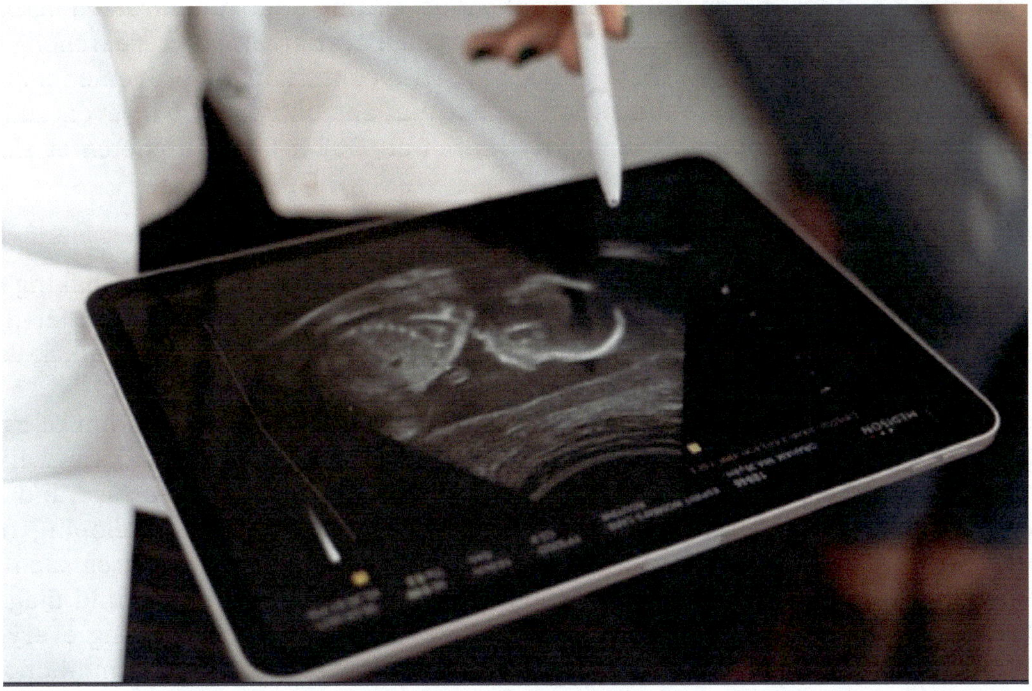

Source: https://media.licdn.com/dms/image/v2/D4D12AQHxnkZ4VVwV3g/article-cover_image-shrink_600_2000/article-cover_image-shrink_600_2000/0/1689655692211?e=2147483647&v=beta&t=_vNFxfOTPDfzV6VnhNHUTGiqInLFVWd5ZXOGhr04kBU.

5.5.2. Integration with Artificial Intelligence (AI)

Ultrasound imaging is getting a boost thanks to AI, and it is clear this isn't just a trend. New techniques in deep and machine learning help make sense of ultrasound data in ways that – quite frankly – are faster and more on-target than before. You might see, for example, that these AI routines now handle multiple organ checks, covering everything from gynecological exams to liver and bile duct evaluations. Studies suggest that when these tools are mixed into routine imaging, identifying abnormalities gets a definite lift (Cai et al., 2024). With ultrasound studies booming around the globe, many think that these smart solutions could ease the workload on radiologists while keeping patient care both prompt and precise. Bringing AI into the ultrasound room isn't just about sharper diagnosis; it is also shaking up how we do monitoring and drafting reports. Natural language processing (NLP) and automation in report making mean that data management now feels a bit more, well, manageable. By letting machines handle the routine bits, doctors can devote more time to those complex cases that need individual attention. Generating full reports with almost no human help stands as a major step forward – especially as more studies back these systems and the FDA, in most cases, gives its approval (Chansangpetch et al., 2024). This shift is slowly but surely nudging us toward a day when AI isn't just an add-on but a core part of every ultrasound workflow. Of course, the road to making AI work seamlessly in ultrasound isn't completely smooth. There's the real concern over bias in these systems, along with a desperate need for robust, multi-center validation—factors that, more often than not, keep these tools from being trusted across all clinical settings. While initial findings are promising, a lot of AI applications are still held back by limited testing on different fronts. Plus, getting data standardized across various platforms remains a tricky hurdle. It seems that closer collaboration among researchers, clinicians, and tech experts is key to ironing out these kinks. Still, with continuous improvements in AI-driven technology, the hope is that ultrasound practices and patient outcomes will eventually hit that target of both enhanced precision and reliability (Cai et al., 2024; Chansangpetch et al., 2024).

5.5.3. Potential for Portable Ultrasound Devices

Medical diagnostics have changed a lot lately—portable ultrasound devices are shaking things up. You see these little machines popping up in busy emergency rooms as well as in far-flung areas where standard imaging isn't available. Recent studies suggest that mixing these quick-use devices with conventional methods can bump up the accuracy of a diagnosis, which helps docs decide on the right course of action sooner. It is notable how having a tool right at the point of care speeds up condition assessments, a feature that's especially vital in high-pressure situations like trauma or obstetrics. These devices aren't just for hospitals anymore. Their ease-of-use and adaptable design mean they're finding a place in home health visits and even in developing regions—a real game-changer for making healthcare more accessible. Adding smart features such as AI and remote connectivity only ramps up their potential; clinicians can now consult and diagnose even when distances would normally get in the way. In many cases, it is about giving everyone a fair shot at quality care, blending traditional practices (think Ayurveda, where time-honored ideas meet modern modifications (Das et al., 2024) with up-to-date technology. Looking ahead, portable ultrasound technology is evolving in unexpected ways that might redefine imaging and patient care. Engineers and researchers are busy tweaking these gadgets to sharpen their resolution and widen their diagnostic capabilities, making them a surprisingly viable alternative for complex cases. Some studies even point out that in evaluating musculoskeletal issues, these portable devices perform nearly on par with conventional systems (Chen et al., 2024). With healthcare systems increasingly focused on efficiency and cost-effectiveness, the affordability of these ultrasounds makes them an attractive option, allowing high-quality imaging services to reach communities that might otherwise be overlooked.

Test Your Knowledge

1. How is artificial intelligence integrated into ultrasound imaging to improve diagnostic accuracy and efficiency?
2. What is the potential impact of portable ultrasound devices on healthcare delivery, especially in remote or underserved areas?

Summary

Ultrasound imaging has come a long way—it has changed prenatal care in more ways than one. Healthcare professionals now spot and manage pregnancy complications with fresh eyes, thanks in part to recent deep learning breakthroughs. Convolutional neural networks, specially tuned for the job, now tackle tasks like finding the right plane and segmenting the cerebellum. In most cases, these techniques help in identifying neurodevelopmental issues early on. The new models, which some might say are pretty impressive, boast accuracy levels near 98.6% and even a dice coefficient of about 0.956% for key tasks. Overall, these gains don't just represent a tech upgrade; they mark a crucial move toward better patient outcomes in prenatal care (Vetriselvi et al., 2025). Ultrasound isn't just for prenatal checks, either. It is proving to be a strong ally in spotting other conditions as well—take, for instance, the detection of endometrial carcinoma in postmenopausal women with abnormal bleeding. By mixing clinical details with ultrasound findings, clinicians can now put together a risk scoring system that speaks to a patient's situation. Critical signs like endometrial thickness and the way blood flows through vessels are used again and again as hints toward malignancy. The ultrasound-based model shows high sensitivity and specificity, making it a dependable, non-invasive option that helps cut down on unnecessary invasive procedures. This approach not only smooths out patient management but also boosts the overall standard of care for women in tough health spots. Looking at everything together, the steady advances in ultrasound imaging reveal its expanding role in healthcare. Both in prenatal and gynecological fields, the tool proves that it can hit the mark with both precision and the less intrusive approach many appreciate. The blending of smart algorithms and intuitive scoring systems reflects a broader trend toward personalized medicine, where every patient's details truly matter. The future seems promising—ongoing improvements are set to impact a variety of healthcare fields, leading to earlier detections and faster interventions. In most cases, keeping pace with these innovations is key to refining diagnostic accuracy and enhancing outcomes. Ultimately, all of these efforts drive home the fact that ultrasound imaging is a vital part of modern, holistic patient care.

Ultrasound imaging shines in the world of medical imaging. It is a non-invasive and safe tool that does a ton in different situations. High-frequency sound waves are used to capture live images of soft tissues and organs, which makes it indispensable for things like prenatal care and checking out various conditions. Quick, real-time images mean that doctors can make decisions fast, a real bonus when timing is critical. New modifications on the technology—think Doppler ultrasound—let you see blood flow, which is super helpful when evaluating vascular or cardiac issues. All these improvements show how ultrasound is becoming more and more central in healthcare, giving detailed views that help drive clinical decisions while cutting down on exposure to ionizing radiation. In using ultrasound effectively, sticking to clear, evidence-based protocols matters. Every step—from snapping the first image to interpreting details and managing what comes next—is crucial to getting things right for the patient. Generally speaking, proper training is key; if healthcare providers aren't well-prepped, misreads might lead to misdiagnoses or less-than-ideal treatment plans. Recent recommendations from professional groups highlight that following these practical guidelines can catch issues early and reduce mistakes in judgment. In most cases, this adherence underscores how essential ultrasound has become in diagnostics. Ultrasound's widespread use makes it clear that ongoing research and steady tech improvements aren't just nice to have—they're necessary. The field isn't standing still; new innovations like three-dimensional ultrasound and portable devices are on the rise, promising better image quality and easier access for patients. These technological leaps don't just improve resolution and reliability, they open up even more possibilities in different medical areas. This evolution also serves as a reminder that continual education (and sometimes a bit of trial and error) is vital for keeping pace with these advances. Overall, combining solid guidelines, constant training, and fresh technology forms the backbone of ultrasound imaging's essential role in today's healthcare landscape (Cosentino et al., 2019; Mathijssen, 2020).

KEY TERMS FROM THIS CHAPTER

- 3D ultrasound
- Acoustic impedance
- Contrast-enhanced ultrasound (CEUS)
- Doppler ultrasound
- Fetal health
- Musculoskeletal ultrasound
- Reflection
- Super-resolution ultrasound (SRUS)
- 4D ultrasound
- Blood vessels
- Doppler effect
- Echo patterns
- High-frequency sound waves
- Real-time imaging
- Refraction
- Transducer

Critical Thinking Questions

1. **What type of waves are used in ultrasound imaging?**
   a. X-rays
   b. Radio waves
   c. Sound waves
   d. Gamma rays
2. **What is the typical frequency range used in diagnostic ultrasound?**
   a. 2–15 Hz
   b. 2–15 MHz
   c. 20–40 kHz
   d. 100–500 MHz
3. **Which of the following structures is best visualized using ultrasound imaging?**
   a. Lungs
   b. Bones
   c. Soft tissues and organs
   d. Teeth
4. **What is the role of ultrasound gel in imaging?**
   a. It reduces radiation exposure
   b. It acts as a disinfectant
   c. It improves sound wave transmission
   d. It cools the transducer
5. **Which of the following is a common use of Doppler ultrasound?**
   a. Imaging bones
   b. Assessing blood flow
   c. Detecting dental caries
   d. Measuring body fat

Short Answer Questions

1. What are the basic principles behind ultrasound technology and how are sound waves used to create images?
2. What are the different types of ultrasound imaging, such as Doppler and 3D ultrasound, and how do they differ in use?
3. In what ways is ultrasound imaging commonly applied in medical diagnostics and patient care?
4. What are the key advantages and limitations of using ultrasound compared to other imaging techniques?
5. What are some expected future developments in ultrasound technology that could enhance diagnostic capabilities?

Answers to Critical Thinking Questions

1. (c); 2. (b); 3. (c); 4. (c); 5. (b)

References

1. Abhimanyu, F., Orekhov, A., Galeotti, J., & Choset, H. (2024). Learning to register needles in ultrasound images during tissue insertion. *Proceedings of the 16th Hamlyn Symposium on Medical Robotics 2024*. https://www.semanticscholar.org/paper/41f13fc2cb849c9240bcdcce07d0e76dab536673 (accessed on 23 May 2025).
2. Bao, X., & Tatel, G. (2025). Micro-structured and telecom fibers for acoustic and ultrasound sensing and imaging. *Journal of Lightwave Technology, 43*, 1581–1594. https://www.semanticscholar.org/paper/75e598c454a763a271229010660572bc1ed9c354 (accessed on 23 May 2025).
3. Bastola, S., & Tekes, C. (2024). Vector-quantization variational autoencoder based data rate reduction for wireless ultrasound imaging systems. *SoutheastCon 2024*. https://www.semanticscholar.org/paper/2f23a33500bf1c3687ff1600948d342b5a0783d2 (accessed on 23 May 2025).
4. Boostani, M., Hamilton-Meikle, P., Bozsányi, S., Farkas, K., Szabó, B., Bánvölgyi, A., et al. (2025). Novel imaging techniques for tumor margin detection in basal cell carcinoma: A systematic scoping review of FDA and EMA-approved imaging modalities. *International Journal of Dermatology, 64*(2), 287–301. https://doi.org/10.1111/ijd.17496.
5. Cai, L., & Pfob, A. (2024). Artificial intelligence in abdominal and pelvic ultrasound imaging: Current applications. *Abdominal Radiology (New York), 50*, 1775–1789. https://www.semanticscholar.org/paper/55314a35acef6c9e235b37b28972c8abfbcc0089 (accessed on 23 May 2025).
6. Carnazzo, S., Nasikas, S., & Comisi, F. F. (2024). Lung ultrasound in neonates: A narrative review along with diagnostic insights and early postnatal applications. *Cureus, 16*. https://www.semanticscholar.org/paper/46f868324cfc1be6efd5f4c7954795d85c7633c8 (accessed on 23 May 2025).
7. Chansangpetch, S., Ittarat, M., Cheungpasitporn, W., & Lin, S. (2024). Artificial intelligence and big data integration in anterior segment imaging for glaucoma. *Taiwan Journal of Ophthalmology, 14*, 319–332. https://www.semanticscholar.org/paper/87411bde6a4021e056b65b4b9af0f7f4332b710d (accessed on 23 May 2025).
8. Chen, W., Zhang, Y., Wang, X., & Liu, J. (2024). Comparative analysis of imaging modalities for diagnosing musculoskeletal disorders. *Journal of Innovations in Medical Research, 3*(1), 45–53. Retrieved from: https://www.paradigmpress.org/jimr/article/view/1073 (accessed on 23 May 2025).
9. Cheong, I. (2025). Diagnosis of lung abscess and pancreatic collection using transesophageal and trans gastric point-of-care ultrasound in a critically ill patient. *Journal of Clinical Ultrasound: JCU, 53*(2), 373–376. https://doi.org/10.1002/jcu.23856.
10. Chinene, B., Mutandiro, L., Mushosho, E., Khumbula, L., Zanga, A., Banhwa, J., & Bwanga, O. (2024). Role of radiographers in the provision of diagnostic medical ultrasound services in Zimbabwe: Past, present and way forward. *Medical Journal of Zambia*. https://www.semanticscholar.org/paper/ee6160e1b7bdea72820bea4f1c829301b05fd358 (accessed on 23 May 2025).
11. Chitra, N. T., Gogula, S., & Satapathy, S. (2025). A survey of advanced algorithms and experimental

approaches for kidney abnormality detection in ultrasound imaging. *2025 International Conference on Electronics and Renewable Systems (ICEARS)*. https://www.semanticscholar.org/paper/6e8b1ca82e6fa74cb0dd9452f25fa58cb0243fe2 (accessed on 23 May 2025).

12. Cho, J., Lee, S., & Yi, J. (2025). Ultrasound standard liver section classification independent of imaging device. *2025 19th International Conference on Ubiquitous Information Management and Communication (IMCOM)*. https://www.semanticscholar.org/paper/2d1ef41560ba3c2708cb8c65bfe6affd9659f622 (accessed on 23 May 2025).

13. Cosentino, F., Grant, P. J., Aboyans, V., Bailey, C. J., Ceriello, A., Delgado, V., Federici, M., et al. (2019). 2019 ESC guidelines on diabetes, pre-diabetes, and cardiovascular diseases developed in collaboration with the EASD. *European Heart Journal, 41*, 255–323. https://doi.org/10.1093/eurheartj/ehz486.

14. Das, N. K., & Panday, S. D. (2024). Integrating radiological diagnostic tools in Shalya Tantra: Advancements and clinical applications. *International Journal for Multidisciplinary Research*. https://doi.org/10.36948/ijfmr.2024.v06i03.23395.

15. De Cassai, A., Zarantonello, F., Pistollato, E., Pettenuzzo, T., Busetto, V., Sella, N., & Boscolo, A. (2025). Regional anesthesia in obese patients: Challenges, considerations, and solutions. *Saudi Journal of Anaesthesia, 19*, 221–226. https://www.semanticscholar.org/paper/2a27c02fb5b29766439c1b5d923af1a646b10566 (accessed on 23 May 2025).

16. Deán-Ben, X. L. (2023). Editorial: Advances in image formation methods for optoacoustic and ultrasound imaging. *Frontiers in Physics, 10*, 1115390. https://doi.org/10.3389/fphy.2022.1115390.

17. Domínguez, M., Velikova, Y., Navab, N., & Azampour, M. F. (2024). Diffusion as sound propagation: Physics-inspired model for ultrasound image generation. https://www.semanticscholar.org/paper/99055351da3cd76d4f455b33870daae74e42029b (accessed on 23 May 2025).

18. Gamarra, A., Salamanca, J., Díez-Villanueva, P., Cuenca, S., Vázquez, J., Aguilar, R., Diego, G., et al. (2025). Ultrasound imaging of congestion in heart failure: A narrative review. *Cardiovascular Diagnosis and Therapy, 15*, 233–250. https://www.semanticscholar.org/paper/1a9c01d8df04709e9d76aed32a22483a72e9eba3 (accessed on 23 May 2025).

19. Gambo, N., & Shehu, M. (2024). The role of diagnostic medical physics in medicine: An overview. *Sahel Journal of Life Sciences FUDMA*. https://www.semanticscholar.org/paper/372a33a3ed2cd5bb3d645657730b8c7801785d41 (accessed on 23 May 2025).

20. Geetha, R., Rani, D. J., & Anbarasu, K. (2024). Applying deep learning methods to non-alcoholic fatty liver disease management. *2024 5th International Conference on Circuits, Control, Communication and Computing (I4C)*. https://www.semanticscholar.org/paper/57869e5db46971d258731e10bcd86028db2ea617 (accessed on 23 May 2025).

21. Ghosh, D., & Hoyt, K. (2025). Advancements in three-dimensional super-resolution ultrasound imaging. *Journal of Ultrasound in Medicine*. https://doi.org/10.1002/jum.16682.

22. Gnanaraj, V. T., J, C., Amanullah, M., & I, F. (2024). Cross-domain application of deep learning techniques for improved diagnostic and phenotyping accuracy in medical and agricultural imaging. *2024 International Conference on Emerging Research in Computational Science (ICERCS)*. https://www.semanticscholar.org/paper/c96db13ca72b965b0eb313fba37fcb6568626752 (accessed on 23 May 2025).

23. Gupta, S., Joshi, M., Handa, P., Yadav, R., & Goel, N. (2024). Revolutionizing medical imaging: Unveiling ChatGPT's potential in diagnostics. *2024 2nd World Conference on Communication & Computing (WCONF)*. https://www.semanticscholar.org/paper/4fc26967176e3c7a8d9d8e695c1b0e78312b4002 (accessed on 23 May 2025).

24. Gusev, A. A. (2025). What neural networks and how a urologist can utilize in his routine tasks: Practical tips. *Urology Herald (Vestnik Urologii)*, *13*(1), 99–109.

25. Hama, H. K., Majeed, H. D., & Nariman, G. S. (2025). Enhanced kidney stone detection and classification using SVM and LBP features. *UHD Journal of Science and Technology*. https://www.semanticscholar.org/paper/5e79ed23ed21e6f4c60b6c372727d307facfcb1c (accessed on 23 May 2025).

26. Hattori, S., Saggar, R., Heidinger, E., Qi, A., Mullen, J., Fee, B., Brown, C. L., et al. (2024). Advances in ultrasound-guided surgery and artificial intelligence applications in musculoskeletal diseases. *Diagnostics, 14*. https://www.semanticscholar.org/paper/a89c8c3c284522840c49c28888ead5ac70b57ac7 (accessed on 23 May 2025).

27. Joshi, S. V., Sadeghpour, S., Kuznetsova, N., Wang, C., & Kraft, M. (2025). Flexible micromachined ultrasound transducers (MUTs) for biomedical applications. *Microsystems & Nanoengineering, 11*. https://www.semanticscholar.org/paper/2faddb0d43fe9d204db80855387f590788a7f134 (accessed on 23 May 2025).

28. Kamel, R. J., Naeem, S. A., Musa, M. M., & Karim, S. N. (2024). Advancements in medical imaging technologies: Ultrasound, X-ray, and MRI. *European Journal of Theoretical and Applied Sciences*. https://www.semanticscholar.org/paper/97b5f5f89673779203ab0ee5742c614500c2a960 (accessed on 23 May 2025).

29. Kapoor, A., & Singh, T. (2017). A brief review: Speckle reducing filtering for ultrasound images. In *2017 International Conference on I-SMAC (IoT in Social, Mobile, Analytics and Cloud) (I-SMAC)*. https://www.semanticscholar.org/paper/f21b73d38f85bc162475c2ab8427ed8c2b4e0d41 (accessed on 23 May 2025).

30. Manske, R., Voight, M. L., Wolfe, C., & Page, P. (2024). Utilizing diagnostic musculoskeletal ultrasound for assessment of the infraspinatus muscle and tendon: Implications for rehabilitation professionals. *International Journal of Sports Physical Therapy, 19*, 935–941. https://www.semanticscholar.org/paper/e01332b79d6ebb8830f46339ec198f461f7837ff (accessed on 23 May 2025).

31. Mathijssen, I. M. J. (2020). Updated guideline on treatment and management of craniosynostosis. *Journal of Craniofacial Surgery, 32*, 371–450. https://doi.org/10.1097/scs.0000000000007035.

32. Memon, K., Yahya, N., Yusoff, M. Z., Remli, R., Mustapha, A. W. M. M., Hashim, H., Ali, S. S. A., et al. (2024). Edge computing for AI-based brain MRI applications: A critical evaluation of real-time classification and segmentation. *Sensors (Basel, Switzerland), 24*. https://www.semanticscholar.org/paper/16dfca58bf4fb2c2ada5e956a48b19f7636e8290 (accessed on 23 May 2025).

33. Miller, J. P., Carney, M., Lim, S., & Lindsey, J. (2018). Ultrasound and plastic surgery: Clinical applications of the newest technology. *Annals of Plastic Surgery, 80*, S356–S361. https://www.semanticscholar.org/paper/62b97b7b92d490d79a4719c1dc073363ff762362 (accessed on 23 May 2025).

34. Monika, Dr. (Mrs.), & Kumar, C. (2025). Improved medical image enhancement by optimized

features and parameters using convolution with grey wolves' approach. *Communications on Applied Nonlinear Analysis, 32*(8s). https://doi.org/10.52783/cana.v32.3718.

35. Nanthini, S., Maindola, M., R, M., Ravishankar, M. D., Gandhi, J., & Patil, H. (2024). A DL-DeNoiseNet framework for robust image denoising and artifact reduction in medical image diagnostics. *2024 International Conference on Integrated Intelligence and Communication Systems (ICIICS)*. https://www.semanticscholar.org/paper/3a6e8703f0846313a0ea6aed15d1531e723fa742 (accessed on 23 May 2025).

36. Nyakairu, D. G. (2025). Ultrasound engineering: Innovations in non-invasive diagnostics. *Research Output Journal of Biological and Applied Science*. https://www.semanticscholar.org/paper/97fc7196325b073358e04569591f08cf0bcc01e1 (accessed on 23 May 2025).

37. Oglat, A. A., & Abukhalil, T. (2024). Ultrasound elastography: Methods, clinical applications, and limitations: A review article. *Applied Sciences*. https://www.semanticscholar.org/paper/0bc80b40eaf5c4e7484d0c0537133c7ebebe57e9 (accessed on 23 May 2025).

38. Pilz, N., Heinz, V., Ax, T., Fesseler, L., Patzak, A., & Bothe, T. (2024). Pulse wave velocity: Methodology, clinical applications, and interplay with heart rate variability. *Reviews in Cardiovascular Medicine, 25*. https://www.semanticscholar.org/paper/c7bee884a5a8464e87ada1c81cb5a4b8cd16b25f (accessed on 23 May 2025).

39. Pooh, R. K. (2015). First trimester scan by 3D, 3D HDlive and HDlive silhouette/flow ultrasound imaging. *Donald School Journal of Ultrasound in Obstetrics and Gynecology, 9*(4), 361–371.

40. R, M. (2024). Enhancing diagnostic accuracy in breast ultrasound imaging through deep learning and image augmentation techniques. *2024 International Conference on Emerging Research in Computational Science (ICERCS)*. https://www.semanticscholar.org/paper/423439701360c41bc17085e01de27ccaf8f5845b (accessed on 23 May 2025).

41. Recker, F., Gembruch, U., & Strizek, B. (2024). Clinical ultrasound applications in obstetrics and gynecology in the year 2024. *Journal of Clinical Medicine, 13*. https://www.semanticscholar.org/paper/84dcd3f0a3d22ab805936891cac8912e637ac903 (accessed on 23 May 2025).

42. Shen, E., Fan, K., Lu, Y., Chen, X., Li, C., Ma, X., Wu, T., et al. (2024). 3D multi-modality free-hand ultrasound imaging for medical research. *2024 IEEE International Symposium on Biomedical Imaging (ISBI)*. https://www.semanticscholar.org/paper/c7cb411fca2eac22c3bd4390192e5713512f0554 (accessed on 23 May 2025).

43. Shi, D., & Li, L. (2025). Advancements in ultrasound imaging for assessing the biological behavior of hepatocellular carcinoma. *International Journal of Biology and Life Sciences, 9*(1), 63–67. https://doi.org/10.54097/geg0bx51.

44. Shi, X., Zhao, F., Feng, L., Liu, Y., & Zhou, X. (2025). Predicting the high intensity focused ultrasound focus *in vivo* using acoustic radiation force imaging. *Medical Physics, 52*(3), 1728–1745. https://doi.org/10.1002/mp.17564.

45. Silverman, R. H. (2023). Principles of ophthalmic ultrasound. *Expert Review of Ophthalmology, 18*, 379–389. https://www.semanticscholar.org/paper/8121a8aceee821223ef8d8c9f03bf0b912e84640 (accessed on 23 May 2025).

46. Tonni, G., Grisolia, G., Tonni, S., Lacerda, V. A., Ruano, R., & Sepulveda, W. (2024). Fetal face: Enhancing 3D ultrasound imaging by postprocessing with AI applications: Myth, reality, or legal concerns? *Journal of Clinical Ultrasound: JCU*. https://www.semanticscholar.org/paper/e21278e49cdd3b6d77c04b242d14a3458b5da189 (accessed on 23 May 2025).

47. Verhoef, L., Soloukey, S., Mastik, F., Generowicz, B. S., Bos, E. M., Schouten, J., Koekkoek, S., et al. (2025). Freehand ultrafast Doppler ultrasound imaging with optical tracking allows for detailed 3D reconstruction of blood flow in the human brain. *IEEE Transactions on Medical Imaging (in press)*. https://www.semanticscholar.org/paper/87a348d9bc57c87e90e81c30d3ff93c30d7d8145 (accessed on 23 May 2025).

48. Vetriselvi, D., & Thenmozhi, R. (2025). Prenatal diagnostics using deep learning: A dual approach to plane localization and cerebellum segmentation in ultrasound images. *Journal of Clinical Ultrasound (JCU)*. https://www.semanticscholar.org/paper/7dc5369a6319c2b6adf9d499fa2d5c9a09c6a1ea (accessed on 23 May 2025).

49. Wolder, D., Swat, A., Wolak, P., Zmelonek-Znamirowska, A., Białek, K., Rokita, W., Kaczmarek, P., et al. (2024). Enhanced diagnostic capabilities: Ultrasound imaging of fetal alimentary tract obstruction with advanced imaging technologies. *The American Journal of Case Reports, 25*, e943419-1–e943419-7. https://www.semanticscholar.org/paper/7545be3cecd451b530536e256bbe063f26abac18 (accessed on 23 May 2025).

50. Wu, W. T., Onishi, K., Mezian, K., Naňka, O., Wang, B., Su, D., Ricci, V., et al. (2024). Ultrasound imaging of the posterior lateral corner of the knee: A pictorial review of anatomy and pathologies. *Insights into Imaging, 15*. https://www.semanticscholar.org/paper/16de5332b3166d0aa224fd7fa34bc50bc5c9445c (accessed on 23 May 2025).

51. Yang, F., Mao, Q., Shi, M., Xie, F., & Cheng, K. (2024). Enhancing ultrasound imaging through convolutional neural networks: A health informatics approach. In A. Morales, J. Laparra, & J. Kalra (Eds.), *Health Informatics and Biomedical Engineering Applications. AHFE International Conference* (Vol. 142). AHFE Open Access. http://doi.org/10.54941/ahfe1005073.

52. Zhang, B., Liu, L., Meng, D., & Kue, C. (2024a). Medical imaging technology: Principles and systems. *INNOSC Theragnostic and Pharmacological Sciences*. https://www.semanticscholar.org/paper/292a65058f9459d7f883ae88d285cb8e5b82c439 (accessed on 23 May 2025).

53. Zhang, J. X., Li, L. F., Zhong, H. W., & Xiao, J. Y. (2024b). Miniaturized endoscopic probe for photoacoustic and ultrasound molecular imaging of deep tissues. *Acta Physica Sinica, 73*(21), 214203. https://doi.org/10.7498/aps.73.20241076.

54. Zhang, L., Du, W., Kim, J. H., Yu, C., & Dagdeviren, C. (2023). An emerging era: Conformable ultrasound electronics. *Advanced Materials, 36*. https://www.semanticscholar.org/paper/9539ee78c26ca6aa919c7efc7fc8ead2397e8cc7 (accessed on 23 May 2025).

55. Zhang, Q., Chen, J., Wang, J., Wang, H., He, Y., Li, B., Zhuang, Z., et al. (2025). Needle tracking and segmentation in breast ultrasound imaging based on spatio-temporal memory network. *Frontiers in Oncology, 14*. https://www.semanticscholar.org/paper/80bdcf9bd9019a734f1ee04b6b88073d6ef34e53 (accessed on 23 May 2025).

56. Zhang, R., Rabia'tul A'dawiah, Choo, T. W. J., Li, X., Balasundaram, G., Qi, Y., Goh, Y., et al. (2024c). Navigating challenges and solutions in quantitative photoacoustic imaging. *Applied Physics Reviews*. https://www.semanticscholar.org/paper/12692f76112c542ce2d358f282877effbb42100e (accessed on 23 May 2025).

57. Zotov, D., Dmitriev, K. V., & Rumyantseva, O. D. (2024). Reconstruction of sound speed and absorption coefficient of soft biological tissues by ultrasound tomography. *Journal of Physics: Conference Series, 2822*, 012002.

NUCLEAR MEDICINE IMAGING

6

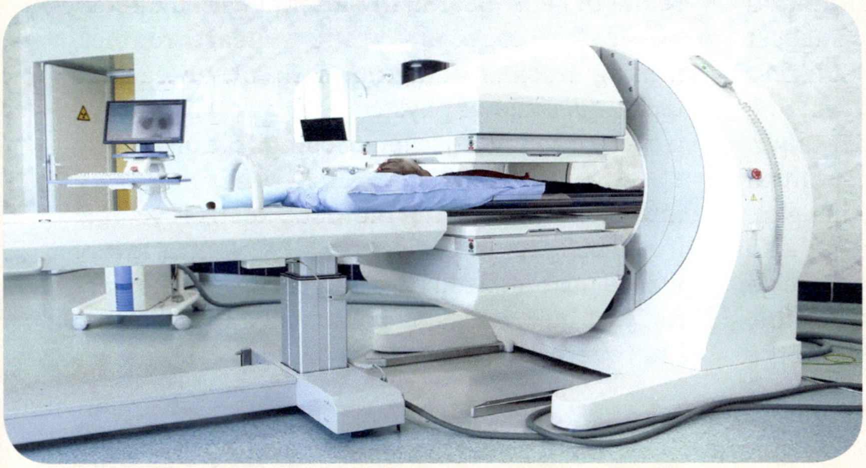

LEARNING OBJECTIVES

After studying this chapter, you will be able to:

1. Understand the principles of nuclear medicine.
2. Explore various imaging techniques used in nuclear medicine.
3. Examine the role of nuclear medicine in diagnostic procedures.
4. Identify the safety and regulations of nuclear medicine imaging.
5. Evaluate the advantages, challenges and limitations of nuclear medicine imaging.

Introduction

Imaging technology has come a long way, reshaping how we tackle medical diagnosis – and nuclear medicine imaging now plays a pretty central role. Instead of following a neat, step-by-step procedure, this approach uses small amounts of radioactive material to shed light on bodily functions in ways that traditional scans just can't. Researchers are, in many cases, mixing these time-tested methods with newer ideas like machine learning and AI, all aimed at boosting accuracy and speeding things up. When you start to understand what nuclear medicine imaging is about, you also begin to see its potential to change modern healthcare in a big way. In oncology, things get even more interesting. Nuclear medicine imaging isn't just an add-on; it has become a cornerstone for both diagnosing and planning treatments. PET and SPECT scans, for instance, give clinicians a peek at a tumor's metabolic activity, which often leads to earlier detection and better treatment options. The introduction of PSMA-based PET imaging has, generally speaking, improved early prostate cancer diagnosis quite a bit. Traditional imaging techniques seem to be getting combined with these emerging methods, nudging us toward a more personalized approach where each patient's treatment can be uniquely tailored. The latest twist involves deep learning algorithms that are reshaping how medical images are processed - from the moment they're captured to the automated diagnosis that follows. Recent studies suggest that these advanced techniques help address a range of challenges across different imaging modalities, often highlighting details that might slip by a human observer. Integrating artificial intelligence (AI) into nuclear medicine imaging not only ramps up speed and precision but also catches subtle anomalies that could otherwise go unnoticed. Overall, watching nuclear medicine, machine learning, and personalized care merge together offers an intriguing glimpse of where this innovative field is headed.

Definition of Nuclear Medicine Imaging

Radiopharmaceuticals let us peek into the body's inner workings in a way that mixes the fields of radiology and molecular biology. Doctors inject tiny amounts of radioactive material that give off gamma rays, and through techniques like PET and SPECT, images are produced that reflect how organs function rather than just showing us shapes and structures. This method, which is especially handy for identifying diseases early on, finds itself at the heart of diagnostics in areas such as oncology, cardiology, and neurology. It is pretty useful that these scans can also produce numerical data, helping to shape treatment choices and keep an eye on how therapies fare over time. Tech is never standing still, and in most cases, people are now looking at AI and machine learning to breathe new life into nuclear imaging. Recent studies suggest that smart algorithms can ease the burden on clinicians by automating parts of the interpretation process—even if, sometimes, the automation isn't perfect—and thereby reducing errors and speeding up diagnosis. Convolutional neural networks, for example, have shown a knack for spotting the subtle hints of disease that might slip by unnoticed with standard methods, boosting both the sensitivity and specificity of tests (Tapper et al., 2024). Beyond cancer, nuclear imaging is also proving its worth in the realm of heart health. In patients with diabetes, who can be especially prone to heart troubles, mixing nuclear imaging with other cardiac techniques allows physicians to discern between ischemic and non-ischemic complications pretty effectively (Wamil et al., 2022). Ongoing work into blending imaging methods keeps revealing fresh insights into disease, hinting at a future where personalized care and early detection are not just buzzwords but practical approaches to improve patient outcomes (Figure 6.1).

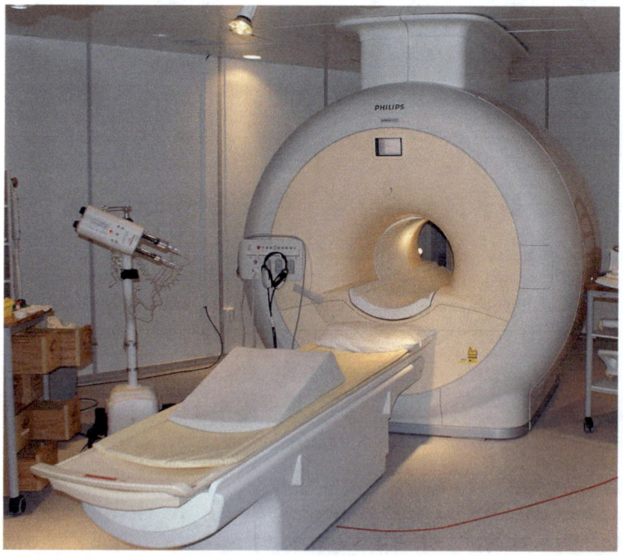

Figure 6.1. A patient having a nuclear medicine imaging scan after administration of radioactive tracer material.

Source: By Jan Ainali - Own work, CC BY 3.0, https://commons.wikimedia.org/w/index.php?curid=3546051.

Historical Development of Nuclear Medicine

Back in the mid-20th century, things started to change in how we peeked inside the human body. Nuclear medicine stepped into the spotlight with a breakthrough device—the Anger camera. It used sodium iodide crystals and photomultiplier tubes to capture images of radiopharmaceuticals, giving doctors clearer and more sensitive pictures. This clever bit of tech, almost by accident, opened the door for later tools like SPECT. SPECT, by tweaking collimator designs to catch photons at just the right angles, let clinicians observe lively biological processes as they happened. You could say its ripple effect stretched from heart check-ups to cancer scans, subtly reshaping patient care in ways that still matter today (Alqahtani, 2022). Soon enough, positron emission tomography (PET) waltzed onto the scene, blending the anatomical details from CT scans with the functional charm of PET imaging. In most cases, this mix allowed doctors to hit a level of diagnostic precision they hadn't seen before.

Techniques like absorption correction—and even time-of-flight (TOF) advancements—helped sharpen the images, making it easier to spot malignancies or metabolic oddities. This synergy also put a new spotlight on picking the right radiopharmaceuticals, an often underrated decision that turned out to be essential. In real terms, the combined PET/CT setup became a key player in exploring lung cancer, brain tumors, and a host of cardiovascular issues, firmly planting nuclear medicine in the landscape of modern healthcare (Alqahtani, 2022). On a more nuanced note, nuclear medicine didn't just focus on fancy images; it also began to probe the very roots of disease. Researchers gradually turned their attention to how conditions like atherosclerosis develop, with endothelial cell misbehavior emerging as a major factor in heart problems. As insights into cellular and molecular mechanics came to light, nuclear imaging began offering a window into vascular health. This blend of everyday clinical data with next-level imaging not only deepened our grasp of disease but also sparked fresh ideas for treatment. By linking signs of endothelial dysfunction with what the scans revealed, practitioners started spotting early warning signals and new approaches to therapy—an evolution that has, generally speaking, reshaped how cardiovascular issues are tackled today (Figure 6.2).

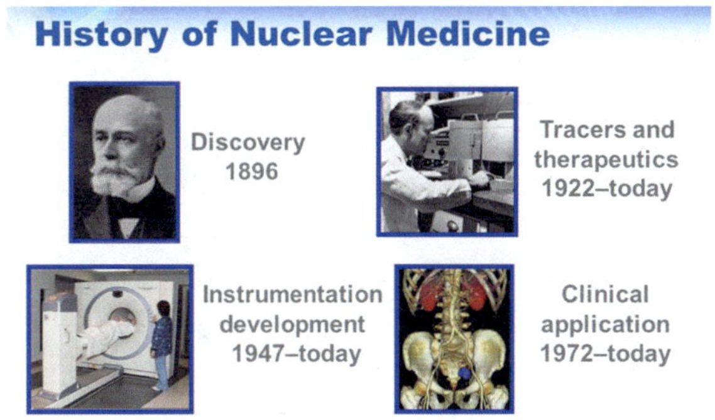

Figure 6.2. History of nuclear medicine.

Source: https://images.slideplayer.com/16/4883552/slides/slide_5.jpg.

Importance in Modern Medical Diagnostics

Nuclear medicine has reshaped medical diagnostics lately, thanks in large part to innovative radiopharmaceuticals. Gallium-68, for instance, is now the star of PET imaging—it is a fleeting positron emitter that comes off generator systems like 68Ge/68Ga and pops up all over clinical settings. It can be tagged with small molecules and peptides, which in most cases opens up targeted imaging routes for different diseases. This element not only sharpens diagnostic accuracy but also lays the foundation for combined imaging and treatment (theranostic) strategies, making its role in modern healthcare hard to overlook (Mehmonov et al., 2025). Scintillation crystals, on the other hand, are the unsung heroes behind many diagnostic tools. They're essential for detecting gamma-rays and bring about high-resolution images that clinicians rely on. Interestingly, between 1992 and 2022, research shows a big surge in patents for scintillation materials—with American companies leading the charge with a hefty number of patents. Whether we're talking about BGO, NaI or other variants, these materials keep evolving and, in most cases, not only boost current diagnostic methods but also set the stage for new applications. Their ongoing development underscores how vital scintillation technology is in today's diagnostic landscape (Danylenko et al., 2023). Beyond boosting accuracy in diagnoses, nuclear medicine imaging is stepping up the game in personalized care. It is now more about tailoring treatments to each patient—theranostics, for example, blends imaging with therapy to help manage diseases like cancer more effectively. With advanced imaging techniques, clinicians can closely monitor treatment responses and make timely adjustments, which is pretty crucial in our fast-evolving healthcare scene. Overall, nuclear medicine goes well past just spotting disease; it champions a more holistic approach to patient care that promises to shape the future of both diagnostics and treatment strategies across various health settings (Mehmonov et al., 2025).

6.1. Principles of Nuclear Medicine

Learning Outcome

1. Understand the basic concepts of radioactivity.
2. Discuss the types of radiopharmaceuticals.
3. Explain the mechanism of action in imaging.

Modern nuclear medicine depends on the interplay between imaging and patient diagnosis – a link that drives the field. Clinicians increasingly turn to various imaging methods, and at the heart of it all are radiotracers that emit bursts of radiation, which specialized cameras pick up so we can see what's happening inside. Techniques like PET and SPECT give us real-time images that reveal not only unusual areas but also how organs operate on the fly. Generally speaking, when you mix in advances in radiopharmaceuticals, you end up with a deeper, more molecular view of complex conditions; this change, in many cases, reinforces nuclear medicine's growing role in healthcare. It is not a neat, step-by-step process – the ideas jumble together, almost like a casual conversation about cutting-edge science. Step into nuclear medicine today and you'll notice that digital image processing makes a world of difference by boosting both clarity and meaning. The field has shifted away from old film techniques; now, digital methods easily kick aside issues like poor contrast or film that just can't keep up over time. For example, advanced algorithms handle noise reduction, rebuild images from scratch, and even switch between modalities in ways that help sharpen diagnostic outcomes. This digital transformation not only smooths out the everyday workflow but also gives radiologic technologists more room to get creative with complicated analyses, showing that nuclear medicine is always evolving (Seeram, 2018). Even if the changes seem subtle, they're changing the game in practical and surprising ways. On top of that, AI – with tools like generative adversarial networks (GANs) – is making its mark as a transformative force in imaging. These AI techniques bring fresh ideas like data augmentation, which thickens up training datasets that machine learning needs to work well. The fact that GANs can spin high-quality images from low-quality inputs is a real breakthrough, especially in de-noising steps that may help lower radiation exposure for patients. Moreover, these models assist with increasing image resolution and adapting visuals across different domains, addressing some of the inherent limits in certain imaging methods.

As these technologies continue evolving, they promise, in most cases, to broaden their reach in tackling complicated clinical puzzles and, by extension, solidify nuclear medicine's key role in precision diagnostics (Koshino et al., 2021).

6.1.1. Basic Concepts of Radioactivity

Grasping how radioactivity works is pretty important—it lays the groundwork for new advances in nuclear medicine imaging. At its core, radioactivity means that unstable atomic nuclei break down all on their own, releasing energy in forms like alpha particles, beta particles, and gamma rays. One way to keep track of this decay is by using half-lives, which tell us how long it takes for half of a radioactive sample to fade away. In nuclear medicine, having isotopes with well-known half-lives helps fine-tune imaging and treatment, so doctors can be more precise. For example, Technetium-99m often finds its way into diagnostic imaging because its short half-life and gamma ray output work well for methods like SPECT and PET imaging (Landsberger, 2006). Radiation's interaction with our tissues adds even more depth to its role in medical imaging. When radioactive isotopes are administered, they emit signals that external devices can detect, giving us a closer look at what's happening inside the body. Gamma cameras, for instance, pick up these emissions from radiopharmaceuticals—compounds that carry radioactive isotopes into patients—delivering detailed views of inner structures. This technique not only aids in diagnosing a range of diseases, cancer being a common one, but it also reveals functional activity within organs. Generally speaking, understanding how radiation mingles with human biology is key to making imaging safer; it helps us gauge potential risks like radiation sickness or, over the long haul, an increased chance of cancer from repeated exposure (Landsberger, 2006). Radioactivity isn't just a tool for diagnosis, though—it plays a huge part in treatments too. In targeted radiation therapy, radioisotopes are used to zap cancer cells while sparing as much normal tissue as possible, which is no easy feat. The success of these treatments depends on knowing the ins and outs of radioactivity, like dose rates and how different types of radiation affect biological tissues. In many cases, ongoing research into these effects drives improvements in therapy. Over time, a blend of imaging and treatment – often called theranostics – has come into play, allowing doctors to personalize a patient's treatment based on how their tumor lights up on scans. This mix shows just how tightly linked radioactivity is with nuclear medicine in boosting clinical outcomes and patient care (Kane, 2002) (Figure 6.3).

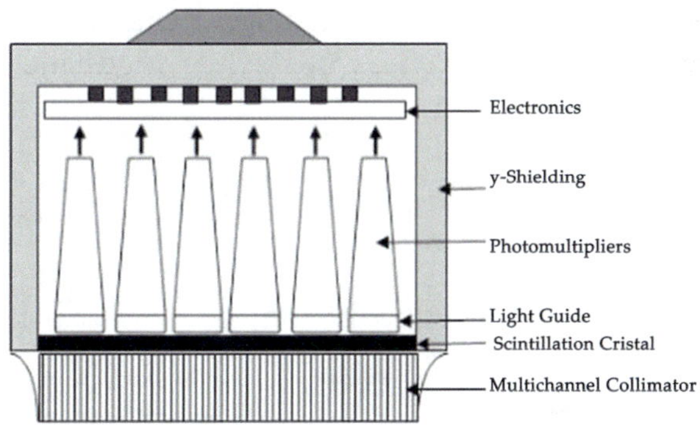

Figure 6.3. Main components of a gamma-camera.

Source: Kharfi F. Principles and Applications of Nuclear Medical Imaging: A Survey on Recent Developments [Internet]. Imaging and Radioanalytical Techniques in Interdisciplinary Research - Fundamentals and Cutting Edge Applications. InTech; 2013. Available from: http://dx.doi.org/10.5772/54884.

6.1.2. Types of Radiopharmaceuticals

Radiopharmaceuticals are at the heart of nuclear imaging. They help us see inside the body in ways that are both precise and versatile—often playing a dual role in diagnosing and even treating various conditions. For example, scans like PET and SPECT rely on compounds tagged with radioactivity that light up key biological processes in real time. Lately, improvements in these agents—especially in cancer care—have made it easier to catch metabolic signals that guide treatment decisions. New, sharper imaging compounds mean doctors can tailor approaches to each patient, generally leading to better outcomes. On the treatment side, radiopharmaceuticals don't just stop at giving us images. In targeted radionuclide therapy the same principles used for diagnosis are applied to deliver measured doses of radiation directly into tumors. For instance, radioligand therapy zooms in on specific biomarkers found in cancer cells, which helps focus the treatment while sparing most of the surrounding healthy tissue. There's also theranostics—a blend of imaging and therapy—that marks a shift toward more personalized care in nuclear medicine. In most cases, these methods, bolstered by insights from molecular imaging, are key in crafting treatment plans that address a patient's unique situation (Barca et al., 2021). Bone metastases, however, remain a particularly tough challenge. Nowadays, modern imaging techniques—like advanced PET/CT scans paired with novel radiolabeled agents—are changing how we spot and track these complications, especially in cancers such as breast and prostate. Guidelines from leading medical bodies usually stress the need for these cutting-edge modalities to stage and monitor metastasis accurately. While traditional methods had their merits, next-generation imaging now makes assessing treatment response and planning further steps much more effective. By embracing these breakthroughs, radiopharmaceuticals continue to play an indispensable role in managing the complex realities of metastatic disease, ultimately boosting the overall effectiveness of nuclear medicine imaging (Orcajo-Rincón et al., 2022) (Figure 6.4).

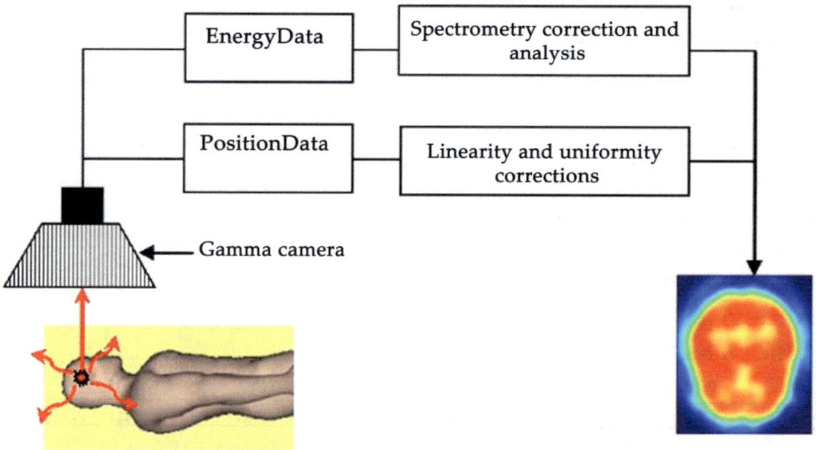

Figure 6.4. Illustration of data acquisition in planer gamma scintigraphy.

Source: Kharfi F. Principles and Applications of Nuclear Medical Imaging: A Survey on Recent Developments [Internet]. Imaging and Radioanalytical Techniques in Interdisciplinary Research - Fundamentals and Cutting Edge Applications. InTech; 2013.

6.1.3. Mechanism of Action in Imaging

Advanced imaging has changed nuclear medicine. Radiopharmaceuticals – those compounds that emit radiation and are picked up by specialized equipment – let doctors see what's happening on a tiny, molecular level inside the body. This fresh approach helps diagnose and track diseases by offering key insights into how tissues and organs work, especially regarding their metabolism.

For example, PET takes advantage of the natural decay in radiolabeled compounds to sketch out metabolic routes in issues like cancer or certain brain disorders. Such detailed imaging sharpens treatment choices, aligning therapies with the actual biological activity found in patients. In many cases, effective imaging forms the very backbone of nuclear medicine, directly influencing patient care with more tailored interventions. Diagnostic accuracy isn't the only win here—nuclear medicine's imaging tools also lean on basic principles that boost their usefulness. Think about it: localization, uptake, and clearance form the core ideas behind how radiopharmaceuticals behave in our tissues. Understanding these biological pathways is essential, since radiotracers tend to bind to specific receptors or enzymes, which often mirrors what's going wrong inside the body. For instance, using PET to look at the serotonin system is a huge help when assessing major depressive disorder, showing just how deep nuclear medicine can reach into understanding mental health. Ongoing advancements in imaging require continuous research and careful checks to set up baseline data that guide clinical interpretation, ensuring that results are as reliable as possible. This mix of tech and biology ups the impact of nuclear medicine imaging. As the field marches forward, innovative AI applications are promising to shake up how images are interpreted. Advanced algorithms now jump in to process complex imaging data, which not only boosts detection accuracy but also cuts down on delays in diagnosis. Take tumor detection in PET scans, for example – early evidence suggests AI can fine-tune this process, potentially reducing human mistakes linked to optimism bias in diagnostic reasoning (Forsting, 2017). Meanwhile, current studies are diving into how genetic differences mingle with imaging findings, narrowing the gap between molecular genetics and radiological assessments (Chen et al., 2016). Blending these new tech elements with traditional imaging keeps nuclear medicine at the cutting edge of clinical innovation, all in the service of smarter diagnostic moves and better treatment decisions for patients (Figure 6.5).

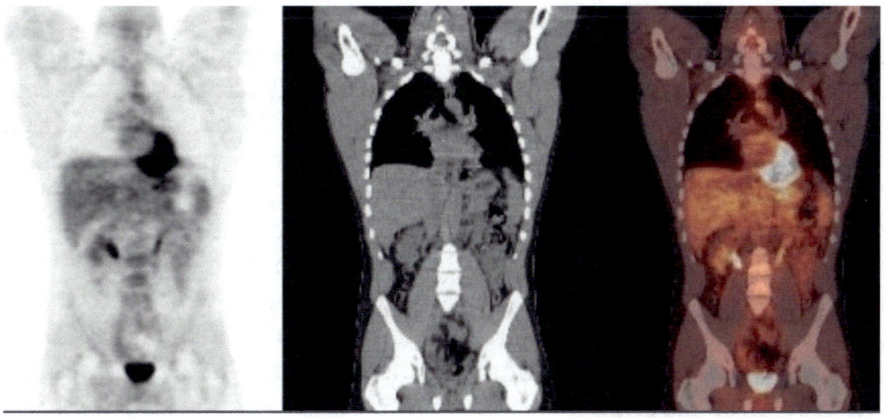

Figure 6.5. Mechanism of Action in Imaging

Source: https://stanfordhealthcare.org/medical-tests/n/nuclear-imaging/_jcr_content/tab-nav-component/tab-nav-parsys/imagewithcaption/image.img.full.high.jpg/1474753976313.jpg.

Test Your Knowledge

1. What are the basic concepts of radioactivity that are important for understanding nuclear medicine imaging?
2. What are radiopharmaceuticals, and how do different types serve specific diagnostic or therapeutic purposes?

6.2. Imaging Techniques

Learning Outcome

1. Understand the principles and clinical applications of positron emission tomography (PET).
2. Discuss about single photon emission computed tomography (SPECT).
3. Explain the hybrid imaging techniques.

Imaging in nuclear medicine goes far beyond simply spotting diseases—it drives how we manage and treat a whole range of conditions. Take radionuclide renal scintigraphy, for example; it is incredibly useful for collecting the functional data needed to diagnose problems with the kidneys, ureters, and bladder. Radiopharmaceuticals, picked to match various clinical needs, can yield several quantitative markers, and generally speaking, that lets the nuclear medicine team tailor protocols to address the specific clinical question at hand, boosting the accuracy of the renal study (Taylor, 2020). In essence, these techniques not only help identify issues but also play a key role in guiding treatment decisions. Bone scintigraphy, meanwhile, stands out as a go-to test for screening suspected bone metastases, thanks to its sensitivity, ready availability, and cost-effectiveness. Its roots date back to early radionuclide experiments, when researchers were just beginning to explore skeletal imaging, and over time it has become a trusted standard for identifying skeletal metastatic disease. Initial studies using isotopes—first experiments with 32phosphorus (32P) and later with 99mTc-labeled compounds—gave pretty valuable insight into skeletal metabolism and pathophysiology. With continuing improvements in gamma camera tech and the jump to modalities like SPECT, bone scintigraphy's usefulness has only grown. Even though modern cross-sectional imaging techniques like computed tomography (CT) and magnetic resonance imaging (MRI) have come a long way, nuclear medicine still holds a strong, significant role in evaluating complex skeletal disorders (Gnanasegaran et al., 2020). On top of the traditional agents, PET has been gaining traction for more focused investigations of bone diseases. When PET is teamed with specific tracers, it often offers enhanced visualization—especially in detecting bone metastases where older methods sometimes fall short. As this field continues to evolve, blending PET with well-established nuclear practices tends to raise diagnostic accuracy, offering functional insights that might be missed by anatomical imaging alone. This expanding mix of imaging options, in many cases, gives healthcare providers the flexibility to pick the method best suited to each patient's unique set of clinical needs. Consequently, with advances in radiopharmaceuticals and imaging technology continuing at a rapid pace, nuclear medicine remains a dynamic and essential part of modern diagnostic and therapeutic strategies.

6.2.1. Positron Emission Tomography (PET)

Imaging technology has changed the game in medicine; it's not just about looking at structures anymore. PET, or Positron Emission Tomography, jumps out as a tool that gives us clear, 3D images of the body's active processes—almost like peeking into cells. Regular scans usually stick to anatomy, but PET shows us the inner chemical buzz, which, in most cases, helps spot tumors early and gauge treatment responses in oncology. As medical practice evolves, adding PET to everyday diagnostics underlines how important it is to check body functions rather than just shapes. Digging a bit deeper, PET works by using radiopharmaceuticals— molecules with a bit of radioactive label that emit positrons. When these compounds enter the body, they tend to gather in spots where metabolism is high, such as in cancer areas. Once positrons meet electrons, gamma rays pop out; these are then picked up by the scanner to build detailed pictures. Often, this sharp imaging helps not only with identifying cancers but also with exploring conditions like neurodegenerative issues or heart problems. Generally speaking, this ability to notice changes in function before any visible structure shifts is a big deal for early diagnosis and tailoring personalized treatments in nuclear medicine. Researchers have been looking into various radiopharmaceuticals and their benefits, as seen in recent literature (Park et al., 2024). Interestingly enough, PET's reach extends beyond human medicine into areas like veterinary care, especially with horses. It has been shown to offer high-resolution views of a horse's lower limb—vital for pinpointing lameness or subtle injuries that might slip by on regular X-rays. Sure, scintigraphy is still common for whole-body scans in horses, but PET can detect injuries sooner and with more precision. This knack for telling apart fresh injuries from old scars adds a nice layer of detail when planning treatments in vet practice. As the field moves forward, blending PET with other imaging methods in a multi-modal approach looks set to boost diagnostic accuracy and improve outcomes for people and animals alike (Spriet et al., 2024) (Figure 6.6).

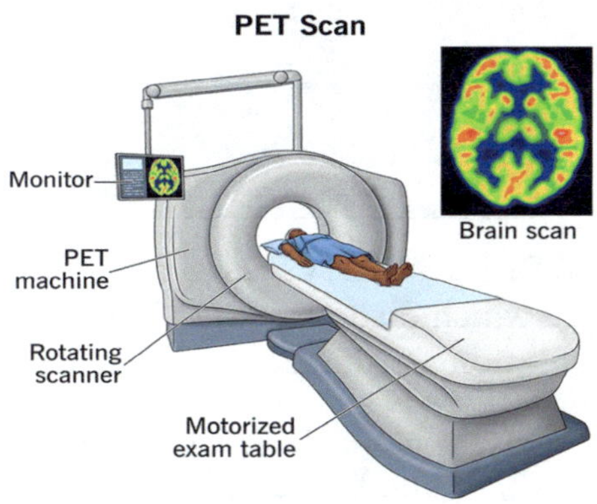

Figure 6.6. A positron emission tomography (PET) scan uses a safe injectable radioactive chemical called a radiotracer and a device called a PET scanner to show images of your organs and tissues at work.

Source: https://my.clevelandclinic.org/health/diagnostics/10123-pet-scan.

6.2.2. Single Photon Emission Computed Tomography (SPECT)

Doctors these days benefit from new imaging breakthroughs that let them pick up all sorts of diseases. There's SPECT—which is fast becoming a go-to method in nuclear medicine. It uses radiopharmaceuticals that emit gamma rays to give a pretty detailed look at organ work and tissue metabolism. This non-invasive method helps in flagging conditions like cancers and inflammatory diseases, issues that used to be quite a headache for diagnosis and treatment. In most cases, by making disease detection more spot-on, SPECT also helps pave the way for targeted treatments like theranostics, offering care plans tailored to each patient's needs (Kaur et al., 2020). When you compare SPECT with older imaging techniques like PET, its evolution is hard to miss. Traditional SPECT systems – those that rely on collimated cameras – run into problems with detection efficiency and spatial resolution. Still, new ideas such as Compton cameras are being checked out to overcome these limits. These advanced detectors can boost imaging quality by sharpening energy resolution and even letting clinicians use higher-energy radioisotopes, something the older systems often can't handle very well. Several studies (Fontana et al., 2017) show that these fresh approaches lead to noticeably better detection efficiency, improved spatial detail, and overall stronger diagnostic capability. Generally speaking, this progress underscores why ongoing research in nuclear medicine imaging remains so important. On the treatment front, SPECT isn't just about diagnosing—it is crucial for treatment planning, too. By capturing dynamic images of live biological processes, SPECT lets doctors monitor therapeutic responses almost in real time, so they can tweak treatment protocols as needed. This near-immediate feedback is key for managing complex cases, whether it is fighting various cancers or handling cardiovascular issues. As SPECT keeps merging improved imaging techniques with better radiopharmaceuticals, it promises not only higher diagnostic accuracy but also better treatment results. All of this points to an evolving approach in nuclear medicine that puts the patient first and relies on solid, evidence-based care—which firmly cements SPECT's role as a modern imaging cornerstone (Kaur et al., 2020) (Figure 6.7).

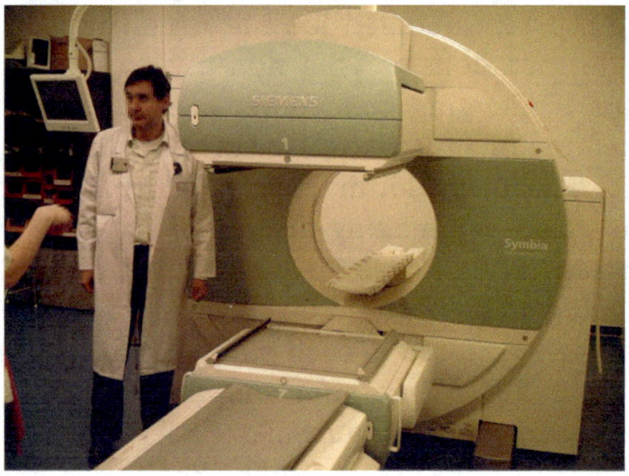

Figure 6.7. Single photon emission computed tomography (SPECT) scan.

Source: By Jejecam - Own work, CC BY-SA 3.0, https://commons.wikimedia.org/w/index.php?curid=8398156.

6.2.3. Hybrid Imaging Techniques

Various imaging techniques are merging in ways that are reshaping nuclear medicine—making diagnoses sharper and treatment plans more on point. Take PET-CT, for example; it ties together functional insights with anatomical sketches in a way that not only brings cellular details into focus but also paints an overall picture of the body. You see, this mix-up isn't just about pretty images—it is also about making sense of complex processes, whether in oncology, cardiology, neurology, or other domains. Yet, one must note that these cutting-edge systems, for reasons like tight budgets, lacking infrastructure, and even the availability of radiopharmaceuticals, often don't reach low-resource places such as Bangladesh, underscoring a noticeable gap in global healthcare access (Das et al., 2025). When we look at how hybrid imaging is used clinically, the benefits seem clear in guidelines and expert tips, especially in cardiovascular cases. A recent literature review brought forward a multitude of recommendations for options like SPECT(/CT), PET(/CT), and PET(/MRI)—each playing a role in early diagnosis and later treatment checks. Still, the review also flagged some real issues: only about 7.9% of these guidelines lean on systematic reviews, and nearly a quarter offer no solid evidence at all. Generally speaking, this patchiness in how these recommendations are set up complicates their everyday use, which then ripples out to impact patient outcomes (Besson et al., 2024).

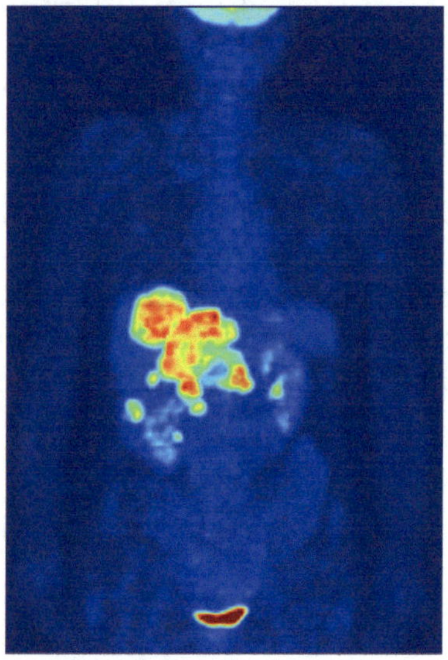

Figure 6.8. FDG-PET/CT is a hybrid imaging technique which fuses functional PET data with high-resolution CT datasets.

Source: By Jens Maus (https://jens-maus.de/) - Own work, Public Domain, https://commons.wikimedia.org/w/index.php?curid=801896.

Looking ahead, emerging tech in hybrid imaging might well upend the future of nuclear medicine. Advancements keep cropping up, with interconnected systems easing the capture and reading of images, which in turn pumps up diagnostic accuracy. There's also a growing buzz about AI and machine learning—their entry into hybrid imaging is promising, as they pave the way for automated analyses and even lend a hand in clinicians' decision-making. In most cases, it is now crucial to ensure that our evidence-based guidelines evolve alongside these new tools so that hybrid imaging can be maximized across different clinical settings. Balancing tech innovation with the bedrock principles of evidence-based care is clearly vital to driving the continued growth of nuclear medicine imaging—and ultimately, to boosting patient care and outcomes (Besson et al., 2024) (Figure 6.8).

Test Your Knowledge

1. What is the key difference between Positron Emission Tomography (PET) and Single Photon Emission Computed Tomography (SPECT) in terms of imaging technique and tracer use?
2. How are PET and SPECT used to detect and monitor diseases such as cancer and neurological disorders?

6.3. Applications in Diagnosis

Learning Outcome

1. Explore using nuclear medicine imaging in cancer detection and monitoring.
2. Understand the application of nuclear imaging techniques in evaluating cardiovascular conditions.
3. Examine the role of nuclear medicine in Neurological Disorders Assessment.

Nuclear imaging has shaken up how we tackle cancer diagnoses, especially in issues in women's reproductive systems. Endometrial and ovarian cancers can be pretty tricky because their locations are complex and tumors sometimes progress unusually fast. A PET scan using fluorine-18 fluorodeoxyglucose (18F-FDG PET) is often employed to check both how tissues use energy and what the anatomy looks like, which usually bumps up the accuracy of early stage assessments and lymph node evaluations. When this scan is paired with CT or MRI, the details become even clearer—helping doctors decide on better ways to treat patients. Lymphoscintigraphy with technetium 99m radiotracers has also come to the forefront, offering a smart way to pinpoint sentinel lymph nodes; this technique can reduce the need for bigger, more invasive node dissections, ultimately leading to improved outcomes (Khessib et al., 2024). Nuclear imaging isn't just confined to cancer care, either. It has become a critical tool in understanding and managing strokes. Despite many advancements in stroke treatment, getting a quick and accurate diagnosis often remains a challenge. In most cases, these imaging methods can separate real cases of ischemia from other stroke-like conditions. Radiopharmaceutical tracers—which have generally proven useful in rapidly determining the type of stroke—play a crucial role when every minute counts. Mobile stroke units even have started to integrate nuclear imaging techniques to help cut down delays in care.

Blending approaches like SPECT with MRI gives doctors a more in-depth look at both blood flow and the tissue's metabolic activity, thus fostering a broader understanding of how the brain is affected during a stroke (Azhari, 2024). This mix of techniques highlights how central advanced imaging has become in modern medicine's approach to stroke management. Beyond just diagnostics, nuclear imaging now bridges into therapeutic areas as well, giving patients a more personalized treatment journey. Its double-edged ability lets clinicians not only see what's going wrong but also directly tailor therapies. In the realm of gynecologic cancers, emerging theragnostic agents are identifying a lot of attention; these agents help in both locating problematic tissues and then targeting them specifically, which might be especially promising for patients with advanced or recurring disease. The process relies on detecting particular radiotracer uptakes within tumors and then using that information to guide treatment choices.

Likewise, in stroke care, new radiotracers are being experimented with to zero in on areas with impaired blood flow and metabolic disturbances—even though results can sometimes be a bit surprising. By merging diagnostic findings with targeted treatments, nuclear medicine finds itself at a pivotal junction in today's patient-centered care—where imaging and treatment are woven together to improve overall outcomes (Azhari, 2024; Khessib et al., 2024).

6.3.1. Cancer Detection and Monitoring

Cancer detection and ongoing monitoring isn't simple these days; imaging techniques have come a long way and play an ever more important role in everyday clinical settings. Since more types of cancer seem to be emerging, identifying them as early as possible is vital for better patient outcomes. Nuclear medicine imaging, in many cases, has become a key player for tracking disease progression and checking how treatments are doing. Tools like PET and single-photon emission computed tomography (SPECT) give us a unique window into tumor behavior—they show us metabolic activity in a way traditional scans might not, often highlighting malignancies that could otherwise be missed.

This deeper look into cancer helps doctors decide on timely interventions that, in most cases, can affect survival rates. AI, especially deep learning algorithms, has also been shaking up the field of cancer imaging. These algorithms sift through enormous amounts of data from different imaging methods to sharpen diagnoses and cut down on human mistakes. One review even notes AI's role in breast cancer imaging, showing how deep learning helps with lesion classification and risk prediction in breast cancer detection and monitoring (Balkenende et al., 2022). Even though these new tech capabilities seem promising, more extensive studies are generally needed to see how well they work across all imaging types, nuclear medicine included. As AI continues to merge with everyday clinical routines, there are naturally some questions about regulatory standards, legal matters, and ethical concerns that need careful checking. Beyond the leaps in imaging technology, there's still a strong need to nail down standard methods for spotting complications like bone metastases. Early detection of these secondary issues is pretty much essential not just for boosting survival but also for improving patients' quality of life overall. Most experts tend to agree that next-generation techniques—think whole-body diffusion-weighted MRI and PET/CT—should be put before older methods when monitoring metastases for breast and prostate cancers (Rincón et al., 2022). Getting ahead of these problems with early intervention usually paves the way for better management strategies that lessen skeletal-related issues. And as researchers keep exploring fresh ways to detect and monitor these challenges, combining nuclear medicine imaging with advanced technologies should ultimately strengthen the overall approach to cancer care (Figure 6.9).

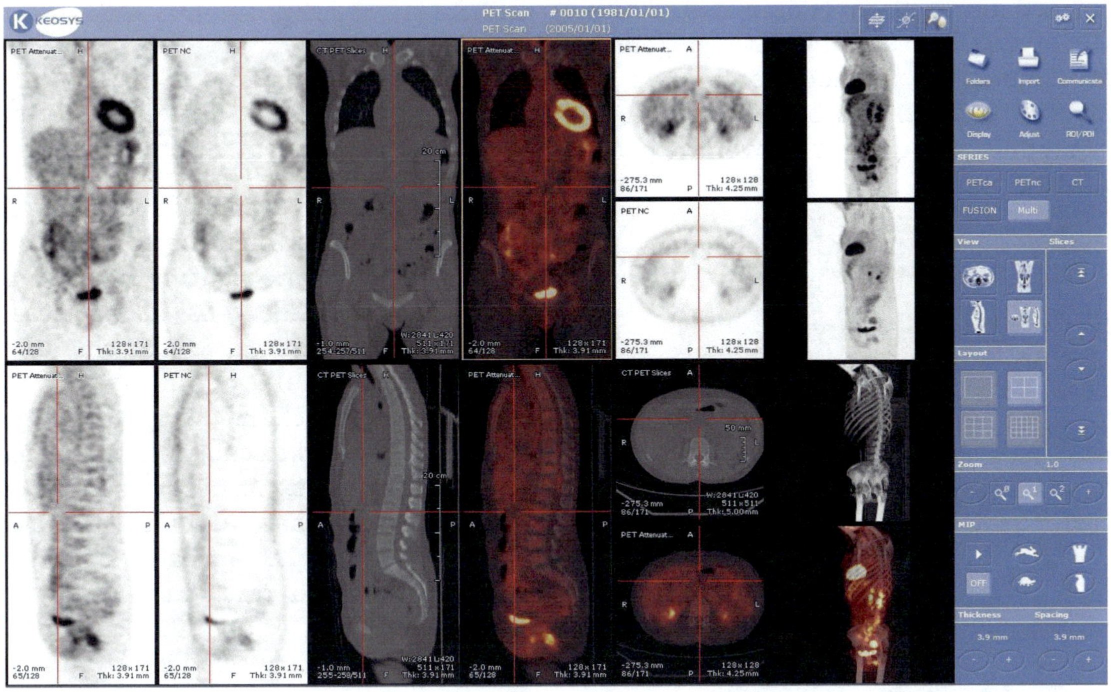

Figure 6.9. Fused CT-PET scans more clearly show tumors and are therefore often used to diagnose and monitor the growth of cancerous tumors.

Source: By Mco44 - Own work, Public Domain, https://commons.wikimedia.org/w/index.php?curid=3732977.

6.3.2. Cardiovascular Imaging

Nuclear medicine breakthroughs have shaken up how we view heart conditions. Ischemic heart disease keeps rising around the world, and imaging now plays a key, almost frontline role in spotting areas with weak blood flow, especially when using myocardial perfusion imaging (MPI). In most cases, a better grasp of heart problems has come along with new imaging tools—tools that let doctors see things in a more down-to-earth, detailed way. These improvements, blending with older techniques, change how we pin down heart issues and tweak patient treatment plans. AI is now mixing things up in nuclear medicine too. Smart algorithms, including deep learning and other machine learning methods, now dig into loads of data from different scans, MPI included, to sort out details that might elude us otherwise. Generally speaking, these AI tricks help in reducing the time spent on image processing while keeping diagnoses on track, especially for patients with coronary artery disease (CAD). It is like a fresh, innovative twist that not only sharpens our diagnostic tools but also nudges nuclear medicine and AI closer together—each adding its own flavor to patient care in cardiovascular disease. Doctors usually rely on a mix of imaging techniques to get the full picture of a heart's health, and no single method tells the whole story. Often, an echocardiogram kicks things off, and then nuclear medicine—thanks to its knack for capturing blood flow and viability—fills in those finer details. Cardiac computed tomography and cardiovascular magnetic resonance (CMR) join the conversation too, especially when dealing with tough cases such as in Marfan syndrome. In most cases, this kind of multi-pronged approach leads to a more complete diagnosis and quicker, well-informed interventions (Golub et al., 2025; Perrone et al., 2025). Overall, by tossing together a variety of imaging methods, our grasp of cardiovascular complexities becomes richer—even if sometimes it feels a bit all over the place (Figure 6.10).

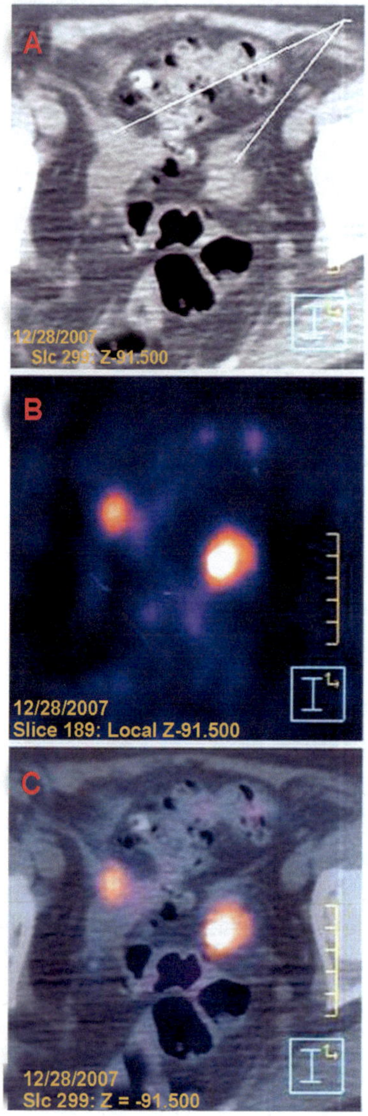

Figure 6.10. Imaging.

Source: By Renato M.E. Sabbatini, PhD - http://en.wikipedia.org/wiki/Image:Pet-ct-images.jpg, CC BY 3.0, https://commons.wikimedia.org/w/index.php?curid=5008797.

6.3.3. Neurological Disorders Assessment

Imaging tech has come a long way and changed how we look at neurological disorders. Take sodium MRI as an example—this method, which picks up on changes in cell sodium levels, taps into the idea that when the sodium-potassium pump doesn't work right, it leads to a build-up of sodium inside cells. In most cases, this tweak in sodium balance is a clue to various brain ailments like epilepsy or multiple sclerosis. Researchers, using single quantum images at different echo times, have managed to spot differences in decay rates (mono and biexponential) that bump up the ability of sodium MRI to pick up early signs of neural degeneration and track how well treatment is working (Qian et al., 2024). Another angle comes from nuclear medicine imaging, with PET leading the charge. Generally speaking, PET has been a rock-solid tool in brain research for years, especially now with advanced multiring systems offering high-res, 3D views.

Even though it sometimes struggles with spatial resolution and sensitivity, its knack for identifying real-time changes in brain function is nothing short of invaluable. When you mix PET with structural scans like CT or MRI, you get a more precise picture—this merge helps link metabolic markers with anatomical uniqueness, which is key for conditions like Alzheimer's or even spotting tumors; it's all about getting a clearer diagnosis and better therapy planning (Heiss, 2016). More recently, simultaneous PET/MRI acquisition has opened up a whole new approach. This method lets doctors gather functional and structural details at the same time, which helps dodge the mix-ups that can happen when scans are taken one after the other. Beyond just saving time, this combined technique makes it easier to figure out the exact spot of trouble—say in cases of focal epilepsy—by offering a sharper look at lesions and treatment responses. In most cases, this richer, intertwined data gives us a better grasp on what's going on inside the brain, ultimately paving the way for more tailored and effective interventions (Heiss, 2016) (Figure 6.11).

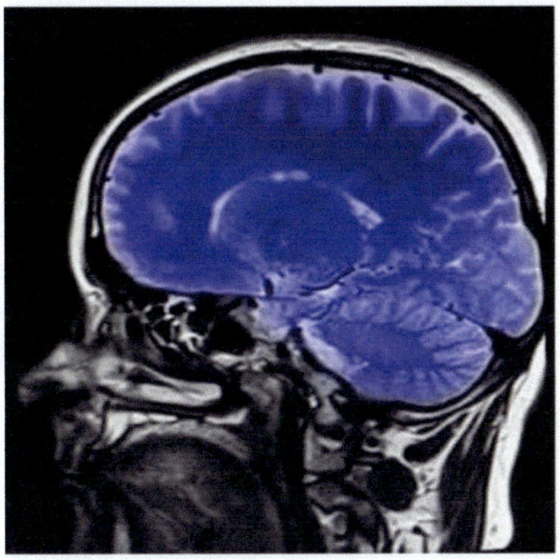

Figure 6.11. Imaging tech has come a long way and changed how we look at neurological disorders.

Source: https://openmedscience.com/nuclear-neurology-a-significant-advancement-to-diagnose-brain-disorders/.

Test Your Knowledge

1. How is nuclear imaging used to diagnose conditions such as cancer, heart disease, and thyroid disorders?
2. What role does nuclear imaging play in assessing organ function and detecting abnormalities at an early stage?

6.4. Safety and Regulations

Learning Outcome

1. Understand the radiation safety protocols.
2. Explain the regulatory bodies and guidelines.
3. Define patient consent and ethical considerations.

Nuclear medicine deals with plenty of built-in risks, so clear safety rules become a must. These guidelines aren't just about looking out for patients—they also help guard healthcare staff and our environment. International groups like the IAEA have long pressed that sticking to these safety practices is key to keeping harmful radiation effects at bay. Hospitals, for example, run regular audits; these little checks help build a safety-first vibe by showing how closely the protocols are followed, spurring ongoing improvements in nuclear imaging practice (Giammarile et al., 2024). When people talk about nuclear medicine, they sometimes mix up its benefits with the hazards. Many misunderstandings crop up, which is why having a firm grasp of safety rules, as discussed in current literature, is so important. Sure, nuclear medicine has seriously transformed how we diagnose diseases, but it also calls for strict safety measures to keep patients from unnecessary radiation exposure. This blend of pros and cons naturally sparks debates about ethics and the need for good patient education.

Repeating these points helps professionals explain to patients and their families why following the safety protocols is so essential (Othman et al., 2024). Looking back at the progress in safety measures, it is clear that the field has come a long way—both in technology and in everyday practice. Regulatory bodies keep tweaking the rules as fresh innovations improve imaging precision and put patient safety first, which, in most cases, shows a collective commitment to top-notch care driven by both ethical and scientific concerns. International collaborations, where experts share best practices and insights, further ensure that everyone stays up-to-date with changing rules and emerging technology. Mixing these guidelines into everyday routines creates a safety-first atmosphere that naturally cuts down on the risks linked with nuclear imaging (Giammarile et al., 2024). This ongoing back-and-forth between new ideas and established rules is a key factor in moving nuclear medicine forward while keeping health outcomes secure (Figure 6.12).

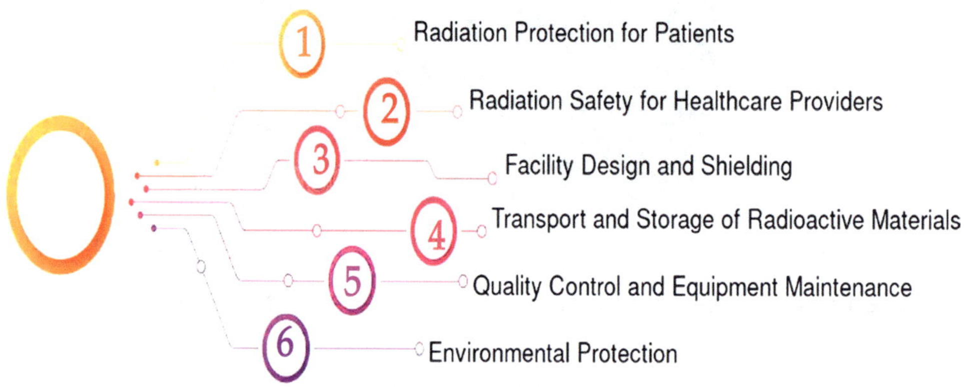
1
Radiation Protection for Patients
2
Radiation Safety for Healthcare Providers
3
Facility Design and Shielding
4
Transport and Storage of Radioactive Materials
5
Quality Control and Equipment Maintenance
6
Environmental Protection

Figure 6.12. Safety issues.

Source: https://fastercapital.com/topics/nuclear-medicine-equipment.html.

6.4.1. Radiation Safety Protocols

Nuclear medicine imaging puts patient and staff safety first – a fact that's hard to overstate. The idea behind it is pretty simple: follow the ALARA principle, meaning keep radiation exposure as low as possible while still getting clear diagnostic images. In practice, that means carefully planning each step so only the needed amount of radioactive material is used. Training sessions are held regularly, too, so everyone stays on top of what to do if something goes awry. Hospitals also check their own rules from time to time, making sure they're in line with guidelines, which becomes extra important during high-pressure moments like echocardiography in crises such as COVID-19 (Kirkpatrick et al., 2020).

Another big piece of the puzzle is using personal protective equipment (PPE) – and this isn't just a box to tick. Depending on the situation, whether you're talking gloves, surgical masks, or even those high-tech air-purifying respirators, the gear is picked based on how risky the procedure might be. For example, some procedures – say, transesophageal echocardiography – can kick up more airborne particles, meaning stricter airborne precautions are needed. With guidelines constantly shifting and resource issues cropping up, keeping everyone in the loop is key. When the team understands the specific risks of a procedure, it not only safeguards the healthcare workers but also builds a trust with patients that things are being done right. Listening to the latest expert opinions helps merge official protocols with what's happening on the ground, ultimately boosting patient care (Turner, 2018). Keeping track of radiation exposure through proper documentation isn't just paperwork – it builds a safety culture in imaging departments. Detailed records let staff spot exposure trends over time and adjust procedures when needed. This number-driven method often highlights why ongoing improvements in safety practices are so crucial for protecting both patients and workers. It also opens the door for more honest conversations about risks and the best ways to tackle them. Sometimes a bit of extra training goes a long way in showing everyone why following safety rules matters. And as new imaging innovations roll out, staying alert and ready to update safety measures ensures that accurate diagnoses go hand in hand with protecting both patients and staff (Kirkpatrick et al., 2020) (Figure 6.13).

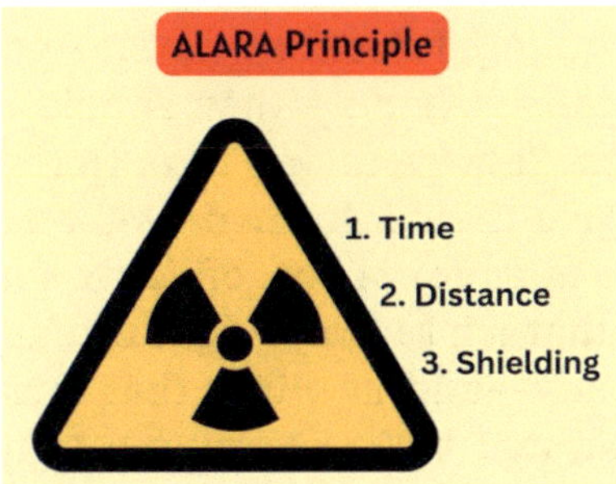

Figure 6.13. ALARA principle radiation protection.

Source: https://i.pinimg.com/736x/3a/21/4f/3a214f487d0fa186d449ed81c43ba7d3.jpg.

6.4.2. Regulatory Bodies and Guidelines

In the realm of nuclear medicine imaging, having a set of well-thought-out guidelines from regulatory groups is key to keeping practices safe and effective. It's not just theoretical – agencies like the American Association of Physicists in Medicine (AAPM) are central to offering clear advice that everyday medical physicists lean on when they work with radiation. The AAPM updates its practice recommendations roughly every five years, which kind of shows they're serious about keeping up with new developments and ensuring professionals always have fresh know-how. By stressing the need for proper training and essential skills, these guidelines (yep, even if repeated at times) aim to set a more consistent standard that boosts patient care and builds public confidence across the States. Nuclear medicine isn't static these days; things are shifting as theranostics—a mix of diagnostics and therapy—makes its mark.

The International Atomic Energy Agency (IAEA) noticed early on that specialists need more than basic training to handle these new techniques. In 2023, a consultancy meeting sparked the creation of a harmonized training program intended to ensure a level of global proficiency in theranostics. This initiative lays out straightforward guiding ideas that back both high-quality imaging and treatment methods while also making sure practitioners come away with the right set of know-how, ultimately helping to smooth out global variations in practice. Getting these guidelines to work in the real world calls for genuine teamwork among regulatory bodies and educational institutions. As the field morphs with rapid changes in healthcare technology, blending insights from groups like the AAPM and IAEA becomes pretty essential to keeping nuclear imaging at a high standard. They offer more than just a checklist – they create a conversation space where professionals can keep tinkering with best practices (and maybe even throwing in a few grammatical uniqueness along the way). By following these recommendations, nuclear medicine experts can sharpen their quality checks and stick closer to safety protocols, ultimately shaping a future in which patient care remains the top priority (Figure 6.14).

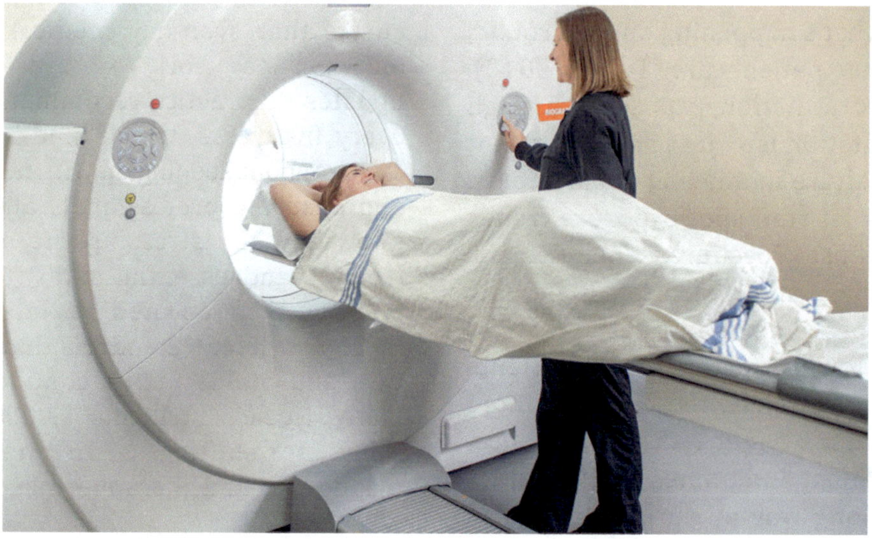

Figure 6.14. In the realm of nuclear medicine imaging, having a set of well-thought-out guidelines from regulatory groups is key to keeping practices safe and effective.

Source: https://cdn.pharmiweb.com/media/18818/nuclear-medicine-market.jpg.

6.4.3. Patient Consent and Ethical Considerations

In nuclear medicine imaging, getting a patient's okay is everything. Patients who face procedures with radioactive substances need to have all the relevant details at hand – they should know the risks as well as the benefits. Clear talk helps them grasp what they're diving into. Rules ask that before any procedure involving ionizing radiation, patients give their informed nod, and in most cases, that's non-negotiable. The mix of patient rights and the need for sharp, effective diagnostics often forces healthcare individuals into a balancing act, one that isn't always neat or easy. This is why building a system where patients are educated consistently—and in a way that invites open, ongoing dialogue—becomes a must. Ethical worries aren't limited to just getting a signature on a form. Patients might wonder about long-term issues when nuclear medicine steps in, especially among groups like pregnant women or little ones. healthcare providers must sit down and chat about these ethical puzzles, not just count the immediate imaging upsides but also consider the lingering uncertainties tied to radiation exposure. In many cases, the promise of precision medicine comes into the picture here. By tailoring choices to individual situations, providers aim to get the best outcomes possible. New guidelines from different health bodies even suggest adding thorough risk checks into the consent conversation (Vlachothanasi, 2024). Recent shifts in the way we train medical professionals show that ethical thinking and patient consent are central to what they learn. Training now frequently mixes simulation-based drills that tackle tricky ethical choices in emergency and nuclear medicine settings. These efforts not only sharpen clinical abilities but also underline why knowing how to talk with patients matters so much. Studies have pointed out that residents differ widely in handling ethical issues—so, continuous education (and a bit of self-checking) becomes key. Simulation exercises, for instance, give new practitioners a chance to face ethical dilemmas in a hands-on way, promoting a kind of everyday ethical alertness in nuclear medicine imaging. This overall strategy isn't merely about dumping facts; it is designed to pull healthcare teams into a lively, ongoing conversation about best practices and the ethical standards they need to live up to (Aydin, 2024) (Figure 6.15).

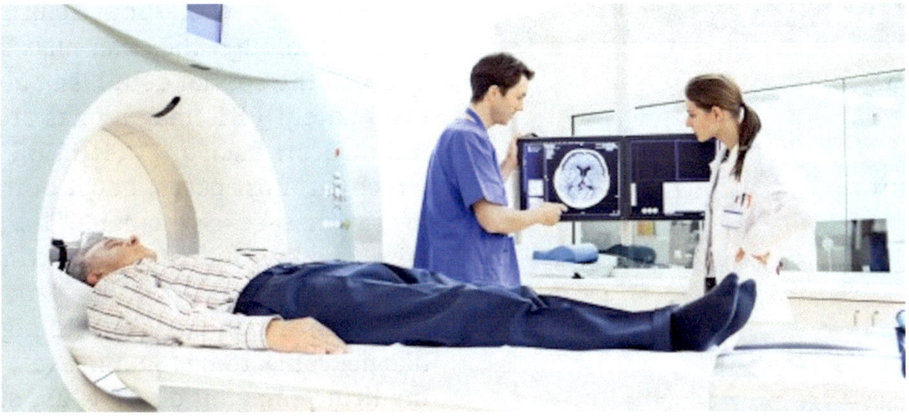

Figure 6.15. Patient Consent.

Source: https://d3njjcbhbojbot.cloudfront.net/api/utilities/v1/imageproxy/https://images.ctfassets.net/wp1lcwdav1p1/aVZqx6vjvCOUG2bqpLJy1/b3aa51304f2dca2d11d927d02e8ccade/GettyImages-155539853.jpg?w=1500&h=680&q=60&fit=fill&f=faces&fm=jpg&fl=progressive&auto=format%2Ccompress&dpr=1&w=1000.

t

Test Your Knowledge

1. What are some key radiation safety protocols followed in nuclear medicine to protect patients and healthcare workers?
2. Which regulatory bodies oversee using radioactive materials in medical imaging, and what guidelines do they provide?

6.5. Advantages, Challenges and Limitations of Nuclear Medicine Imaging

Learning Outcome

1. Identify and evaluate the key advantages of nuclear medicine imaging in clinical diagnostics.
2. Analyze the challenges and limitations associated with nuclear medicine imaging.

6.5.1. Advantages of Nuclear Medicine Imaging

Advanced imaging techniques have changed how doctors diagnose and track different cancers. For example, in neuroblastoma, about 50% of patients already show signs of metastasis at diagnosis, making nuclear medicine not just helpful but absolutely essential. Traditional methods like meta-[123I]iodobenzylguanidine ([123I]mIBG) whole-body scintigraphy are still in play, although they can miss smaller lesions because the spatial detail isn't always up to the task. Lately, PET imaging has stepped in using radiotracers such as [124I]mIBG and [18F]FDG, which, in most cases, boost both accuracy and overall disease assessment. This progress helps with staging and quickly setting up targeted treatment plans, which proves especially important when dealing with high-risk cancers like neuroblastoma (Samim et al., 2021). Nuclear medicine imaging doesn't just stop at refining diagnosis—it also plays a big role in identifying and monitoring breast cancer. In the United States, roughly one in eight women faces breast cancer, and mixing nuclear imaging with other techniques has improved early detection.

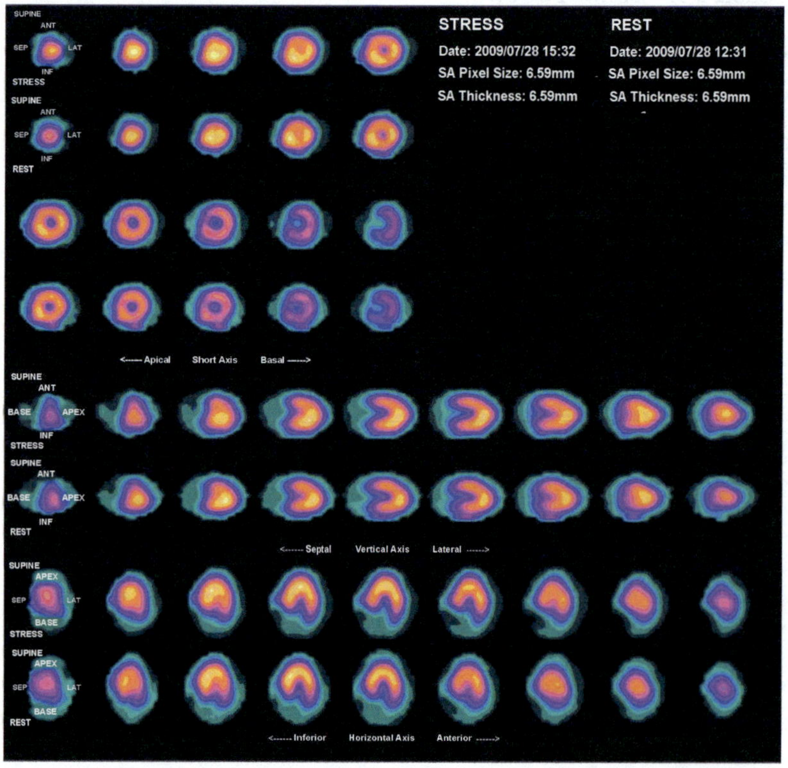

Figure 6.16. The advantages of nuclear medicine.

Source: CC BY 3.0, https://commons.wikimedia.org/w/index.php?curid=116435073.

Radiotracers add extra sensitivity and specificity, meaning that even those smaller spots a typical mammogram might overlook can sometimes be picked up. Early detection has, time and again, been linked with much higher survival rates; this, in turn, underlines just how valuable nuclear medicine is. Its adaptability in staging and evaluating treatment responses makes it a cornerstone in designing personalized care plans (Iranmakani et al., 2020). Beyond detection, nuclear medicine imaging can steer treatment decisions and patient management strategies. When doctors can see metabolic processes—not just static anatomical structures—it gives them a better idea of how the disease is evolving. Take, say, the assessment of treatment response in complex cases like neuroblastoma or breast cancer; here, nuclear methods often shine by offering a more precise view than traditional approaches. PET imaging, for instance, generally outperforms its older counterparts in showing whether a therapy is doing its job or if the disease is moving on. This shift toward a more individualized approach means that care becomes tailored to each patient's unique response, ultimately raising both the quality of care and overall patient outcomes (Iranmakani et al., 2020; Samim et al., 2021) (Figure 6.16).

6.5.1.1. Non-Invasive Nature

Imaging technology has turned the tide in medicine. Nuclear medicine shows off how non-invasive methods can be a game changer - you don't need surgery to get a clear picture of what's going on inside the body. Doctors can learn about both normal and abnormal processes simply through a quick radiopharmaceutical injection during tests like PET or SPECT, and this usually means fewer aches and less worry for patients. It is pretty neat that we can peek into the body's inner workings without messing much with it, which keeps everything as intact as possible while still gathering vital details. Beyond just making patients more comfortable, these techniques boost diagnostic accuracy in unexpected ways. Rather than depending solely on pictures of structure, nuclear imaging taps into the body's own markers—allowing conditions to be flagged earlier than with some other methods. Take cancer detection: radiotracers can be aimed at specific cellular behaviors, giving us a more detailed look at metabolic processes. This kind of early insight often means better outcomes because treatments can kick in sooner. Plus, since the process is non-invasive, doctors can repeat the tests over time to track how things evolve without piling on the risk that comes with repeated invasive procedures. Relying on methods that don't require cutting into the body fits well with today's push for personalized medicine. As tech advances, we're finding more ways to tailor tests to how diseases show up uniquely in each person. This is especially true in cancer care, where imaging can guide treatment choices based not just on size or location but on the tumor's underlying biology. New techniques — like using gadobenate dimeglumine in breast MRI (Kirchin et al., 2015) — highlight ongoing efforts to make these exams even more sensitive while sticking to non-invasive means. Overall, this trend puts patient safety and comfort right at the center and represents a big leap forward in the field of diagnostic imaging.

6.5.1.2. Functional Imaging Capabilities

Imaging tech has come a long way, shaking up how we do diagnoses—especially in nuclear methods. Now, doctors and researchers can essentially see and measure the body's metabolism in real time, a trick that old imaging just didn't pull off. Take, for example, combining PET with MRI; this mix gives us a peek into the biochemical hustle inside tissues, which helps when checking on stuff like cancer or those brain diseases that slowly sneak up on us. It all kind of shows how vital these hands-on imaging techniques are for getting a grip on disease and even understanding how treatments are doing their job. Lately, fresh imaging breakthroughs have thrown open doors to catch conditions earlier with unexpectedly sharp tools. New tricks, such as blending near-infrared fluorescence spectroscopy with traditional nuclear methods, seem to pick up on tiny, subtle changes at both a brain and molecular level.

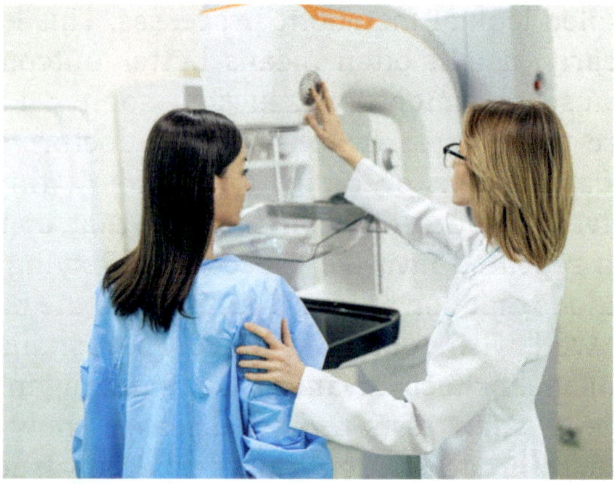

Figure 6.17. Functional Imaging Capabilities.

Source: https://www.oncologysystems.com/wp-content/uploads/2023/11/iStock-1314466012-1.jpg.

This matters a lot, especially when thinking about Alzheimer's—one of those cases where timing can change the game. By tracking the live, dynamic shifts in our bodies, these advancements not only boost our diagnostic smarts but also feed research into what makes diseases tick. In a way, this detailed view is opening up paths for more targeted therapies and, hopefully, better outcomes for patients. It is not just about early spotting either; keeping tabs on a disease as it unfolds has become a lot more concrete now. With real-time glimpses of what's happening deep inside, clinicians can sort of gauge whether a treatment's working as planned. For instance, watching how tumors handle glucose via PET scans can clue us in on how effective chemotherapy might be. Plus, newer imaging methods can hint at how different treatments may affect the brain or other key organs, steering the move toward more personalized care. As ongoing studies reveal even more possibilities, it seems clear that these imaging tools will keep building our understanding of complex illnesses and, in most cases, help lift the overall quality of patient care (Baianu et al., 2011) (Figure 6.17).

6.5.1.3. Early Detection of Diseases

New diagnostic approaches are changing how we handle health issues these days. Nuclear medicine imaging, for example, is one of those breakthroughs that's identifying problems early. It uses radiopharmaceuticals so that doctors can see what's happening at a nearly molecular level. This means illnesses like cancer, heart disease, and brain disorders tend to be spotted sooner and with better accuracy than before. Early detection, in most cases, gives clinicians a chance to start treatments that work better, which naturally leads to improved patient outcomes—clearly a big win for modern healthcare. In heart health, this imaging technique helps reveal myocardial fibrosis, a red flag for deeper issues. Fibrosis happens when fibroblasts kick into gear and produce too much collagen, a situation that, if missed, can eventually lead to serious problems like heart failure. Generally speaking, detecting myocardial fibrosis early can open the door to targeted treatments aimed at reversing unwanted changes in the heart's structure. While methods like cardiac magnetic resonance (CMR) do provide useful details, nuclear medicine shines by offering a non-invasive peek that pushes forward innovative treatment ideas, addressing a pressing need in cardiovascular care (Zhu et al., 2024). Over in the bone field, SPECT imaging shows real promise in identifying metastases and conditions like arthritis at their onset. By offering a detailed look at metabolic activity in bone tissue, this method lets clinicians notice abnormal patterns linked with cancer or inflammation. Using advanced algorithms to build targeted classifiers not only ups the accuracy but also deepens the overall diagnostic picture. In many cases, finding arthritis early paves the way for interventions that reduce long-term damage and, ultimately, enhance quality of life. With its notably high accuracy and recall rates, SPECT imaging is a clear example of how nuclear medicine keeps evolving into an indispensable tool for early diagnosis and better patient care (Wang et al., 2021).

6.5.2. Challenges and Limitations

Integrating nuclear medicine imaging into everyday clinical work isn't a walk in the park—it brings a host of challenges that demand thoughtful reflection. Sometimes, the tools simply don't give enough detail, especially when patients come in with a tangled medical history or multiple conditions at once. Take pregnant women, for instance; when scanning them, both maternal and fetal well-being need to be considered simultaneously, which calls for a team effort across different specialties. Several experts, speaking from various medical circles, have generally noted that dealing with cancer during pregnancy forces us to design protocols that look after both parties without sacrificing the clear results we need—an issue that exposes some inherent limits in current nuclear imaging methods (Cubillo et al., 2020). Patient safety is another matter that can't be brushed aside. Using radioactive isotopes naturally comes with risks, particularly for vulnerable groups like kids and expecting mothers. That's why sticking to strict safety checks and performing careful risk-versus-benefit reviews is absolutely critical; even a small imaging error can delay a diagnosis and throw off treatment. With imaging technology evolving so quickly, healthcare providers pretty much have to stay in a state of continuous learning—balancing innovative new techniques with well-established safety guidelines. Hybrid imaging methods, which mix different modalities, offer an intriguing promise yet also introduce some extra layers of complexity that underline the challenges and limitations present in today's nuclear medicine imaging (Sohns et al., 2017).

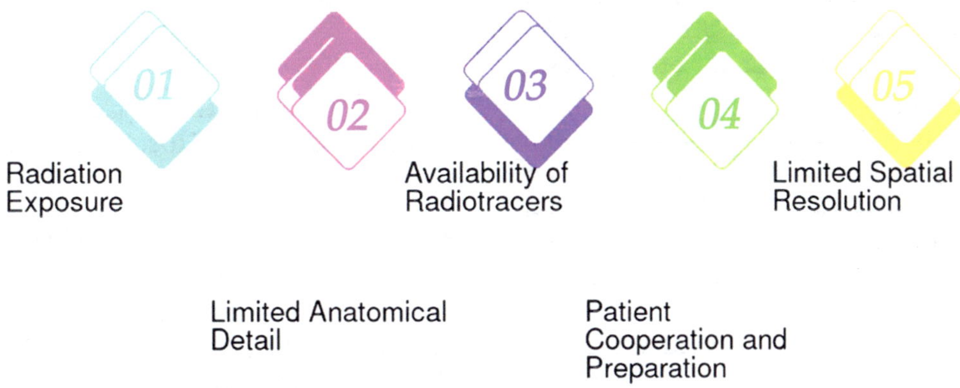

Figure 6.18. Limitations of nuclear medicine.

Source: https://fastercapital.com/content/Nuclear-Medicine-Unit--What-is-Nuclear-Medicine-and-How-Does-It-Help-in-Diagnosis-and-Treatment.html#Advantages-and-Limitations.

Beyond issues directly tied to patients, rolling out new technology in the field faces its own set of practical roadblocks. Specialized equipment, a well-trained crew, and solid institutional backing are not always on hand, and that can slow the spread of advanced imaging techniques. Budget constraints and uneven access only make these disparities worse, leading to real gaps in healthcare delivery. Meanwhile, the whole field must keep pace with a regulatory maze that governs using radiopharmaceuticals—a constant balancing act between innovation and compliance. Even as fresh advancements come into play, sticking to these evolving rules without dropping care standards remains one of the field's toughest challenges. All these factors, taken together, highlight the uphill battle nuclear medicine professionals face when trying to improve patient outcomes (Figure 6.18).

6.5.2.1. Availability of Radiopharmaceuticals

Radiopharmaceutical availability drives how well nuclear imaging works—it is something that often goes unnoticed until you compare it with more common scans. CT and MRI, for example, show up everywhere, but they just don't give you that precise detail you get from nuclear methods. Radiopharmaceuticals like [99mTc]-methyl diphosphonate ([99mTc]Tc-MDP) and [18F]sodium fluoride ([18F]NaF) are pretty much the core of SPECT and PET scans; having more of these agents around could, in most cases, boost our ability to catch issues like bone metastases early on (Ashhar et al., 2024). Even with all the progress in nuclear medicine, many parts of the world still wrestle with getting these crucial agents. It isn't just about having the technology—the methods used to make them, like generators and cyclotrons, end up being a big stumbling block in a lot of regions. A look at practices in 35 countries shows that many are stuck relying on a single provider, tangled up in tough regulations and reimbursement challenges (Cutler et al., 2020). Such hurdles tend to widen the gap in healthcare, especially in low- and middle-income areas where the nuclear infrastructure might still be a work in progress. Generally speaking, solving these issues needs cooperation on a global scale, working together to make sure everyone gets fair access. Over the past few years, a number of initiatives have popped up, trying to break down the barriers to radiopharmaceutical access. For instance, organizations like the Nuclear Medicine Global Initiative have been busy pinning down what holds back these agents from reaching more patients. They gather loads of data on both diagnostic and therapeutic isotopes, pointing out the need for smoother supply chains and new partnerships—sometimes even repeating the same point to drive it home. Some efforts also lean on standardizing procedures and boosting education for providers, hoping to make better use of what's already available. Among the ideas floated are changes to tighten up the regulatory landscape and to tweak reimbursement practices, all aimed at making nuclear medicine procedures more accessible worldwide (Cutler et al., 2020).

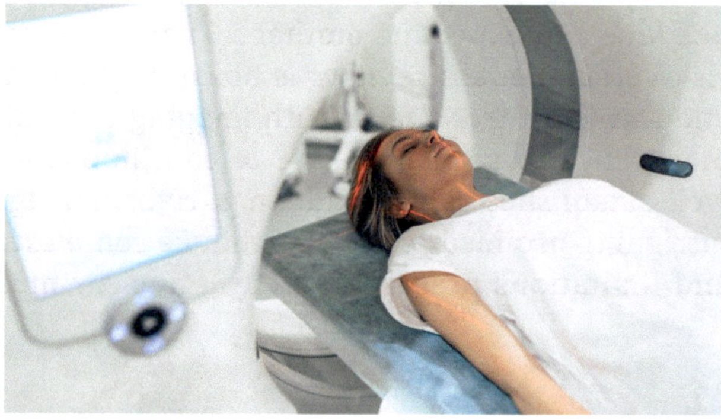

Source: https://www.medpace.com/wp-content/uploads/2023/02/iStock-1314466766.jpg.

6.5.2.2. Cost and Accessibility Issues

Nuclear medicine imaging in hospitals is a tough nut to crack. It usually needs a hefty financial outlay for not just the machines but also for setting everything up. Many hospitals, faced with limited resources, often lean toward more common techniques like CT scans or MRIs, sometimes leaving out tougher methods such as PET. Smaller or less urban centers tend to feel this pinch even more, meaning patients there might not get the same opportunities for these advanced scans, and this can slow down research simply because key groups aren't represented as they should be. Then there are those sneaky extra costs beyond the expensive equipment. In most cases, training staff to handle and interpret nuclear scans eats up a lot of time and money, as does buying specialized radiopharmaceuticals repeatedly. In a way, hospitals might find themselves low on both funds and qualified people, leading to longer waits for patients who need these services. Sometimes it seems like even if you've got the tech, the support just isn't there to make full use of it. And, of course, insurance rules come into play as well. Quite often, insurers impose strict limitations and high co-payments that further close the door on access to nuclear imaging. Because of these financial restrictions, people might delay or even skip essential diagnostic tests, potentially letting treatable conditions slip by. Generally speaking, rethinking insurance policies and exploring creative funding options is key to making sure everyone gets a fair share of the benefits these advanced imaging methods promise.

6.5.2.3. Patient Safety Concerns

In healthcare, patient safety tops the list—especially in nuclear medicine imaging. Radiation exposure, which is a common topic of debate, affects people differently, particularly those undergoing scans like PET or SPECT. Kids and patients needing multiple sessions tend to be more vulnerable. In most cases, it is vital that the benefits clearly outweigh the risks. That's why medical teams often stick to strict but evolving practices: they work to keep doses as low as possible while picking the right imaging option. Ongoing learning about radiation hazards and protection methods helps cut down on problems and builds trust in nuclear imaging (Chen et al., 2024). Quality assurance is another big piece of the puzzle, especially in ensuring that diagnoses and treatments are on point. Sometimes, errors in imaging show up either from human mistakes or from equipment glitches, and these can lead to misdiagnoses or treatments that miss the mark. False positives or negatives might set patients on unwanted—and sometimes stressful—therapeutic detours. Generally speaking, comprehensive training for healthcare professionals helps create a safety-first culture in which errors are spotted and fixed quickly. Regular checkups, calibration, and upkeep of the machinery also play a critical role in avoiding any misreads that could hurt patient care (Khessib et al., 2024). New imaging advances, while boosting our ability to diagnose, also bring fresh safety challenges. Innovations like hybrid techniques—where functional and anatomical details mix together—demand extra attention on how they might impact patient safety. Sure, these technological leaps can sharpen diagnostic precision, but if not handled correctly, they might also bump up the radiation exposure. Plus, the complexity of newer methods sometimes means that interpretations can vary, influencing clinical decisions in unexpected ways. For these reasons, it remains crucial to keep tweaking imaging protocols and to study the long-term effects of radiation, ensuring a balance between great diagnostics and safe practices in nuclear medicine (Chen et al., 2024).

Test Your Knowledge

1. What are the main advantages of nuclear medicine imaging compared to other diagnostic techniques?
2. What challenges and limitations are associated with nuclear medicine imaging in terms of cost, availability, and radiation exposure?

Summary

Nuclear medicine imaging is changing in ways that force us to rethink old educational routines and tech tools. Lately, people have started mixing up teaching with fresh ideas like the multi-interactive teaching mode, a style that brings everyone into the conversation. This method builds a hands-on atmosphere—students get involved and even improve their clinical skills along the way. By jumping on digital platforms such as We Chat and other multimedia bits, we're gradually moving away from the boring one-way info dump of the past. All these shifts show how important it is to rework our teaching approaches so that future pros can handle the modifications in nuclear medicine imaging (Danylenko and Nepokupna, 2023).

Then there's machine learning (ML), which is pretty much flipping the script in our field. In most cases, ML is seen as a powerful data-crunching tool, speeding up image captures, boosting image quality and even cutting down those annoying artifacts. But its benefits don't stop there; ML also brings together data from different imaging methods—a move that works especially well in oncology settings. This layered strategy not only helps in making smarter decisions but also plays a key part in developing imaging biomarkers, promising to ultimately revamp patient care and change the way clinical routines play out in nuclear medicine (Kuestner et al., 2022).

To wrap it up, merging fresh teaching ideas with new-tech breakthroughs is placing nuclear medicine imaging right at the forefront of modern medicine. With an ongoing back-and-forth between interactive learning and ML innovations, educators and clinicians alike are being nudged to keep up with this fast-paced change. As these developments continue rolling in, it is becoming more and more obvious that creating spaces that support complete learning and smart tech use isn't just a bonus—it is essential.

This drive for continuous progress will no doubt raise the standard of care in nuclear medicine, equipping new healthcare professionals with the tools they need to tackle an ever-evolving medical world (Danylenko and Nepokupna, 2023; Kuestner et al., 2022). Nuclear medicine imaging has come into its own over the past few decades—it's changed how we spot illnesses and figure out treatments. Radiopharmaceuticals are not just a new gadget in clinics; they've popped up across many different organ systems and disease processes. Take theranostics, for example—it is where treatment and diagnosis kind of blend together. It all started with radioiodine for thyroid issues, but these days new agents are combined with targeting cancers like neuroendocrine tumors and even prostate cancer.

This fresh direction not only sharpens treatment precision but also forges a closer link between pinpoint health and personalized care (Jadvar, 2021). Learning resources, too, have taken on a whole new vibe. Textbooks—like Nuclear Medicine Textbook: Methodology and Clinical Applications—have grown into vital tools for everyone from newbies to seasoned pros. They break down the core science, explain clinical applications, and outline procedural tips in a way that sometimes feels almost conversational. Topics jump from radiopharmaceutical basics to quality checks, showing just how vast the knowledge base can be. Plus, the inclusion of real-life case examples helps bring theory into the messy world of everyday practice, bridging that gap between academia and the clinic (Jadvar, 2021). At its heart, nuclear medicine imaging is all about changing patient care and streamlining how treatments are planned. Its advanced methods let doctors diagnose with pinpoint accuracy while crafting treatment plans that fit individual needs. With new radiopharmaceuticals and techniques emerging non-stop, this field keeps adapting to our ever-shifting healthcare landscape. In my view, the steady flow of updated resources gives both practitioners and researchers the edge they need to stay safe and innovative. And, generally speaking, as the field gets more complex, a commitment to ongoing learning and research isn't just nice to have—it is essential.

KEY TERMS FROM THIS CHAPTER

- Cardiology
- Collimator
- Fluorodeoxyglucose (FDG)
- Gamma camera
- Gamma rays
- Molecular imaging
- Myocardial perfusion imaging
- Oncology
- Positron emission tomography (PET)
- Radioisotope
- Radionuclide
- Radiopharmaceuticals
- Scintigraphy
- Technetium-99m

Critical Thinking Questions

1. **What is the primary principle behind nuclear medicine imaging?**
   a. X-rays are used to capture images
   b. Radioactive tracers are injected or ingested to produce images
   c. Magnetic fields and radio waves are used to create images
   d. Ultrasound waves are used to create images
2. **Which of the following is the most commonly used radioactive isotope in nuclear medicine imaging?**
   a. Technetium-99m
   b. Iodine-131
   c. Carbon-14
   d. Uranium-235
3. **What does a PET (Positron Emission Tomography) scan primarily measure?**
   a. Bone density
   b. Blood flow and metabolism
   c. Soft tissue damage
   d. Electrical activity of the heart
4. **In a typical nuclear medicine scan, where are the radioactive tracers detected?**
   a. In the patient's blood
   b. By an external gamma camera
   c. Inside a magnetic resonance field
   d. By a computer in the form of sound waves
5. **What is the primary advantage of nuclear medicine imaging over other imaging techniques?**
   a. It provides real-time imaging
   b. It requires no radiation
   c. It allows functional and molecular imaging
   d. It is cheaper than other imaging modalities

Short Answer Questions

1. What are the basic principles of nuclear medicine and how do radioactive tracers help in imaging?
2. What are the common imaging techniques used in nuclear medicine, such as PET and SPECT?
3. How is nuclear medicine used in the diagnosis of conditions like cancer, heart disease, or infections?
4. What safety measures and regulations are in place to ensure the safe use of nuclear medicine imaging?
5. What are the advantages, challenges, and limitations of nuclear medicine imaging compared to other imaging modalities?

Answers to Critical Thinking Questions

1. (b); 2. (a); 3. (b); 4. (b); 5. (c)

References

1. Al-Ibraheem, A., Baum, R. P., Ben-Haim, S., Blay, J., et al. (2024). Guiding principles on the education and practice of theragnostic. https://core.ac.uk/download/611825231.pdf (accessed on 23 May 2025).

2. Alqahtani, F. F. (2022). SPECT/CT and PET/CT, related radiopharmaceuticals, and areas of application and comparison. *Saudi Pharmaceutical Journal, 31*(3), 312–328. https://doi.org/10.1016/j.jsps.2022.12.013.

3. Anders, J., Lanzafame, R., & Arany, P. (2015). Low-level light/laser therapy versus photobiomodulation therapy. *Photomedicine and Laser Surgery, 33*(4), 183–184. https://www.semanticscholar.org/paper/8081502f20f81428b9744e276a961e4ae51747dc (accessed on 23 May 2025).

4. Ashhar, Z., Fadzil, M. F. A., Hassan, H., Othman, M. F., Md Hassan, M. B., Vui, V. Y. C., Choo, C. G., et al. (2024). The potential of radiolabeled bisphosphonates in SPECT and PET for bone imaging. *Current Medical Imaging, 20*(1), e15734056270935. https://www.semanticscholar.org/paper/af9a85cf61303c38f604e90c755122d093659dd0 (accessed on 23 May 2025).

5. Aydin, M. (2024). Exploring clinical competencies and ethical reflections: A multi-patient simulation-based training program for emergency medicine residents. *Journal of Pioneering Medical Science*. https://www.semanticscholar.org/paper/24d0ab4edaa5e8bd1d9cb00524de906fd93c3e76 (accessed on 23 May 2025).

6. Azhari, H. (2024). Advancing stroke diagnosis and management through nuclear medicine: A systematic review of clinical trials. *Frontiers in Medicine, 11*. https://www.semanticscholar.org/paper/898add660c34a11dc4b9f33000d37473ef009fba (accessed on 23 May 2025).

7. Baianu, I. C. (2011). Early diagnosis of Alzheimer's disease by NIRF spectroscopy and nuclear medicine. https://core.ac.uk/download/pdf/332860.pdf.

8. Balkenende, L., Teuwen, J., & Mann, R. M. (2022). Application of deep learning in breast cancer imaging. *Seminars in Nuclear Medicine, 52*, 584–596. https://doi.org/10.1053/j.semnuclmed.2022.02.003.

9. Barca, C., Griessinger, C. M., Faust, A., Depke, D. A., Essler, M., Windhorst, A. D., Devoogdt, N., et al. (2021). Expanding theragnostic radiopharmaceuticals for tumor diagnosis and therapy. *Pharmaceuticals, 15*(1), 13. https://doi.org/10.3390/ph15010013.

10. Besson, F. L., Treglia, G., Bucerius, J., Anagnostopoulos, C., Buechel, R., Dweck, M., Erba, P. A., et al. (2024). A systematic review for the evidence of recommendations and guidelines in hybrid nuclear cardiovascular imaging. *European Journal of Nuclear Medicine and Molecular Imaging, 51*, 2247–2259. https://www.semanticscholar.org/paper/7ac8acb8e92da6252fee12d24edd3b21434d6fd1 (accessed on 23 May 2025).

11. Bonnard, B., Cots, O., Glaser, S. J., Lapert, M., et al. (2012). Geometric optimal control of the contrast imaging problem in nuclear magnetic resonance. *arXiv*. http://arxiv.org/abs/1208.2794 (accessed on 23 May 2025).

12. Chen, L., Chen, F. Y., Jiang, T., Deng, Y., & Shi, G. Q. (2024). Endoscopic injection of Lauro macrogol foam sclerotherapy for rectal cavernous hemangioma: A case report. *Medicine, 103*. https://www.semanticscholar.org/paper/9caa89a37de23559a59901b2b9cc6d1178fe2c9d (accessed on 23 May 2025).

13. Chen, Z., Peng, W., Sun, H., Kuang, W., WenBin, L., Jia, Z., & Gong, Q. (2016). PS184. Biophysical alterations of the brain in first-episode, drug-naïve patients with major depressive disorder: A magnetization transfer imaging study. *International Journal of Neuropsychopharmacology, 19*(Suppl 1), 66–67. https://www.semanticscholar.org/paper/d83a701b8626a58447f740d31a4e7c75b0be2bc8 (accessed on 23 May 2025).

14. Clements, J. B., Baird, C. T., de Boer, S. F., Fairobent, L. A., Fisher, T., Goodwin, J. H., Gress, D. A., et al. (2018). AAPM medical physics practice guideline 10.a.: Scope of practice for clinical medical physics. *Journal of Applied Clinical Medical Physics, 19*(6), 11–25. https://doi.org/10.1002/acm2.12469.

15. Cubillo, A., Echaverria Morales, S., Goñi, E., Matute Teresa, F., Muga Muñoz, J. L., Pérez-Díaz, D., de Santiago, J., et al. (2020). Multidisciplinary consensus on cancer management during pregnancy. *Clinical & Translational Oncology, 23*, 1054–1066. https://doi.org/10.1007/s12094-020-02491-8.

16. Cutler, C., Bailey, E., Kumar, V., Schwarz, S., Bom, H., Hatazawa, J., Paez, D., et al. (2020). Global issues of radiopharmaceutical access and availability: A Nuclear Medicine Global Initiative Project. *The Journal of Nuclear Medicine, 62*(3), 422–430. https://www.semanticscholar.org/paper/8a69fcee8108151f71a2f52549c1f1aed06afc8b (accessed on 23 May 2025).

17. Danylenko, Y., & Nepokupna, T. (2023). Analysis of scintillation materials for nuclear medicine on the basis of patent analytics. *Science and Innovation*. https://www.semanticscholar.org/paper/206d612274d284bc16b6bb7b0affa5150136fe27 (accessed on 23 May 2025).

18. Das, S., Alam, M. J., Ahmed, K. R., Nusrat, M., Sultana, J., Tabassum, I., Rashid, M. B., et al. (2025). Challenges in accessing and operating PET-CT: Patient experiences and institutional hurdles in a newly established nuclear medicine institute in Bangladesh. *Bangladesh Journal of Nuclear Medicine*. https://www.semanticscholar.org/paper/d0c163085f28263d8514bac3389bc8e4b198fdc1 (accessed on 23 May 2025).

19. Decuyper, M., Maebe, J., Van Holen, R., & Vandenberghe, S. (2021). Artificial intelligence with deep learning in nuclear medicine and radiology. *EJNMMI Physics, 8*. https://www.semanticscholar.org/paper/e609b4777cea0cc8eefeed7d0a8365aef593c497 (accessed on 23 May 2025).

20. Fontana, M., Dauvergne, D., Létang, J. M., Ley, J., & Testa, É. (2017). Compton camera study for high efficiency SPECT and benchmark with Anger system. *Physics in Medicine and Biology, 62*, 8794–8812. https://doi.org/10.1088/1361-6560/aa926a.

21. Forsting, M. (2017). Machine learning will change medicine. *The Journal of Nuclear Medicine, 58*, 357–358. https://www.semanticscholar.org/paper/5dda2add82869318e5e4f5b3146cccd3dc530bab (accessed on 23 May 2025).

22. Giammarile, F., Knoll, P., Kunikowska, J., Paez, D., Lobato, E. E., Mikhail-Lette, M., Wahl, R. L., et al. (2024). Guardians of precision: Advancing radiation protection, safety, and quality systems in nuclear medicine. *European Journal of Nuclear Medicine and Molecular Imaging, 51*, 1498–1505. https://www.semanticscholar.org/paper/ba4d477a381f2da0df6fce2b8d911cea6808681d (accessed on 23 May 2025).

23. Gimbrone, M. A., & García-Cardeña, G. (2016). Endothelial cell dysfunction and the pathobiology of atherosclerosis. *Circulation Research, 118*(5), 620–636. https://doi.org/10.1161/circresaha.115.306301.

24. Gnanasegaran, G., & Cook, G. (2020). Nuclear medicine imaging techniques of the musculoskeletal system. In *Clinical Nuclear Medicine*. https://doi.org/10.1007/978-3-030-39457-8_10.

25. Golub, I. S., Thummala, A. R., Morad, T., Dhaliwal, J., Elisarraras, F., Karlsberg, R. P., & Cho, G. W. (2025). Artificial intelligence in nuclear cardiac imaging: Novel advances, emerging techniques, and recent clinical trials. *Journal of Clinical Medicine, 14*. https://www.semanticscholar.org/paper/ad5f9cc5b538c9b30df9ca0c29da1f45fbeed2c9 (accessed on 23 May 2025).

26. Heiss, W. (2016). Hybrid PET/MR imaging in neurology: Present applications and prospects for the future. *The Journal of Nuclear Medicine, 57*(7), 993–995. https://www.semanticscholar.org/paper/66536fabc37cad2512e2ff7aa6c830ecdaad8933 (accessed on 23 May 2025).

27. Iranmakani, S., Mortezazadeh, T., Sajadian, F., Fazel Ghaziani, M., Ghafari, A., Khezerloo, D., & Musa, A. E. (2020). A review of various modalities in breast imaging: Technical aspects and clinical outcomes. *The Egyptian Journal of Radiology and Nuclear Medicine, 51*. https://doi.org/10.1186/s43055-020-00175-5.

28. Jadvar, H. (2021). *Nuclear Medicine Textbook: Methodology and clinical applications. The Journal of Nuclear Medicine, 63*, 967. https://www.semanticscholar.org/paper/41a4a89bd4ad93a5f6b9322ba02d4fe42b719974 (accessed on 23 May 2025).

29. Kane, S. (2002). Introduction to physics in modern medicine. https://www.semanticscholar.org/paper/73e6cda683edcb60d6295e9fa42e67e5769151e7 (accessed on 23 May 2025).

30. Kaur, C. D., Mishra, K., Sahu, A. K., Panik, R., Kashyap, P., Mishra, S. P., & Kumar, A. (2020). Theragnostic: New era in nuclear medicine and radiopharmaceuticals. In *Intech Open eBooks*. https://doi.org/10.5772/intechopen.91868.

31. Khessib, T., Jha, P., Davidzon, G., Iagaru, A., & Shah, J. (2024). Nuclear medicine and molecular imaging applications in gynecologic malignancies: A comprehensive review. *Seminars in Nuclear Medicine*. https://www.semanticscholar.org/paper/12384f33dfe04b676cfe3f9518d113c4869bb6d5 (accessed on 23 May 2025).

32. Kirchin, M., Luciani, M. L., Pediconi, F., Telesca, M., et al. (2015). Clinical utility of gadobenate dimeglumine in contrast-enhanced MRI of the breast: A review. https://core.ac.uk/download/141692117.pdf (accessed on 23 May 2025).

33. Kirkpatrick, J. N., Mitchell, C., Taub, C., Kort, S., Hung, J., & Swaminathan, M. (2020). ASE statement on protection of patients and echocardiography service providers during the 2019 novel coronavirus outbreak: Endorsed by the American College of Cardiology. *Journal of the American Society of Echocardiography, 33*, 648–653. https://doi.org/10.1016/j.echo.2020.04.001.

34. Koshino, K., Werner, R. A., Pomper, M. G., Bundschuh, R. A., Toriumi, F., Higuchi, T., & Rowe, S. P. (2021). Narrative review of generative adversarial networks in medical and molecular imaging. *Annals of Translational Medicine, 9*, 821. https://doi.org/10.21037/atm-20-6325.

35. Kuestner, T., Hepp, T., & Seith, F. (2022). Multiparametric oncologic hybrid imaging: Machine learning challenges and opportunities. *RoFo: Fortschritte auf dem Gebiete der Rontgenstrahlen und der Nuklearmedizin*. https://www.semanticscholar.org/paper/3ddf3e7a72bc3283303d54f13ddcead4a7012fea (accessed on 23 May 2025).

36. Landsberger, S. (2006). Radiation and modern life: Fulfilling Marie Curie's dream. *Journal of Clinical Investigation, 116*(2), 286. https://www.semanticscholar.org/paper/2f9d37a6b4b27b15c5815e8432d08ee7d929b1b6 (accessed on 23 May 2025).
37. Mehmonov, G., Khujaev, S., & Egamediev, S. (2025). Gallium 68 production and its expanding role in nuclear medicine. *Uzbek Journal of Physics*. https://www.semanticscholar.org/paper/6b0c6be2e7a984fe5c76c5fddb04d000d936aac3 (accessed on 23 May 2025).
38. Orcajo-Rincón, J., Muñoz-Langa, J., Sepúlveda-Sánchez, J. M., Fernández-Pérez, G. C., Martínez, M., Noriega-Álvarez, E., Sanz Viedma, S., et al. (2022). Review of imaging techniques for evaluating morphological and functional responses to the treatment of bone metastases in prostate and breast cancer. *Clinical & Translational Oncology, 24*, 1290–1310. https://doi.org/10.1007/s12094-022-02784-0.
39. Othman, S. A., Radzi, N. A. S. M., & Jalil, M. A. M. (2024). Radiation risk in nuclear medicine–A short review. *Journal of Advanced Research Design*. https://www.semanticscholar.org/paper/e064f63b3d7c9b8d9841c7ee4724762133b88d0d (accessed on 23 May 2025).
40. Park, J. Y., Park, S. M., Lee, T. S., Lee, S. J., Kim, J. Y., Oh, S. J., Yoon, H., et al. (2024). Innovations in nuclear medicine imaging for reactive oxygen species: Applications and radiopharmaceuticals. *Antioxidants, 13*. https://www.semanticscholar.org/paper/e50a26ba3b98f8a6fa5429faf06cd0c96ad14055 (accessed on 23 May 2025).
41. Perrone, M., Moscatelli, S., Guglielmi, G., Bianco, F., Cappelletti, D., Pellizzon, A., Baggiano, A., et al. (2025). Advances in cardiovascular multimodality imaging in patients with Marfan syndrome. *Diagnostics, 15*. https://www.semanticscholar.org/paper/99ad5c26f0dfb8d989c53825a6c1eeab57cd4fd9 (accessed on 23 May 2025).
42. Qian, Y., Lin, Y. C., Chen, X., Ge, Y., Lui, Y. W., Boada Bernard, F. E., & Schwartz Center for Biomedical Imaging, et al. (2024). Multi-TE single-quantum sodium (23Na) MRI: A clinically translatable technique for separation of mono- and bi-T2 sodium signals. https://www.semanticscholar.org/paper/fd548d761df2ec239d7e7b86db89300f4b01501f (accessed on 23 May 2025).
43. Samim, A., Tytgat, G. A. M., Bleeker, G., Wenker, S. T. M., Chatalic, K. L. S., Poot, A. J., Tolboom, N., et al. (2021). Nuclear medicine imaging in neuroblastoma: Current status and new developments. *Journal of Personalized Medicine, 11*(4), 270. https://doi.org/10.3390/jpm11040270.
44. Seeram, E. (2018). *Digital Image Processing*. CRC Press. https://doi.org/10.1201/9781315152325-4.
45. Sohns, J. M., Bavendiek, U., Roß, T. L., & Bengel, F. M. (2017). Targeting cardiovascular implant infection. *Circulation: Cardiovascular Imaging, 10*. https://doi.org/10.1161/circimaging.117.005376.
46. Spriet, M., & Vandenberghe, F. (2024). Equine nuclear medicine in 2024: Use and value of scintigraphy and PET in equine lameness diagnosis. *Animals, 14*. https://www.semanticscholar.org/paper/2774334ddf6883c7c3debab676526ae9e47fc6de (accessed on 23 May 2025).
47. Tapper, W., Carneiro, G., Mikropoulos, C., Thomas, S. A., Evans, P. M., & Boussios, S. (2024). The application of radiomics and AI to molecular imaging for prostate cancer. *Journal of Personalized Medicine, 14*. https://www.semanticscholar.org/paper/0e3bafe8aa1895605ab9dc95a9dada411e11c81f (accessed on 23 May 2025).

48. Taylor, A. (2020). Nuclear medicine imaging techniques of the kidney. In *Clinical Nuclear Medicine*. https://doi.org/10.1007/978-3-030-39457-8_8.

49. Turner, J. H. (2018). An introduction to the clinical practice of theragnostic in oncology. *British Journal of Radiology, 91*. https://doi.org/10.1259/bjr.20180440.

50. Vlachothanasi, E. (2024). Navigating precision medicine within European law: Ethical considerations and legal challenges. *Bioethical*. https://www.semanticscholar.org/paper/b81fcf3fd331a5f29550a08b82236140c8652964 (accessed on 23 May 2025).

51. Wamil, M., Goncalves, M., Rutherford, A., Borlotti, A., & Pellikka, P. (2022). Multi-modality cardiac imaging in the management of diabetic heart disease. *Frontiers in Cardiovascular Medicine, 9*. https://www.semanticscholar.org/paper/aeca880a99e109ede26bdac4e137e1b38c2bdc14 (accessed on 23 May 2025).

52. Wang, W., Cao, Y., Lin, Q., Man, Z., & Li, T. (2021). Research on arthritis detection method for SPECT nuclear medicine bone imaging. *2021 International Conference on Communications, Information System and Computer Engineering (CISCE)*. https://www.semanticscholar.org/paper/3f6dc1fb362aa105c546a58f8d3a94a34f744b38 (accessed on 23 May 2025).

53. Zhu, H., Xie, K., Qian, Y., Zou, Z., Jiang, M., & Pu, J. (2024). Recent progresses in the multimodality imaging assessment of myocardial fibrosis. *Reviews in Cardiovascular Medicine, 25*. https://www.semanticscholar.org/paper/1e3c8eb57392e07edfa3dc2a755c0973a477db44 (accessed on 23 May 2025).

MAMMOGRAPHY

7

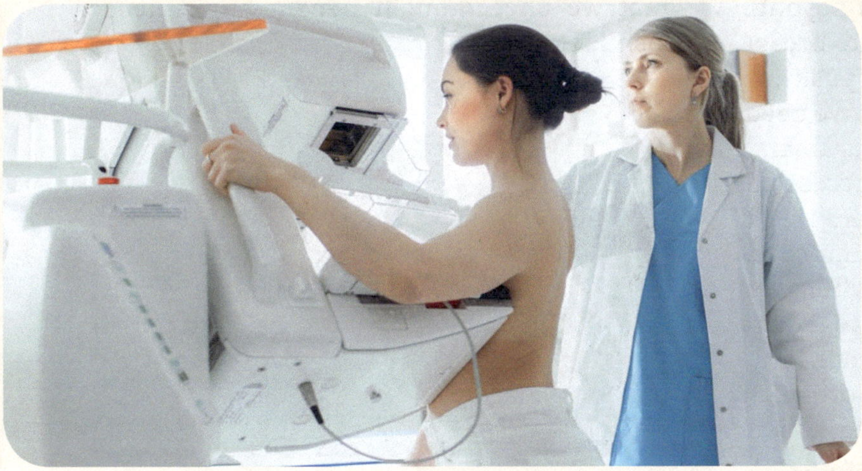

LEARNING OBJECTIVES

After studying this chapter, you will be able to:

1. Understand the historical development of mammography.
2. Explore the different types of mammography techniques.
3. Examine the mammography procedure, including preparation, imaging process, and interpretation.
4. Identify the key benefits of mammography.
5. Evaluate the risks and limitations associated with mammography.

Introduction

Early detection of breast cancer is absolutely crucial—this disease still ranks as one of the top killers among women worldwide. Mammograms, trusted almost without question by doctors, help catch the problem before it escalates; regular check-ups generally raise the chances of beating the illness. People often note that social factors matter too: women facing economic or other hardships tend to skip screenings more often. In short, studies repeatedly point to the fact that a person's social standing is tightly linked to health outcomes, making it clear that we must address these gaps in access to care, especially in under-served communities (Jhumkhawala et al., 2024). Even when you glance over the research, the message is the same—a routine screening can be a real game changer. Breast cancer screening can sometimes do double duty by offering clues about heart health as well. For example, a routine mammogram might unexpectedly reveal signs like Breast Arterial Calcification (BAC), which hints at possible cardiovascular issues. Researchers, in most cases, are starting to see these incidental findings as a useful bonus, suggesting that mammograms can provide a broader picture of a woman's overall health. Several studies have nudged the field toward considering more expansive screening protocols that look at both cancer and certain heart conditions, especially among women with specific risk factors (Yuvabalakumaran. et al., 2024). This extra insight could, over time, help evolve our approach to health checks for women, particularly for those in their 40s and beyond. Dealing with the many challenges tied to breast cancer screening means it is time to push for targeted, evidence-based interventions. We need to zero in on the socioeconomic, cultural, and systemic hurdles that block timely access to mammography—because if these barriers aren't managed, screening rates just won't improve. Research consistently shows that when we understand how these factors mesh together, we're in a better position to craft public health strategies that lift early detection and promote health fairness. Recent studies even point out that better healthcare access and higher quality of care boost screening utilization, reinforcing the importance of policies aimed at helping the uninsured (Jhumkhawala et al., 2024). As the conversation around mammography continues to evolve, it becomes clear that blending insights from multiple studies is key to creating practices that not only catch breast cancer early but also meet the diverse needs of women from all walks of life.

Definition of Mammography

Medical imaging has come a long way, changing how we catch health issues early. Mammography is one example—a type of X-ray that focuses on breast tissue using a low dose of radiation to capture detailed images. This allows doctors to spot abnormal growths or changes that might otherwise go unnoticed. Sometimes, routine screening tests are done on women without symptoms, while other times a more focused, diagnostic approach follows an unusual finding. Identifying differences in tissue density or small calcifications is key in diagnosing breast cancer early—a step that often improves outcomes for diverse groups of patients. Still, mammography isn't solely about finding breast cancer. Newer studies suggest that what shows up on these images—like breast arterial calcification (BAC)—might also hint at heart trouble. For example, Jaing et al. found a notable link between BAC and coronary artery disease, which implies that what we once thought benign might need a fresh look.

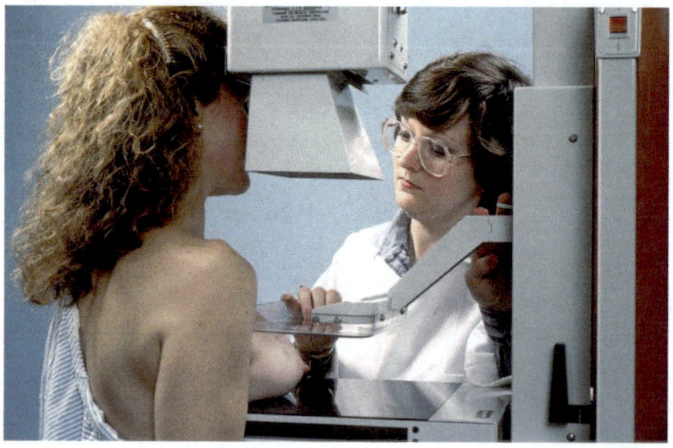

Figure 7.1. A mammogram can identify breast abnormalities that could lead to cancer.

Source: By National Cancer Institute - US National Institutes of Health - National Cancer Institutehttp://www.cancer.gov/cancertopics/pdq/screening/breast/Patient/page3http://www.cancer.gov/images/cdr/live/CDR415525-750.jpg, Public Domain, https://commons.wikimedia.org/w/index.php?curid=601035.

Generally speaking, this emerging insight nudges us to view mammography results more broadly, since carefully noting BAC could lead to earlier interventions for cardiovascular issues. As healthcare moves toward a more interconnected model, it is becoming clear that various risk factors are more intertwined than we used to think. Beyond individual care, mammography also shapes public health policies and screening recommendations. Data-driven guidelines emphasize regular imaging for women, particularly those at higher risk, and many experts believe that pairing mammography with ultrasound fills in gaps left by X-rays alone. It is also important that public education highlights not only the need for routine screenings but also the significance of understanding one's personal and family medical history. In the end, whether it is identifying cancer early or assessing broader health risks, mammography remains a vital part of modern healthcare, driving improvements in clinical practices and patient outcomes (Barlow, 2015; Dixon, 2014) (Figure 7.1).

Importance of Mammography in Breast Cancer Detection

Awareness and how individuals act in health shape whether women decide on mammograms. Research generally suggests that when a woman senses she might be at risk, she's more inclined to get screened. In communities where knowledge about breast cancer and its possible fallout is higher, participation in screening programs tends to go up. For example, one study with Malaysian women found that a stronger feeling of vulnerability—and a clear nod to the benefits of clinical breast exams—often lined up with a greater chance of having a mammogram (Kandiah et al., 2010). When care providers work on boosting overall understanding of breast cancer, it leads to more screenings, which usually means identifying the disease earlier and achieving better outcomes. Mammograms do more than just detect issues; they also play a big role in cutting down breast cancer deaths. In most cases, research has shown that spotting tumors early—when treatment is more effective and less of a burden financially—is key. Interestingly, one investigation among Iranian women indicated that having a genuine drive toward healthful habits, including undergoing mammograms, noticeably improved screening numbers. When policymakers take into account the mix of psychological and social factors that shape women's attitudes toward these exams, they can design interventions that improve both access and education. In that sense, highlighting how important early detection is through mammography remains central to wide-ranging public health plans. Removing the hurdles to getting a mammogram is just as crucial as encouraging the screening itself. Many women point to issues like financial limits, poor access to healthcare, and not having enough clear info about the test as major stumbling blocks. Some effective ways to tackle these barriers include local education programs, free or low-cost screening options, and policies that put women's health first. Studies across various groups suggest that when women feel more confident about managing their health and when those barriers are reduced, they're way more likely to go for a mammogram. In the end, if we all pitch in to make mammography more understandable and easier to access, not only do screening rates improve, but lives are also saved by identifying breast cancer early enough for more efficient treatment (Figure 7.2).

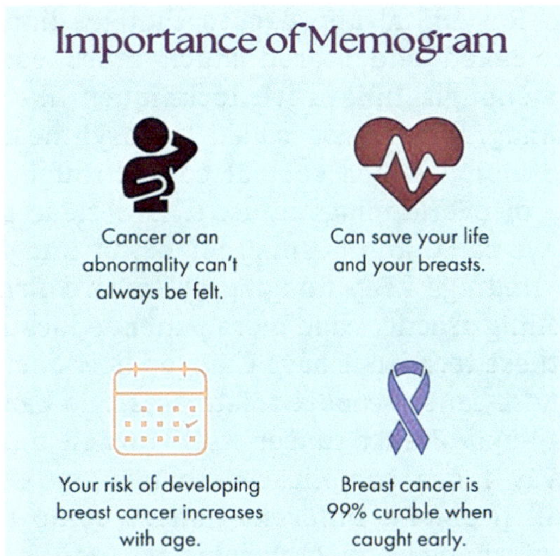

Figure 7.2. Importance of memogram.

Source: https://www.instagram.com/drnirmalgujarathi/p/C9wK-97O0ss/.

7.1. History of Mammography

Learning Outcome

1. Understand the development of early mammography techniques.
2. Explore the key milestones in mammography technology.
3. Examine the evolution of guidelines and recommendations.

Mammography changed things for women by identifying breast cancer early. Back in the day, cancer was usually spotted way too late - doctors often only found it once it was advanced, which left few options. In the 1960s, though, when X-ray imaging of breast tissue came into play, that all shifted. Doctors suddenly had a tool to see tiny lumps that you wouldn't catch by touch alone. Regular checkups using this new method started popping up everywhere, sparking public campaigns and reshaping what women's health meant in everyday life. Over time, the way we do mammography got a makeover too. The old film-screen methods slowly faded out, making room for digital approaches that let images be tweaked and stored much more easily. Soon enough, innovative techniques like 3D mammography - also called tomosynthesis - came along, which sort of cuts through the mess of overlapping tissue. It is a clear sign that we can't stop pushing for better imaging. New findings keep nudging us toward firmer screening practices and more patient education, and these tech leaps have changed how doctors diagnose cancer, choose treatments, and handle follow-ups. Breast cancer itself turned out to be way more complicated than a one-size-fits-all problem. Different tumors come in a mix of shapes and molecular makes, so the usual screening methods needed a twist. Today, merging molecular tests with traditional imaging lets practitioners pinpoint specific cancer types, matching up with each person's unique risk factors. Even artificial intelligence (AI) is stepping in to help sort through tumor traits—a move that, in most cases, speeds up detection and guides treatment choices. This nuanced, targeted style is key for early intervention and can boost survival rates (Kashyap et al., 2022; Sergiusz Łukasiewicz et al., 2021) (Figure 7.3).

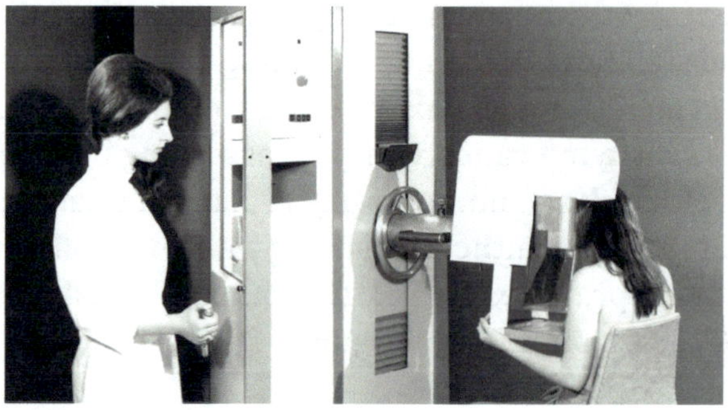

Figure 7.3. X-ray imaging of breast tissue.

Source: https://www.medmuseum.siemens-healthineers.com/en/stories-from-the-museum/history-mammography.

7.1.1. Development of Early Mammography Techniques

Back in the mid-1900s, breast cancer detection got a serious kickstart as rising rates of illness and death forced a reevaluation of old methods. People were mostly relying on physical check-ups and plain X-rays back then, and frankly, they just weren't doing the job of identifying tiny, early tumors. Then came mammography—a real game changer that used low-dose X-rays to peek inside the breast in a non-invasive way. This new method, which could spot little anomalies that traditional methods often missed, not only bumped up early detection but also nudged public health policies toward regular screenings. Overall, it set off a chain reaction that eventually led to more complex imaging techniques and truly transformed how breast cancer was diagnosed. As time wore on, it became clear that even mammography had its limits. Generally speaking, the early techniques produced two-dimensional images that sometimes made tissues overlap, which could hide potential tumors, especially in those with denser breasts. When digital mammography rolled in during the late 20th century, things began to shift—images could now be tweaked more effectively, and diagnostic confidence got a boost. The digital approach not only sharpened image clarity but also cut down on radiation, making it safer for patients.

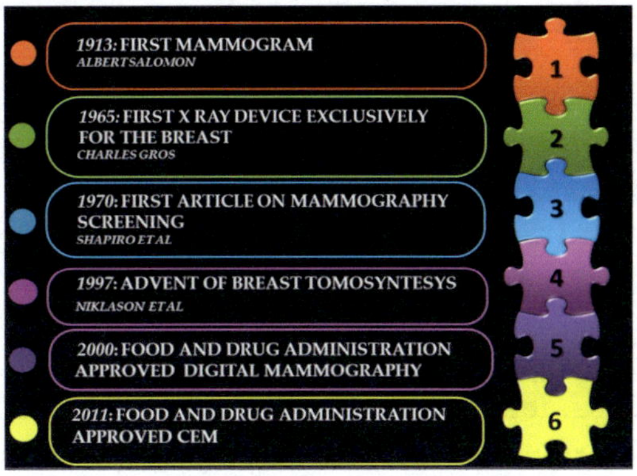

Figure 7.4. Some of the main achievements of mammography over time.

Source: Nicosia, Luca, Giulia Gnocchi, Ilaria Gorini, Massimo Venturini, Federico Fontana, Filippo Pesapane, Ida Abiuso, Anna Carla Bozzini, Maria Pizzamiglio, Antuono Latronico, and et al. 2023. "History of Mammography: Analysis of Breast Imaging Diagnostic Achievements over the Last Century" *Healthcare* 11, no. 11: 1596. https://doi.org/10.3390/healthcare11111596.

Plus, the arrival of computer-aided detection systems, which flagged areas that might need a closer look, further lifted the accuracy of readings. In most cases, these upgrades underscored how critical it was for technology to keep evolving, as researchers and clinicians started to appreciate more fully just how diverse breast tissue can be. More recently, adding AI to mammography has ushered in what many call a whole new era in breast cancer detection. With AI in the mix, advanced algorithms now take on the task of analyzing images, often identifying details that even experienced radiologists might miss. Thanks to breakthroughs in machine learning—and deep learning on top of that—AI has begun automating parts of image analysis, which, in turn, has meaningfully cut down false-positive alerts. By offering extra tools to help interpret mammograms, AI directly tackles challenges posed by dense tissue and streamlines overall screening. Ongoing trials in real-world clinical settings also show that these systems could be key in shaping what breast imaging trends look like in the future. Eventually, as techniques evolve further, these innovations promise not only to boost detection rates but also illustrate the need for smooth integration into existing healthcare systems, a vital step in advancing efforts to prevent breast cancer (Pachana et al., 2024; Zieminska et al., 2025) (Figure 7.4).

7.1.2. Milestones in Mammography Technology

Mammography technology has come a long way in the fight against breast cancer—playing a huge role in both detection and treatment. In the early days, the go-to method was film-based mammography; it offered a simple way to capture images of the breast. Its shortcomings, like a lower ability to pick up details in dense tissue, pushed developers to try something different in the late 1990s. Digital mammography emerged, generally speaking, with crisper images and the handy option to tweak them afterwards. Radiologists found themselves spotting unusual areas with greater ease and sharing images digitally (which often made the whole process run more smoothly), contributing to better outcomes for patients. Overall, these steady improvements remind us that adapting our diagnostic tools is key as clinical needs evolve. Then came a major twist: three-dimensional mammography, also known as breast tomosynthesis. Instead of relying on a single image, this method obtains several shots from different angles to build a layered, almost tangible view of the breast's inner workings. This approach seems particularly useful for women with dense breast tissue, as it tends to cut down on both false alarms and missed cancers compared to traditional 2D images. In many cases, recent AI research for medical imaging is weaving into this process, with algorithms under trial to smooth out the interpretation of these complex views. Overall, this breakthrough shows that when we mix fresh imaging techniques with emerging tech, we start to shift the standards in breast cancer screening. AI's role in mammography marks a transformative leap in healthcare technology, going beyond simply capturing an image. With deep learning algorithms at its core, AI digs through enormous amounts of data to flag and sort out abnormalities with impressive accuracy—even if the process can sometimes feel a bit unpredictable. This speed in analyzing images often results in lighter workloads for clinicians and generally better diagnostic results. Moreover, employing AI can help tailor treatment plans based on the specifics of what's detected, which in most cases leads to more personalized patient care. At the same time, there are still important ethical issues to sort out, like data privacy and informed consent, which means careful implementation remains a must. In the final analysis, blending AI with mammography reflects a broader trend where ongoing innovation reshapes diagnostic practices and paves the way for a new era in medical imaging (Coelho, 2023; Karalis, 2024).

7.1.3. Evolution of Guidelines and Recommendations

Clinical guidelines for mammography have been moving forward for a long time, always with an eye on improving how we screen for breast cancer. In the old days, the rules were shaped a lot by what was happening in medicine and technology – things that sometimes made practices vary a good bit. Over time, experts have been gathering all sorts of research and opinions, trying to mold them into recommendations that boost patient care. For example, as ideas about what good screening means shifted, individuals began to question age limits and how often screenings should occur. If you look back at past guidelines, it is pretty clear that taking a mixed, almost hands-on approach is key to handling the different risks patients face – it all points to the need for more personalized screening practices (Ingleby, 2023). Tech has played a huge role in changing mammography, and believe it or not, every new gadget has pushed us to rethink and update the guidelines. Digital mammography, tomosynthesis, and even AI are examples of these leaps forward that need a fresh look within current frameworks. Their aim is generally to ramp up detection rates while cutting down on false alarms, making our screening efforts both sharper and more efficient. At the same time, guidelines have started leaning more into patient-focused care – a balance between what the tech can offer and what patients prefer, in most cases. This ongoing chatter about fitting new technology into the mix meshes pretty well with the older recommendations, showing that experts are continually rechecking and rethinking best practices based on new evidence (Servin et al., 2023). These days, there's been a noticeable shift toward shared decision-making that has changed the conversation around mammography guidelines. Healthcare providers are waking up to the fact that every patient's story is unique, which means that guidelines have slowly morphed from strict orders into more flexible plans. This change opens the door for real talk about the risks and benefits of screening, giving women the chance to choose what fits best with their own lives. Overall, this trend shows that healthcare is gradually putting more emphasis on personal involvement rather than one-size-fits-all solutions. And, as discussions about mammography keep evolving, it's crucial that guidelines continue to adapt in step with both scientific breakthroughs and shifting patient expectations (Ingleby, 2023) (Figure 7.5).

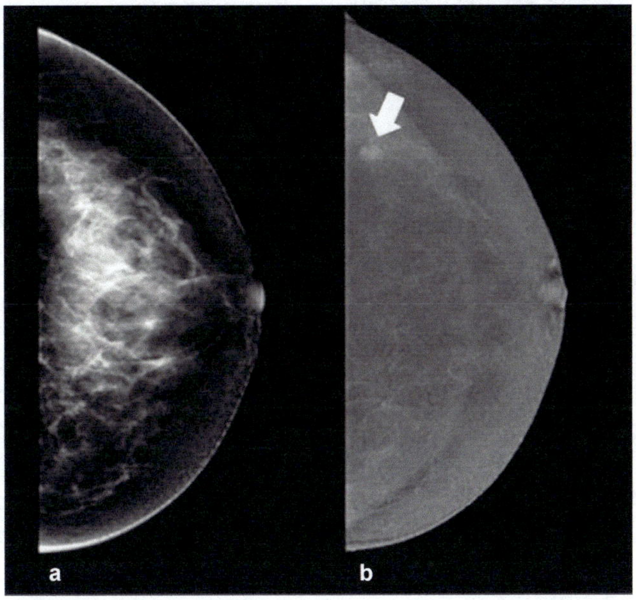

Figure 7.5. A CEM recombined image (after injection of contrast medium) from a 48-year-old woman with dense breasts.

Source: Nicosia, Luca, Giulia Gnocchi, Ilaria Gorini, Massimo Venturini, Federico Fontana, Filippo Pesapane, Ida Abiuso, Anna Carla Bozzini, Maria Pizzamiglio, Antuono Latronico, and et al. 2023. "History of Mammography: Analysis of Breast Imaging Diagnostic Achievements over the Last Century" *Healthcare* 11, no. 11: 1596. https://doi.org/10.3390/healthcare11111596.

Test Your Knowledge

1. What were the key developments in early mammography techniques that contributed to the detection of breast cancer?
2. What are some significant milestones in the evolution of mammography technology, and how have they improved diagnostic accuracy?

7.2. Types of Mammography

Learning Outcome

1. Explain the conventional film mammography.
2. Define digital mammography and 3D mammography (tomosynthesis).

Breast cancer screening techniques have come a long way. Film mammography was once the backbone of detecting both invasive and non-invasive tumors, a method relied upon for decades. Yet, over time, its limits in sensitivity pushed experts to try something new—digital mammography, which ups the image clarity and even lets doctors adjust images more freely. Digital records also speed up how quickly images are pulled up and shared among clinicians, thereby easing the diagnostic process. As we learn more about breast cancer, it becomes pretty clear: better imaging does matter for early detection, and that, in turn, has a big impact on patient outcomes and survival rates. 3D mammography, often called tomosynthesis, has burst onto the scene in an almost surprising way. This method snaps several slices of breast tissue, letting radiologists view the breast in layers rather than a single flat picture. Research generally suggests that, especially for women with denser breast tissue (where older methods sometimes miss tumors), this layered approach catches more cancers. It also seems to cut down on false positives, which can ease the worry and extra testing that come with them. Some preliminary findings even hint at a reduction in callbacks for follow-up exams, meaning less needless intervention and a more efficient use of medical resources. Then there's contrast-enhanced breast MRI—a notable step forward for women deemed high risk. Studies show that this technique can hit sensitivities between 81% and 100%—roughly twice as good as classic film-based methods—demonstrating its knack for spotting more aggressive cancers. It is particularly useful for those with a family history, as it not only catches cancers earlier but also picks up various types that might slip past standard imaging. As the imaging landscape keeps shifting, grasping the differences and unique perks of each technique is key; doing so helps refine screening protocols and, ultimately, improves how we manage breast cancer (Akram et al., 2017; Mann et al., 2019).

7.2.1. Conventional Film Mammography

Breast imaging has come a long way and changed how we look after women's health, especially when talking about spotting cancer early on. Film mammography, even though it has been around forever, still tends to be the first test many doctors rely on. It works by taking two-dimensional X-ray pictures of the breast so that, in many cases, radiologists can hunt for signs like calcifications or lumps. Identifying these signals early has a huge impact on treatment success, yet the method isn't perfect—it can mix up overlapping tissues and sometimes give a false alarm or miss something important (Sinclair et al., 2015). One of the big frustrations with film mammography is how its reliance on physical film can muddy details, especially in denser breasts where layers of tissue end up hiding potential issues. In many situations, the film's sensitivity to exposure creates inconsistent image quality across different types of breast compositions, leaving doctors struggling to pin down a solid diagnosis. Often, that means more imaging tests are needed to get a clear picture. Generally speaking, this isn't just a minor hiccup but a reminder we need to keep fine-tuning our techniques—healthcare pros must catch onto these uniqueness to better serve their patients (Sinclair et al., 2015). Because of these drawbacks, many new imaging technologies have started to take center stage. Newer methods, like digital mammography and even digital breast tomosynthesis, offer sharper images and give radiologists more ways to adjust and explore the pictures. This fresh approach not only makes it easier to see what's going on inside the breast but also fits better with today's expectations from both practitioners and patients. Still, the old film method isn't thrown out entirely; blending the traditional approach with digital insights helps smooth over the rough edges and ultimately leads to more accurate diagnoses and improved breast care (Figure 7.6).

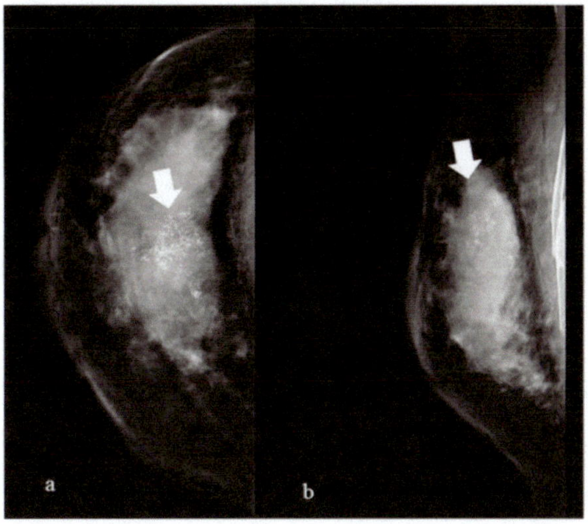

Figure 7.6. A 45-year-old woman with infiltrating ductal carcinoma of the right breast. In the figure, we can observe a craniocaudal (**a**) and mediolateral oblique projection (**b**) radiogram of the right breast with the presence of polymorphic microcalcifications extended to the upper sectors (arrow).

Source: Nicosia, Luca, Giulia Gnocchi, Ilaria Gorini, Massimo Venturini, Federico Fontana, Filippo Pesapane, Ida Abiuso, Anna Carla Bozzini, Maria Pizzamiglio, Antuono Latronico, and et al. 2023. "History of Mammography: Analysis of Breast Imaging Diagnostic Achievements over the Last Century" *Healthcare* 11, no. 11: 1596. https://doi.org/10.3390/healthcare11111596.

7.2.2. Digital Mammography

Mammography has come a long way and completely reshaped how breast cancer screening happens today. The old film methods have largely been swapped out for modern digital techniques that not only boost image quality but also make it much easier for doctors to spot subtle details in breast tissue. Digital systems use electronic sensors to capture images which then appear on high-resolution screens – giving radiologists the flexibility to tweak contrast or brightness on the fly to highlight potential issues. In most cases, these improvements have been linked to better early-stage cancer detection, paving the way for quicker treatments and overall improved patient outcomes. Plus, the newfound ease of storing and sending digital images makes second opinions and remote consultations more accessible, underlining the widespread benefits of this technology in current healthcare setups. Machine learning and AI have emerged as standout innovations, further elevating the diagnostic accuracy of digital mammography. Recent studies generally show that enormous datasets – like those from the Curated Breast Imaging Subset of the Digital Database for Screening Mammography (CBIS-DDSM) – are now used to train clever algorithms that can pick up even the most subtle shifts in an image. Predictive analytics pulls out critical details such as texture and shape, which play a key role in distinguishing between benign and malignant findings. For example, one deep learning study reported a mass lesion detection accuracy of 99.24%—a striking figure that highlights the potential of these approaches. Overall, the integration of advanced computational methods suggests a move toward a future with more efficient and reliable breast cancer screening. Open-access mammography databases have also become a key asset in pushing research and sparking innovation in breast cancer detection. These large data repositories give researchers the raw material they need to develop and fine-tune new algorithms, especially those driven by AI and deep learning. Well-known collections like the Digital Database for Screening Mammography (DDSM) and Mini-DDSM serve as essential resources, fueling collaborative efforts that refine computer-aided diagnosis tools. Such shared environments encourage a free flow of ideas—an aspect that is absolutely vital for improving these systems. Importantly, the continuous development of these databases is boosting both accuracy and efficiency in mammography, which in turn plays a crucial role in lessening the global impact of breast cancer (Figure 7.7).

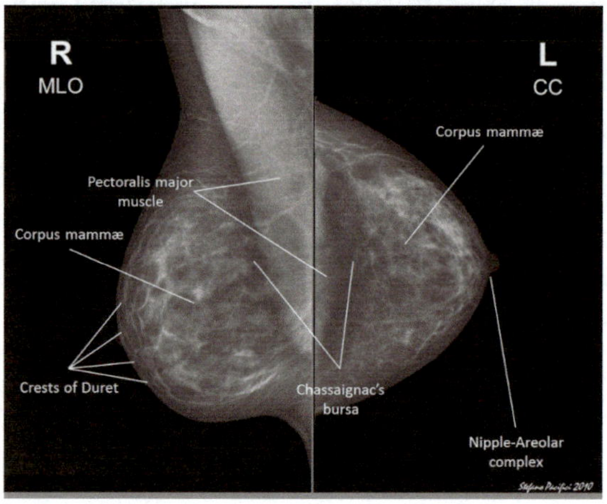

Figure 7.7. Digital mammography.

Source: https://www.wikidoc.org/index.php/File:Normal_mammograms.jpg.

7.2.3. 3D Mammography (Tomosynthesis)

3D mammography—often known as tomosynthesis—has changed the game in breast cancer screening. It obtains multiple images of the breast from all kinds of angles, instead of just offering that plain 2D view. This richer imaging, which can be a real help when the breast tissue is especially dense and spotting tumors turns into a challenge, seems to boost detection rates while cutting down on those nerve-wracking recalls from false alarms. People have been testing this out in lots of screening programs, and generally speaking, its effect on finding cancers is getting a good amount of attention. Researchers are still digging into what 3D mammography means long term, especially in those cancers that emerge between regular tests—often called interval cancers. Studies are trying to figure out if the extra images bring the rate of these in-between cancers down, which in most cases would make the overall screening process more effective. Early results hint that even though 3D chances to uncover more cancers, there's some worry about overdiagnosis, particularly spotting slow-growing tumors that might not need any treatment (Brawley et al., 2023).

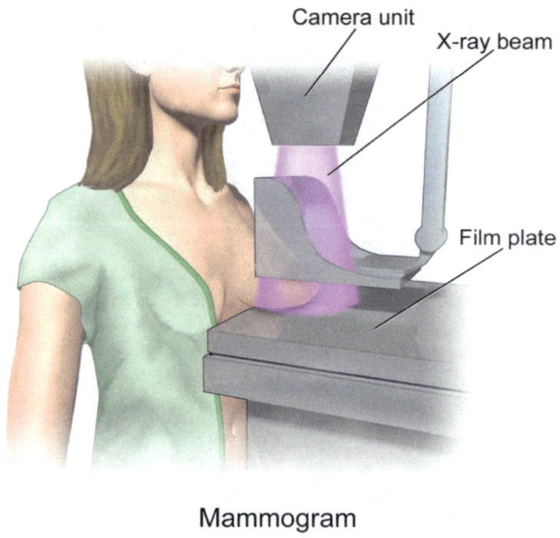

Figure 7.8. 3D mammogram or tomosynthesis.

Source: By BruceBlaus. When using this image in external sources it can be cited as:Blausen.com staff (2014). "Medical gallery of Blausen Medical 2014." WikiJournal of Medicine 1 (2). DOI:10.15347/wjm/2014.010. ISSN 2002-4436. - Own work, CC BY 3.0, https://commons.wikimedia.org/w/index.php?curid=30462648.

This situation leaves us with some tricky questions about how to balance better detection with the risk of overtreatment. Public health messages about mammography have had to keep up with these new advances, too. While individuals still stress the importance of regular screenings, it's important to also talk about the downsides—like the chances for overdiagnosis and overtreatment that come along with this heightened sensitivity (Brawley et al., 2023). The ongoing TMIST trial is looking into both sides of the coin by diving into the real-world benefits and possible issues with tomosynthesis when used in population screening (Houssami et al., 2017). As more centers adopt 3D mammography, clear and straightforward communication is key so that women get the scoop on both the benefits and the risks when making decisions about their breast health (Figure 7.8).

Test Your Knowledge

1. How does conventional film mammography work, and what are its advantages and limitations compared to newer technologies?
2. What are the key differences between digital mammography and conventional film mammography in terms of image quality and diagnostic efficiency?

7.3. The Mammography Procedure

Learning Outcome

1. Understand the preparation for a mammogram.
2. Examine the step-by-step process of the mammogram.
3. Identify post-procedure care and considerations for patients.

Mammography isn't only about snapping images—it is equally about keeping things safe and sound. The process is set up so that screenings work well while cutting down on unnecessary radiation. There's a focus on these safety checkpoints recorded during certification that kind of act as a net, identifying risks before they become issues. Looking closely at these barriers gives insights for tweaking the design to boost patient safety, and it shows how the whole procedure might be fine-tuned for both better performance and a safer experience. As noted in the literature, getting a good grip on these safety measures not only explains how mammography works but also builds trust in its overall reliability and results (Zheng et al., 2004). On the technical side, recent upgrades in image processing have seriously upped the diagnostic game. For example, using a Bayesian maximum entropy method (MEM) for radiological image deconvolution has led to crisper spatial details while still keeping noise levels in check. This method fixes issues like geometric blurring—especially when magnification is involved—making it easier to spot critical details. Radiologists benefit from these clearer shots, which in turn sparks more honest chats with patients about what might come next. Generally speaking, these innovations could ease our dependence on older imaging techniques and reshape how screenings are done (Birch et al., 2004).

Patient experience also plays a huge role in how mammography is perceived. The emotional and psychological sides of the process—like anxiety or discomfort—can sometimes get in the way of a smooth screening. A little upfront, genuine communication about what to expect can do wonders in cutting through that unease. Healthcare providers are encouraged to offer both reassurance and clear pre-procedure guidance, even if it means letting a few small inconsistencies slip in here and there. When patients feel understood and a bit more at ease, they're more likely to cooperate fully, which ultimately leads to better outcomes. In short, blending smart tech with real human care is essential for making the whole experience work well (Figure 7.9).

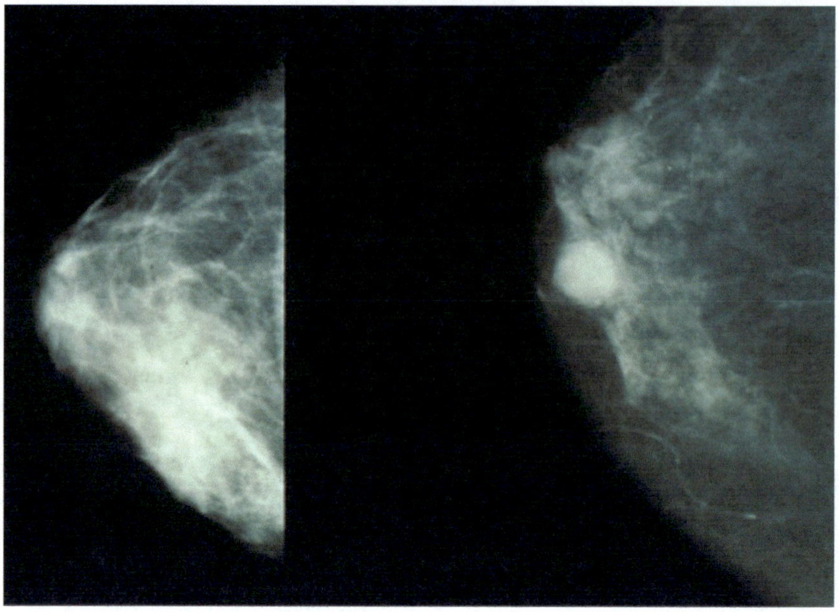

Figure 7.9. Procedure of mammography.

Source: Public Domain, https://commons.wikimedia.org/w/index.php?curid=812249.

7.3.1. Preparation for a Mammogram

Getting ready for a mammogram matters—it can change how useful the screening turns out. People often suggest planning the appointment around your cycle, usually scheduling it just after your period to help ease breast soreness. Skipping deodorants, lotions, or perfumes on the day is another tip since even a little residue might mess with the images. And if you happen to have older records, bringing them along gives the radiologist a chance to spot any shifts in your breast tissue. Knowing these simple steps before you go can improve the whole process and catch issues early. Being mentally ready is just as important as sorting out the details. Many women end up feeling nervous about the test, anxious over what the results might imply, so figuring out what to expect can ease those jitters a bit. Medical professionals keep pointing out that early detection is key—it might open the door to better treatment options. They also invite you to speak your mind if you have any concerns before the exam. Creating an environment of support makes a big difference in how the experience feels, reinforcing why regular screenings are worth it. At the end of the day, putting patient-first practices in place pays off for everyone involved. Hospitals and clinics need to offer clear, easy-to-follow information about the mammogram process, including what happens during the test, its benefits, and what comes next. Research generally shows that when patients know what's going on and feel empowered, they're more likely to stick with their appointments (Rasaq et al., 2024). Spreading awareness on proper preparation can help ease anxiety and improve overall experiences. Programs that reach out to underserved communities also play a part in making sure every woman gets screened. All these efforts together build a solid approach that leads to better detection—and eventually, better health outcomes—for women across the country (Alkureishi et al., 2009) (Figure 7.10).

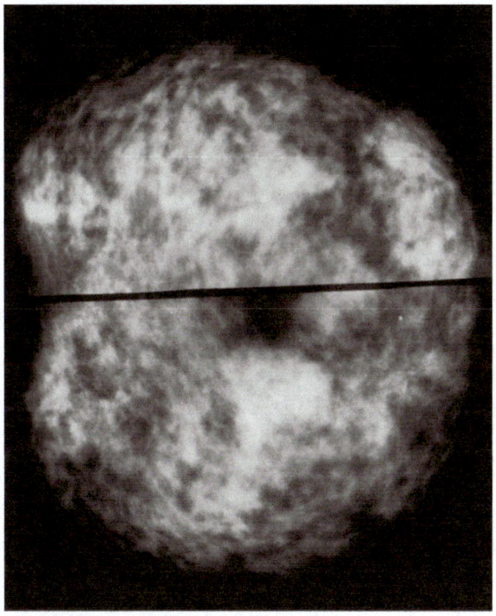

Figure 7.10. A mammogram.

Source: By Unknown photographer - This image was released by the National Cancer Institute, an agency part of the National Institutes of Health, with the ID 2695 (image) (next)., Public Domain, https://commons.wikimedia.org/w/index.php?curid=24052336.

7.3.2. Step-by-Step Process of the Mammogram

Effective mammography starts well before the actual imaging takes place. Patients usually get a rundown of what to expect, so by the time they step into the center they're fairly informed and ready—a little conversation here and there sets the stage. At the center, a technician helps guide whoever's there through paperwork and all the necessary steps. Often, the patient is asked to change into a simple gown to keep things smooth. Creating a relaxed atmosphere and spelling things out in advance helps dial down the usual nerves; this early prep builds a kind of foundation that makes the whole process work more effectively. When it is time to take the images, getting the breast positioned just right is key. The technician carefully places the breast on the mammography plate and uses a paddle to compress it. This squeeze not only keeps the breast from moving but also spreads the tissue to yield a clearer picture. Sure, the compression might feel a bit uncomfortable for a short moment, but it is a trade-off for high-quality images. Usually, each breast gets captured from two different views so that the radiologist ends up with a fuller picture of the tissue. Technologies like digital mammography come in handy here, boosting the clarity of the images and helping in the fine-tuning of lesion analysis. After those images are taken, they go through a pretty intense evaluation phase. First, any extra parts—say, the pectoral muscle—are removed to make the image cleaner. Then, some enhancement methods are applied to bump up the contrast and overall visibility, which in most cases helps pinpoint areas that might be suspect. This stage is crucial to tease apart benign from more worrisome aspects of the tissue. In the final step, automated classification tools, driven by machine learning algorithms, take the stage. These algorithms have shown impressive accuracy—typically between 92% and 97% in detecting breast lesions—highlighting the value of a careful and well-planned approach (Almalki et al., 2022; Avcı and Karakaya, 2023). (Figure 7.11).

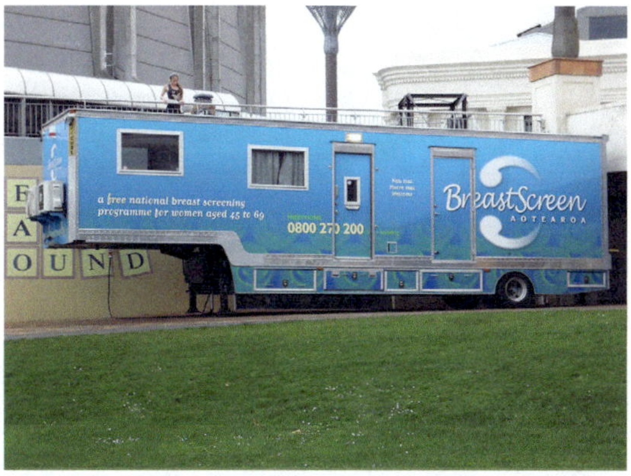

Figure 7.11. Importance of a mammogram.

Source: By William Stadtwald Demchick - Own work, CC BY 3.0, https://commons.wikimedia.org/w/index.php?curid=34458224.

7.3.3. Post-Procedure Care and Considerations

A mammogram can stir up a mix of feelings that end up influencing what happens next. Many women, after the exam, might feel uneasy about what the results could show—which sometimes even discourages getting follow-up care or future screenings. It's important, in most cases, to offer some reassurance and create a warm, supportive setting. Taking care of how patients feel helps them grasp the process better and understand why regular check-ups matter. Simple, clear information about what to expect afterward—not just the steps but also addressing issues like minor pain or discomfort—can ease their worries (Kalsta et al., 2012). It is not just about comfort, though; practical tips after the exam are equally crucial. Some women may end up with tenderness or a bit of swelling, so recommendations like using ice packs or even over-the-counter pain relievers can work wonders. Doctors should let patients know what side effects might be normal versus signs that need a closer look, giving them the tools to spot complications early and feel more in control of their recovery. A well-rounded care plan means women get not only top-notch care during the screening but also proper guidance for handling any aftereffects (Bravo et al., 2014). Staying connected after a mammogram plays a big part in long-term breast health. Quick follow-up messages can make sure patients get their results without delay and know what steps to take next. Digital tools—mHealth apps, for example—offer a handy way to access results, find educational info, and get reminders for future screenings. Many women have mentioned that these digital options help, especially for those who might struggle with face-to-face access. Research generally shows that the simplicity of using mobile apps encourages ongoing involvement in breast health programs and nudges patients to be more proactive about their wellbeing. Overall, solid post-procedure care and regular support are essential for a screening program that truly puts women's health first (Bravo et al., 2014).

Test Your Knowledge

1. What preparations should a patient make before undergoing a mammogram to ensure accurate results?
2. What is the step-by-step process involved in performing a mammogram, from positioning to imaging?

7.4. Benefits of Mammography

Learning Outcome

1. Understand the role of early detection in improving breast cancer outcomes.
2. Examine the impact of mammography on reducing breast cancer mortality rates through early intervention.
3. Explore the psychological benefits for patients.

Breast cancer is still a major issue worldwide, and finding ways to catch it early can make a difference. Mammography, which has long been relied upon as an early-detection method, keeps showing its worth. Studies tell us that women who stick with regular mammograms see a big drop in their risk of dying from the disease. Identifying tumors when they're in a milder, more manageable stage is key—even if, generally speaking, later stages can be far more troublesome. As our grasp of individual risks gets sharper, tweaking screening plans seems to help even more women get the timely care they need (Alshamrani et al., 2024).

A lot has changed with how we look at breast cancer detection these days. New imaging techniques have teamed up with classic mammography, and the result isn't hard to see. For example, blending in tools like ultrasound and digital breast tomosynthesis has noticeably upped the detection game. Early findings from the Personalized, Integrated, Network, Knowledge (P.I.N.K.) study even hint at a roughly 35.5% boost in diagnostic accuracy when extra imaging joins the mix. This kind of extra sensitivity means that pinpointing malignancies gets a bit easier, and, in most cases, patients end up with better treatment prospects. As more data trickles in, it wouldn't be surprising if screening moves toward approaches that are more personalized to each woman's risks (Franchini et al., 2021). It is also worth noting the mental boost that routine screenings provide. Many women mention feeling a bit more at ease knowing they're keeping an eye on their breast health—like they're actively managing their own risks. This proactive stance, while sometimes sounding repetitive, builds a sense of empowerment that encourages ongoing care. With growing awareness of what increases breast cancer risks, more women seem to be diving into discussions about their own health choices. So really, mammography isn't just about finding cancer early—it is part of a broad push to improve overall wellness and nudge women toward taking better charge of their lives (Alshamrani et al., 2024) (Figure 7.12).

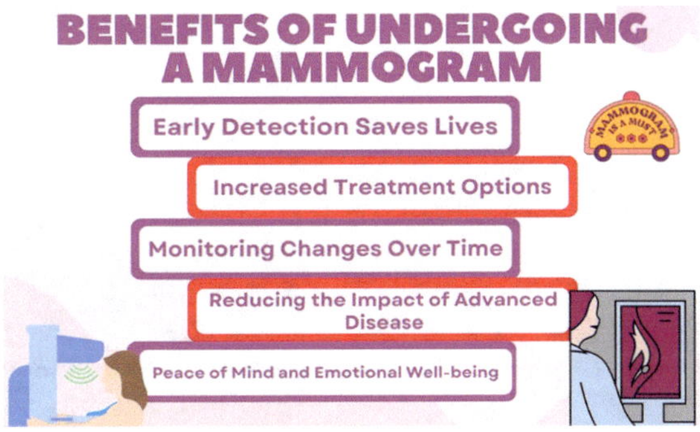

Figure 7.12. Benefits of mammography.

Source: https://www.gardenobgyn.com/cdn-cgi/image/format=webp,width=1200,height=630/https://www.gardenobgyn.com/sms/dashboard/blog_img/241790762.png.

7.4.1. Early Detection of Breast Cancer

Medical imaging tech has changed how we catch breast cancer early. Tools like mammography and breast ultrasound are key in spotting oddities that might hide cancer—sometimes in unexpected ways. In Ghana, for instance, a study found that not many hospitals offer mammography (only 21, in fact), even though a good number of women live within about an hour's drive of these services; this points to untapped opportunities for early warning systems (Price et al., 2024). Psychosocial factors also play a big role in whether women decide to get checked early. Generally speaking, when researchers looked into this using the Health Belief Model (HBM), they saw that regular breast self-exams (BSE) boosted awareness of personal risk. A study in Iraq revealed that women who did BSE on a regular basis were more tuned in to their vulnerability, which often pushed them to get a mammogram (Taher et al., 2023). This kind of observation shows that focused educational programs—ones that talk about both the risks and benefits—can create a ripple effect, nudging more women toward proactive screening. Cutting down the obstacles to screening is vital, especially in communities where medical resources are scarce. Women often face a mix of hurdles—not just issues like transportation and service availability, but also the weight of fear and misinformation about breast cancer. Strengthening the radiology workforce and ramping up community outreach might just be the way to ease these challenges. More widespread access to tests like mammography and ultrasound could lift early detection rates, which is crucial for effective treatment and better outcomes. Finally, teaming up with healthcare providers, local leaders and schools can help spread the word and build a support system for women's health initiatives (Figure 7.13).

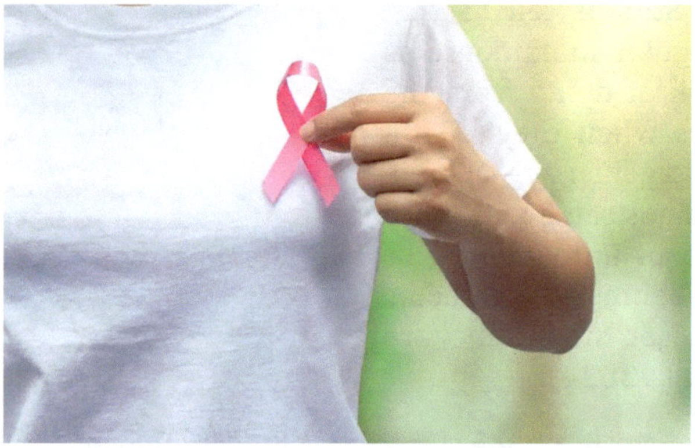

Figure 7.13. Medical imaging tech has changed how we catch breast cancer early.

Source: https://etimg.etb2bimg.com/thumb/msid-95077250,imgsize-35636,width-1200,height=765,overlay-ethealth/health-it/advanced-technologies-that-aid-in-early-detection-and-prognosis-of-breast-cancer.jpg.

7.4.2. Reduction in Mortality Rates

Improved mammogram screening has shifted the game against breast cancer. For example, looking at one set of simulations from the Valencia Region shows that when women aged 45 to 74 were included, mortality dropped by about 32.2% – a bit more impressive than the roughly 30.6% reduction seen when only the 45–69 age group was screened (Pinto-Carbó et al., 2024). These numbers, in most cases, suggest that simply widening the age range can work wonders by identifying issues earlier and ultimately saving lives. Sticking to the screening guidelines also seems to boost benefits even more. Even a modest increase in participation, say around 5%, consistently tied into better outcomes, with more cases being spotted earlier and death rates gradually declining (Pinto-Carbó et al., 2022). When more individuals get involved in these programs, it turns out that the added benefit compounds over time, highlighting again the vital role early detection plays. That said, expanding the age limits isn't without its downsides. Broadening the criteria often brings along a surge in false positives and even overdiagnosis – risks that can weigh heavily both psychologically and financially on patients and the healthcare system. In those same real-world tests, the higher likelihood of false alarms became an additional concern, meaning that while the promise of widespread screening is appealing, optimizing protocols to minimize these risks is absolutely crucial (Pinto-Carbó et al., 2022) (Figure 7.14).

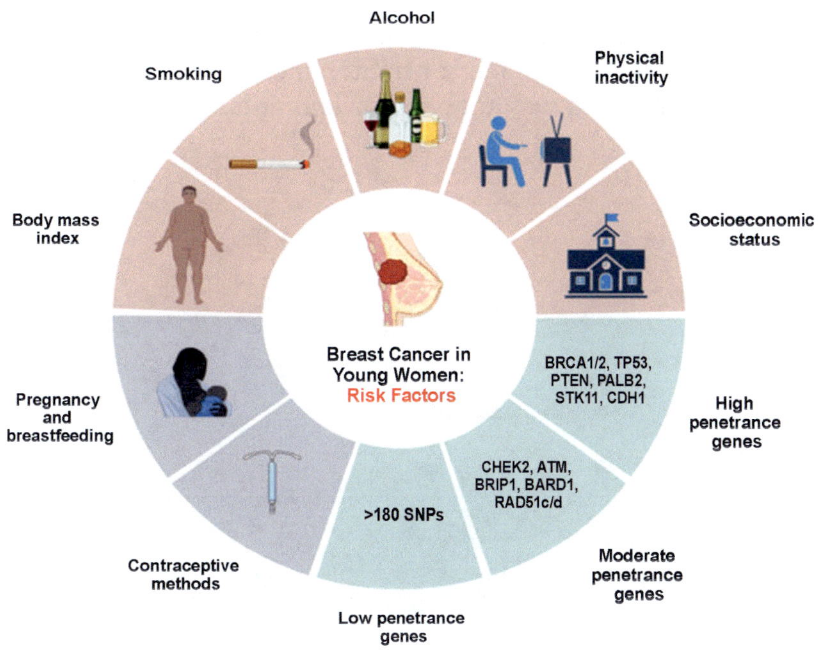

Figure 7.14. Annual reduction in the breast cancer mortality rate, relative to a situation without screening.

Source: Zhu JW, Charkhchi P, Adekunte S, Akbari MR. What Is Known about Breast Cancer in Young Women? *Cancers*. 2023; 15(6):1917. https://doi.org/10.3390/cancers15061917.

7.4.3. Psychological Benefits for Patients

Psychological rewards and the whole experience of getting a mammogram mix together in ways that aren't always straightforward. Many women see going in for a mammogram as more than just a check-up—it becomes a sign they're taking their health seriously, boosting their sense of control and even a touch of empowerment. In most cases, this active step helps calm those uneasy feelings about a possible breast cancer diagnosis because it feels like they're doing something definitive. Routine screenings, as odd as it sounds, also lighten the emotional weight of not knowing exactly how their health is holding up. When you keep up with these tests, it is almost like you're doubling down on self-care, which in turn cuts down anxiety and lifts overall well-being. Then, there's the whole issue of skepticism that can add stress into the mix. Sometimes, doubts about mammography don't just spring from a dislike for the idea of screening—they often stem from conflicting views on its benefits versus the possible downsides. Generally speaking, when patients get consistent, clear messages about what a mammogram can do, those nagging doubts tend to ease up. It appears that when the information flows naturally and isn't too jumbled, people start to feel more at ease and even more willing to stick with regular checks. A straightforward sharing of the science might help individuals sort out their mixed beliefs, crafting a more informed and confident approach to screening (Scherer et al., 2024). Looking past the procedure itself, the impact on how one feels can extend well beyond the screening room. Early detection does more than just spot issues—it can take the edge off the fear of a surprise diagnosis. Even though there's a chance for false positives and a few extra tests along the way, for many, the peace of mind that comes from knowing their status just makes up for it. The calm that results from understanding where one stands health-wise tends to foster a brighter, more balanced outlook, underscoring the need to weigh risks and benefits in a way that supports mental health (Muhammed Sütçü, 2023).

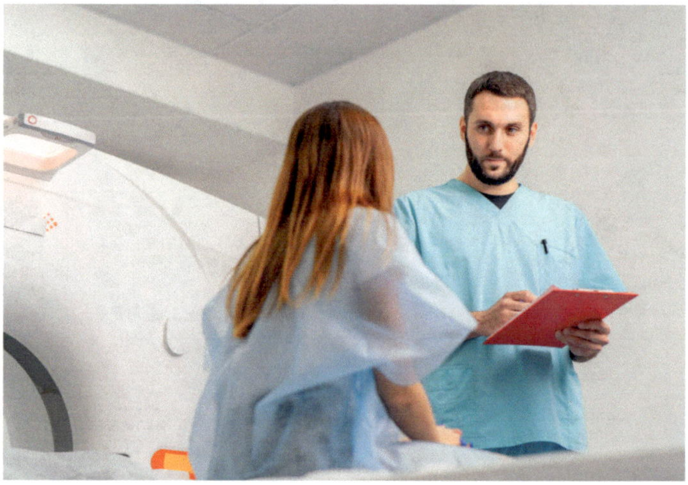

Source: https://precisionimagingcenters.com/wp-content/uploads/2024/07/early-cancer-detection.jpg.

t

Test Your Knowledge

1. What are the key benefits of mammography in detecting breast cancer at an early stage?
2. How does mammography help in reducing the risk of death from breast cancer by enabling early intervention?

7.5. Risks and Limitations

Learning Outcome

1. Understand the implications of false positives and false negatives in mammography.
2. Examine the concerns related to radiation exposure in mammography.
3. Analyze the limitations of mammography in specific populations.

Breast cancer screening sparks a lot of debate. Mammograms are seen as the top way to catch cancer early, but they come with some real issues. Overdiagnosis, for example, might lead to treatments that aren't needed, putting patients through unnecessary physical and mental stress. Even though the radiation from a mammogram is pretty small, there's still worry about what repeated exposure might mean in the long run—especially for younger women and those who get screened several times (Bell, 2022). Then there's the whole mix of other imaging techniques. MRI, along with methods like dynamic contrast-enhanced MRI, can be a better fit for some high-risk cases. Still, these alternatives sometimes miss the mark with low specificity and higher costs that make them less accessible in everyday practice. On top of that, people are looking into AI to boost mammogram results. AI shows promise, but its real impact on clinical outcomes and how accurately it screens still needs a closer look. A big factor here is the quality of data—bad data can easily swing things into producing too many false positives or negatives (Bell, 2022). In most cases, it seems like a fresh look at current mammography practices is overdue. New tech and fresh methods keep changing how we weigh the benefits against the risks. Ropers et al. even point out that the scales can tip over time, so rather than ditching screening altogether, tweaks like adjusting how often one screens or focusing on those at higher risk might do the trick. Recognizing these risks and limits is important if we want to build a screening approach that is safer and fairer to everyone (Bell, 2022) (Figure 7.15).

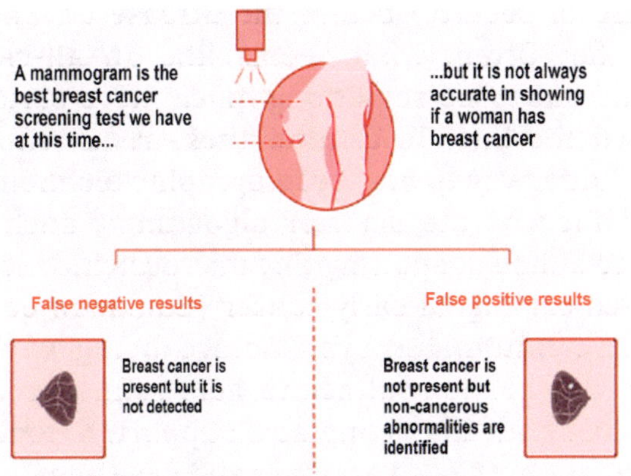

Figure 7.15. Limitations of breast screening.

Source: https://www2.hse.ie/conditions/breast-screening/benefits-limitations/.

7.5.1. False Positives and Negatives

Mammographic screening can be a real maze with lots of hidden complications that mess with how accurately we diagnose things. False positives, For example, are a major headache – sometimes a mammogram wrongly points to cancer, which creates extra worry, leads to unnecessary invasive tests like biopsies, and hikes up healthcare bills. Research generally shows that radiographers, even with their intensive training, tend to match seasoned radiologists in picking up true positives, but they also bring along a higher chance of false alarms. For example, a group of Mexican radiographers had a median false-positive rate of 49.5% (Torres-Mejía et al., 2015) – a clear sign that even a test with decent sensitivity can mix things up. This has people wondering about the effectiveness of training programs for non-physician readers and highlights the pressing need for better-designed screening systems, especially in places where radiologists are few and far between. On the other hand, false negatives are equally worrisome because they can hold up a cancer diagnosis, letting the disease go unchecked. Early-stage breast cancers might be so quiet on a mammogram that they barely make a blip, leaving patients with a false sense of security before the disease advances too far. Often, what seems like an all-clear turns out to be something much more serious down the line. To counter these risks, efforts are underway to boost radiographic technology and incorporate smarter algorithms, such as those aimed at spotting tiny microcalcifications, which can signal early cancer (Bankman et al., 1993). Automated systems are being woven into diagnostic routines to help refine overall accuracy, ideally acting as a supportive tool to decrease both false positives and false negatives. When you look at the bigger picture, the tug-of-war between false alarms and missed cases has a real impact on patient care and health policy. The desire to ramp up sensitivity sometimes inadvertently triggers a surge in false positives, setting off a chain reaction of anxiety and extra testing, not to mention piling more financial pressure on healthcare systems. With radiographers already showing some promise, there's growing interest in rethinking training methods and harnessing new technologies to strike a better balance. In most cases, carefully reviewing these approaches is essential, particularly in areas grappling with a radiologist shortage, so that screening programs continue to work effectively while keeping the pitfalls of mistaken interpretations to a minimum (Torres-Mejía et al., 2015).

7.5.2. Radiation Exposure Concerns

Radiation risks in mammography continue to worry both patients and clinicians. The test's benefits get weighed against the chance for harm, and many studies, in most cases, hint that professionals, especially women, are uneasy about long-term exposure affecting reproductive health. Some female experts in fields like urology or electrophysiology even mention that current policies just don't cut it during pregnancy. Outdated data mixed with anecdotal stories often holds back progress, revealing a real need for fresh, research-driven safety guidelines (Wenzel et al., 2024). Ionizing radiation doesn't just live in theory; it pops up in many real-life ways that can ripple into future generations. Quite a few medics, particularly women, have voiced concerns that the radiation they face might mess with their fertility or even compromise their children's well-being. One study of electrophysiology staff showed about 67.1% felt uneasy about radiation's effects on their reproductive abilities – a sentiment echoed in other high-exposure areas.

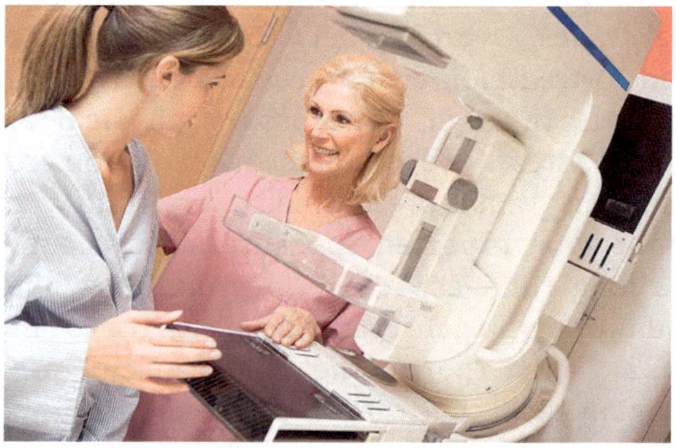

Source: https://www.eehealth.org/-/media/images/modules/blog/posts/2018/4/hdcancermammogramradiation.jpg.

This persistent worry calls, generally speaking, for improved training and more secure working conditions, including specific adjustments for pregnant professionals in the mammography realm (Adeliño et al., 2023). All this evidence makes it clear that tougher safety protocols for mammography are urgently needed. Building awareness through education can give healthcare providers the know-how for safer practices, particularly for those most at risk, such as pregnant women. When a work culture values safety and sticks with current guidelines, the benefits of mammograms can be balanced more fairly against radiation hazards. This hands-on, proactive approach not only helps ease present fears but also fosters a more informed and trusting patient experience – a sign of genuine commitment to top-notch healthcare for women (Wenzel et al., 2024).

7.5.3. Limitations in Certain Populations

Mammography uptake isn't just about having the screening available—there's a tangled mix of factors at play that hit some communities harder than others. Culture, For example, carries a lot of weight. Take the case of the KIM-CHI program among Korean Americans; rather than just pushing for mammograms, this initiative got couples involved, sparking conversation about health in a way that resonated. By tuning into the specific cultural health beliefs, the effort led to a noticeable, statistically significant rise in screening over time. This shows that when messages are shaped to fit a community's unique views, they tend to work better—especially for groups like immigrant women who traditionally participate less in these programs (Cho et al., 2014). On the other side of the coin, socio-economic factors add another layer of complexity. Women facing financial challenges often run up against obstacles like high costs, lack of insurance, and few nearby healthcare centers. Sometimes, issues like limited transportation options and chaotic work or family schedules only amplify the problem. There's also that common mix of not knowing why regular mammograms matter and even feeling uneasy about medical procedures—a reality supported by various studies. While targeted education campaigns can help clear up misunderstandings and encourage screening, if the deeper economic hurdles aren't tackled, a simple push for more awareness won't be enough (Schwartz et al., 2011). All these factors play a part in why breast cancer survival rates suffer among underserved groups. When access is uneven, diagnosis and treatment tend to come too late, leading to poorer outcomes compared to places with smoother screening systems. To move the needle on mammography rates, healthcare policies need to focus on breaking down these access barriers and offering financial help to those who need it. Getting communities involved in designing health initiatives can also build trust and boost participation. Initiatives like KIM-CHI illustrate that blending cultural sensitivity with solutions to economic challenges can make a big difference. The ongoing task is to put together strategies that mix clear educational efforts with real systemic changes, ensuring that everyone gets a fair shot at breast cancer screening (Cho et al., 2014).

Test Your Knowledge

1. What are the potential risks associated with mammography, particularly concerning radiation exposure?
2. What are some of the limitations of mammography, including false positives and false negatives, and how do they affect patient care?

Summary

Mammography's impact on cutting breast cancer deaths isn't just about the technology—it also depends on how easily individuals can get screenings and follow-up care. In many cases, communities with fewer resources run into unexpected roadblocks that keep them from regular check-ups, which messes with early detection. Look at New York State's Cancer Services Program (CSP) as one example; a study showed that only about 3.5% of people using CSP missed their follow-up visits compared to 16.5% among insured patients (Dineen et al., 2023). This gap points to a need for more focused steps, so more people stick with their follow-up care and chances for identifying cancer early improve. On another note, noticing the social and economic gaps in cancer care turns out to be pretty crucial for making good health policies. The European Cancer Inequalities Registry (ECIR) tells us that differences in who gets a mammogram aren't the same everywhere—they often depend on things like education, income, and even whether someone lives in a busy urban area. In fact, ECIR found that in some EU countries a surprisingly high number of women, especially those with less schooling, report never having had a mammogram. Generally speaking, these findings call for more determined measures to handle such imbalances, which could boost early detection and, eventually, the survival rates for breast cancer patients across a variety of backgrounds. All things considered, tackling the challenges of mammography requires a mix of new imaging advances along with strong policy moves that make sure care isn't reserved only for some. It means crafting wide-ranging strategies—ones that blend community outreach and patient education with precise interventions to ease problems of cost and access. Lessons from programs like the CSP and insights from the ECIR, in most cases, serve almost like a roadmap for policymakers trying to build health programs that work for everyone. Ultimately, if more people get into regular screenings and proper follow-up care, it could lower breast cancer deaths and help create a fairer health system for all, no matter one's background or financial situation (Piccolo et al., 2024).

Mammography has come a long way, changing how we find breast cancer in ways that aren't always neat and tidy. Contrast-Enhanced Mammography (CEM) has been stirring curiosity lately, since it might have some clear upsides over old-school digital methods. Research generally shows that CEM mixes what you see with how things behave—a combo that can sharpen diagnosis and steer treatment decisions. Some studies, for instance, have pointed out links between certain CEM traits and factors like tumor grade and molecular markers, hinting that this method could help personalize treatment plans. Sure, most write-ups mention issues like small sample sizes or some technical limits, but overall, the promise of CEM in advancing screening remains pretty compelling in the broader conversation on better imaging and oncology care (Piccolo et al., 2024). It doesn't stop at just spotting a problem, either. Mammographic results, when done right, seem to do more than flag cancer—they can shape treatment paths and even touch on a patient's mental well-being. Studies generally say that better imaging leads to earlier steps in treatment, which is key for survival. Improved techniques aren't solely about identifying a malignancy; they also help in examining tumors more deeply, which is useful when weighing surgery against other therapies. For example, CEM has been tied to revealing traits that might shift treatment plans based on how a tumor behaves or shows its biological markers. This mix of details underscores why adding advanced imaging into everyday care routines is so important, even if it sometimes feels a bit all over the place (Kyryk, 2024). In the broader realm of breast cancer screening, discussions keep popping up about new mammography methods and their chance to tweak clinical guidelines. As

CEM and other fresh imaging tools are put under the microscope, it seems vital to build protocols that look at sensitivity and specificity—but also consider how patients feel and what costs might come into play. Exploring these new techniques is all about balancing innovative ideas with what can work across different healthcare settings. Ongoing research, with its fair share of experimental bumps and limitations, is essential if we're to figure out the best ways to use these tools. Ultimately, the aim is to ensure women get top-notch care for detection and treatment, hopefully leading us toward a more individualized approach in oncology (Piccolo et al., 2024).

KEY TERMS FROM THIS CHAPTER

- 3D mammography
- Breast cancer screening
- Contrast-enhanced mammography
- Digital mammography
- Mammogram
- Public health plans
- X-ray imaging
- Breast arterial calcification (BAC)
- Breast imaging
- Dense breast tissue
- Early detection
- Microcalcifications
- Screening guidelines

Critical Thinking Questions

1. **What is the primary purpose of mammography?**
   a. To detect lung cancer
   b. To visualize the heart and blood vessels
   c. To screen for breast cancer
   d. To assess bone fractures
2. **Which type of radiation is used in mammography?**
   a. Alpha radiation
   b. X-rays
   c. Radio waves
   d. Ultrasound waves
3. **What is the common term used to describe a mammogram that shows no signs of abnormality?**
   a. Negative mammogram
   b. Positive mammogram
   c. Benign mammogram
   d. Abnormal mammogram
4. **Which of the following factors is commonly associated with an increased risk for breast cancer, and thus may lead to more frequent mammograms?**
   a. Smoking
   b. Age over 40 years
   c. Having a high-fat diet
   d. Family history of breast cancer
5. **How is a mammogram typically performed?**
   a. By injecting a contrast agent into the breast tissue
   b. By using a CT scan to view the breast tissue
   c. By compressing the breast between two plates to obtain an image
   d. By using ultrasound waves to visualize the tissue

Short Answer Questions

1. What is the history of mammography, and how has it evolved over time in breast cancer detection?
2. What are the different types of mammography, such as digital and film-screen, and how do they differ in imaging quality?
3. What is the general procedure for performing a mammogram, and what should patients expect during the process?
4. What are the key benefits of mammography in early breast cancer detection and prevention?
5. What are the potential risks and limitations of mammography, especially related to false positives and radiation exposure?

Answers to Critical Thinking Questions

1. (c); 2. (b); 3. (a); 4. (d); 5. (c)

References

1. Adeliño, R., Małaczyńska-Rajpold, K., Perrotta, L., Manninger, M., Vanduynhoven, P., Nesti, M., Goanta, E., et al. (2023). Occupational radiation exposure of electrophysiology staff with reproductive potential and during pregnancy: An EHRA survey. *Europace, 25*(4). https://www.semanticscholar.org/paper/7364f59748764d13c6e8f850d3724b2fe3f8bcfa (accessed on 23 May 2025).
2. Akram, M., Iqbal, M., Daniyal, M., & Khan, A. U. (2017). Awareness and current knowledge of breast cancer. *Biological Research, 50*. https://doi.org/10.1186/s40659-017-0140-9.
3. Alkureishi, L. W., Burak, Z., Alvarez, J. A., Ballinger, J., Bilde, A., Britten, A. J., Calabrese, L., et al. (2009). Joint practice guidelines for radionuclide lymphoscintigraphy for sentinel node localization in oral/oropharyngeal squamous cell carcinoma. *Annals of Surgical Oncology, 16*, 3190–3210. https://www.semanticscholar.org/paper/629282a768d78c130e2f4f26b9cbc7a1e356866f (accessed on 23 May 2025).
4. Almalki, Y. E., Soomro, T. A., Irfan, M., Alduraibi, S. K., & Ali, A. (2022). Computerized analysis of mammogram images for early detection of breast cancer. *Healthcare, 10*(5), 801. https://doi.org/10.3390/healthcare10050801.
5. Alshamrani, A., Alshahrani, J., Alshehri, F., & Alhathiq, A. (2024). Benefits and risks of mammography screening in women ages 40 to 49 years. *Journal of Advances and Scholarly Researches in Allied Education, 21*, 80–82. https://doi.org/10.29070/1hzsnb29.
6. Avcı, H., & Karakaya, J. (2023). A novel medical image enhancement algorithm for breast cancer detection on mammography images using machine learning. *Diagnostics, 13*, 348. https://doi.org/10.3390/diagnostics13030348.
7. Bankman, I. N., Brody, W. R., Christens-Barry, W. A., Gatewood, et al. (1993). Automated system for early breast cancer detection in mammograms. https://core.ac.uk/download/pdf/10448014.pdf (accessed on 23 May 2025).
8. Barlow, D. (2015). Breast arterial calcification and cardiovascular risk. *Menopause*. https://www.semanticscholar.org/paper/eead5e7b96bb7f2424e11e4cdd82f1ca57ceff5b (accessed on 23 May 2025).
9. Bell, R. (2022). Changes to health screening–we need to remain vigilant. *Climacteric, 25*(3), 319–320. https://www.semanticscholar.org/paper/9574f81a776830aa794f5d08ff53b1dc5b3fc351 (accessed on 23 May 2025).
10. Birch, I. P., Jackson, J. C., Jannetta, A., Kotre, et al. (2004). Mammographic image restoration using maximum entropy deconvolution. https://core.ac.uk/download/4148343.pdf (accessed on 23 May 2025).
11. Bravo, C., O'Donoghue, C., Kaplan, C. P., Luce, J., & Ozanne, E. (2014). Can mHealth improve risk assessment in underserved populations? Acceptability of a breast health questionnaire app in ethnically diverse, older, low-income women. *Journal of Health Disparities Research and Practice, 7*(4), 6.
12. Brawley, O., & Ramalingam, R. (2023). Understanding the varying biological behaviors of breast and other types of cancer to avoid overdiagnosis. *Annals of Internal Medicine, 176*(9), 1273–1274. https://www.semanticscholar.org/paper/048f3f2dfc538e9493aa4bd11f686b52631e0bdb (accessed on 23 May 2025).

13. Cho, Y., Kviz, F., Lee, E., Menon, et al. (2014). The effect of a couple's intervention to increase breast cancer screening among Korean Americans. https://core.ac.uk/download/287623823.pdf.

14. Coelho, L. (2023). How artificial intelligence is shaping medical imaging technology: A survey of innovations and applications. *Bioengineering, 10*, 1435. https://doi.org/10.3390/bioengineering10121435.

15. Dineen, P. J., & Williams, M. M. (2023). Abstract C134: Efficacy of mobile mammography and state-funded cancer services in reducing disparities in follow-up adherence: A retrospective analysis. *Cancer Epidemiology, Biomarkers & Prevention.* https://www.semanticscholar.org/paper/0f772a458034c7b617caebb2810360b8b1a453c5 (accessed on 23 May 2025).

16. Dixon, A. (2014). *Diagnostic Breast Imaging: Mammography, Sonography, Magnetic Resonance Imaging, And Interventional Procedures* (3rd ed., Vol. 22, pp. 182–183). *Ultrasound.* https://www.semanticscholar.org/paper/b2951fc6e0cc1e7c3ada8aae356e223c7f8d2671 (accessed on 23 May 2025).

17. Franchini, M., Pieroni, S., Montrucchio, E., Cucchiari, J. N., di Maggio, C., Cassano, E., Di Nubila, B., et al. (2021). The P.I.N.K. study approach for supporting personalized risk assessment and early diagnosis of breast cancer. *International Journal of Environmental Research and Public Health, 18.* https://www.semanticscholar.org/paper/562c050414317e80889a64cd3d6d1dd6617645fb (accessed on 23 May 2025).

18. Houssami, N., Lång, K., Hofvind, S., Zackrisson, S., Bernardi, D., Hunter, K., Askie, L., et al. (2017). Effectiveness of digital breast tomosynthesis (3D-mammography) in population breast cancer screening: A protocol for a collaborative individual participant data (IPD) meta-analysis. *Translational Cancer Research, 6*, 869–877. https://www.semanticscholar.org/paper/cad52793aa02c4167b7e79009097f62387b4a86a (accessed on 23 May 2025).

19. Ingleby, A. (2023). The evolution of leg ulcer guidelines and recommendations. *British Journal of Community Nursing, 28*(Suppl 12), S22–S30. https://www.semanticscholar.org/paper/7ec680736b2f600057fb9208f2ffd9d400279aab (accessed on 23 May 2025).

20. Jaradat, J. H., Amro, R., Hamamreh, R., Musleh, A., & Abdelgalil, M. (2024). From data to diagnosis: Narrative review of open-access mammography databases for breast cancer detection. *High Yield Medical Reviews.* https://www.semanticscholar.org/paper/44e0ebb0f6e3a6bcf9a56451c2790a5e5eb9c10e (accessed on 23 May 2025).

21. Jhumkhawala, V., Lobaina, D., Okwaraji, G., Zerrouki, Y., Burgoa, S., Marciniak, A., Densley, S., et al. (2024). Social determinants of health and health inequities in breast cancer screening: A scoping review. *Frontiers in Public Health, 12.* https://www.semanticscholar.org/paper/1f9cbb51b7deba91b0f30865533506227d6d1fab (accessed on 23 May 2025).

22. Kalsta, K., Cox, K., Holloway, A., & Kalokerinou, A. (2012). Mammography screening in Greece: An exploratory survey of women's views, experiences and behaviours. *International Journal of Caring Sciences, 5*(2), 147–156.

23. Kandiah, M., & Parsa, P. (2010). Predictors of adherence to clinical breast examination and mammography screening among Malaysian women. https://core.ac.uk/download/153800246.pdf (accessed on 23 May 2025).

24. Karalis, V. (2024). The integration of artificial intelligence into clinical practice. *Applied Biosciences, 3*(1), 14–44. https://doi.org/10.3390/applbiosci3010002.

25. Kashyap, D., Pal, D., Sharma, R., Garg, V. K., Goel, N., Koundal, D., Zaguia, A., et al. (2022). Global increase in breast cancer incidence: Risk factors and preventive measures. *BioMed Research International, 2022*, 1–16. https://doi.org/10.1155/2022/9605439.

26. Kim, T., & Kim, S. (2024). Predictive analysis of breast cancer from full-field digital mammography images using residual network. *Scalable Computing: Practice and Experience, 25*. https://www.semanticscholar.org/paper/5309865bed1850b136339381b92ba86540d48d51 (accessed on 23 May 2025).

27. Kyryk, V. (2024). Stem cell therapy for cardiac regeneration: Key points. *Cell and Organ Transplantology*. https://www.semanticscholar.org/paper/6a1b536f3691ad0d162e4187a4a2e2ffd1507b5f (accessed on 23 May 2025).

28. Łukasiewicz, S., Czeczelewski, M., Forma, A., Baj, J., Sitarz, R., & Stanisławek, A. (2021). Breast cancer—Epidemiology, risk factors, classification, prognostic markers, and current treatment strategies—An updated review. *Cancers, 13*(17), 4287. https://doi.org/10.3390/cancers13174287.

29. Mann, R. M., Kühl, C., & Moy, L. (2019). Contrast-enhanced MRI for breast cancer screening. *Journal of Magnetic Resonance Imaging, 50*(2), 377–390. https://doi.org/10.1002/jmri.26654.

30. Noroozi, A., & Tahmasebi, R. (2011). Factors influencing breast cancer screening behavior among Iranian women. https://core.ac.uk/download/33099150.pdf (accessed on 23 May 2025).

31. Olaosebikan, R. R., Crowgey, E. L., Abdullahi, S., Wudil, B. J., Gambo, S., Ramakrishnaiah, R., Bello, M., et al. (2024). Genetic and clinical determinants of stroke in sickle cell patients: Insights from a Nigerian cohort. *Blood*. https://www.semanticscholar.org/paper/54cb5a9a2deaedf79fdc737ab304206b40acb3f2 (accessed on 23 May 2025).

32. Pachana, M., Piersiak, M., Sawczuk, H., Tomasiewicz, A., Zabierowski, J., Kukuła, P., Marschollek, J., & Ziomek, M. (2024). Mammography in breast cancer screening–Current knowledge, challenges, the impact of artificial intelligence, and effectiveness with a focus on Poland. *Quality in Sport, 31*, 55967. https://doi.org/10.12775/QS.2024.31.55967.

33. Piccolo, C., Celli, I., Bandini, C., Tommasiello, M., Sammarra, M., Faggioni, L., Cioni, D., et al. (2024). The correlation between morpho-dynamic contrast-enhanced mammography (CEM) features and prognostic factors in breast cancer: A single-center retrospective analysis. *Cancers, 16*. https://www.semanticscholar.org/paper/14025ffeebddb35c1353fdd560bea84f739a3f25 (accessed on 23 May 2025).

34. Pinto-Carbó, M., Vanaclocha-Espí, M., Martín-Pozuelo, J., Romeo-Cervera, P., Hernández-García, M., Ibañez, J., Castán-Cameo, S., et al. (2024). Impact of different age ranges on the benefits and harms of the breast cancer screening programmed by the EU-TOPIA tool. *The European Journal of Public Health, 34*, 806–811. https://www.semanticscholar.org/paper/16cae362e1766578a0314321eae8434b524f9262 (accessed on 23 May 2025).

35. Pinto-Carbó, M., Vanaclocha-Espí, M., Martín-Pozuelo, J., Romeo-Cervera, P., Hernández-García, M., Ibañez, J., Castán-Cameo, S., et al. (2022). Age ranges in breast cancer screening: Simulated scenarios and analysis of benefits and harms. *The European Journal of Public Health, 32*. https://www.semanticscholar.org/paper/1c911086d7e6bad82a78f655dfc30b392778ed2c (accessed on 23 May 2025).

36. Price, M. D., Mali, M., Dedey, F., Dzefi-Tettey, K., Li, Y., Almeida, C., Brownson, K., et al. (2024).

Mammography and breast ultrasonography services in Ghana, availability, and geographic access. *JCO Global Oncology, 10*, e2400218. https://www.semanticscholar.org/paper/0f7cda5da9b8a10940781722b2dd19ab67a65f1c (accessed on 23 May 2025).

37. Rakowski, J., & Dennis, M. J. (2006). A comparison of reconstruction algorithms for C-arm mammography tomosynthesis. *Medical Physics, 33*(8), 3018–3032. https://www.semanticscholar.org/paper/bc9fc9ec4ec2425d9c2ed18d6e3705ace2314e56 (accessed on 23 May 2025).
38. Scherer, L. D., Lewis, C. L., Cappella, J., Hersch, J., McCaffery, K., Tate, C., Smyth, H. L., et al. (2024). Skeptical reactions to breast cancer screening benefits and harms: Antecedents, consequences, and implications for screening communication. *Health Psychology*. https://www.semanticscholar.org/paper/74ab8b4a21170f64012b611622a3e9c3bc769301 (accessed on 23 May 2025).
39. Schwartz, P. H. (2011). Questioning the quantitative imperative: Decision aids, prevention, and the ethics of disclosure. https://core.ac.uk/download/131214164.pdf (accessed on 23 May 2025).
40. Servin, C., Hawthorne, E. K., Postner, L., Tang, C., & Tucker, C. S. (2023). Mathematical considerations in two-year computing degrees: The evolution of math in curricular guidelines. *Proceedings of the 24th Annual Conference on Information Technology Education*. https://www.semanticscholar.org/paper/e82f30b1404a56beb452ca6fba4fa02fab526390 (accessed on 23 May 2025).
41. Sinclair, P., Kable, A., & Levett-Jones, T. (2015). The effectiveness of internet-based e-learning on clinician behavior and patient outcomes: A systematic review protocol. *JBI Database of Systematic Reviews and Implementation Reports, 13*(2), 52–64. https://www.semanticscholar.org/paper/9e4406273c0fc9033c3a879e664d2bb5683e9237 (accessed on 23 May 2025).
42. Sütçü, M. (2023). Optimal time intervals between personal mammogram test decisions. *International Journal of Advanced Natural Sciences and Engineering Researches, 7*(4), 196–202. https://doi.org/10.59287/ijanser.650.
43. Taher, T. M. J., Saadi, R., & Sarray, F. (2023). The health belief model attitudes of Iraqi women towards breast cancer and its early detection methods. *Ethiopian Journal of Reproductive Health.* https://www.semanticscholar.org/paper/f7f164eed42f4c990a84b72f9a1d7346a02fc629 (accessed on 23 May 2025).
44. Torres-Mejía, G., Smith, R. A., Carranza-Flores, M. d. l. L., et al. (2015). Radiographers supporting radiologists in the interpretation of screening mammography: A viable strategy to meet the shortage in the number of radiologists. *BMC Cancer, 15*, 410. https://doi.org/10.1186/s12885-015-1399-2.
45. Wenzel, J. L., Seideman, C. A., & Semins, M. J. (2024). Occupational radiation exposure during pregnancy: A survey of urologists on perception, experience, and practice patterns. *Journal of Endourology, 38*(7), 682–689. https://doi.org/10.1089/end.2024.0029.
46. World Health Organization (WHO) Epidemic and Pandemic Prevention. (2023). Monitoring inequalities in cancer prevention and care in Europe. *The European Journal of Public Health, 33*. https://www.semanticscholar.org/paper/9bd68ffb7d9b9c8150cdf4f8f29228489b66971f (accessed on 23 May 2025).

47. Yuvabalakumaran, G., Selvakumaran, A., Sidhesh, R. M., & Nishanth, N. (2024). Breast arterial calcification in screening mammograms and its correlation with carotid intima media thickness: A cross-sectional study. *Frontiers in Health Informatics, 14*(2), 11–18.

48. Zheng, B., Dhillon, B. S., Boggis, C. R. M., Johnson, C. W., Reason, J., Strigini, L., Storey, N., et al. (2004). How explicit are the barriers to failure in safety arguments? https://core.ac.uk/download/65876.pdf.

49. Ziemińska, D., Motolko, K., Burczyk, R., Duszyński, K., Tokarczyk, E., Michalska, M., & Łabuda, A. (2025). The role of artificial intelligence in detecting breast lesions using ultrasound. *Quality in Sport, 37*, 57301. https://doi.org/10.12775/QS.2025.37.57301.

FLUOROSCOPY

8

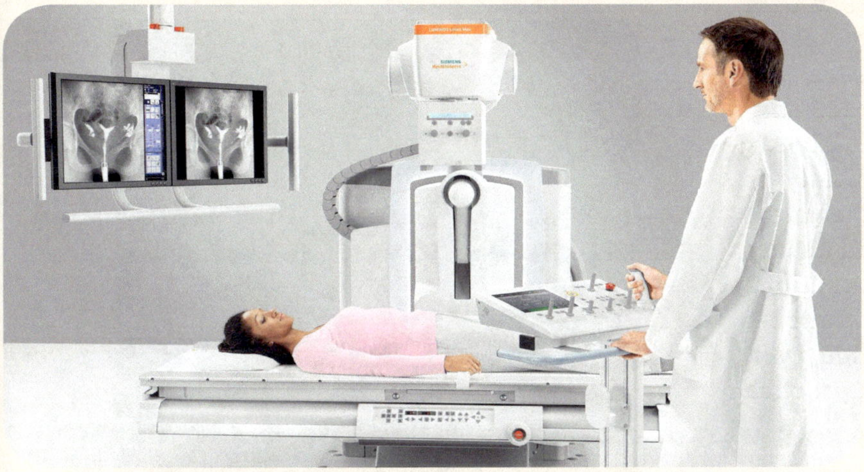

LEARNING OBJECTIVES

After studying this chapter, you will be able to:

1. Understand the principles underlying fluoroscopy.
2. Explore the various applications of fluoroscopy in medical diagnostics and procedures.
3. Analyze the advantages, risks, and limitations associated with fluoroscopy in clinical practice.
4. Identify and apply safety protocols in fluoroscopy to minimize patient.

Introduction

Medical imaging has changed how doctors diagnose conditions. One standout method is fluoroscopy—it uses X-rays to deliver live views of what's happening inside the body. This approach has shaken up old diagnostic routines, offering quicker, more accurate guidance during procedures that navigate tricky anatomical spots. Real-time feedback from fluoroscopy means clinicians can steer through complex areas more confidently. With more practitioners leaning on this technique, they must understand its inner workings, its real benefits, and even its limits so that they get the best results while keeping risks low. Digging into how fluoroscopy functions, we see it depends on nonstop X-ray imaging to capture moving images of internal organs. The process is pretty straightforward—a device called a fluoroscope, which pairs an X-ray source with either a fluorescent screen or a digital detector, does the trick. This setup lets healthcare providers watch bodily processes as they unfold rather than relying on static images from conventional radiography. Its flexibility has meant that fluoroscopy finds its way into many different areas, from gastrointestinal studies to tweaks in the musculoskeletal system and even vascular imaging. In many cases, its dual role in diagnosis and treatment has helped make it a central component in modern medicine, spurring ongoing tweaks and improvements in both technique and technology. Still, fluoroscopy isn't without challenges. The biggest concern, generally speaking, is radiation exposure—a risk that persists even as new tech tries to trim down the dose. There's always a worry about long-term effects from repeated exposure, and misusing this tool can lead to extra, unnecessary radiation and other unwanted outcomes. Experts suggest that using fluoroscopy carefully is critical, so staying up-to-date with the latest safety guidelines and incorporating solid quality checks is a must. By keeping these precautions in place, clinicians can better protect patients while using this powerful imaging method, even if occasionally small inconsistencies in practice slip through.

Definition of Fluoroscopy

Fluoroscopy is a key method in medicine that lets doctors see inside the body live. Regular X-rays just give you a still shot, but this technique uses a continuous X-ray beam to create a sort of moving video that shows how things work inside. It is used for all kinds of checks—locating stray objects, examining the digestive tract, or guiding catheters during minimally invasive surgeries—and technology has come a long way. Better images and lower radiation levels mean that as procedures get trickier, keeping up with safety rules becomes extra important (Fisher et al., 2022). Medical physicists, with their specialized know-how, are often on hand to make sure things run safely and effectively (Vahanian et al., 2021). At the heart of this technique is the fluoroscope, a device that mixes an X-ray source with either a fluorescent screen or a digital system. In plain terms, X-rays go right through a patient and then get turned into light that you can see, so doctors can watch movement happen in real time. This live action is super helpful for procedures like barium swallows, angiography and various interventional radiology tasks. Since these exams might mean longer exposure to radiation, keeping an eye on things like cumulative air kerma and peak skin dose is critical for balancing clarity with safety (Fisher et al., 2022).

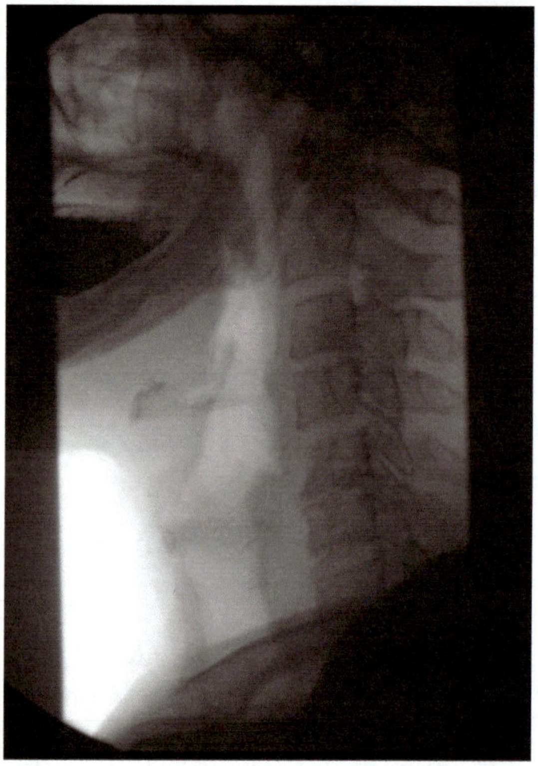

Figure 8.1. Fluoroscopy can show how parts of your body work, how blood flows through them, or help place medical devices.

Source: By Normaler_Schluck-00.jpg (and others): Hellerhoffderivative work: Anka Friedrich (talk) - 34 files:Normaler_Schluck-00.jpg[...]Normaler_Schluck-33.jpg, CC BY 4.0, https://commons.wikimedia.org/w/index.php?curid=15333554.

It is one reason why ongoing education and training in these practices is taken so seriously

(Vahanian et al., 2021). Using fluoroscopy has boosted how accurately conditions are diagnosed, but it is not without its risks—namely, extra radiation exposure. As the tech behind it keeps evolving, medical centers must regularly rethink how they manage radiation doses. They often set up detailed systems to track exposure, keep records, and even arrange follow-up care when needed. Over time, as we've learned more about the effects of cumulative radiation, there's been a stronger push toward patient safety through clear communication and informed consent. This way, the benefits of fluoroscopy are meant to more than outweigh the risks (Fisher et al., 2022). Organizations like the American Association of Physicists in Medicine agree with guidelines that help keep practices safe, effective, and ethically sound (Vahanian et al., 2021) (Figure 8.1).

Historical Background of Fluoroscopy

Fluoroscopy changed how doctors peek inside the body. Back in the late 1800s, Wilhelm Conrad Roentgen discovered X-rays in 1895 – a bit of an accident that stirred up the entire field of radiology. That little spark eventually led to a whole suite of imaging methods, with fluoroscopy emerging in the early 1900s as a game changer. Suddenly, doctors could watch live, moving images of what was going on inside patients, which was especially eye-opening in gastrointestinal cases where real-time views of organs and their functions turned guesses into facts. There was, however, a darker side. Early on, many practitioners weren't fully clued in on the dangers of ionizing radiation; they leaned on the technique a bit too heavily without proper safety checks. Studies eventually flagged some worrying trends – like a strikingly higher incidence of left-sided head and neck tumors among interventionalists (Burkland, 2020). In most cases, as the risks became clearer, professionals started to adopt safer practices. Enter the ALARA principle –, keeping radiation "as low as reasonably achievable" while still getting the diagnostic benefits. This shift, generally speaking, marked a more balanced mindset, blending new tech with caution. By the late 20th and early 21st centuries, fresh technological strides reshaped the fluoroscopy scene once again. Newer devices, such as advanced electroanatomic mapping systems, even let doctors operate with pinpoint accuracy and, in some cases, without leaning too hard on traditional fluoroscopy at all. There are reports of ablation procedures that skipped extensive fluoroscopic guidance, a move that not only protected patients but also lightened the radiation load for staff (Karimian et al., 2024). As research continues and these techniques evolve further, the promise is clear: better imaging tools that still keep safety front and center—even if sometimes the way things are expressed looks a little rough around the edges (Figure 8.2).

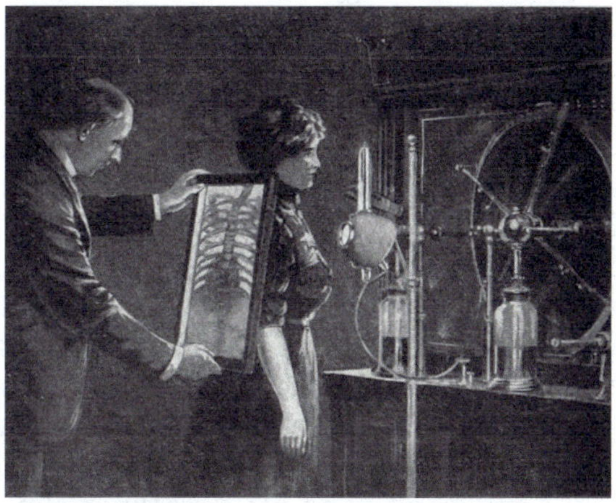

Figure 8.2. Thoracic fluoroscopy using handheld fluorescent screen, 1909. No radiation protection is used, as the dangers of X-rays were not yet recognized.

Source: https://en.wikipedia.org/wiki/Fluoroscopy#/media/File:Fluoroscopy_procedure_1909.jpg.

Importance of Fluoroscopy in Modern Medicine

Interventional radiology has come a long way, largely thanks to imaging advances—fluoroscopy in particular. It gives doctors a live view inside the body, which helps them get into a procedure with as little invasion as possible while boosting patient results. Sometimes the boundaries blur when fluoroscopy works hand-in-hand with other imaging tricks; its mix with X-ray radiography and computed tomography (CT) lets clinicians handle tasks with a level of precision and safety that wasn't seen before. In many cases, image-guided therapies have turned our usual approach on its head—fluoroscopy is at the heart of that change (Brock et al., 2023). There's a subtle repetition here: the more we use it, the more its ability to transform patient care stands out. Fluoroscopy is also a go-to tool for diagnosing and treating a wide range of conditions that impact patient management. It pops up in diverse settings, from gastroenterology to orthopedics and even cardiovascular interventions—truly a versatile player. By offering dynamic, real-time images, it lets healthcare providers see how organs work; this is especially useful when applying contrast-enhanced methods that might reveal what still pictures miss. The ongoing tweaks and innovations in fluoroscopy, generally speaking, help lift both diagnosis accuracy and therapy effectiveness, and thus keep it solidly within the domain of modern medical imaging (Bhuiyan et al., 2023). Newer iterations of fluoroscopy have also helped us untangle some of those more complicated conditions while making clinical workflows smoother. Take digital fluoroscopy, for instance—it delivers sharper images while cutting down on radiation, which has long been a safety worry. Such developments not only broaden what doctors can do diagnostically but also bolster translational research; in effect, they enrich patient care. As fluoroscopy continues to evolve, its knack for guiding interventions, checking if treatments are working, and spotting issues early remains undeniable. All that clearly underlines why ongoing investment—in both training and technology—is needed to fully tap into its potential in enhancing healthcare outcomes (Brock et al., 2023) (Figure 8.3).

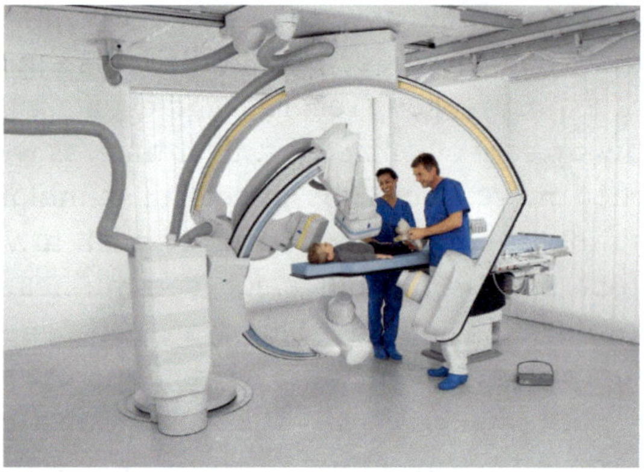

Figure 8.3. Interventional radiology has come a long way, largely thanks to imaging advances—fluoroscopy.

Source: https://media.licdn.com/dms/image/v2/D4E12AQFdSItOJfhT-w/article-cover_image-shrink_720_1280/article-cover_image-shrink_720_1280/0/1681465452343?e=2147483647&v=beta&t=mEus74l1Tpt7j48bIlMh0suJX0S41xdqokxVi9k16Ac.

8.1. Principles of Fluoroscopy

Learning Outcome

1. Understand the mechanism of action of fluoroscopy.
2. Explore the different types of fluoroscopic imaging.
3. Describe the role of X-rays in fluoroscopy.

Fluoroscopy changes the game in medical imaging—it gives us live shots of what's going on inside the body without much fuss. It works by beaming continuous X-rays that whip up images on the fly, letting doctors catch processes as they unfold. The whole idea boils down to how X-rays slip through tissues in different ways: denser parts slow them down more while lighter areas let them pass, which creates a natural contrast. That contrast is then tuned up by imaging software so that every detail of the body's inner workings pops out more clearly. Sure, it is a fantastic diagnostic tool, but there's a flip side: all that radiation exposure needs careful management. More often than not, it comes down to striking the right balance between crisp, clear images and keeping patient risks low. Artificial Intelligence (AI) has now jumped in to help sort out those radiation worries, marking a neat shift in the field. AI is gradually making fluoroscopy procedures smarter by focusing the X-rays only on the important spots. For example, clever algorithms can pick out the region of interest, meaning nearby tissues get a break from unnecessary exposure.

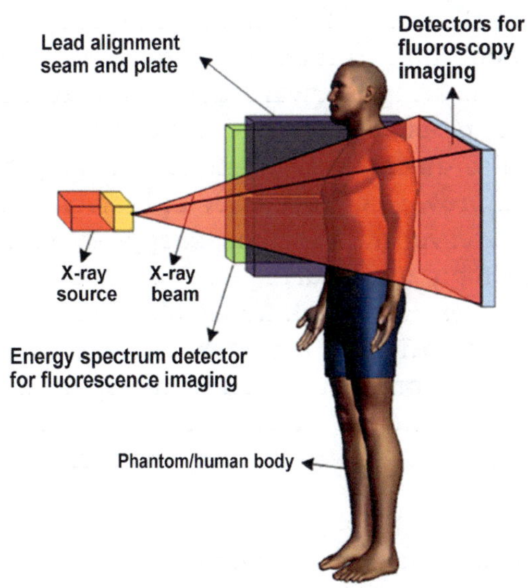

Figure 8.4. The diagram shows the components of a fluoroscopic imaging chain.

Source: Yan Z, Li L, Qiu R, Chen Z. Research on X-ray Fluorescence Enhanced Fluoroscopy Imaging Technology. *Photonics*. 2021; 8(10):441. https://doi.org/10.3390/photonics8100441.

The result? Diagnostic images get sharper and patient safety gets a boost, as current studies are now pointing out the urgent call for modern methods in radiation protection in fluoroscopy (Fiagbedzi et al., 2022). In many cases, it is that nuanced use of AI that makes the whole process feel more targeted and safe. Quality checks aren't left out of the picture either. Regular maintenance and spot-checks of fluoroscopic equipment help keep everything humming along safely and at peak performance. Older X-ray machines, for instance, can be a real hassle—outdated tech often ups radiation exposure and muddies the picture quality. By tackling these issues head-on, healthcare centers are now shifting to more advanced systems, many of which come with AI capabilities that fine-tune imaging practices while chopping down on radiation doses (Li et al., 2023). Overall, making sure everyone on the team stays up to speed with these advancements is key to boosting patient outcomes and building a culture where safety comes first (Figure 8.4).

8.1.1. Mechanism of Action

Fluoroscopy works like a live-window into the body—a steady burst of X-rays lets doctors catch a glimpse of moving tissues and anatomy in real time. Its power comes partly from how radiation interacts with different tissues, often prompting small biological responses that help sharpen images. Sometimes a carefully aimed dose brightens up details like bones, making it easier to spot issues such as fractures or arthritis. New treatment methods now mix this imaging trick into procedures like injections or ablations, meaning clinicians can maneuver through tricky anatomical areas with greater ease and, in most cases, boost patient outcomes. It all comes together in a way that often feels both practical and, frankly, a bit unsung. The way our bodies show up under the X-ray beam is pretty fascinating too. In procedures like arthrography, a contrast agent is injected right into a joint, which helps lift the internal details into better view. When that contrast mixes with

X-rays, you get different absorption patterns that make those hidden structures pop. This dynamic look at joint spaces can even offer early hints of problems like rheumatoid arthritis or other degenerative issues. These clearer images feed into better patient care and more tailored treatments. Its role in guiding joint injections, for instance, helps focus on areas that need extra attention, reinforcing treatment plans suited to each patient's unique situation. Linking imaging with treatment has taken some exciting modifications recently (Sparks, 2018). Consider merging advanced fluoroscopic methods with new modalities like extracorporeal shockwave therapy (ESWT).

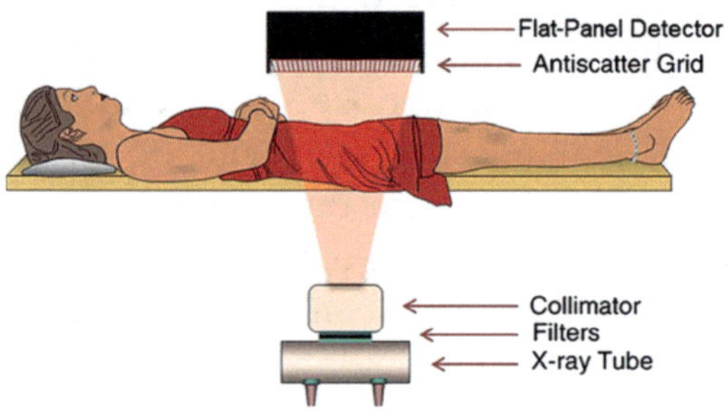

Figure 8.5. Diagram of a fluoroscopic system. The fluoroscopic imaging chain is illustrated, with the patient in the supine position. This system includes a flat-panel detector. The X-ray system includes a collimator with motorized blades that automatically adjust to conform to the current field of view (FOV) and source to image distance (SID).

Source: https://radiologykey.com/fluoroscopy-3/.

In most cases, when ESWT delivers pinpoint energy, it may even trigger cellular processes—mechanotransduction, as some call it—that boost natural healing in the musculoskeletal system. The real-time view from fluoroscopy, paired with targeted energy, gives clinicians a way to zero in on exactly where a boost is needed, thereby upping the overall therapeutic effect. Though this combination might seem a bit off the beaten path at times, it shows an evolving understanding of both how we see and treat internal issues. Researchers are continuously exploring these fresh approaches, hoping to fine-tune healing protocols across a range of challenging clinical scenarios (Tenforde et al., 2022) (Figure 8.5).

8.1.2. Types of Fluoroscopic Imaging

Fluoroscopy has many roles in modern medicine and its applications often blend diagnostic and therapeutic needs in ways that aren't always laid out in a fixed order. Consider gastrointestinal fluoroscopy, which lets doctors watch the digestive tract working in real time – you see, for instance, how swallowing and the natural push of peristalsis play out live. In an upper GI series, the patient drinks a contrast agent, usually barium, that makes the esophagus, stomach, and duodenum stand out. This approach brings forward details about ulcers, tumors, or blockages that static images might just miss; in most cases, newer imaging tools have improved both accuracy and safety. There's also interventional fluoroscopy—a method increasingly used during less-invasive surgical procedures. Here, techniques like fluoroscopic-guided biopsies or catheter placements offer immediate, sometimes even on-the-spot, visuals, helping physicians steer instruments through the body while gently avoiding important areas.

Doctors, generally speaking, find this real-time feedback vital; such images not only lower patient risk but also act as a check during the operation. Recent studies, as seen in some spinal surgery research (Ueda et al., 2025), show that enhanced three-dimensional models paired with these methods have been pretty useful in refining both training and outcomes. Then there's the field of vascular fluoroscopy, which changed the game for angiography. By using contrast agents to light up blood vessels, clinicians can get a detailed look at conditions like atherosclerosis and aneurysms. Techniques such as angioplasty and stenting lean on this continuous imaging to allow precise, targeted interventions. Moreover, innovative quality assurance measures—thanks to advanced algorithms and neural networks that flag imaging discrepancies and even dead detector elements (Box et al., 2022)—continue to push the envelope. All these advancements, when taken together, underscore the evolving and critical role of fluoroscopy in today's medical diagnostics and interventions (Figure 8.6).

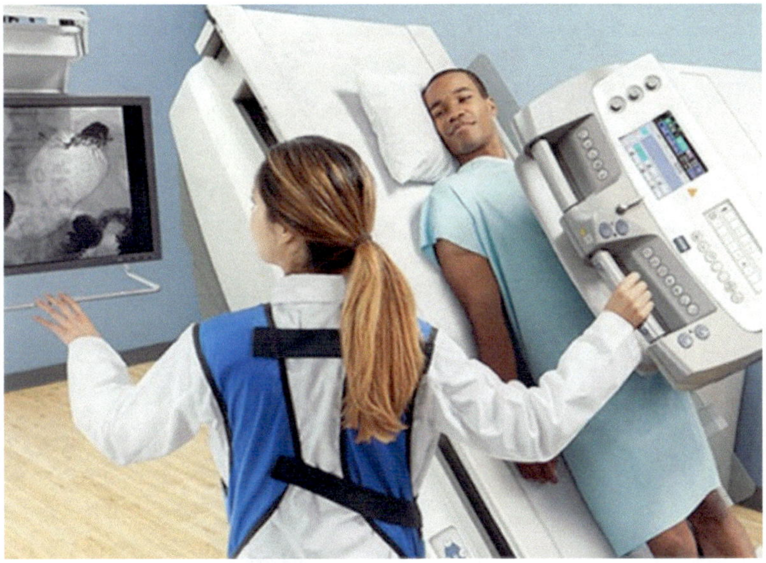

Figure 8.6. Fluoroscopic Imaging.

Source: https://coshoctonhospital.org/wp-content/uploads/2023/04/Fluoroscopy-%E2%80%93-Digital-X-ray-Imaging.jpg.

8.1.3. Role of X-Rays in Fluoroscopy

X-ray tech mixed with fluoroscopy has changed up medical imaging by letting us see processes live as they happen. It is not just a neat trick—doctors now get to watch organs and structures in motion during procedures, whether they're placing a catheter, checking on gut movement, or doing interventional work. A steady stream of X-ray images gives clinicians more room to decide on the spot, and, in many cases, this progress has combined with less invasive surgeries that help patients heal faster and better. Sure, there's a flip side here. Using X-rays in fluoroscopy also brings up some real concerns about patient safety and radiation exposure. Ionizing radiation has its risks, especially for individuals who need frequent imaging because of chronic issues. Generally speaking, finding that sweet spot between top-notch images and keeping radiation low is a big deal. Recent tweaks in imaging protocols—and a bit of AI thrown in—are showing promise in softening those risks. Low-dose imaging techniques, although not perfect, can sometimes help healthcare teams safeguard patients without losing too much diagnostic punch. The march of X-ray innovations in fluoroscopy keeps opening up new paths to clarity and speed. Digital imaging and real-time processing are now part of the scene, turning blurry images into crisp, reliable pictures that boost diagnostic confidence. As noted in some recent papers, integrating AI into these protocols may help optimize contrast and cut down on artifact interferences, making exams both sharper and smoother. These advances also tend to streamline busy clinical workflows, so doctors can jump in quicker when needed. In most cases, ongoing research remains key to tackling the current hurdles and gradually expanding what fluoroscopy can achieve (David-Olawade et al., 2025; Kim et al., 2015) (Figure 8.7).

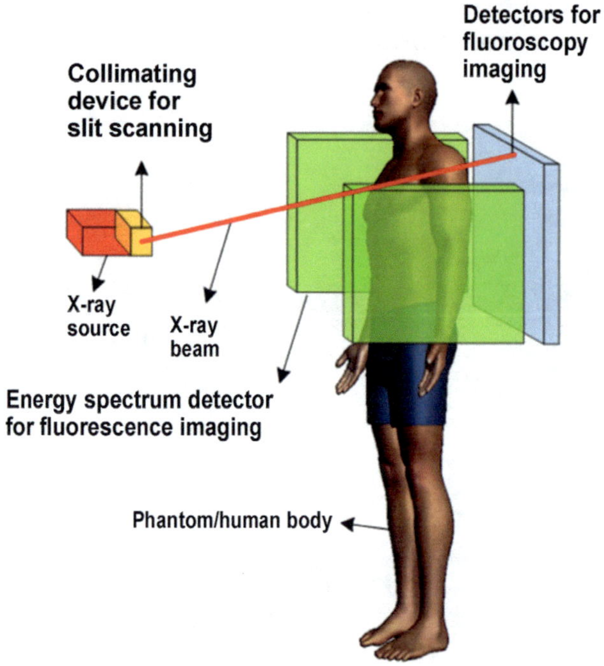

Figure 8.7. X-ray fluoroscopy system.

Source: Yan Z, Li L, Qiu R, Chen Z. Research on X-ray Fluorescence Enhanced Fluoroscopy Imaging Technology. *Photonics*. 2021; 8(10):441. https://doi.org/10.3390/photonics8100441.

Test Your Knowledge

1. What are the different types of fluoroscopic imaging, and how are they used in medical diagnostics?
2. What role do X-rays play in fluoroscopy, and how is continuous imaging achieved during a procedure?

8.2. Applications of Fluoroscopy

Learning Outcome

1. Explore the diagnostic applications of fluoroscopy across various medical specialties.
2. Understand using fluoroscopy in guiding interventional procedures with real-time imaging.
3. Examine the role of fluoroscopy in gastrointestinal studies for functional and structural assessment.

Fluoroscopy is a crucial tool in modern medical care. It lets doctors watch internal movements live using X-rays, which comes in handy in fields like gastroenterology, orthopedics, and even heart procedures. Think about how it helps when placing a stent—the images guide a doctor's every move. It is also a go-to method for checking swallowing issues, since physicians can see the mechanics in action and catch any oddities. The live view not only sharpens diagnoses but makes procedures more precise, reducing the need for invasive interventions. Adding a layer of AI to fluoroscopy is changing things up quite a bit. These smart algorithms, which are kind of complex, help clear up images, cut down on background noise, and boost how accurately issues are spotted. Generally speaking, this means clinicians can work with lower-dose imaging protocols to ease worries over radiation exposure. In many cases, studies show that AI-enhanced imaging ups both safety and effectiveness during exams—so doctors might not have to repeat scans because the quality's already there, making the whole process safer and more efficient. Fluoroscopy isn't confined to typical diagnostic work either; it has proven its worth in crises like the COVID-19 pandemic. In hospitals, the technique sped up pneumonia diagnoses, guiding quick treatment decisions. And with the rapid rollout of AI tools, radiologists could even tease apart COVID-19 pneumonia from community-acquired pneumonia—despite their similar looks on images (David-Olawade et al., 2025). All of this means that patients get the right treatment faster, and overall, the steady tweaks in fluoroscopy (especially those AI additions) hint at an exciting, if sometimes unpredictable, future for medical imaging (Figure 8.8).

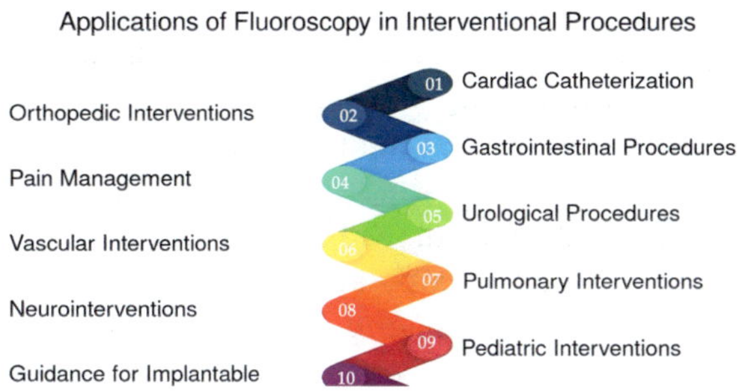

Figure 8.8. Applications of fluoroscopy in interventional procedures.

Source: https://fastercapital.com/topics/benefits-and-advantages-of-fluoroscopy-in-interventional-procedures.html.

8.2.1. Diagnostic Uses in Various Medical Fields

Medical imaging has come a long way—doctors now can look at complex issues with a clarity that was once hard to imagine. Fluoroscopy, for example, finds itself at the heart of many routines in interventional radiology and cardiology; it uses ionizing radiation to deliver real-time visuals that help with tasks like placing catheters or studying the gastrointestinal system. A neat addition is a radiation dose summary page, which in most cases gives a quick rundown of the exposure levels, thereby helping manage the health risks tied to ionizing rays (Zhao et al., 2024). In short, fluoroscopy isn't just about seeing inside the body; it is also a tool for guiding therapy and keeping patients safe. For practitioners in gastroenterology, fluoroscopy stands as a go-to method in uncovering issues within the digestive tract. Sometimes, you'll see it used in swallow studies or during barium enemas, where these tests let clinicians check for motility hiccups or even structural uniqueness in the esophagus and intestines. The beauty here is its ability to capture real-time actions—watching how contrast moves or how a swallow unfolds can boost diagnostic accuracy in ways that traditional images just can't match. And then there's the rise of AI—machine learning operations (MLOps) are now being married to these imaging techniques, generally improving data quality and model resilience so that eventually, outcomes become more reliable in GI diagnostics (Moskalenko and Kharchenko et al., 2024). In many ways, the blend of fluoroscopy and AI signals a fresh chapter in medical imaging. Fluoroscopy's reach doesn't stop at radiology or gastroenterology—it is also a trusted partner in fields like orthopedics and urology. In orthopedics, using fluoroscopic guidance helps during joint injections and even fracture repairs, making sure needles get exactly where they need to be while cutting down on potential mishaps. Meanwhile, in urology, techniques like retrograde pyelography take advantage of fluoroscopic imaging to map the urinary tract and pinpoint obstructions or oddities. Enhanced imaging methods like these work together to offer a more rounded view of patient care. Still, as technology keeps pushing forward, keeping a close eye on radiation safety and dose management remains, in most cases, absolutely critical. Balancing diagnostic brilliance with patient safety is what continues to make fluoroscopy a key player in modern medicine (Zhao et al., 2024).

8.2.2. Interventional Procedures Guided by Fluoroscopy

Advanced imaging plays a huge role in today's practice, especially in interventional radiology. Fluoroscopy now shows up in both diagnostic and therapeutic procedures, giving doctors a kind of live picture as they work through the body's complex layouts. It may sound like a win, but it isn't without its drawbacks; spending extra time in front of the machine and snapping repeated images can mean a lot more radiation for patients—and even for the medical staff. One study, for example, generally reminds us that keeping track of radiation levels isn't optional; it is a must. Overall, this mix of high-tech imaging, required safety checks, and the need for clinical precision shows that walking the line between getting a clear view and staying safe isn't always straightforward (Baron, 2024). At the same time, as more procedures lean on fluoroscopy, there's been a growing buzz about the risks attached. Healthcare individuals now have to be extra careful when choosing patients and carrying out the procedures, otherwise things can go sideways. It is not only about having the right equipment—the operator's skill and ongoing awareness of potential pitfalls weigh in too. Research suggests that while you can't completely erase all risks, a bit of careful planning and the right technique can reduce them a lot, in most cases (Bianco et al., 2023). This layered challenge means that learning never stops, and continuous training is key for anyone involved in these image-driven interventions. Patient safety remains front and center, especially when chronic pain management is on the line. With the help of fluoroscopy, doctors can often target their interventions more precisely, leading to better outcomes for patients. Yet switching from conservative methods to more invasive ones naturally brings extra risks, so a well-informed and cautious approach is needed. Ongoing chats about best practices—and even occasional missteps in technique—help everyone stay on their toes. By mixing thorough pre-procedure check-ups, careful techniques during the interventions, and a watchful eye afterward, healthcare providers can better handle the ups and downs of fluoroscopy-guided care. That balance between doing the job well and keeping patients safe ultimately boosts the quality of overall treatment (Bianco et al., 2023) (Figure 8.9).

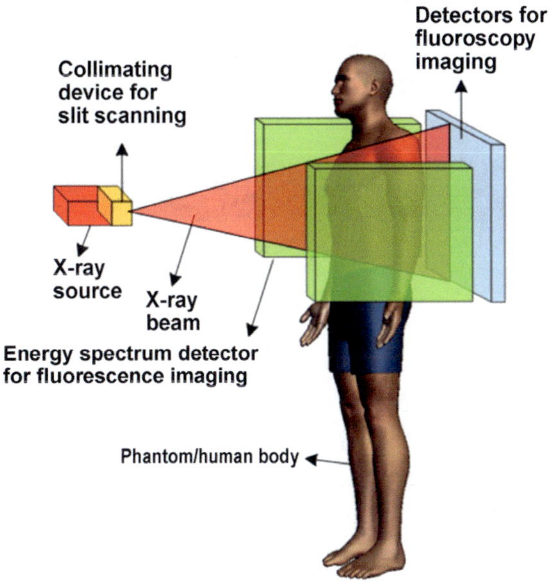

Figure 8.9. Fluorscopic approaches.

Source: Yan Z, Li L, Qiu R, Chen Z. Research on X-ray Fluorescence Enhanced Fluoroscopy Imaging Technology. *Photonics*. 2021; 8(10):441. https://doi.org/10.3390/photonics8100441.

8.2.3. Fluoroscopy in Gastrointestinal Studies

Fluoroscopy jumps in as a versatile tool for checking out digestive problems, offering a lively way to diagnose and manage issues along the gut. Real-time images let doctors spot both shape and movement uniqueness in the GI tract, and mixing in procedures like enterography or barium studies has shown to help pinpoint things such as tumors, narrow spots, or inflammation. Using a contrast dye, this method lights up the system in a way that mere static pictures just can't match. Generally speaking, tech upgrades have boosted the clarity of these images and, in many cases, even cut down how much radiation gets to patients, adding another layer of benefit to these studies. Beyond the usual fluoroscopy work, new methods have popped up that stretch what these examinations can do. Take, for instance, single operator peroral cholangiopancreatoscopy (SOPCP)—this procedure leans on fluoroscopy to improve the view when handling tricky work on the bile and pancreas. In recent studies, blending fluoroscopy with other imaging tricks tends to sharpen diagnostic precision and even enhance treatment results when dealing with biliopancreatic issues. It is important, too, to keep an eye on risks like post-procedure pancreatitis after SOPCP, since these details still steer the decision-making process for patient care. With such an all-around approach, gastroenterologists are getting more chances to fine-tune treatment plans for better outcomes (Hansson et al., 2022).

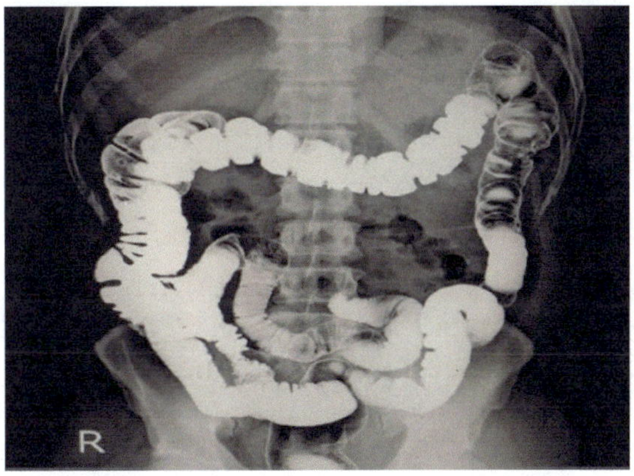

Figure 8.10. Gastrointestinal fluoroscopic examination.

Source: https://d2jx2rerrg6sh3.cloudfront.net/image-handler/picture/2019/3/shutterstock_1098970352.jpg.

Still, while fluoroscopy brings a lot to the table, there's a need to be mindful of the risks—especially the radiation part, which remains a real concern. Even though tech improvements have generally pushed doses lower, the overall exposure over time can still add up, posing challenges in everyday practice. Doctors have to juggle the clear benefits of a live, detailed view against the potential downsides of radiation exposure. Experimenting with other imaging tools and smarter dose management techniques is becoming ever more important, particularly as our understanding of radiation effects grows. Overall, this mixed approach shows why ongoing research and creative tweaks are vital—to keep patient safety in check while still making the most of what fluoroscopic imaging can do for gastrointestinal studies (Hansson et al., 2022) (Figure 8.10).

Test Your Knowledge

1. How is fluoroscopy used to guide interventional procedures such as angioplasty or catheter insertion?
2. In what ways is fluoroscopy applied in gastrointestinal studies to assess conditions like blockages or reflux?

8.3. Advantages of Risks and Limitations of Fluoroscopy

Learning Outcome

1. Explain the advantages of fluoroscopy.
2. Define the risks and limitations of fluoroscopy.

8.3.1. Advantages of Fluoroscopy

Fluoroscopy's knack for showing live images is key in many medical procedures. It gives doctors a chance to see body parts and processes as they naturally unfold, which ups the precision in treatments. In many cases, this quick view becomes critical, especially when adjustments need to happen on the fly. Take cardiac catheterization, for example - operators can watch blood flow and check the heart's structure in real time. That kind of live feedback not only boosts the assessment of heart conditions but also helps in managing them more effectively, making fluoroscopy a must-have tool in these settings. As some studies note, mixing in modern imaging techniques tends to enhance overall safety and outcomes in medicine, particularly in interventional cardiology (Ali et al., 2011).

On another note, using fluoroscopy also cuts down on both complications and procedure time. Its continuous imaging means that unexpected issues can be spotted early, letting surgeons jump in with fixes before things go sideways. This is especially vital in endoscopic work, where navigating the turns of the body's interior can be quite challenging. I recall one study on CT-based navigation for endoscopic spinal surgeries where researchers mentioned that while fluoroscopy usually guides the process reliably, its downsides do include radiation exposure and occasional positioning hassles (Assaker et al., 2001), being able to keep an eye on the operative field all the time helps lower the risk of mistakes that might extend surgery—helping overall efficiency in minimally invasive techniques.

Fluoroscopy isn't just a one-trick pony either—it finds its way into many medical specialties. You can see it in orthopedic surgeries, gastroenterology procedures, and even in vascular interventions, which shows how adaptable it is for different clinical needs. This wide-ranging usability gives healthcare professionals a sort of universal imaging tool, one that supports both diagnosis and treatment. For instance, in orthopedics, it plays a role in guiding the accurate placement of screws or other hardware, while in gastroenterology it assists in procedures like barium swallows by revealing the inner workings of the gastrointestinal tract. Overall, its combined strengths across various fields solidify fluoroscopy's status as a cornerstone in modern medical practice (Ali et al., 2011) (Figure 8.11).

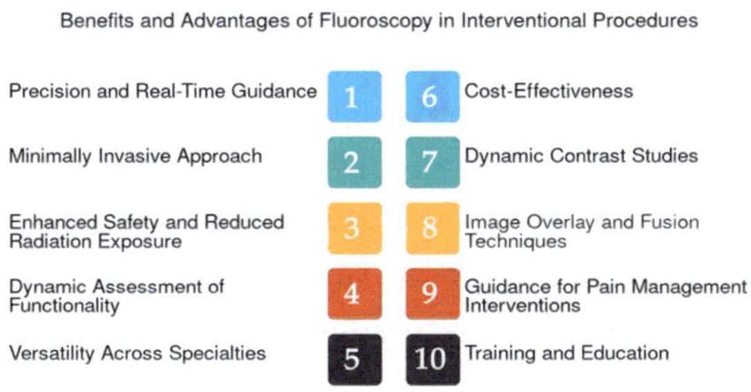

Figure 8.11. Benefits and advantages of fluoroscopy in interventional procedures.

Source: https://fastercapital.com/topics/benefits-and-advantages-of-fluoroscopy-in-interventional-procedures.html.

8.3.1.1. Real-Time Imaging Capabilities

Fluoroscopy changed the game in medical imaging. Imaging technology, which has come a long way, now captures the human body's inner workings exactly as they happen. Traditionally, doctors used film-based methods, but switching to digital approaches has speed things up and boosted accuracy. Real-time viewing now let's healthcare pros make split-second decisions that tend to improve outcomes directly—cutting back on extra imaging sessions and streamlining workflows overall. This progress, generally speaking, means more efficient patient care (Rayyani et al., 2024). AI is starting to mix with real-time imaging in interesting ways. With fluoroscopy now paired with AI, clinicians find they have extra tools for interpreting live visuals. In most cases, AI algorithms scan images quickly for any abnormalities, helping to spot potential issues early. They even contribute, in a somewhat subtle way, to tailoring treatment plans by sorting risks in real time—think of those complex cardiovascular interventions, for example. This blend of everyday tech and specialized practice pushes the quality of care a step further (Duplaga et al., 2024). The improved fluoroscopic techniques also have a big impact on interventional procedures. Right-now imaging gives doctors clear, immediate feedback during minimally invasive operations like catheter placements or biopsies, which often reduces complications and bumps up success rates. Such instant visuals, though not perfectly uniform in every case, help guide these delicate procedures. Step by step, this steady improvement in imaging means more accurate diagnoses and new, innovative therapeutic strategies, marking a transformative shift in modern clinical practice (Rayyani et al., 2024) (Figure 8.12).

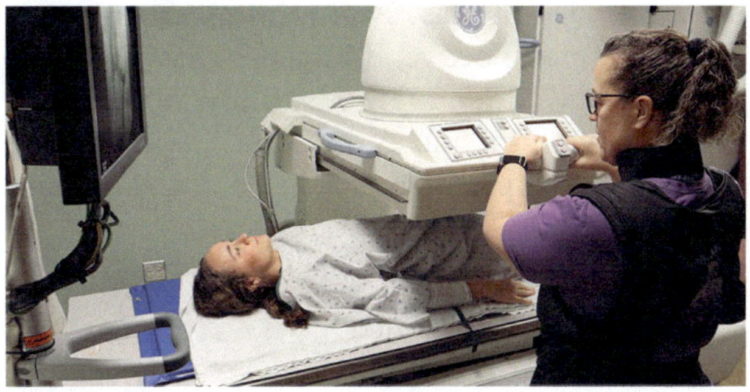

Figure 8.12. Real-Time Imaging Capabilities.

Source: https://www.brookingshealth.org/sites/default/files/media/images/articles/Brookings%20Health%20Buzz/Fluoroscopy.jpg.

8.3.1.2. Minimally Invasive Procedures

Modern surgical practices have slowly shifted away from highly invasive operations, leaning instead toward techniques that cut down on harm while still getting the job done. Small-cut surgeries—what many call minimally invasive procedures—stand out as a clear departure from traditional open methods. In many cases, tapping into real-time fluoroscopy lets doctors see what matters, boosting both precision and safety. I remember a study on adolescent idiopathic scoliosis where using fluoroscopy during MIS helped achieve notable curve corrections, minimized blood loss, and sped up recovery times. This mix of smart imaging and hands-on skill offers a glimpse into a future where operations are gentler on the patient's body and recovery comes with fewer bumps along the way (Ho et al., 2024). Fluoroscopic guidance in these less invasive approaches reaps a host of benefits by giving surgeons a live, detailed view of important body structures without the need for heavy-handed tactics. Instead of relying on clunky, traditional visuals, real-time imaging presents a sort of instant roadmap of key anatomical features. Take, for example, an intriguing midfoot study that put together fluoroscopic heatmaps to trace out crucial neurovascular routes—an innovation that helped lower the risks of unintended injuries. This fresh perspective, though not flawless, fills gaps left by older methods, allowing doctors to navigate a bit more intuitively and cutting down on postoperative hiccups (Karaismailoğlu et al., 2024).

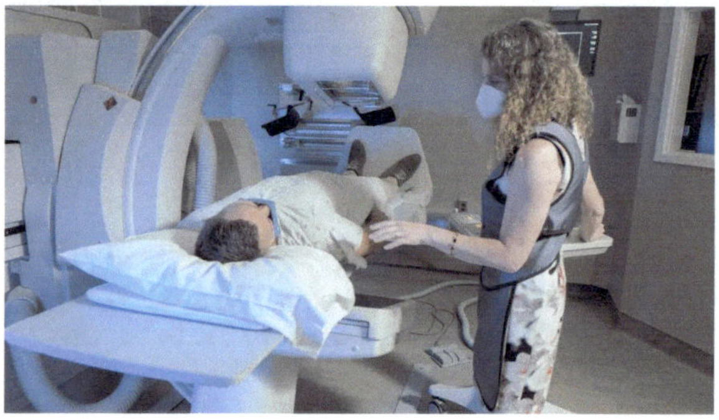

Figure 8.13. Modern surgical practices have slowly shifted away from highly invasive operations.

Source: https://www.gritman.org/wp-content/uploads/Advanced-Technology-Flouroscopy-Dominant.jpg.webp.

These smaller, nimble techniques do more than just improve immediate surgical results; they're beginning to reshape entire healthcare systems. Generally speaking, when patients undergo these refined procedures, they often find themselves spending less time in the hospital and needing fewer opioids afterwards—a real win for patient-focused care. Plus, a shorter time in surgery means less exposure to anesthesia and a smarter use of hospital resources overall. As our understanding of these methods deepens, tools like fluoroscopy keep becoming indispensable in spurring new, innovative practices in the operating room. Overall, this steady push toward improved minimally invasive strategies signals an encouraging outlook for the future of surgical care (Ho et al., 2024; Karaismailoğlu et al., 2024) (Figure 8.13).

8.3.1.3. Enhanced Diagnostic Accuracy

Medical imaging has come a long way, shifting how doctors can pinpoint problems. CT and MRI have been the usual tools to reveal what's going on inside the body, even though their images sometimes lack the resolution needed and some procedures can be invasive. Newer methods, like 3D C-arm fluoroscopy, now step in as a fresh alternative by giving real-time images with better spatial cues. Blending these 3D images with pre-operative MRI generally gives a tighter match than older setups, in turn cutting down the risk of mistakes when targeting tricky spots—especially in deep brain stimulation. This combo lets clinicians check out conditions more thoroughly and jump to interventions faster. Fluoroscopy isn't just about sharper pictures; it also smooths out how work gets done while lowering the radiation that patients face. Research shows that 3D C-arm fluoroscopy tends to involve lower average radiation levels than standard CT scans, which is a pretty big deal for keeping patients safe, and it also gives docs more confidence in their call-making. Portable fluoroscopy units, being so adaptable, can fit into a variety of clinical setups, making enhanced imaging more available across different healthcare settings. All this points to a drive to boost diagnostic performance and patient care overall (Manfield et al., 2024). Bringing improved diagnostic accuracy into everyday clinical practice isn't a one-and-done deal—it takes tech upgrades, cross-field research, and ongoing professional learning. Mixing different imaging approaches, especially with fluoroscopy in the mix, means getting a handle on how visual info ties in with clinical decisions. Ongoing studies—drawing insights from physics, psychology and neuroscience—are slowly refining these methods. These blended research efforts, though a bit uneven at times, help trim down errors and ease the understanding of tricky images. In most cases, as the medical community gets a better feel for how all these visual cues interact, diagnostic accuracy should improve, ultimately raising the bar for patient care (Manning, 2005).

8.3.2. Risks and Limitations of Fluoroscopy

Fluoroscopy has changed how we do imaging and interventions. It is amazing what it can do, yet as its use keeps growing, so do the worries about radiation exposure. Patients often get different amounts of radiation – sometimes enough that, if the dose gets too high, they might suffer immediate issues like skin burns or even develop cataracts. There's also the nagging possibility of long-term effects, like a higher chance of cancer, which generally becomes more of a concern as doses keep adding up over time. Even low doses, accumulated over years, can have implications, so balancing the benefits against the risks is a must. In most cases, this is why ongoing training and a constant refresh on radiation safety for healthcare workers is so important (Modarai et al., 2022). It is not only the patients who have to watch out; healthcare workers too must deal with these hazards. Increasingly sophisticated endovascular methods and longer fluoroscopy sessions mean that staff can get hit with higher cumulative doses. Even with advances in protective gear – think lead aprons and shields – the risk of radiation injuries remains, and in practice, operators of the equipment aren't just there to run the show. They're also keeping an eye on radiation for everyone involved, themselves included. Sometimes, lapses in following safety steps can unexpectedly lead to damaging exposure events. Usually, sticking strictly to the ideas of justification and optimization is key, especially as new technologies start showing up in everyday use (Lorusso et al., 2021). While fluoroscopy offers clear advantages, it isn't without its hurdles. The need for live, real-time imaging often means procedures drag on longer, which directly boosts radiation exposure. Plus, factors like not-so-perfect equipment calibration, unexpected patient movements, and the messy reality of complicated anatomy can throw off the clarity of images. Conditions such as obesity or a history of surgery can also throw a wrench into getting the best picture possible. So, operators have to juggle these challenges – making sure imaging is effective while keeping radiation down. In most cases, streamlined protocols, ongoing research, and regular, rigorous training are the way forward to maintain both safety and effectiveness in fluoroscopic practice (Modarai et al., 2022).

8.3.2.1. Radiation Exposure Concerns

Fluoroscopy is increasingly common in many medical procedures, and this trend has sparked a lot of chatter about radiation risks. Patients who have to undergo multiple imaging sessions sometimes worry about how those repeated doses might add up over time. In scenarios like ERCP—endoscopic retrograde cholangiopancreatography—the stakes are even higher since both the mother and fetus can face serious complications, especially in pregnant women. Even if ERCP tends to be technically demanding, some non-radiation methods are popping up as real alternatives. A review covering 27 studies on ERCP in pregnant patients underscores how crucial it is to limit radiation for those most at risk. Shifting gears, technological advances in surgery have also brought new discussions about fluoroscopic exposure (Azab et al., 2019). Computer-assisted orthopedic surgery (CAOS) now often uses fluoroscopy where precision is the name of the game for treating musculoskeletal problems. The mix of volumetric CT scans with fluoroscopic images has raised eyebrows about just how much radiation patients endure during surgical planning. Generally speaking, as CAOS moves forward, it is pretty critical to keep radiation levels in check while still getting accurate outcomes. This balancing act between harnessing high-tech capabilities and protecting patient health has driven ongoing work on alternative imaging methods that cut exposure without sacrificing quality (Kalová et al., 2019). The talk around radiation doesn't stop with immediate procedure concerns; it extends to long-term health effects too. Chronic, low-dose exposure has sometimes been linked to a higher risk of cancers and other health issues, leading many institutions to adopt strategies aimed at reducing this risk. Hospitals now use measures like lead shields and tweak their fluoroscopy protocols—steps that are seen as essential in managing exposure. Plus, when patients grasp both the risks and benefits of these exams, it makes for more relaxed, informed chats with doctors about available imaging options. Ultimately, even though fluoroscopy remains a key diagnostic tool, keeping a constant eye on radiation levels is vital to protect patient health and secure responsible medical practices (Figure 8.14).

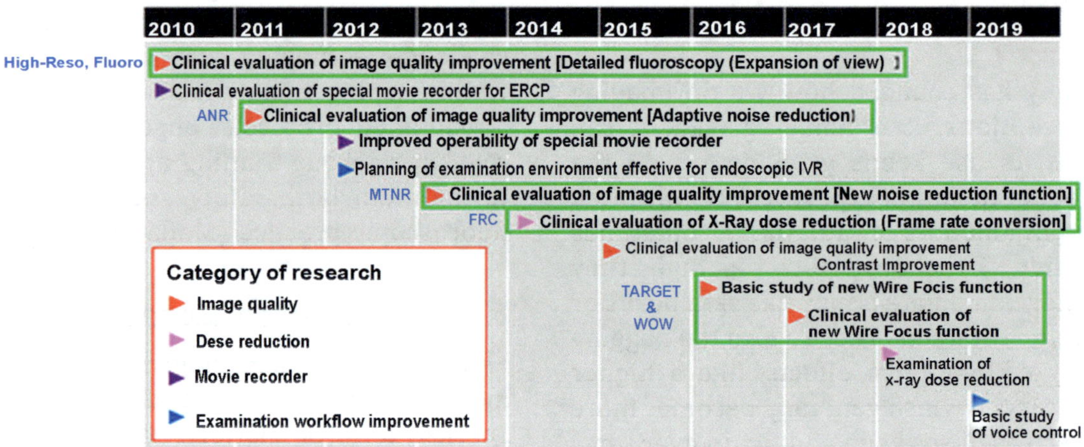

Figure 8.14. Scattered radiation during anterior-posterior fluoroscopy, with the patient in ventral decubitus. A, When the X-ray source is positioned above the patient, the radiation spreads upwards in the room. B, The best practice in terms of surgeon's exposure is when the X-ray source is positioned below the table directing the distribution of the radiation to the floor.

Source: Fukuma, Taito, Shigeto Ishii, Toshio Fujisawa, Keiko Takahashi, Tadashi Nakamura, Futoshi Shibata, Ko Tomishima, Yusuke Takasaki, Akinori Suzuki, Sho Takahashi, and et al. 2025. "Development of a Dedicated X-Ray Fluoroscopic Apparatus for Therapeutic Pancreatobiliary Endoscopy: A Review" *Journal of Clinical Medicine* 14, no. 4: 1214. https://doi.org/10.3390/jcm14041214.

8.3.2.2. Potential for Allergic Reactions to Contrast Agents

Contrast agents used in fluoroscopy can be a real mixed bag. They boost imaging clarity but sometimes come with an unwelcome side—allergic reactions that can range from minor hives to downright severe anaphylaxis. Many patients, generally speaking, handle these agents fine, yet those with a past of allergies, asthma, or even earlier contrast exposure often face higher risks.

Often the culprit seems to be hypersensitivity to iodine-based compounds that set off mediators like histamine. Knowing these risks lets healthcare providers craft a plan that tries to balance top-notch diagnostics with keeping patients safe. Gadolinium-based contrast agents (GBCA) are another story. These agents have been getting a lot of attention lately because of safety concerns despite their common use in MRI. People tend to praise GBCA for having fewer allergic-like reactions compared to traditional iodine compounds, but recent studies point out that patients with compromised kidney function might not be so lucky. Reports linking GBCA to nephrogenic systemic fibrosis have led some to rethink their dosage and overall use. Researchers have noted, in most cases, that while a build-up of gadolinium doesn't directly lead to clear neurological problems, its retention in certain brain regions calls for further scrutiny (Vymazal et al., 2024). Things keep shifting as newer drugs enter the picture. Take sugammadex, for instance, which has been introduced to reverse neuromuscular blockade; it cuts down on many of the side effects seen with older agents, yet it carries its own risk for hypersensitivity reactions (Banoub et al., 2023). This serves as a reminder, even when using well-trusted innovations, that vigilance is key. Allergic reactions—whether they're mild or quite severe—should always be part of the discussion when planning imaging studies. By having open conversations about these risks and staying curious about pharmaceutical advances, healthcare providers can hope to better manage the ever-changing challenges of patient safety during fluoroscopy.

8.3.2.3. Limitations in Certain Patient Populations

Fluoroscopy has changed how doctors look inside the body—opening up new ways to diagnose and treat conditions that used to seem almost impossible. Still, not every patient fits the typical mold. Children, for example, come with their own set of uniqueness in their bodies. Their smaller frames and special physiological needs mean that even a tiny amount of radiation can hit them harder. It is important to cut back on exposure while still nailing a clear diagnostic image. Throw in challenges like obesity or limited mobility, and suddenly the usual scan protocols might have to be adjusted on the fly just to get decent results. Older patients bring another twist to the picture. They often juggle many issues—arthritis, heart problems, even cognitive lapses—that make holding still during a scan a real challenge.

When even a small movement messes with the image and creates artifacts, it can end up muddying the clinical decision-making process. In many cases, concerns about radiation effects hit this group even harder, and providers sometimes find that getting proper informed consent becomes even more complicated when memory isn't as sharp as it once was. Generally speaking, it is a delicate balancing act: achieving clear images while always keeping the patient's well-being front and center. Then there are patients with other underlying conditions that further complicate matters. People with serious heart issues, for instance, might find themselves at increased risk when contrast agents are used to sharpen up the images—these substances can sometimes trigger abrupt kidney problems, especially if there's preexisting renal weakness. Also, those who struggle with claustrophobia or anxiety can find the enclosed space of the scanning area downright daunting, which only adds to the challenge. All these factors point to the need for more personalized, flexible approaches as imaging technology continues to evolve, helping to lower risks and boost overall efficacy in everyday clinical settings.

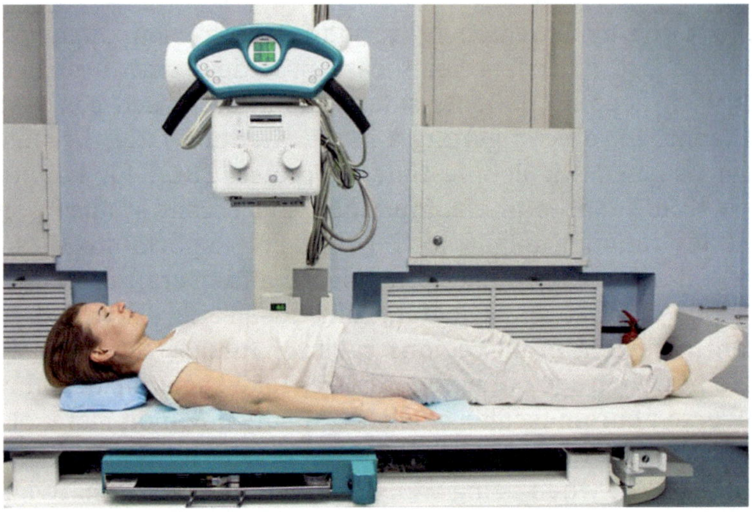

Source: https://s43932.pcdn.co/wp-content/uploads/sites/113/2023/12/Fluoroscopy-FT_1737350537.jpg.optimal.jpg.

t

Test Your Knowledge

1. What are the main advantages of fluoroscopy in providing real-time imaging during medical procedures?
2. What are some risks and limitations of fluoroscopy, especially concerning radiation exposure and prolonged procedure times?

8.4. Safety Protocols in Fluoroscopy

Learning Outcome

1. Understand and apply guidelines for minimizing radiation exposure during fluoroscopic procedures.
2. Recognize the importance of obtaining informed patient consent and providing education about fluoroscopy.
3. Examine the role of radiologic technologists in ensuring safety and adherence to radiation protection protocols.

Fluoroscopy safety measures matter a whole lot to keep both patients and healthcare staff from unnecessary radiation risks. The idea is pretty simple—stick to the ALARA principle, meaning use just as much radiation as needed for a clear picture. It starts with doing routine equipment checks and giving hands-on training to those operating it; things like that help keep procedures on the safe side. Then there's the practical bit of strapping on lead aprons, thyroid collars and the like, which cuts down extra exposure. And, in most cases, staying updated on new tech and safety tactics can make a big difference in everyday clinical settings. Watching radiation levels during procedures is also a key step, almost like an early warning system. Keeping detailed records and monitoring cumulative doses sometimes flags when things might be getting too heavy, nudging the team to make a quick change if needed. With dose-monitoring built into the system, real-time feedback—albeit a bit unexpected sometimes—lets clinicians tweak their techniques on the fly. Also, chatting with patients about how things work can help them understand both the risks and the perks, which in turn builds a kind of shared responsibility for care. Sometimes, trying out advanced imaging methods such as pulsed fluoroscopy or digital subtraction angiography lowers radiation levels while still giving decent image quality, dovetailing neatly with overall safety plans. Following these safety protocols isn't just a box-ticking exercise; it helps foster a genuine culture of care in places where fluoroscopy is used. Regular audits and reviews, even when they seem nitpicky, ensure everyone's following guidelines set by regulatory bodies. Making it easy for staff to call out any issues - even if it means a few awkward moments - speeds up improvements and keeps risks in check. Continuous training that covers not only technical skills but also the real-life impacts of radiation exposure builds a resilient system. In the end, all these efforts help safety practices evolve alongside new tech and best practices, putting the well-being of both patients and healthcare workers first (Stout et al., 2018; Tenforde et al., 2022).

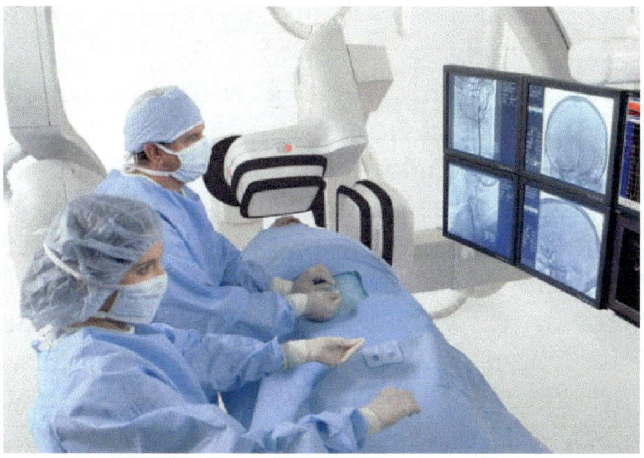

Source: https://pacifichealthusa.com/wp-content/uploads/2021/02/Untitled-design-21.png.

8.4.1. Guidelines for Minimizing Radiation Exposure

Setting up solid rules to cut down radiation during fluoroscopic procedures is vital. Risks tied to radiation in medical settings—especially during both routine diagnostics and more hands-on interventional work—show that having broad, well-thought-out protocols matters a lot. Training teams to use fluoroscopic machines properly, and weaving in simple optimization techniques into everyday routines, goes a long way toward keeping exposures low. Checklists, along with quick pre-procedure time-outs, serve as extra safety nets, reducing needless hazards. Dose alerts that kick in when radiation nears critical levels further boost patient safety. All these forward-looking steps help build a safety-first mindset in healthcare, protecting both patients and staff (Damilakis et al., 2017). On top of that, agreed-upon, consensus-based guidelines have become almost indispensable when handling the tricky sides of fluoroscopy—for example, in gastrointestinal endoscopy.

Generally speaking, these consensus statements, developed through rigorous Delphi methods, offer a more flexible way to address radiation concerns while still keeping procedures sharp and effective. They underscore caring for both healthcare workers and patients by putting safety front and center. In many cases this means keeping education and training ongoing so that everyone stays updated on best practices, risks, and the need for caution. By framing safety tips into categories like general points, continuous learning, and direct patient care, many institutions manage to cut radiation exposure without sacrificing quality (Khalaf et al., 2024). Besides routine protocols, it is pretty important that healthcare facilities also review any radiation overexposure incidents systematically. This review should dig into what went wrong, checking if the proper policies were followed, and making evidence-based tweaks to procedures. Looking closely at these mishaps can often give teams insights that help stop future issues. The guidelines also push for honest communication and transparency among staff, creating an atmosphere where radiation concerns are openly discussed—even if sometimes the discussion gets a bit messy. That collaborative feel not only makes professionals feel more personally responsible for safety but also ultimately boosts overall patient care. In sum, sticking with well-defined guidelines is key to continuously trimming radiation risks in fluoroscopy, leading to better safety outcomes in healthcare settings (Damilakis et al., 2017).

8.4.2. Importance of Patient Consent and Education

Healthcare ethics isn't a neat checklist—it is more like a jumbled conversation where patients need to know what's coming their way, especially when advanced imaging like fluoroscopy is involved. Patients should be clued in about any procedure by getting a proper rundown of what to expect; in most cases, this means understanding both the potential upsides and the risks before moving ahead. When people are allowed to weigh these factors, it builds a kind of trust and gives them control over what happens next. Forgetting to secure real consent can break that trust and even open up legal issues. Taking the time to explain what fluoroscopy might mean for someone ensures they're not just passive receivers of care, but active participants—this idea even shows up in current ethical guidelines (Ye, 2024). Talking about procedures like fluoroscopy, where the technical bits might seem overwhelming, requires plain, everyday language. A good educational approach doesn't just stick to a few words; it uses visuals, printed materials, and sometimes even casual explanations to make sure everyone gets the point. When doctors and nurses take a moment to clear up confusing details, it not only makes consent more meaningful but also eases some of the fear that comes with uncertainty. And as the world of nursing starts embracing new tech—say, AI, for instance—the need to keep patients updated on these changes becomes all the more important (Badawy et al., 2024). This balancing act between clear consent and genuine education makes patients feel respected, valued, and right at home in their decision-making process. On top of that, when the whole vibe around fluoroscopy is about open and ongoing dialogue, it naturally sets up a space where patients and providers can chat freely about whether a test is needed. This kind of atmosphere encourages patients to share doubts or preferences, which in turn helps clear up any misunderstandings—like those about radiation exposure—that might be floating around. Regular, maybe even slightly offbeat, training for healthcare teams on these ethical concerns plays a big part in keeping things grounded and effective. Staying committed to ongoing education and checking in on how well ethical guidelines are followed can make the patient-provider bond stronger and ensure that recommended imaging studies are done right (Ye, 2024). In the end, putting patient consent and education first isn't just an ethical must—it is the key to making fluoroscopy safer and more efficient in everyday practice.

8.4.3. Role of Radiologic Technologists in Safety

Radiologic techs working with fluoroscopy do a lot more than just run the imaging gear. They're busy making sure that both patients and themselves face as little radiation as possible. Following simple, yet effective, safety rules, they tackle risks head-on—this kind of hands-on care shows when studies point out that proper safety measures can cut down workplace exposure substantially (Shubayr, 2024). It is interesting how getting everyone in the healthcare crew more clued in about safety can change how individuals follow the rules. Their steady, sometimes even slightly imperfect, approach helps build an overall safer healthcare vibe. Using protective gear is key in these procedures. Techs are trained firmly to push for using lead aprons, thyroid shields, and even gonadal shields—gear that's meant to be used every time a procedure happens. Research from different hospital settings often shows that radiologic staff stick to these guidelines pretty well (Nisar et al., 2024). This isn't just about patient care; using the right apparel helps protect all healthcare personnel from potential radiation risks. In the end, their role in both encouraging and putting these protective steps into play shapes a safer work area. Keeping up-to-date with radiation safety isn't optional—it is a vital part of a tech's professional journey. As imaging tools evolve, so do the ways to handle safety, and continuous learning helps them stay ahead even when new challenges pop up. Studies have even noted lapses in safety awareness among some nursing staff, pointing to a need for more focused training on understanding and managing risk (Shubayr, 2024). By jumping into training sessions and other educational opportunities, radiologic techs not only fine-tune their own skills but also gift their colleagues with extra know-how, creating a shared sense of safety during fluoroscopic procedures (Nisar et al., 2024) (Figure 8.15).

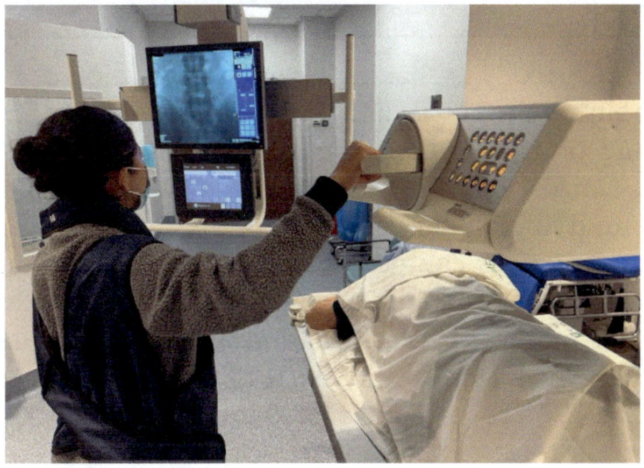

Figure 8.15. Role of Radiologic Technologists in Safety.

Source: https://www.laiic.com/cdn/shop/articles/fluoroscopy_los_angeles_explained_2100x.webp?v=1682966034.

Test Your Knowledge

1. What safety protocols are implemented to minimize radiation exposure during fluoroscopic procedures?
2. How do lead shielding and proper equipment settings contribute to safety in fluoroscopy?

Summary

Fluoroscopy is shaking up modern medicine in ways that aren't always expected. Our recent findings point out that this imaging method isn't just another tool—it is changing how doctors both diagnose and treat patients. Researchers have looked at how bones move by analyzing joint motion during a simple walk; for example, the way talocrural and subtalar joints shift now gives us a glimpse into living, dynamic body motion. In many studies, this method's speed and sharpness have shown that doctors can get vital details—details that more traditional scans might miss—helping guide surgeries and tough decisions. Fluoroscopy also makes a big mark beyond diagnosis by influencing how medical professionals train. New endovascular methods demand a level of coordination and teamwork that can be hard to master; as a result, virtual reality (VR) simulations are stepping in as a neat complement to real-life imaging insights. Such simulations, often seen as a safe practice ground, let teams rehearse both technical moves and softer skills without putting patient safety at risk. Generally speaking, this mix of high-tech imaging with hands-on training shows a lively, almost unexpected, interplay between pulling insights from the screen and learning in a simulated space. As advancements with fluoroscopy continue, so do the challenges that come along. High error rates during complex endovascular procedures remind us that there's still room to improve training protocols—sometimes using simulations that lean on fluoroscopic data. Looking ahead, it seems plausible that newer, more refined assessment tools may eventually pair well with these training methods, boosting both procedure accuracy and patient safety. In the end, the blend of advanced imaging with innovative training approaches holds a lot of promise for upping clinician skills and overall patient care; it is an exciting time that reinforces why fluoroscopy remains central in today's medical practices.

Fluoroscopy techniques have come a long way in medical imaging, changing how surgeries get done by boosting precision and safety. These days, it is not just about the static image anymore—the rise of smart, live-imaging systems has become key, especially in those minimally invasive procedures. Take, for example, a tricky operation like catheter ablation for cardiac arrhythmia; here, these fluoroscopy-assisted setups prove indispensable. They use contact force sensing not only to ramp up the ablation's effectiveness but also to check how well the catheter interacts with nearby tissues. And, in most cases, various methods—ranging from direct sensor techniques to surrogate markers—are employed to keep electrode-to-tissue contact just right, which is crucial for a successful outcome (Yu et al., 2019). In complex surgeries such as Transcatheter Aortic Valve Implantation (TAVI), fluoroscopic guidance takes center stage. Surgeons lean on these live visuals to get real-time looks at anatomical structures, helping them place devices with remarkable accuracy. In a neat leap forward, some systems mix in three-dimensional aortic mesh models with the live feed, automatically estimating the valve's target zone. Generally speaking, such insights streamline the whole procedure and even cut back on the need for contrast agents—a definite bonus for patient safety. Plus, using template-based tracking methods further fine-tunes prostheses placement, adapting smoothly to the aortic root's natural movements during surgery. Practical tests back up these improvements, showing clear contributions to better surgical outcomes (Karar et al., 2012). Recent advancements in fluoroscopy, broadly speaking, are part of a larger trend toward image-guided techniques that stress safety and efficiency. It is not merely about snapping pictures anymore; the whole system now aids surgeons in making decisions throughout the operation. For instance, the interactive graphical user interface allows doctors to manually tweak visual overlays, which not only adds a personal touch but also boosts overall confidence and precision. Retrospective studies even reveal that errors in device placement stay within clinically acceptable bounds—pretty reassuring if you ask me. Ultimately, blending advanced imaging with robust computational models is paving the way for newer, more patient-centered image-guided therapies, continually reshaping surgical methods (Karar et al., 2012).

KEY TERMS FROM THIS CHAPTER

- Angiography
- Barium swallow
- Cardiac catheterization
- C-arm
- Catheter placement
- Continuous imaging
- Conventional radiography
- Extracorporeal shockwave therapy (ESWT)
- Fluoroscopic guidance
- Heart conditions
- Interventional radiology
- Machine learning operations (MLOps)
- Radiation exposure
- Real-time imaging
- Upper GI series
- X-ray beam

Critical Thinking Questions

1. **What is the primary use of fluoroscopy in medical imaging?**
   a. To obtain detailed images of soft tissues
   b. To produce real-time moving images of the inside of the body
   c. To measure bone density
   d. To visualize the brain's electrical activity
2. **In fluoroscopy, which of the following is used to visualize the internal structures?**
   a. High-frequency sound waves
   b. X-rays
   c. Magnetic fields
   d. Radioactive tracers
3. **Fluoroscopy is commonly used in which of the following procedures?**
   a. Mammography
   b. Colonoscopy
   c. Barium swallow and other GI imaging procedures
   d. MRI scanning
4. **What is the key advantage of fluoroscopy over traditional X-ray imaging?**
   a. It does not use radiation
   b. It provides static images
   c. It allows for continuous monitoring of a patient's movement and function
   d. It requires no contrast agents
5. **During a fluoroscopic procedure, the patient is typically exposed to which type of radiation?**
   a. Radioactive particles
   b. High doses of ionizing radiation
   c. Non-ionizing radiation
   d. Sound waves

Short Answer Questions

1. What are the basic principles of fluoroscopy, and how does it differ from other imaging techniques like X-ray?
2. How is fluoroscopy applied in various medical procedures, such as guiding catheter placements or monitoring the digestive tract?
3. What are the advantages of using fluoroscopy in real-time imaging, and how does it enhance diagnostic and therapeutic procedures?
4. What are the main risks and limitations associated with fluoroscopy, particularly concerning radiation exposure and image quality?
5. What safety protocols are typically followed during fluoroscopic procedures to minimize radiation exposure to patients and healthcare workers?

Answers to Critical Thinking Questions

1. (b); 2. (b); 3. (c); 4. (c); 5. (b)

References

1. Acharya, A. J., Reddy, K., Ullur, P., J, P., & T, P. (2024). Technological advances in cancer imaging: A transformative impact. In *2024 4th Asian Conference on Innovation in Technology (ASIANCON)*. https://www.semanticscholar.org/paper/343e64b6740ac19bca2967324ac24ee73e1e2431 (accessed on 23 May 2025).
2. Ali, S., George, L. K., Das, P., & Koshy, S. (2011). Intracardiac echocardiography: Clinical utility and application. *Echocardiography, 28*. https://www.semanticscholar.org/paper/dd45241437e1914f11ba20bf52dbe9186b684609 (accessed on 23 May 2025).
3. Assaker, R., Reyns, N., Pertruzon, B., & Lejeune, J. P. (2001). Image-guided endoscopic spine surgery: Part II: Clinical applications. *Spine, 26*(15), 1711–1718. https://www.semanticscholar.org/paper/bae2ea7f4a8dc7fd1f57557db11103b4893f0f55 (accessed on 23 May 2025).
4. Azab, M., Bharadwaj, S., Jayaraj, M., Hong, A. S., Solaimani, P., Mubder, M., Yeom, H., Yoo, J. W., & Volk, M. L. (2019). Safety of endoscopic retrograde cholangiopancreatography (ERCP) in pregnancy: A systematic review and meta-analysis. *Saudi Journal of Gastroenterology, 25*(6), 341–354. https://doi.org/10.4103/sjg.SJG_92_19.
5. Badawy, W., Zinhom, H., & Shaban, M. (2024). Navigating ethical considerations in the use of artificial intelligence for patient care: A systematic review. *International Nursing Review*. Advance online publication. https://doi.org/10.1111/inr.13059.
6. Banoub, R., Alalade, E., Bryant, J., Winch, P., & Tobias, J. D. (2023). Allergic reactions to sugammadex: A case series and review of the literature. *The Journal of Pediatric Pharmacology and Therapeutics, 28*(4), 374–379. https://www.semanticscholar.org/paper/283b90eee304fbf2382100fe8c8adf5cc0dc9d9d (accessed on 23 May 2025).
7. Baron, K. (2024). Evaluating the radiation dose involved in interventional radiology procedures. *The Arab Journal of Interventional Radiology*. https://www.semanticscholar.org/paper/71215e72727e611e49ebbbb18e6a5226f8d81df0 (accessed on 23 May 2025).
8. Bhuiyan, M. M. H., Gupta, K. D., Hossain, I., et al. (2023). Introduction of medical imaging modalities. *arXiv*. https://arxiv.org/abs/2306.01022 (accessed on 23 May 2025).
9. Box, J., Salazar, A., Johnson, D., & Rutel, I. (2022). Dead detector element detection in flat panels using convolutional neural networks. *Medical Physics*. https://www.semanticscholar.org/paper/07fdfcd574be9264ccfbba81628b4a765b96a534 (accessed on 23 May 2025).
10. Brock, K. K., Chen, S. R., Sheth, R. A., Siewerdsen, J. H., et al. (2023). Imaging in interventional radiology: 2043 and beyond. https://core.ac.uk/download/622991664.pdf (accessed on 23 May 2025).
11. Burkland, D. (2020). Zero-fluoroscopy ablation at the Texas Heart Institute. *Texas Heart Institute Journal, 47*(1), 53–56. https://www.semanticscholar.org/paper/6bc0dab14b1ca9e8cdb75c8712d99e219a67375b (accessed on 23 May 2025).
12. Cao, P. (2024). Optimizing computer-aided design for multi-modal perception calculation of tourism landscape images. In *2024 5th International Conference on Image Processing and Capsule Networks (ICIPCN)*. https://www.semanticscholar.org/paper/9b2e3027eeb5e8299ef89ca0c6b0c3841d121b27 (accessed on 23 May 2025).
13. Dagnino, G., & Kundrat, D. (2024). Robot-assistive minimally invasive surgery: Trends and future directions. https://core.ac.uk/download/613613924.pdf (accessed on 23 May 2025).

14. David-Olawade, A. C., Olawade, D. B., Vanderbloemen, L., Rotifa, O. B., Fidelis, S. C., Egbon, E., Akpan, A. O., Adeleke, S., Ghose, A., & Boussios, S. (2025). AI-driven advances in low-dose imaging and enhancement—a review. *Diagnostics, 15*(6), 689. https://doi.org/10.3390/diagnostics15060689.

15. Duplaga, T. A., Krasnoborska, J., Samojedny, S., Superson, et al. (2024). Revolutionizing cardiovascular treatments with using AI: Current status and future prospects. https://core.ac.uk/download/620863037.pdf (accessed on 23 May 2025).

16. Fiagbedzi, E., Gorleku, P. N., Nyarko, S., Atuwo-Ampoh, V., Fiagan, Y. A. C., & Asare, A. (2022). The role of artificial intelligence (AI) in radiation protection of computed tomography and fluoroscopy: A review. *Open Journal of Medical Imaging*. https://www.semanticscholar.org/paper/3a9d2f5c94fdd954eb344524d92c3c1a3acd82a2 (accessed on 23 May 2025).

17. Fisher, R., Applegate, K. E., Berkowitz, L. K., Christianson, O., Dave, J. K., DeWeese, L., Harris, N., et al. (2022). AAPM medical physics practice guideline 12.a: Fluoroscopy dose management. *Journal of Applied Clinical Medical Physics, 23*. https://doi.org/10.1002/acm2.13526.

18. Ho, Y. J., Chiang, W. C., & Lin, Y. C. (2024). Advancements in minimally invasive surgery for adolescent idiopathic scoliosis: A case series and literature review. *Tzu-Chi Medical Journal, 37*(2), 80–85. https://www.semanticscholar.org/paper/6a06a41b1fb84592df841ceb7d5ab9d2375bff1f (accessed on 23 May 2025).

19. Hu, L., Chen, J., Vaughan, J., Yang, H., Wang, K., Sudjianto, A., & Nair, V. (2020). Supervised machine learning techniques: An overview with applications to banking. *International Statistical Review, 89*(4), 573–604. https://www.semanticscholar.org/paper/83687fc501f64a852c57c45d708084abf2182d06 (accessed on 23 May 2025).

20. İn, E., Altıntop Geçkil, A., Kavuran, G., Şahin, M., Berber, N., & Kuluöztürk, M. (2022). Using artificial intelligence to improve the diagnostic efficiency of pulmonologists in differentiating COVID-19 pneumonia from community-acquired pneumonia. *Journal of Medical Virology, 94*, 3698–3705. https://www.semanticscholar.org/paper/1f4ac79f69b6e1f3a01ae2f8ac664059dcb8de18 (accessed on 23 May 2025).

21. Kalová, M., Kubíček, J., Oczka, D., et al. (2019). Recent trends, technical concepts and components of computer-assisted orthopedic surgery systems: A comprehensive review. https://core.ac.uk/download/287649034.pdf (accessed on 23 May 2025).

22. Karaismailoğlu, B., Peiffer, M., Raduan, F., Hollander, J., Knebel, A., Kwon, J. Y., Bejarano-Pineda, L., et al. (2024). Heatmaps on radiological safety in minimally invasive midfoot fusion: A cadaver study. *Foot & Ankle Orthopedics, 9*. https://www.semanticscholar.org/paper/5422a8fba71eb1376d56fcf4c96680f5e0e4d009 (accessed on 23 May 2025).

23. Karar, M. E. A. R. H. (2012). Development of a surgical assistance system for guiding transcatheter aortic valve implantation. https://core.ac.uk/download/226099340.pdf (accessed on 23 May 2025).

24. Karimian, M., Rahmatizadeh, S., Kohzadi, Z., Kohzadi, Z., Madadi, F., & Dabbagh, A. (2024). Analyzing patterns in anesthesiology residents' exam performance using data mining techniques. *Anesthesiology and Pain Medicine, 14*. https://www.semanticscholar.org/paper/67ee1fcf87843328ab231289ae764c09d7e55883 (accessed on 23 May 2025).

25. Khalaf, K., Pawlak, K. M., Adler, D. G., Alkandari, A. A., Barkun, A. N., Baron, T. H., Bechara, R., Berzin, T. M., Binda, C., Cai, M. Y., Carrara, S., Chen, Y. I., de Moura, E. G. H., Forbes, N., Fugazza,

A., Hassan, C., James, P. D., Kahaleh, M., Martin, H., Maselli, R., & Causada Calo, N. S. (2024). Defining standards for fluoroscopy in gastrointestinal endoscopy using Delphi methodology. *Endoscopy International Open, 12*(11), E1315–E1325. https://doi.org/10.1055/a-2427-3893.

26. Kim, K. D., Kim, S. B., Lee, D. J., et al. (2015). Stereotactic guidance for navigated percutaneous sacroiliac joint fusion. https://core.ac.uk/download/323069173.pdf.

27. Li, W., Bi, S., Liang, Y., & Zhu, H. (2022). [Retracted] Construction of rheumatoid arthritis risk prediction and medical image applications from rheumatoid factor levels. *Computational and Mathematical Methods in Medicine, 2022*, 8617467. https://doi.org/10.1155/2022/8617467.

28. Li, Y., Liao, Y. P., Wang, J., Lu, W., & Zhang, Y. (2025). Patient-specific MRI super-resolution via implicit neural representations and knowledge transfer. *Physics in Medicine and Biology, 70*(7). https://doi.org/10.1088/1361-6560/adbed4.

29. Lo Bianco, G., Tinnirello, A., Papa, A., Marchesini, M., Day, M., Palumbo, G., Terranova, G., et al. (2023). Interventional pain procedures: A narrative review focusing on safety and complications. Part 2: Interventional procedures for back pain. *Journal of Pain Research, 16*, 761–772. https://www.semanticscholar.org/paper/82aa4f7693b4d84659473aeb8b2a27beb75be1d7 (accessed on 23 May 2025).

30. Lorusso, R., Shekar, K., MacLaren, G., Schmidt, M., Pellegrino, V., Meyns, B., Haft, J. W., et al. (2021). ELSO interim guidelines for Veno arterial extracorporeal membrane oxygenation in adult cardiac patients. *ASAIO Journal, 67*(8), 827–844. https://doi.org/10.1097/mat.0000000000001510.

31. Manfield, J., Martin, S., Green, A. L., & FitzGerald, J. J. (2024). Evaluation of 3D C-Arm fluoroscopy versus diagnostic CT for deep brain stimulation stereotactic registration and post-operative lead localization. *Stereotactic and Functional Neurosurgery, 102*(3), 195–202. https://doi.org/10.1159/000536017.

32. Manning, D. J. (2005). 'Do you see what I see?' Medical imaging: The interpretation of visual information. Inaugural Professorial Lecture, University of Cumbria, Lancaster, UK.

33. Martin, C. J., Vassileva, J., Vano, E., Mahesh, M., Ebdon-Jackson, S., Ng, K. H., Frush, D. P., Loose, R., & Damilakis, J. (2017). Unintended and accidental medical radiation exposures in radiology: Guidelines on investigation and prevention. *Journal of Radiological Protection, 37*(4), 883–906. https://doi.org/10.1088/1361-6498/aa881e.

34. McHenry, B. D., Exten, E. L., Long, J., Law, B., Marks, R. M., & Harris, G. (2015). Sagittal subtalar and talocrural joint assessment with weight-bearing fluoroscopy during barefoot ambulation. *Foot & Ankle International, 36*(4), 430–435. https://doi.org/10.1177/1071100714559540.

35. Modarai, B., Haulon, S., Ainsbury, E. A., Böckler, D., Vañó-Carruana, E., Dawson, J., Farber, M. A., et al. (2022). Editor's choice–European Society for Vascular Surgery (ESVS) 2023 clinical practice guidelines on radiation safety. *European Journal of Vascular and Endovascular Surgery, 65*, 171–222. https://doi.org/10.1016/j.ejvs.2022.09.005.

36. Moskalenko, V., & Kharchenko, V. (2024). Resilience-aware MLOps for AI-based medical diagnostic system. *Frontiers in Public Health, 12*, 1342937. https://doi.org/10.3389/fpubh.2024.1342937.

37. Nandakumar, A., Nanjappa, S. H., N S, L. P., & S, Y. (2025). Oral wafer technology: Revolutionizing drug delivery for enhanced patient compliance and bioavailability of specific low dose drug categories. *Journal of Advances in Medical and Pharmaceutical Sciences, 27*(5), 8–32. https://doi.org/10.9734/jamps/2025/v27i5775.

38. Nisar, Z., & Bano, S. (2024). Assessment of practice of radiation protection devices in fluoroscopy in SKIMS SOURA Hospital Srinagar J&K. *South Asian Research Journal of Nursing and Healthcare*. https://www.semanticscholar.org/paper/0f75348058c8fb1bc203f005f6a9904b5fce4b93 (accessed on 23 May 2025).

39. Rayyani, A. A., Shalalni, A. A., Radwan, A. H., Shibli, K. A., Jabin, J. Y., Mokli, M. A. Y., Mabuj, J. M., et al. (2024). Digital X-ray imaging: Emphasis on developments in digital X-ray technologies and their applications in diagnosis and treatment. *Journal of Positive Psychology and Wellbeing, 6*(4). https://core.ac.uk/download/616775625.pdf (accessed on 23 May 2025).

40. Reuterwall Hansson, M. (2022). New technologies for the further advancement of ERCP (Doctoral dissertation, Karolinska Institutet). https://hdl.handle.net/10616/47900 (accessed on 23 May 2025).

41. Rudarakanchana, N., Van Herzeele, I., Desender, L., & Cheshire, N. J. (2015). Virtual reality simulation for the optimization of endovascular procedures: Current perspectives. *Vascular Health and Risk Management, 11*, 195–202. https://doi.org/10.2147/VHRM.S46194.

42. Sayed, A. N., Ramahi, O. M., & Shaker, G. (2024). Frequency-modulated continuous-wave radar perspectives on unmanned aerial vehicle detection and classification: A primer for researchers with comprehensive machine learning review and emphasis on full-wave electromagnetic computer-aided design tools. *Drones, 8*(8), 370. https://doi.org/10.3390/drones8080370.

43. Sharma, P., Kumar, M., Sharma, H., & Biju, S. M. (2024). Generative adversarial networks (GANs): Introduction, taxonomy, variants, limitations, and applications. *Multimedia Tools and Applications, 83*, 88811–88858. https://www.semanticscholar.org/paper/f850330bcc7b207ac8fe6d4aa5d4e5bcba7fdb47 (accessed on 23 May 2025).

44. Shubayr, N. (2024). Operating room radiation safety measures: Awareness, compliance, and perceived risks among nurses and other healthcare workers. *International Nursing Review*. https://www.semanticscholar.org/paper/319b9afe07e1c8db4f2b141fa54c649499869bff (accessed on 23 May 2025).

45. Sparks, J. A. (2018). Rheumatoid arthritis. *Annals of Internal Medicine, 170*, ITC1. https://doi.org/10.7326/aitc201901010.

46. Stout, K., Daniels, C. J., Aboulhosn, J., Bozkurt, B., Broberg, C. S., Colman, J. M., Crumb, S. R., et al. (2018). 2018 AHA/ACC guideline for the management of adults with congenital heart disease: A report of the American College of Cardiology/American Heart Association Task Force on Clinical Practice Guidelines. *Circulation, 139*. https://doi.org/10.1161/cir.0000000000000603.

47. Tenforde, A. S., Borgstrom, H., DeLuca, S., McCormack, M., Singh, M., Soo Hoo, J., & Yun, P. H. (2022). Best practices for extracorporeal shockwave therapy in musculoskeletal medicine: Clinical application and training consideration. *PM&R, 14*, 611–619. https://doi.org/10.1002/pmrj.12790.

48. Ueda, H., Inami, S., Moridaira, H., Takahata, M., Iimura, T., Tanaka, N., Takada, S., et al. (2025). The usefulness and potential of high-fidelity three-dimensional models in spine surgery training: Cross-sectional empirical study. *BMC Medical Education, 25*. https://www.semanticscholar.org/paper/e2400b7e7f925a2a378c02dd0584723a7352a046 (accessed on 23 May 2025).

49. Unberath, M., Fotouhi, J., Hajek, J., Maier, A., Osgood, G., Taylor, R., Armand, M., & Navab, N. (2018). Augmented reality-based feedback for technician-in-the-loop C-arm repositioning. *Healthcare Technology Letters, 5*(5), 143–147. https://doi.org/10.1049/htl.2018.5066.

50. Vahanian, A., Beyersdorf, F., Praz, F., Milojevic, M., Baldus, S., Bauersachs, J., Capodanno, D., et al. (2021). 2021 ESC/EACTS guidelines for the management of valvular heart disease. *European Heart Journal, 43*, 561–632. https://doi.org/10.1093/eurheartj/ehab395.

51. Vymazal, J., & Rulseh, A. (2024). MRI contrast agents and retention in the brain: Review of contemporary knowledge and recommendations to the future. *Insights into Imaging, 15*. https://www.semanticscholar.org/paper/2cfe0e02f5eedba101f6869fd9383940def1743c (accessed on 23 May 2025).

52. Ye, H. (2024). Follow informed patient consent in clinical teaching in order to achieve a truly patient-centered approach. *Journal of Patient Experience, 11*, Article 23743735241273669. https://doi.org/10.1177/23743735241273669.

53. Yu, X. (2019). Evaluating electrode-tissue contact force using the moving pattern of the catheter tip and the electrogram characteristics (Doctoral dissertation). https://epublications.marquette.edu/dissertations_mu/858/ (accessed on 23 May 2025).

INTERVENTIONAL RADIOLOGY

9

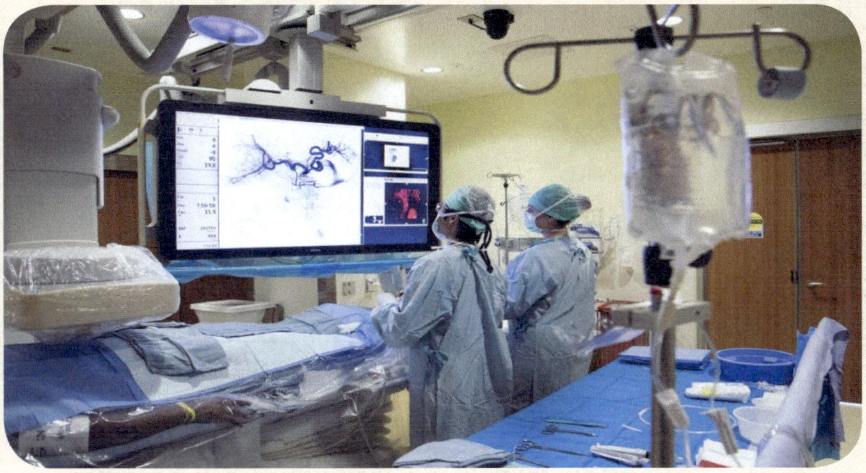

Introduction

Advanced medical practice is changing these days, and new tech is all in. In interventional radiology (IR), where tiny cuts replace big incisions, doctors are now experimenting with tools like augmented reality (AR) and virtual reality (VR)—not just for fancy teaching moments but for making actual procedures smoother. AR and VR help clear up complicated steps, making preoperative planning and real-time decisions a little less daunting, which can even cut down procedure times and boost precision. It is becoming obvious that as these tools evolve, their power to rework IR is pretty significant (Finos et al., 2024). In tricky issues like vascular anomalies, IR shows its strength. Many times, minimally invasive techniques win out over the old-school surgery approach by offering better results with fewer complications. Radiologists are now doing procedures such as embolization and endovenous laser ablation, steps that help lower patient risks. This steady shift towards less invasive methods highlights IR's ongoing growth and its

LEARNING OBJECTIVES

After studying this chapter, you will be able to:

1. Understand the key techniques used in interventional radiology and their clinical applications.
2. Explore common interventional radiology procedures.
3. Examine the specialized equipment and advanced technology utilized in interventional radiology.
4. Identify the steps involved in patient preparation and post-procedure care in interventional radiology.
5. Analyze potential risks and complications associated with interventional radiology procedures.

blend of cutting-edge diagnosis with innovative treatment options for complex vascular problems (Scollan et al., 2023). In a way, these varied approaches remind us just how vital this field has become in boosting patient care. With technology charging forward, it is increasingly important—generally speaking—to keep a close eye on whether these new methods work as promised. Early research is encouraging, but a deeper look at larger sets of data is needed to fully back up the claims. Checking both patient outcomes and practitioner feedback will be key in figuring out which uses of AR and VR are the most helpful. Plus, challenges like cost, ergonomic design, and rapid segmentation still need some ironing out. Once these hurdles are overcome, the full potential of augmented and virtual reality in IR could fundamentally change how procedures are done, making them safer and more efficient (Finos et al., 2024). This whole journey marks not just progress in IR but a pretty transformative approach to modern healthcare delivery.

Definition of Interventional Radiology

Various imaging techniques teamed with procedures that don't require big incisions have reshaped how we care for patients, especially in interventional radiology. This field uses live images to help doctors both diagnose and treat conditions with a high degree of precision. Ultrasound, computed tomography (CT), and fluoroscopy—the tools of the trade—give practitioners the means to ease discomfort and shrink recovery times. In many cases, choosing these less invasive methods cuts the risks often seen with traditional surgery. Interventional radiology, generally speaking, merges advanced imaging with patient-friendly care in a way that feels refreshingly direct. Interventional radiology isn't defined by a single method; instead, it takes a multifaceted approach to both treatment and diagnosis. The specialty covers a wide range of procedures—from vascular fixes and tumor ablation to drainage interventions—that can be mixed and matched to fit an individual's specific needs. This variety often leads to tailored solutions, where the uniqueness of each patient plays a big role. In many cases, the way these procedures adapt reminds one of ideas in functional training, where the focus is on the task and how individuals uniquely respond (Pereira et al., 2025).

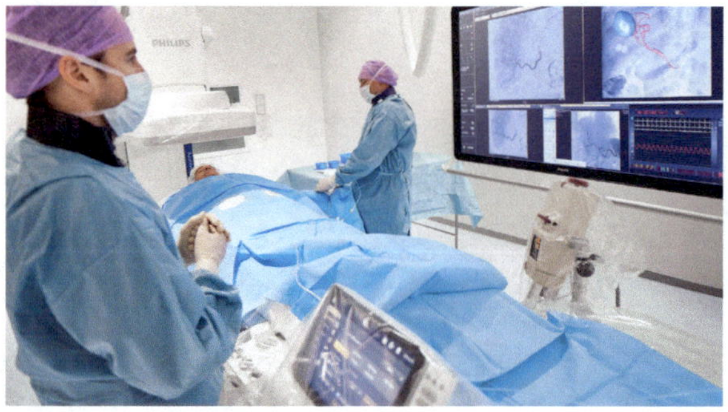

Figure 9.1. Interventional Radiology.

Source: https://www.itnonline.com/sites/default/files/field/image/Screen%20Shot%202019-02-27%20at%202.47.30%20PM.png.

Even though the techniques can be quite intricate, there's an underlying logic that lets practitioners adjust interventions on the fly, bridging classic methods with cutting-edge technology. The result is a field that sits right at the crossroads of tradition and innovation, offering practical as well as forward-thinking solutions. The strides made in interventional radiology signal not only a shift in treatment paradigms but also call for strict standards in safety and efficacy. One key development has been the creation of diagnostic reference levels, which are designed to keep radiation exposure in check during procedures. Different factors in every practice can tweak the radiation dose, and that variability highlights why a more standardized approach is needed. Many countries have taken steps to adopt these reference points, yet variations persist owing to differing criteria and practices (Qian et al., 2023). This uneven situation underscores, in most cases, the need for further research to nail down best practices—practices that bolster patient safety without sacrificing the therapeutic benefits of these innovative methods. As the field continues to evolve, its protocols and regulatory frameworks must adapt in tandem, ensuring that progress always goes hand in hand with safety (Figure 9.1).

Historical Development of the Field

Interventional radiology got its start with leaps in imaging tech that opened new doors for treatments without major surgery. Back when doctors mostly just read pictures, the field began shifting in the mid-1900s. Early on, individuals like Dr. Charles Dotter—one of those daring pioneers—tried out fresh vascular techniques in the 1960s. He and his peers introduced ideas like angioplasty and new catheter tricks that let physicians treat issues without the usual knife work. As people saw these methods worked safely and effectively, the practice gradually earned its space in medicine. Soon after, everything took another turn when newer imaging methods stepped in to mix things up. Digital tech provided real-time views of blood vessels, which meant doctors could target problems more exactly while cutting down on complications. CT scans and MRIs also made their debut, pushing IR beyond just blood vessel treatments. With image-guided biopsies and drainage procedures on the rise, radiologists began teaming up unpredictably with other experts to tackle a wide variety of problems. This jump in using different techniques underscored how crucial interventional radiology had become, sparking a need for focused training and formal recognition in hospitals. Even as IR grew, something else started entering the scene—artificial intelligence (AI). AI began to sneak into the mix, promising to sharpen diagnosis, streamline work, and even tailor treatments for patients in ways that upended routine care. It has shown promise in things like predicting outcomes and helping with computer-aided diagnosis. Sure, there are still bumps in the road with worries over data privacy and the tricky ethics of letting algorithms call the shots. Still, the road ahead for interventional radiology seems bright, driven by steady innovation, growing partnerships between tech gurus and doctors, and a measured commitment to ethical practice (Alowais et al., 2023; Najjar, 2023) (Figure 9.2).

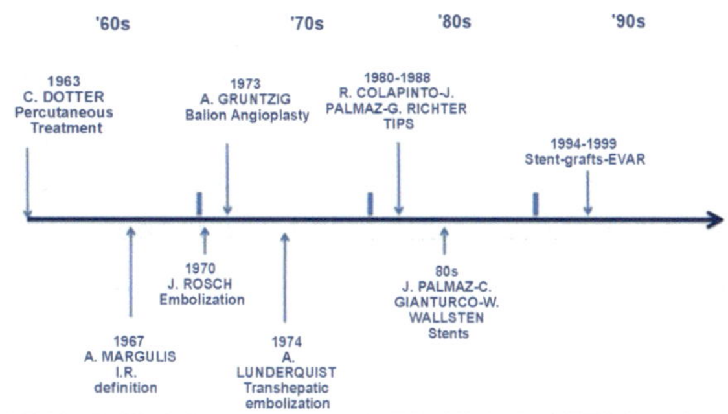

Figure 9.2. The vortical and exciting way of development of the Interventional Radiology: an incredible succession of events, from the first rudimental angioplasty performed in 1964 by Charles Dotter at Oregon University in the USA, to all new therapeutic concepts, treatment modalities, devices, progressively introduced in the modern medical practice.

Source: Marco Midulla, Lorenzo Pescatori, Olivier Chevallier et al. (2019): Future of IR: Emerging Techniques, Looking to the Future... and Learning from the Past: https://jbsr.be/articles/10.5334/jbsr.1727.

Importance in Modern Medicine

Rapid advances in medical technology have turned healthcare on its head, and interventional radiology has come into its own. This field mixes cool imaging methods with tiny, less invasive tweaks so that docs can check out and fix issues without open surgery. Patients tend to recover faster, and there's generally a lower chance for complications than with traditional operations. Treatments like endovenous laser therapy and angioplasty now help handle everything from vascular trouble to tumors, giving individuals more direct access to effective care—an especially big deal in an era that puts patients first. Safety and solid results still steer the ship, even if the perks are obvious. Sure, these procedures shine in many ways, but there's always the lingering risk of radiation exposure if things aren't watched closely. Hospitals keep protocols in place to monitor radiation because any slip-up can be harmful. Recent guidelines even hint that—when staff aren't perfectly trained on the gear and how to fine-tune it—risks can rise (Martin et al., 2017).

That makes detailed training and a few extra checks, like using time-outs, dose alerts, and even checklists, critical for both patient and worker safety. Still, interventional radiology keeps evolving practices to handle these risks while sticking to its essential role in modern care. As healthcare keeps moving forward, teaming up has become more than just a nice idea—it is vital for interventional radiology. Radiologists, surgeons, oncologists, and other specialists coming together leads to more personal treatment plans and better outcomes overall. The ability to see inside the body with real clarity means issues are spotted earlier, allowing for timely action in critical cases. In most instances, this spirit of collaboration nudges continuous learning about the latest tech and teamwork strategies. All of this underscores how interventional radiology remains a key player in today's healthcare systems (Martin et al., 2017).

9.1. Techniques in Interventional Radiology

Learning Outcome

1. Understand the principles and applications of angiography.
2. Examine the different biopsy procedures used in interventional radiology.
3. Explore the techniques and clinical uses of drainage procedures in interventional radiology.

Interventional radiology has taken an unexpected turn lately. High-tech imaging tools - think fluoroscopy, ultrasound, CT, and even MRI - are now front and center in helping doctors get a close-up view of the body. In many cases the clearer picture means complications drop while treatment options broaden, letting clinicians tackle cases that once looked too tricky. It is interesting, - breakthroughs emerging from research groups in France have shown that even a dash of AI can sharpen diagnostics and boost treatment effectiveness (Barat et al., 2024). Machine learning and AI are slowly combined into the mix of routine interventional practice. Recent studies generally speaking point to these smart systems as a way to fine-tune workflow and up the precision in diagnosis. Early on, some researchers have been whispering that analyzing massive amounts of data with radiomics might help predict outcomes, trim procedural mistakes, and even catch complications before they fully emerge. This blend between new technology and classic techniques hints at a future where the care we deliver becomes even more tailored and efficient, especially as investigations uncover creative ways to handle data hiccups (Seah et al., 2022). When you zoom out, it turns out that interventional success isn't just about the skill of the practitioner - it is also bolstered by technology that supports both prevention and treatment. Innovations like dual-energy and photon-counting CT are perfect examples of where the field is leaning into less invasiveness with a big nod to better care. As fresh applications of AI continue to pop up, the promise for even sharper diagnostics and improved therapies just keeps growing. Overall, this steady evolution reminds us that ongoing research and a willingness to adapt are essential for interventional radiology to stand strong against today's complex healthcare challenges (Barat et al., 2024).

9.1.1. Angiography

Imaging has come a long way, and that change has shaken up interventional radiology. In most cases, doctors now use techniques like angiography—a method where X-rays and a contrast dye let you see blood vessels up close—in ways that weren't possible before. This method, which gives a good look at the body's vascular network, helps spot blockages and unusual blood vessel shapes. Sometimes, mixing in digital subtraction methods makes the images sharper, so diagnoses get more reliable and patients end up with better results. Lately, there's been a twist: blending the classic approach with CT scans to boost soft-tissue views has opened up new roles in procedures, especially in cancer care (Taiji et al., 2021). Angiography isn't just for figuring out what's wrong; it is also a handy tool when stepping in to fix problems. For example, it lets specialists deliver less invasive treatments like catheter-directed thrombolysis and targeted embolization—methods that tend to cut down on the risks that come with big surgeries and often help patients recover faster. It is a bit like having a secret map: integrating newer tools such as optical coherence tomography (OCT) offers extra details of arterial walls, guiding treatment decisions even on the fly. Oddly enough, this kind of hands-on imaging keeps proving its worth in patient care management within the radiology field (Gounis et al., 2018). When you dig a bit deeper into interventional radiology, you see that fine-tuning angiographic techniques isn't just routine work—it's essential for tackling complex vascular issues. There's been steady progress, with new imaging tech generally boosting things like resolution and contrast so that the blood vessel details come out true to life. This improvement is critical, say, for tricky procedures like carotid artery stenting or handling an aneurysm, where getting every detail right can make all the difference. As the focus on safety and effectiveness grows, one can say the future of angiography still looks bright, even if sometimes its role seems to shift; after all, as imaging and intervention keep dancing together, angiography isn't going anywhere anytime soon (Taiji et al., 2021) (Figure 9.3).

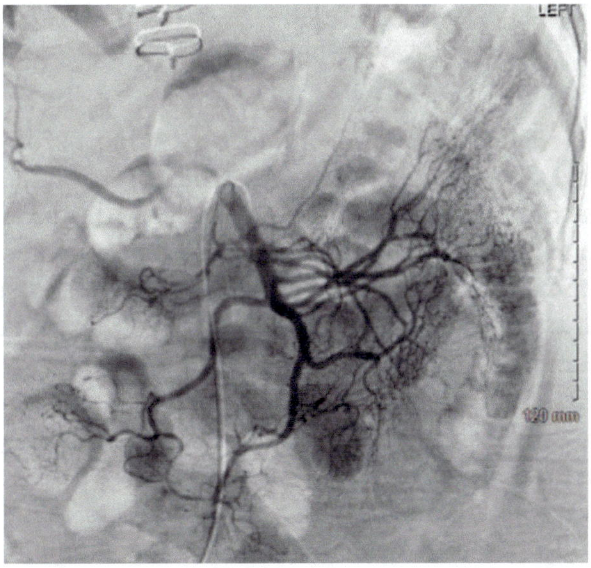

Figure 9.3. Interventional radiology completed angiography of the celiac.

Source: https://www.researchgate.net/figure/Interventional-radiology-completed-angiography-of-the-celiac-a-superior-mesenteric_fig3_354668288.

9.1.2. Biopsy Procedures

Modern medicine today relies on a mix of approaches that help nail a precise diagnosis and treatment plan. Biopsy procedures, for instance, truly emerge as a key way to check out abnormal tissue. They work by carefully snagging small cell samples that can later be examined under a microscope to shed light on what kind of lesion is present. Doctors often use imaging techniques—ultrasound, CT, or

MRI—to guide needles exactly where needed, making sure surrounding tissues are left mostly unharmed. As technology evolves, these image-driven biopsies not only boost accuracy but also make the whole patient experience lighter by cutting down recovery times and reducing issues, which overall lifts the quality of care. Imaging tech breakthroughs have generally had a huge impact on how effective biopsy procedures are in interventional radiology. With the arrival of real-time imaging systems, pinpointing lesions—especially those tricky to spot with older methods—has become much more doable.

The blend of X-ray radiography, fluoroscopy, and other advanced methods has pretty much revolutionized how radiologists see the target area, leading to better patient outcomes. In most cases, emerging technologies offer the promise of even finer precision when collecting tissue samples, sometimes obtaining just the tiniest bits without sacrificing diagnostic quality. As a result, professionals in interventional radiology are now better able to craft personalized treatment plans based on biopsy results, laying solid groundwork for personalized medicine (Brock et al., 2023). Adding another twist, technology and biopsy procedures are now intersecting with AI in ways that could change the picture. AI is stepping in to influence areas like education, risk estimation, and even direct patient care by streamlining parts of the biopsy process.

For example, AI algorithms can crunch through complex imaging data to fine-tune needle targeting and offer improved predictive analytics—improving planning before procedures, accuracy, leading to better outcomes. By automating certain steps, AI might not just boost efficiency but also add to patient safety. Even as interventional radiology welcomes these fresh advances, the future of biopsy procedures seems promising, blending time-tested methods with novel innovations to ultimately benefit both patients and healthcare teams (Nguyen et al., 2024) (Figure 9.4).

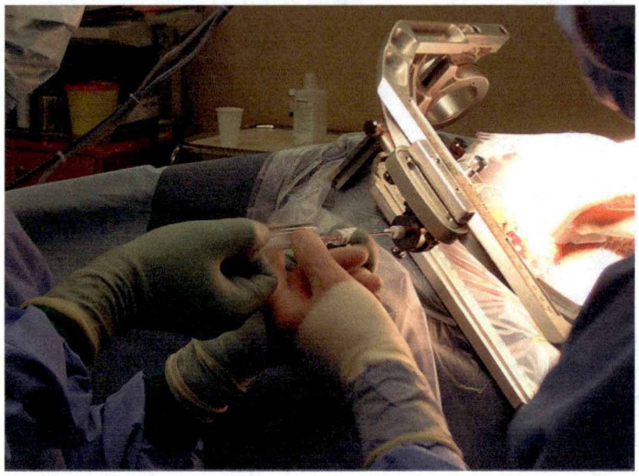

Figure 9.4. Biopsy.

Source: CC BY-SA 2.5, https://commons.wikimedia.org/w/index.php?curid=538919.

9.1.3. Drainage Techniques

Efficient drainage methods in interventional radiology have become a huge deal these days – hardly something you can ignore. They're central to handling conditions from abscesses to pleural effusions, with top-notch imaging helping radiologists zero in on the right spot for drainage. Advanced imaging lets them pinpoint targets so accurately that complications tend to drop while patient outcomes improve. Ultrasound and fluoroscopy, for instance, boost both safety and efficacy, paving the way for minimally invasive approaches. As time goes on, newer tools – think catheter systems and specialized drainage devices – have turned the practice into one that causes less trauma and often makes recoveries faster. Overall, these techniques not only ease symptoms but also help stop underlying conditions from deteriorating. Notably, not every healthcare system offers these drainage services equally. A survey of interventional radiology departments in the UK revealed that while a good number of institutions dabble in interventional oncology (IO) services, only a handful have a designated lead or a formal pathway for drainage initiatives (Alcorn et al., 2017). This uneven setup kind of underscores the need for more centralized referral pathways so that everyone can access these techniques. Institutions without solid networks might inadvertently slow down patient care and limit treatment options. In many cases, building collaborative networks and expanding drainage procedure availability can ensure patients receive timely interventions – improvements that boost clinical outcomes and overall quality of life. The impact of well-executed drainage techniques goes beyond just alleviating immediate symptoms. Advances in these methods reshape the field of interventional radiology, making it easier for radiologists to tackle tougher cases with greater confidence. For instance, various studies indicate that effective drainage can cut down on the need for invasive surgical interventions, nudging the field toward less invasive treatment options (Alcorn et al., 2017). Moreover, when drainage is done right, shorter hospital stays and fewer complications often follow, which can lead to notable economic savings. All things considered, pushing for excellence in drainage approaches not only lifts individual patient care but also helps keep healthcare systems sustainable amid rising demands (Figure 9.5).

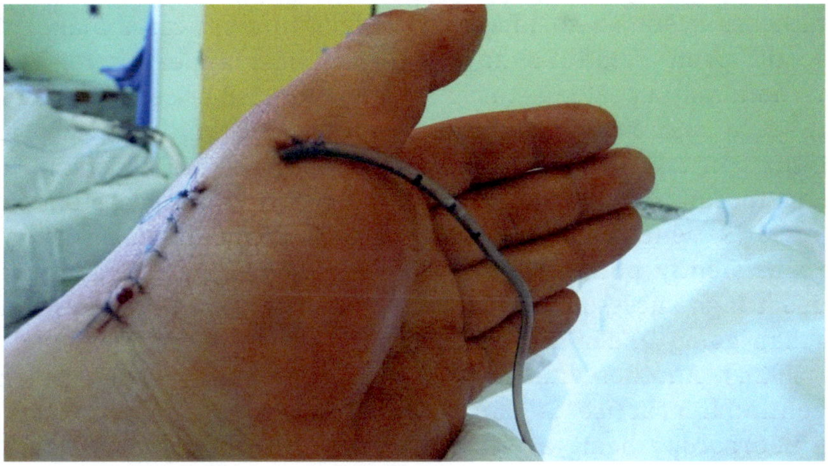

Figure 9.5. Drainage techniques.

Source: By Pavel Ševela, CC BY-SA 3.0, https://commons.wikimedia.org/w/index.php?curid=14688499.

Test Your Knowledge

1. How does angiography work to visualize blood vessels, and in what clinical situations is it commonly used?
2. What are the different types of biopsy procedures, and how are they performed to obtain tissue samples for diagnosis?

9.2. Common Procedures

Learning Outcome

1. Understand the role of stenting in interventional radiology.
2. Define embolization and vertebroplasty.

Minimally invasive methods used in treating many conditions show just how far interventional radiology has come. Lower back pain relief procedures, for example, are becoming a popular choice for those looking to avoid traditional surgery. Spine degeneration—more common among older individuals—is putting quite a dent in our healthcare systems, so image-guided injections and even ablations have steadily caught on. Generally speaking, these techniques not only ease pain and lift quality of life by reducing the constant need for pain meds but also seem to suit individual cases better. Literature reviews, which span a wide range of studies, consistently point out that such approaches boast high success rates and offer a safer path than going under the knife (Tomassoni et al., 2024). Another vital facet of modern interventional practice is using advanced imaging, fluoroscopy being a prime example, which lets clinicians see procedures happening in real time. This method is a real game-changer when guiding interventions and helps doctors navigate through complicated body layouts with a kind of precision that's hard to match. Of course, there are challenges—radiation, for instance, remains a concern for both patients and medical staff. A radiation dose summary page, sometimes easily overlooked, is generated during these procedures to log the overall exposure. This record not only plays a key role in keeping safety checks in line but also deepens our understanding of the technical ins and outs of every intervention, ultimately boosting the overall effectiveness of these approaches (Zhao et al., 2024).

9.2.1. Stenting

Stenting has become a real game changer in interventional radiology—a step forward in handling lots of conditions, both vascular and not. It is a minimally invasive method that, simply put, helps open up blocked pathways, whether those are in big arteries like the aorta, the carotid, or even the smaller peripheral ones, a tiny mesh tube—a stent—is placed right into the trouble spot, keeping it open so blood (or other fluids) can flow freely. This approach is often chosen when more invasive surgery might be too risky, usually meaning quicker recoveries and shorter hospital stays. Plus, with newer techniques and improved materials, there tend to be fewer complications, which in most cases makes the whole process even more appealing for everyday use. When emergencies arise in obstetrics, stenting steps up in a big way, especially for conditions like placenta accrete spectrum disorder (PAS). In most cases, using a stent here gives doctors a way to cut down on heavy bleeding during delivery, helping to better protect both mom and baby. There are several techniques on the table now—such as prophylactic balloon occlusion and even pre-operative arterial embolization—that doctors can choose from when facing PAS. These methods let them manage the blood flow in a fairly controlled way, stepping in where standard treatment might just not cut it; and honestly, that extra control can prevent severe problems. Overall, interventional radiology is broadening its scope, which seems to be steadily improving outcomes in these tough obstetric situations (Deshmukh et al., 2025). Then there's the case of idiopathic intracranial hypertension (IIH), where traditional treatments often just don't do enough for patients with stubborn symptoms. Here, turning to stenting—more specifically, venous sinus stenting (VSS)—has been getting more and more attention. Research, in most cases, shows that VSS can lead to noticeable symptom relief; by inserting stents into narrowed venous sinuses, doctors can not only reduce pressure but also create a better route for cerebrospinal fluid drainage, a key factor in recovery. So, whether it is in obstetrics or neurology, stenting is reshaping treatment options across the board, offering new hope where conventional strategies might fall short (Friso et al., 2024) (Figure 9.6).

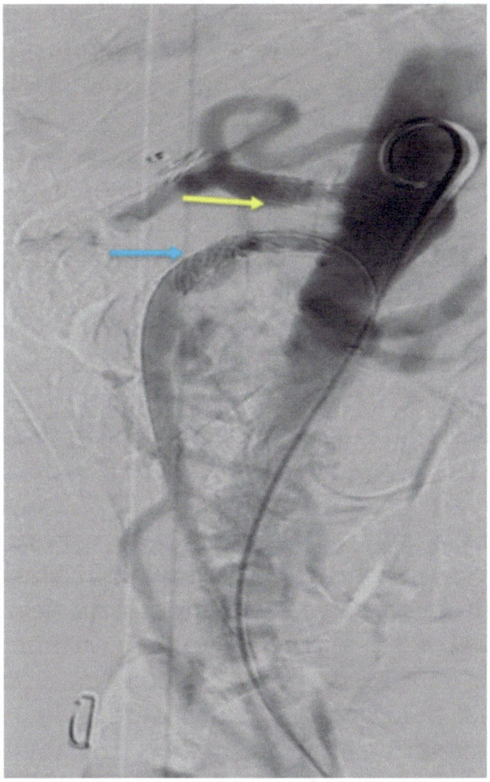

Figure 9.6. Interventional radiology intervention with successful stenting of the critically occluded celiac trunk (yellow arrow) and chronically occluded superior mesenteric artery (blue arrow).

Source: https://www.researchgate.net/publication/373479881/figure/fig3/AS:11431281184386126@1693323946897/nterventional-radiology-intervention-with-successful-stenting-of-the-critically-occluded.ppm.

9.2.2. Embolization

Embolization has transformed interventional radiology – it is a game changer because it avoids open surgery. Instead of more invasive approaches, doctors deliberately block off certain blood vessels to cut the flow where it is causing trouble. New findings generally point to this method tackling tough problems like vascular tumors and arteriovenous malformations—the kind of cases where traditional surgery might be too risky. Radiologists, armed with state-of-the-art imaging (like fluoroscopy and angiography), navigate these procedures with careful precision. Meanwhile, the anesthesia team plays its part by keeping patients stable and still during these delicate interventions, which ups the overall safety and effectiveness (Ahmed et al., 2007). Embolization isn't limited to just one area, either – it is made its mark in obstetrics as well. For example, when abnormal placental placement leads to post-partum hemorrhage, this technique steps in quickly.

In many emergencies, swift action is crucial; during cesarean deliveries with heavy bleeding, pelvic artery embolization (PAE) can avoid the need for a hysterotomy while still controlling the blood loss. In one evaluation, success rates for PAE hit 100% – a pretty strong nod to its reliability (Renzo et al., 2015). When interventional radiology teams work side by side with obstetric specialists, blood loss is minimized and maternal complications tend to drop, which highlights embolization's central role in women's health. Advances in embolization techniques have pushed interventional radiology into a more specialized field capable of handling complex medical challenges. A mix of new technology, hands-on expertise, and innovative procedures produces targeted treatments that are less invasive yet still effective. And as both diagnostic imaging and intervention methods keep changing, the potential uses for embolization are likely to branch out even further, opening up fresh therapeutic avenues in several fields. All things considered, given its proven success in critical situations and its growing role in everyday clinical practice, embolization has firmly established itself as a core element of modern interventional radiology, thereby strengthening comprehensive patient care (Figure 9.7).

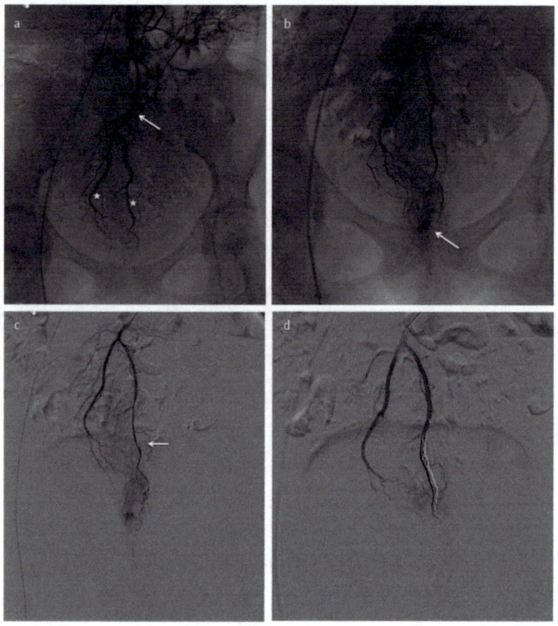

Figure 9.7. A 20-year-old woman (medical student) with a history of Cloves syndrome (venous malformation at the pelvis and left leg), presenting with life-threatening perineal hemorrhage from hemorrhoidal bundles.

Source: Midulla et al. (2019) Future of IR: Emerging Techniques, Looking to the Future... and Learning from the Past; https://jbsr.be/articles/10.5334/jbsr.1727.

9.2.3. Vertebroplasty

Understanding treatments for back problems has come a long way as we learn more about patient care and the messy details of musculoskeletal pain. Vertebroplasty, for instance, is obtaining attention because it eases pain from fractured vertebrae. Patients these days are desperate for any relief, so doctors have to carefully balance its upsides against possible downsides. In recent expert chats among those in interventional radiology, there's been a pretty clear message: don't just look at the quick pain fix, but also consider how the procedure affects long-term well-being and day-to-day quality of life (Anselmetti et al., 2022). This layered way of thinking—taking into account each patient's unique details along with broader clinical factors—drives a more personalized approach. Cutting edge developments in interventional radiology have given rise to less invasive methods like vertebroplasty, which, generally speaking, let doctors target areas of concern without the long recovery that traditional surgeries often demand. This is a game changer for people suffering from metastatic spinal tumors, especially when severe pain and risks like pathologic fractures are on the table (Jeromel et al., 2014). Not only does the technique calm the pain, but it also helps keep the damaged vertebra stable, so patients can move more freely. Its minimally invasive nature—reducing trauma to nearby tissues—makes it a go-to option for those who might not be up for a big, risky surgery. All of these factors underscore a clear move toward care that centers on the patient, where safety and effectiveness shape treatment choices. Advanced imaging plays a crucial role too, refining the accuracy of vertebroplasty and overall patient results. Before the actual procedure, detailed imaging often gives clinicians the lowdown on exactly how a fracture is set-up, which lets them tweak their game plan as needed. It is impressive how interventional radiologists can navigate the nooks and crannies of the vertebral structure—ensuring that the cement is placed just right so it not only eases pain but also bolsters the vertebra against future issues. As more data rolls in on vertebroplasty's effectiveness, ongoing tweaks and assessments will surely fine-tune when and how it should be used, aiming always to maximize benefits. This kind of evidence-based review, in most cases, is key to cementing vertebroplasty's role in modern interventional radiology (Jeromel et al., 2014) (Figure 9.8).

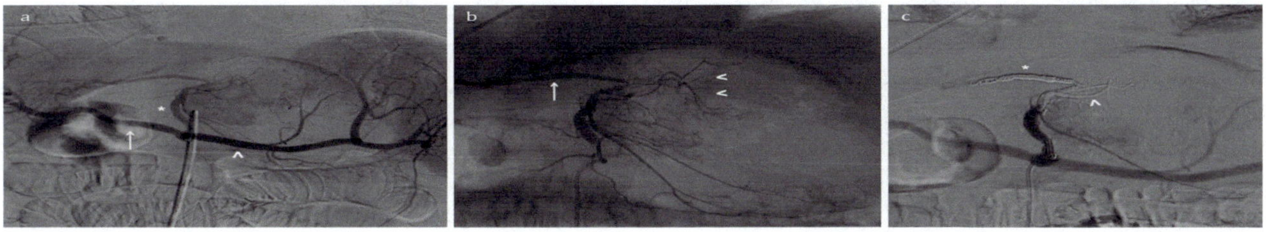

Figure 9.8. Catheterization.

Source: Midulla et al. (2019) Future of IR: Emerging Techniques, Looking to the Future...and Learning from the Past; https://jbsr.be/articles/10.5334/jbsr.1727.

Test Your Knowledge

1. What is the purpose of stenting in interventional radiology, and how does it help maintain vessel patency?
2. How is embolization used to block blood flow to specific areas, and in what clinical conditions is it commonly applied?

9.3. Equipment and Technology

Learning Outcome

1. Understand the imaging modalities used.
2. Define the tools and instruments in interventional radiology.

New gadgets and tech have altered the script in interventional radiology – procedures once seen as impossible are now happening with ease. High-resolution imaging tools, like fluoroscopy and ultrasound, bring a whole new level of clarity to both diagnosing and treating patients. Doctors now work with images in real-time, which lets them navigate our body's intricate corridors with a level of precision that's almost surprising. In many cases, this improved imaging doesn't just guide the procedure; it also cuts down on radiation exposure, a key point in patient safety. With these advanced tools integrated into practice, clinicians can pull off everything from straightforward biopsies to more complex embolization's, thereby broadening the impact of interventional radiology. There's also been a notable push toward constructing dedicated radiology suites. These specially designed rooms, outfitted with the latest machines – digital subtraction angiography systems being a prime example – give a clearer picture that ultimately boosts patient outcomes. Generally speaking, these environments are built to handle an array of procedures while keeping patient comfort and safety in sharp focus. Several guidelines, including those from the American Association of Physicists in Medicine (Clements et al., 2018), underscore the need to hold high standards in medical physics; this insistence drives a continuous cycle of tech updates and strict adherence to best practices. Overall, this blend of cutting-edge imaging and well-planned workspaces helps interventional radiology maintain its vital role in modern healthcare. Beyond the advancements in imaging, the everyday instruments used in interventional radiology have also come a long way. Tools like catheters, guidewires, and specially designed needles are now engineered to be more flexible and adaptable, giving doctors improved maneuverability within even the twistiest vascular routes. Innovations using bioengineered materials have led to instruments that are both lighter and sturdier—crucial factors that help make complex procedures safer. Not to mention, the inclusion of robotic assistance is a pretty big leap, enhancing precision and making it easier to handle intricate interventions.

This ongoing integration of new technology points toward better procedural outcomes and often even shorter recovery times. As the field continues to evolve, regular training and strict adherence to established guidelines will remain the backbone of high-quality patient care (Clements et al., 2018) (Figure 9.9).

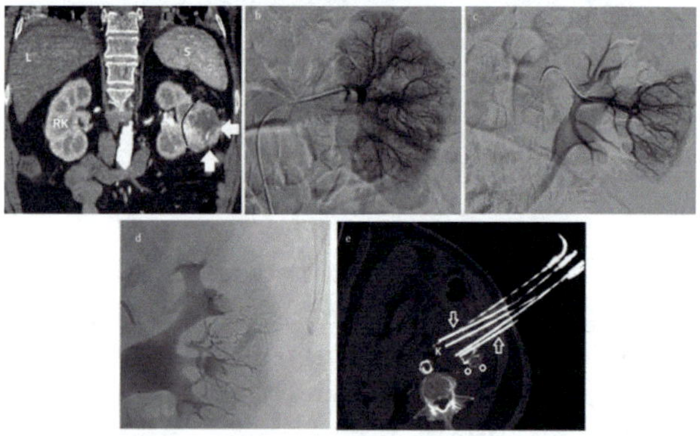

Figure 9.9. Interventional management of a renal mass in an inoperable patient, combined approach: transarterial preoperative embolization is performed through femoral access (b) using selective catheterization (c) and injection of glue (d), thus obtaining devascularization before percutaneous ablation. (e) CT-guided cryotherapy; combination of the percutaneous ablative therapies and the immune-modulating drugs in the so-called "Interventional Immunooncology" becomes an unexplored field of application with a tremendous potential to investigate in the next future.

Source: Midulla et al. (2019) Future of IR: Emerging Techniques, Looking to the Future... and Learning from the Past; https://jbsr.be/articles/10.5334/jbsr.1727.

9.3.1. Imaging Modalities Used

Understanding different imaging techniques is key in interventional radiology. Radiologists use tools like fluoroscopy, ultrasound, CT, and MRI to see inside the body and guide procedures—sometimes with almost a real-time feel that keeps things on track. Fluoroscopy, for example, comes in handy during catheter-based work because it shows the device's path as it moves, while ultrasound does a neat job with needle placements and checking on fluid, cutting down on extra radiation. Each method brings its own perks and uniqueness, so doctors can mix and match what fits a patient's needs best. Cone Beam Computed Tomography (CBCT) has been popping up as an interesting option, especially in musculoskeletal cases.

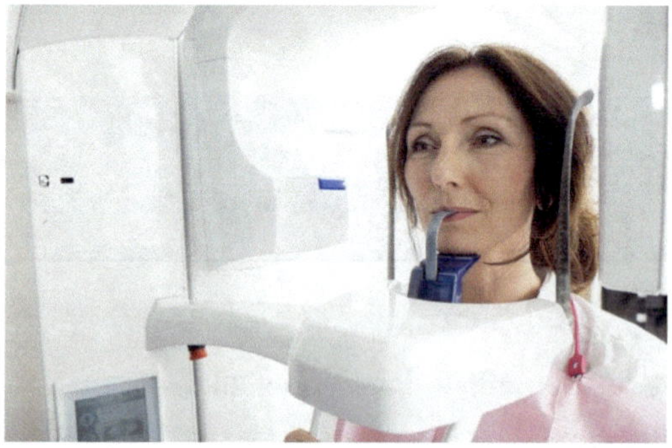

Figure 9.10. Cone beam computed tomography (CBCT) scan.

Source: https://dentalimplantindia.co.in/wp-content/uploads/2021/12/Cone-Beam-Computed-.jpg.

Unlike the usual CT, CBCT gives you sharp, all-around 3D views that make it easier to see both solid bone and softer tissues. This tech is already helping with things like spotting fractures or identifying tiny cartilage issues in joints. It tends to be more affordable and lowers radiation risk, so it often pairs with other methods. There's solid evidence that using CBCT not only sharpens diagnostic accuracy but also helps with planning and follow-up, which can boost patient care overall. Using a mix of imaging methods doesn't just lift the clarity in diagnosis and treatment—it also makes procedures smoother and safer. Combining different approaches can offer a broader picture; for instance, an MRI taken before a procedure might reveal important details about anatomy or an underlying problem, steering the intervention appropriately. Right after a procedure, a quick scan might catch any complications early. With technology constantly evolving—think better digital imaging and even some AI elements—the field is always on the move. In most cases, staying up to date with these developments means interventional radiologists can keep using the best tools available to help their patients (Desimpel et al., 2018) (Figure 9.10).

9.3.2. Tools and Instruments

Specialized tools have pushed interventional radiology forward by making procedures smoother and keeping patients safer. At its center is the catheter—a bendy tube that lets doctors reach deep into blood vessels for both checks and fixes. Instead of being just a plain tube, these catheters come with neat extras like hydrophilic coatings and clever tip tweaks that help them wind through tricky body pathways. Microcatheters, for instance, let physicians zero in on a spot, which usually means less damage to nearby tissues. Generally speaking, that kind of precision matters a lot in urgent cases—take strokes, where quick vessel reopening is crucial for avoiding further issues, as noted in Rohde et al. (2021). In the array of equipment in the field, imaging tools also carry a big load of importance. Fluoroscopy, ultrasound, and CT scans aren't just for guiding the way—they also help shape treatment choices. In many cases, real-time fluoroscopy lets radiologists see exactly where a catheter is placed and check on how the procedure is rolling, cutting down on unexpected problems. Lately, mix-ins like augmented reality and 3D modeling have made planning even tougher cases a bit more manageable. It is interesting how these imaging upgrades have shifted outcomes, especially in procedures like endoscopic retrograde cholangiopancreatography (ERCP) for biliary issues, as mentioned in Almuhaidb et al. (2021). Extra tools beyond the main ones are also popping up, broadening the radiology toolbox. Think stents and embolic agents—they now play a role from handling blockages to addressing tumors. These options provide extra flexibility that can be fine-tuned to a patient's specific needs and body uniqueness. The trend towards less invasive methods, marked by shorter recovery times and quicker hospital exits, emphasizes patient-centered care. Further, emerging tech like robotic-assisted systems is slowly stepping in, promising even finer control during procedures. Overall, by continuously mixing in fresh ideas and fine-tuning their gear, interventional radiology keeps evolving to deliver better outcomes and a smoother patient experience—a real leap forward in modern medicine (Figure 9.11).

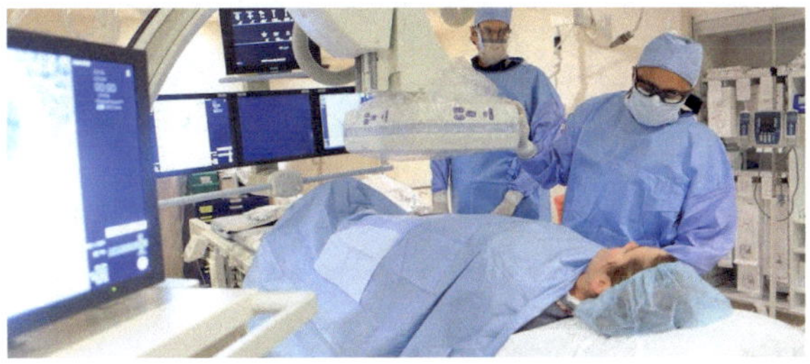

Figure 9.11. Specialized tools have pushed interventional radiology forward by making procedures smoother and keeping patients safer.

Source: https://drjathinsveincenter.com/wp-content/uploads/2022/03/9-Amazing-Procedures-Performed-by-Interventional-Radiologists-1.jpg.

9.3.3. Advances in Technology

Technology has turned the game in medicine—take interventional radiology, for example. Lately, there's been a clear move toward mixing advanced imaging tools that help doctors not only spot issues earlier but also fine-tune treatments on the fly. Radiologists now pull together CT, MRI and ultrasound images to get a fuller, more practical view of what's going on in the body. This kind of blend lets them operate with a level of precision that cuts down the risks usually tied to invasive procedures. In most cases, as IR has carved out its own spot with dedicated training and protocols, the push to keep up with every new tech advance has reshaped what standard care is all about (Nguyen et al., 2024). AI is another big player making waves in interventional radiology. You can't ignore how AI is nudging its way into everything from educational tools to assessing risks and running daily workflows. By digging through massive sets of data, AI starts to pick up on patterns that tweak everything before, during and after procedures. This not only helps smooth out decision-making but also streamlines the whole process, setting up better results for patients. Research keeps hinting that AI amplifies a radiologist's own skills—repeatedly showing its potential to tailor treatments in meaningful ways (Nguyen et al., 2024). As things continue to shift, keeping one's eye on the benefits AI brings along seems pretty key to what comes next in the field. New imaging advances aren't taking a backseat either. Modern techniques like molecular and multimodality imaging now offer a much sharper look at where issues surface, which means doctors can more precisely target problems. Even hybrid setups—those that mix a surgical suite with high-end imaging gadgets—are showing off possibilities that old-school methods never could. Generally speaking, these breakthroughs boost not just how effective procedures can be, but also make treatments a tad safer and more comfortable for patients. As IR leans further into these innovative directions, ongoing collaboration among healthcare pros remains crucial for unlocking these tools' full potential, setting the stage for the future of the discipline (Brock et al., 2023).

Test Your Knowledge

1. What are the essential imaging technologies used in interventional radiology, and how do they assist in guiding procedures?
2. How do tools like catheters, guidewires, and stents contribute to the success of interventional radiology treatments?

9.4. Patient Preparation and Care

Learning Outcome

1. Discuss the pre-procedural assessments.
2. Explain the informed consent process.
3. Examine the procedure post-procedural care.

Patient preparation is key in interventional radiology. The process starts with taking a good look at a patient's history – what medications they use, allergies they might have, and any previous vascular mishaps. In most cases, digging into past conditions helps determine what could complicate things during a procedure. For instance, sometimes an overly aggressive wire maneuver or a device that's too large can lead to an artery getting perforated (Pasecki et al., 2018). It helps a lot when patients understand both the potential benefits and the risks involved. When they are given the lowdown, trust builds naturally, anxiety drops, and everyone's on the same page—which ultimately makes the intervention work out better. It is equally important to care for a patient's state of mind as much as their physical health. Invasive procedures often bring a fair share of worry or uncertainty; simply explaining what's ahead can go a long way in easing that tension. In many situations, a bit of guided imagery or even some mindfulness can help shift their focus to the positive. Further, using checklists and taking a quick pause before getting started (as suggested in some professional guidelines (Martin et al., 2017) reassures both the patient and the team that everything is set, even if the steps sometimes seem a bit scattered. After the procedure, close follow-up care remains essential. Monitoring makes a difference in identifying problems like unexpected bleeding—even when all the necessary precautions were taken (Pasecki et al., 2018). Patients get the heads-up on symptoms they should watch out for, along with clear instructions on what activities to avoid, how to manage their meds, and when to show up for follow-up visits. Handing out simple patient guides that recap key steps and expected outcomes can help a lot too. In this way, linking what was planned with what happens during recovery creates a safer and more confident environment, leading to better outcomes and overall satisfaction (Figure 9.12).

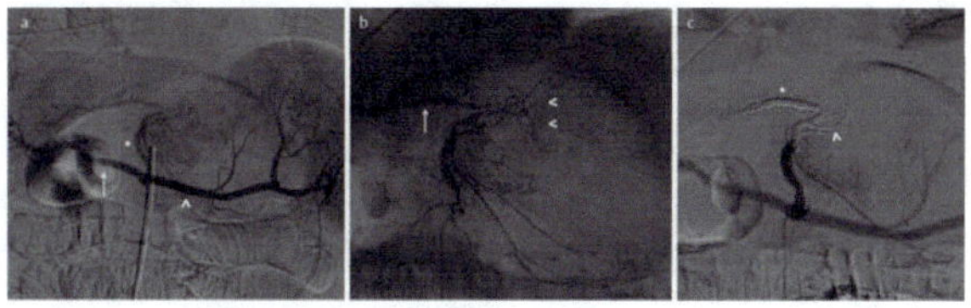

Figure 9.12. Interventional radiology.

Source: Midulla et al. (2019) Future of IR: Emerging Techniques, Looking to the Future and Learning from the Past; https://jbsr.be/articles/10.5334/jbsr.1727.

9.4.1. Pre-Procedural Assessments

Thorough planning underpins safe and effective interventional radiology. Instead of a cookie-cutter approach, experts start by digging into each patient's unique background—medical history, current medications, allergies, and even those details that might seem small at first glance. This deep dive, which isn't always neat and tidy, lets clinicians spot hidden risks, like the possible issues tied to iodinated contrast media that can lead to contrast media-induced nephropathy (CIN) (Indianapolis Coalition for Patient Safety, 2017). In many cases, sizing up these risks not only boosts patient safety but also paves the way for care plans that fit each individual, helping to improve overall procedural outcomes. Beyond just looking at medical history, assessments before the procedure mix in lab tests and imaging studies that offer a snapshot of a patient's broader health. Renal function, for example, is a big deal—especially for those already vulnerable to kidney problems—since contrast agents may complicate things. Radiologists, nurses, and other team members often band together (sometimes in a slightly less formal, more hands-on way) to check every nook and cranny of a patient's well-being (Boone et al., 2012). Sticking to routine protocols during these moments, even if it occasionally feels a bit rigid, can trim down the usual variability across institutions and, in turn, lift the standard of care. Clear, open communication plays a huge role too. Healthcare providers chat with patients about what to expect, making sure that the procedure and its risks come off as understandable rather than intimidating. This kind of straightforward dialogue—despite a few hiccups or even a stray misplaced comma here and there—helps calm nerves and gets patients to follow pre-procedural guidelines, which is pretty critical for the best results. Often, the insights gathered during these discussions hint at how ready a patient is, both physically and emotionally. In the end, these layered assessments weave together meticulous medical reviews, genuine team collaboration, and everyday talk to support the complex world of interventional radiology (Figure 9.13).

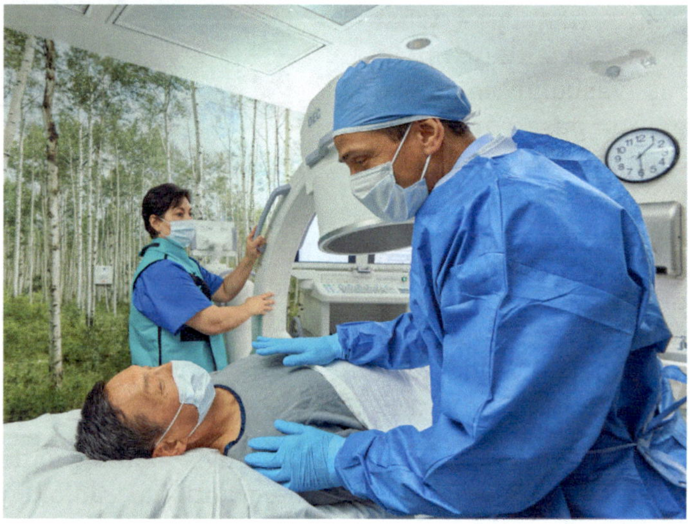

Figure 9.13. Thorough planning underpins safe and effective interventional radiology.

Source: https://www.jeffersonhealth.org/content/dam/health2021/images/photos/photo-shoots/people/clinical/interventional-radiologist-patient-ewc-121721-2055.jpg.

9.4.2. Informed Consent Process

Interventional radiology is tricky, so having a consent process that's both carefully arranged and ethically sound is a must. It isn't just a legal safety net—in most cases it is the way to ensure patients grasp what they're getting into. With such a wide range of procedures and risks like radiation exposure from imaging techniques, sticking to strict standards can help cut down on unexpected issues and build trust between patients and their care providers. Often, when the line between invasive and non-invasive procedures gets a bit blurry, it becomes even more important for doctors to explain both the upsides and the dangers clearly. Overall, this pushes clinicians to be upfront and leave no room for ambiguity in patient care. Because the process in this field is so procedural, healthcare pros end up chatting continuously with patients about their treatment paths. They talk about past outcomes, what might work well, and the possible risks linked with both imaging and intervention. One study that examined the nursing role in interventional radiology suggests that bringing together a mix of expert opinions can boost the consent process (Boone et al., 2012). This collaborative style means patients hear a well-rounded explanation, helping them weigh their options more thoughtfully. And since every patient takes in information differently, care teams need to be flexible—addressing individual concerns and repeating key points here and there so each person can navigate their choices with a clearer picture. If we're aiming to sharpen the informed consent process, it helps to incorporate the latest imaging technologies along with improved radiation safety measures. This approach reassures patients about how safe their procedures are likely to be. Generally speaking, initiatives to improve radiological practices remind us that understanding how radiation might affect the body can empower patients to engage more meaningfully in discussions about their care (Thubab et al., 2024). Clinicians, therefore, should break down this information into plain language, ensuring that patients feel ready to give consent even for procedures that involve significant risks. Taking time to explain things not only boosts patient participation but also keeps everything in line with ethical standards. In the end, a well-executed informed consent process plays a huge role in making interventional radiology work better by centering care on the patient while balancing both ethical and clinical best practices (Figure 9.14).

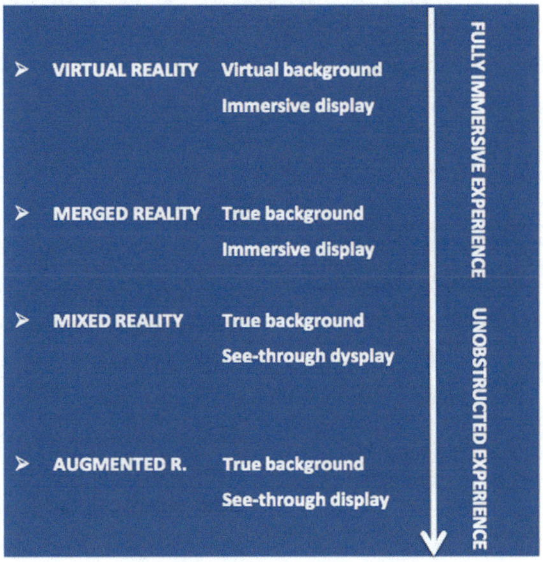

Figure 9.14. Conceptual framework of how to improve consent practices in IR.

Source: Midulla et al. (2019) Future of IR: Emerging Techniques, Looking to the Future...and Learning from the Past; https://jbsr.be/articles/10.5334/jbsr.1727.

9.4.3. Post-Procedural Care

Interventional radiology hinges on what happens afterward—keeping a close eye on patients is key. You don't just check some boxes; you're watching vital signs, inspecting the intervention site, and staying alert for issues like bleeding or infections. Standard observation routines, in most cases, help catch any trouble early on, lowering the chance of big complications. Good training and a thorough checklist before and during procedures play a huge role too, combined with formal policies that clearly sort out who does what when something goes wrong (Martin et al., 2017). Sometimes the care that follows isn't uniform at all—it often has to match each patient's unique situation. Think of it this way: pain management, hydration routines, even patient talks about what to watch for can all come into play. The recovery room after anesthesia is a mishmash of advice and feedback from different healthcare individuals, ensuring nothing slips by. This kind of teamwork is crucial, especially with procedures like catheter-directed thrombolysis (CDT). With CDT, for example, while higher tissue plasminogen activator (t-PA) doses tend to lower pulmonary artery pressure (PAP) effectively, you also have to balance that with bleeding risks, which means being extra careful is just a must (Patel et al., 2019). At the end of the day, neglecting proper follow-up care can ripple out into long-term issues and even affect how efficient healthcare is overall. Generally speaking, a proactive approach lets the team tackle any hiccups fast enough to trim hospital stays and fend off unnecessary readmissions. Ongoing learning about the latest in interventional techniques and recovery strategies is essential; after all, regular updates to protocols based on new evidence help keep the quality of care high. In many cases, emphasizing a solid post-procedural plan isn't just about immediate safety—it is about boosting the entire patient experience and improving clinical outcomes over time (Martin et al., 2017).

t

Test Your Knowledge

1. Why is patient preparation important before undergoing an interventional radiology procedure?
2. What are some common steps involved in preparing a patient for an interventional radiology procedure?

9.5. Risks and Complications

Learning Outcome

1. Understand the common risks associated with procedures.
2. Define the management of complications.
3. Explore the patient safety measures.

Interventional radiology is racing ahead with new techniques, but that progress also brings its own set of challenges. Procedures often get complicated unexpectedly, and with increased complexity come risks—things like bleeding or infections that show up in roughly 9.2% of hospital cases. Ethics come into play when benefits have to be weighed against these potential pitfalls; even routine steps like catheter placements or biopsies remind us that patient care and trust must be protected, even if outcomes aren't always ideal. Digging a bit deeper, complications in these procedures don't just affect individual patients; they ripple into the overall healthcare system. In most cases, a mishap means longer hospital stays and steeper bills. In the UK, for example, some estimates nudge annual costs from complications toward a whopping £2 billion. This huge financial drag has pushed hospitals to rely on careful pre-procedural assessments and regular outcome checks. When you look at the bigger picture, every setback becomes a lesson—helping to build systems that are more accountable and that keep pushing for ongoing improvements in patient care. Patient education in interventional radiology is evolving too, often in surprising ways. Modern tools like GPT-3 and GPT-4 are now part of the mix, offering patients details about procedures that many rate as either completely correct or very good. These advances help patients understand the risks before they give informed consent—although, admittedly, complications can still emerge unexpectedly, keeping the whole consent process dynamic. When both patients and their care teams are thoroughly clued in on the risks, the whole treatment journey tends to be a bit safer and a lot more human, even when things get a little messy.

9.5.1. Common Risks Associated with Procedures

Interventional radiology can be pretty tricky sometimes, with procedures that bring along a mix of challenges affecting patient safety. Take, for example, the risk of injuring blood vessels—this issue crops up especially when doctors have to work near major vessels. Blood vessel variations, often spotted in roughly 35% of people, can make matters even messier if they aren't noticed beforehand. Missing these differences might lead to sudden vascular problems that, in the worst instances, could even cause liver failure. Generally speaking, a thorough pre-procedure check using modern imaging goes a long way in keeping these dangers at bay (Yancey et al., 2025). Radiation exposure is another tough nut to crack with these procedures. It's an unavoidable part of many diagnostic and treatment techniques, yet it is a balancing act between effective care and keeping radiation levels safe. Interestingly, a lot of individuals have little idea about the risks involved—one recent study found that 62.7% of people hadn't even heard of interventional radiology before. This kind of gap in knowledge can muddle the whole process of getting proper patient consent and making informed choices. In most cases, ramping up education for both patients and healthcare providers is essential to better manage these exposures (Alhashim et al., 2024). Then there's the ever-present worry about infections. Whether it is something like placing a catheter or doing a biopsy, the invasive nature of these methods naturally opens the door for germs. The threat of infection after a procedure means that careful, consistently applied sterile techniques—from the very start of preparation to post-care—are absolutely critical. Patients, too, can benefit from knowing the early signs of an infection, which might help nip potential complications in the bud, by keeping an eye on these varied risks, practitioners can not only boost patient safety but also work toward better outcomes in this fast-evolving field (Figure 9.15).

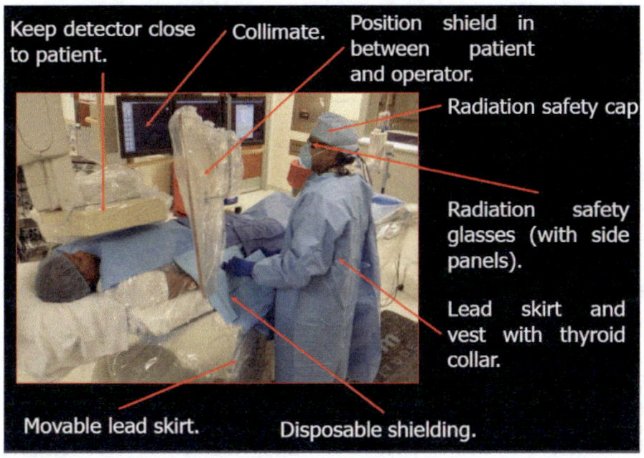

Figure 9.15. Radiation safety for the interventional radiology.

Source: https://radpad.com/wp-content/uploads/2020/09/RADPAD-radiation-protection-cardiology.png.

9.5.2. Management of Complications

Managing complications well makes all the difference in patient care, especially in emergency birth situations with heavy bleeding. Cases involving abnormal placental implantation can be tricky; for instance, a minimally invasive trick like pelvic artery embolization steps in to control bleeding and, in many cases, even helps avoid a hysterectomy. Some retrospective studies, you know, indicate that this approach does a decent job managing postpartum hemorrhage in high-risk deliveries, particularly when an interventional radiology team is hanging around the operating room during emergencies. Having that team present can often mean acting fast enough to curb severe issues like maternal morbidity and mortality. In most cases, taking proactive steps seems key to boosting surgical effectiveness and keeping patients safer (Renzo et al., 2015). Another part of this story involves using specialized devices, bioconvertible inferior vena cava (IVC) filters. These filters are designed to temporarily cut down the risk of pulmonary embolism during the riskiest moments. With some clever innovations that let the filter essentially change state after the danger has passed, clinicians have been able to lower the chances of long-term problems tied to standard retrievable filters. Clinical data generally shows promising results with high rates of successful filter conversion and hardly any reports of symptomatic pulmonary embolism after the procedure. This advance not only bumps up care standards for venous thromboembolic events but also demonstrates how ongoing innovation keeps patient safety at the forefront (Ansel et al., 2019). Working together across specialties also plays a big part in managing complications. Radiology, obstetrics, anesthesia – each surely brings something unique to the table. In particularly complex cases, where issues can crop up unexpectedly, the kind of loosely coordinated collaboration in pre-procedure planning and real-time decision-making seems to boost the team's overall agility. This mix of expertise, even if sometimes a bit scattered in approach, usually helps lower complication rates and builds a culture that values safety and teamwork when every second counts. In most cases, that collaborative spirit is essential for getting the best outcomes possible.

9.5.3. Patient Safety Measures

Interventional radiology (IR) procedures have gotten a lot more tangled over the past few years, and that shift demands we up our patient safety game. Even though these minimally invasive methods usually seem less risky than traditional surgery, they're far from free of mishaps in everyday clinical work. Some numbers suggest that roughly one out of every three radiology incidents involves an IR procedure, a statistic that's hard to ignore. This growing trend points to a need for a more determined push to cut down risks, with many experts now favoring clear-cut protocols to catch mistakes early. Such measures not only help patients get better outcomes but also lift the morale of everyone working in IR departments. After all, a safer environment is something the whole team can rally around. Reducing adverse events in IR depends on mixing hands-on training with practical safety steps. Simulation drills and team exercises have long been celebrated for boosting radiologists' competence, getting them ready for unexpected modifications in complex cases. These sessions help teams deal with tough scenarios while building communication skills that can make all the difference when it counts. Oddly enough, simple checklists have proven to be a powerful tool too, a systematic review even noted that the median error per procedure dropped from about 0.35 to 0.06 in places that embraced these routines. In most cases, such evidence pushes home the idea that structured training and sticking with proven protocols are key for top-notch patient care.

This blend of tactical training and everyday safeguards seems to create not only safer outcomes but also a more confident crew on the job. In specific treatment tweaks, adding extra therapies, like using oxytocin in uterine leiomyoma treatments, has stirred up fresh questions about both safety and effectiveness. Recent studies found that combining oxytocin with high-intensity focused ultrasound (HIFU) didn't improve ablation rates or noticeably cut down treatment times, yet it did lead to more patients reporting pain. This outcome underscores the need to think twice before diving headlong into new combinations, reminding us that every potential benefit has to be weighed against its possible risks. It encourages a more cautious, measured approach when we integrate novel therapies, ensuring that any gains aren't overshadowed by unforeseen downsides. Ultimately, keeping patient safety front and center in IR means continually re-evaluating and adapting treatment protocols to maintain the highest standards of care.

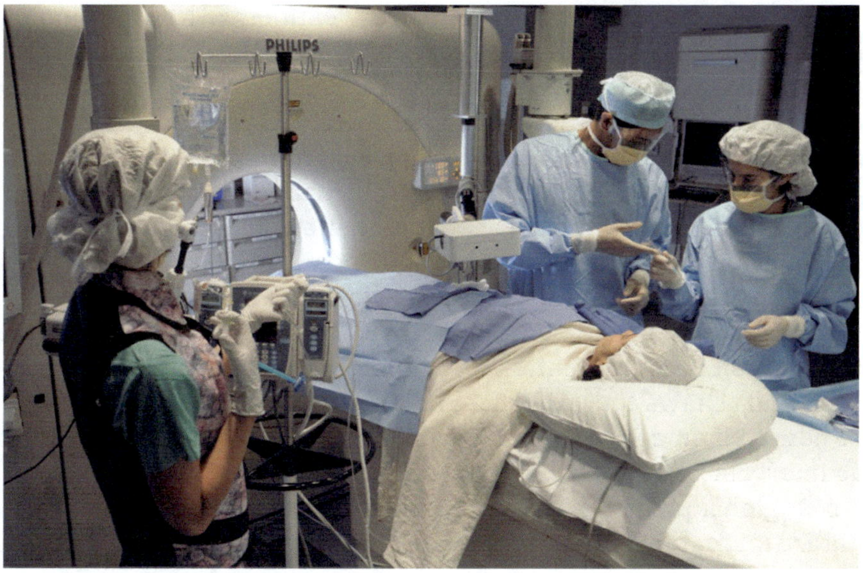

Source: https://live.staticflickr.com/7355/27194104852_ce02bcdfdd_b.jpg.

Test Your Knowledge

1. What are some common risks and complications associated with interventional radiology procedures?
2. How can healthcare professionals minimize and manage complications during interventional radiology treatments?

Summary

Advances in interventional radiology have been reshaping how patients are cared for – almost as if we've entered a new era of minimally invasive treatments. New technology and inventive techniques let doctors now tackle complex procedures with less risk and, quite often, quicker recoveries than we're used to with traditional surgery. This progress, in most cases, not only ups patient safety but also helps hospitals use their resources more wisely. If you take a closer look at radiology training across Europe, the findings reveal that spreading practical knowledge and hands-on skills plays a key role in growing a group of truly capable interventional radiologists; really, this kind of education forms the basic support that ensures professionals stay ready to deal with the ever-changing field of medical imaging and intervention methods (Rehani et al., 2017). When healthcare systems try to mesh advanced medical imaging into their daily operations, the mix of internal structures and outside pressures matters a lot. In fact, hospitals that get these subtle dynamics tend to roll out interventional radiology services more smoothly. Research coming out of Malaysian hospitals shows that external guidance, like that from the Ministry of Health, can significantly shape how well modern imaging tech blends into everyday practice. This kind of insight helps ensure that interventional radiology generally follows national guidelines while matching up with what the best global practices suggest, ultimately bolstering both patient care and overall efficiency in healthcare institutions (Nor et al., 2010). Looking to the future, interventional radiology clearly depends on ongoing learning and a spirit of collaboration. As our health systems evolve, the skills of the professionals within them need to shift too. It's crucial, for many reasons, to improve educational setups and boost teamwork between institutions. When environments encourage open knowledge-sharing, radiologists are better positioned to keep pace with emerging technologies and new techniques. This collaborative approach not only enriches training but also sparks fresh ideas in interventions, benefiting patient outcomes and making the whole delivery process run more smoothly. In short, by embracing these aspects, the field of interventional radiology is poised to make some truly significant strides in global medical care.

Technological progress in Interventional Radiology has upended old diagnostic routines. Take Biomechanical Computed Tomography (BCT), for instance, a tool increasingly being used as an extra check for osteoporosis. Instead of scheduling entirely new scans, doctors now often make use of CT scans taken for other reasons to measure bone strength and mineral density. This clever, almost opportunistic twist means that, in many cases, patients get a more accurate check without throwing off the usual clinical workflow. It also helps catch osteoporosis in individuals who might otherwise slip through the cracks, ultimately showing how fresh radiology techniques can boost patient outcomes while keeping everything running smoothly (Keaveny et al., 2020). Some studies have pointed out that rethinking roles within Interventional Radiology, such as bringing in consultant radiographers, has had a noticeable impact on service delivery. Organizations adopting the Career Progression Framework (CPF) have, generally speaking, managed to modernize imaging practices in ways that patch up old gaps. In practice, this means hospitals are now reassigning advanced practitioner roles in ways that streamline patient care, improve departmental performance, and even help contain costs, all while making better use of their staff's time. This shift, repeated in various settings, has not only improved the way services are delivered, but also raised the overall bar for patient care quality (Miller et al., 2010). Looking more closely, evidence, both numbers and firsthand accounts, suggests that these changes pack a punch. Research shows that adding advanced practitioner roles tends to boost patient throughput without sacrificing safety or quality of care. It appears that even as health systems work harder to meet increased demands, staff morale sees a noticeable lift. Interestingly, introducing consultant roles hasn't led to more errors or extra complaints, which seems to indicate that the added training and responsibility pay off in service quality. Overall, the evolving face of Interventional Radiology keeps adapting to the times, proving over and over again that patient-centered care remains at its very core (Miller et al., 2010).

KEY TERMS FROM THIS CHAPTER

- Angioplasty
- Biopsy
- Blood vessel
- Drainage
- Embolization
- Endovenous laser therapy
- Healthcare systems
- Inferior vena cava (IVC) filter
- Interventional oncology (IO)
- Minimally invasive
- Optical coherence tomography (OCT)
- Pain management
- Thrombolysis
- Tumor ablation
- Virtual reality (VR)

Critical Thinking Questions

1. **What is the main purpose of interventional radiology?**
   a. To perform open surgery on internal organs
   b. To treat medical conditions using non-invasive imaging-guided procedures
   c. To replace traditional X-rays with MRI scans
   d. To treat cancer using high doses of radiation
2. **Which of the following imaging techniques is commonly used during interventional radiology procedures?**
   a. Ultrasound
   b. CT (Computed Tomography)
   c. Fluoroscopy
   d. All of the above
3. **In interventional radiology, what is the role of a catheter?**
   a. To deliver oxygen to the tissues
   b. To collect blood samples for analysis
   c. To access blood vessels and deliver treatments or devices
   d. To block the passage of fluids during procedures
4. **Which of the following is a common procedure performed in interventional radiology?**
   a. Bone marrow biopsy
   b. Angioplasty and stenting
   c. Breast biopsy using ultrasound
   d. Skin lesion removal
5. **What is one of the benefits of interventional radiology compared to traditional surgery?**
   a. It requires a longer recovery time
   b. It involves larger incisions and higher risk
   c. It is minimally invasive with a quicker recovery time
   d. It can only be used for diagnostic purposes

Short Answer Questions

1. What are some key techniques used in interventional radiology to perform minimally invasive procedures?
2. What are the most common interventional radiology procedures, such as angioplasty or embolization, and their primary purposes?
3. What types of equipment and imaging technology are typically used in interventional radiology?
4. How should patients be prepared and cared for before, during, and after an interventional radiology procedure?
5. What are some potential risks and complications associated with interventional radiology, and how are they managed?

Answers to Critical Thinking Questions

1. (b); 2. (d); 3. (c); 4. (b); 5. (c)

References

1. Ahmed Thubab, A. A., Ogdi, K. M., Hezam, S. N., Otaif, A. A., Ogdi, A. M., Al Masoud, S. A., Hamad, M. I., et al. (2024). Challenges and solutions in radiation protection for X-ray procedures. https://core.ac.uk/download/616775622.pdf (accessed on 23 May 2025).
2. Ahmed, A. (2007). Anesthesia for interventional neuroradiology. https://core.ac.uk/download/212883763.pdf (accessed on 23 May 2025).
3. Alcorn, D. J., Atiiga, P., Breen, D. J., et al. (2017). Cross-sectional study of the provision of interventional oncology services in the UK. https://core.ac.uk/download/159994872.pdf (accessed on 23 May 2025).
4. Alhashim, M., Aladel, F., Bukhamseen, M., & Alhariqi, A. (2024). Awareness of interventional radiology and the associated radiation exposure risk among the public population and primary care physicians in Saudi Arabia. *Saudi Journal of Radiology, 3*(1), 16–33. https://doi.org/10.55038/t0h27176.
5. Almuhaidb, A., Olson, D., & Aadam, A. (2021). Advancements in endoscopic biliary interventions by gastroenterology. *Seminars in Interventional Radiology, 38*, 280–290. https://www.semanticscholar.org/paper/92e4a8106989cec2cd736cc45b7541219c1f7976 (accessed on 23 May 2025).
6. Alowais, S. A., Alghamdi, S. S., Alsuhebany, N., Alqahtani, T., Alshaya, A., Almohareb, S. N., Aldairem, A., et al. (2023). Revolutionizing healthcare: The role of artificial intelligence in clinical practice. *BMC Medical Education, 23*. https://doi.org/10.1186/s12909-023-04698-z.
7. Ansel, G. M., Dake, M. D., Johnson, M. S., et al. (2019). The clinical rationale for the Sentry bio convertible inferior vena cava filter for the prevention of pulmonary embolism. https://core.ac.uk/download/228066254.pdf (accessed on 23 May 2025).
8. Anselmetti, G. C., Ardura, F., Beall, D., et al. (2022). Vertebral augmentation: Is it time to get past the pain? A consensus statement from the Sardinia Spine and Stroke Congress. https://core.ac.uk/download/558773495.pdf (accessed on 23 May 2025).
9. Barat, M., Crombé, A., Boeken, T., et al. (2024). Imaging in France: 2024 update. *Canadian Association of Radiologists Journal, 76*(2), 221–231. https://doi.org/10.1177/08465371241288425.
10. Blum, S., & Hoffmann, R. T. (2024). Avoiding adverse events in interventional radiology–A systematic review on the instruments. *CVIR Endovascular, 7*. https://www.semanticscholar.org/paper/3bfbae6363adb51446e1c006cd8fc3d71dc1e56e (accessed on 23 May 2025).
11. Boone, B. (2012). A qualitative descriptive study of the work of nurses in interventional radiology [PhD dissertation]. https://core.ac.uk/download/477678860.pdf (accessed on 23 May 2025).
12. Brock, K. K., Chen, S. R., Sheth, R. A., et al. (2023). Imaging in interventional radiology: 2043 and beyond. https://core.ac.uk/download/622991664.pdf (accessed on 23 May 2025).
13. Clements, J. B., Baird, C. T., de Boer, S. F., Fairobent, L. A., Fisher, T., Goodwin, J. H., Gress, D. A., Johnson, J. L., Kolsky, K. L., Mageras, G. S., Marsh, R. M., Martin, M. C., Parker, B., Pavord, D. C., Schell, M. C., Seibert, J. A., Stevens, D. M., Tarver, R. B., Waite-Jones, C. G., & Wingreen, N. (2018). AAPM medical physics practice guideline 10.a.: Scope of practice for

clinical medical physics. *Journal of Applied Clinical Medical Physics, 19*, 11–25. https://doi.org/10.1002/acm2.12469.

14. Clements, W., & Koukounaras, J. (2023). Complications in interventional radiology: The role of clinical governance and iterative hospital systems in quality improvement. *CVIR Endovascular, 6*(1), 38. https://doi.org/10.1186/s42155-023-00388-5.
15. Deshmukh, U., Pabon-Ramos, W., & Ayyagari, R. (2025). The role of interventional radiology in managing placenta accreta spectrum disorder. *Clinical Obstetrics and Gynecology*. https://www.semanticscholar.org/paper/c64b5614656c7fee8465cc5ceac1267cbc6851a3 (accessed on 23 May 2025).
16. Desimpel, J., Posadzy, M., & Vanhoenacker, F. (2018). Cone beam CT of the musculoskeletal system: Clinical applications. https://core.ac.uk/download/147045015.pdf (accessed on 23 May 2025).
17. Finos, K., Datta, S., Sedrakyan, A., Milsom, J. W., & Pua, B. B. (2024). Mixed reality in interventional radiology: A focus on first clinical use of XR90 augmented reality-based visualization and navigation platform. *Expert Review of Medical Devices, 21*(8), 679–688. https://doi.org/10.1080/17434440.2024.2379925.
18. Friso, S., Giacobbo, V., Toscano, L. M., Baldo, B., Guariento, C., Lacarra, F., Pin, J. N., et al. (2024). A systematic review of surgical and interventional radiology procedures for pediatric idiopathic intracranial hypertension. *Frontiers in Pediatrics, 12*. https://www.semanticscholar.org/paper/e62aace55c94b26bfe848adf0170126acfd48cf8 (accessed on 23 May 2025).
19. Gounis, M. J., Ughi, G. J., Marosföi, M., Lopes, D. K., Fiorella, D., Bezerra, H. G., Liang, C. W., et al. (2018). Intravascular optical coherence tomography for neurointerventional surgery. *Stroke, 50*, 218–223. https://doi.org/10.1161/strokeaha.118.022315.
20. Indianapolis Coalition for Patient Safety. (2017). *Intravascular Iodinated Contrast Media Administration in Adults: A Patient Safety Approach*. ICPS.
21. Jeromel, M., & Salapura, V. (2014). Minimalno invazivno (perkutano) liječenje metastatske spinalne i ekstraspinalne bolesti–pregledni članak. https://core.ac.uk/download/33263780.pdf (accessed on 23 May 2025).
22. Keaveny, T. M., Clarke, B. L., Cosman, F., Orwoll, E. S., Siris, E. S., Khosla, S., & Bouxsein, M. L. (2020). Biomechanical computed tomography analysis (BCT) for clinical assessment of osteoporosis. *Osteoporosis International, 31*(6), 1025–1048. https://doi.org/10.1007/s00198-020-05384-2.
23. Martin, C. J., Vassileva, J., Vano, E., Mahesh, M., Ebdon-Jackson, S., Ng, K. H., Frush, D. P., Loose, R., & Damilakis, J. (2017). Unintended and accidental medical radiation exposures in radiology: Guidelines on investigation and prevention. *Journal of Radiological Protection, 37*(4), 883–906. https://doi.org/10.1088/1361-6498/aa881e.
24. Miller, L., & Price, R. (2010). An evaluation of the impact of implementation of consultant practitioners in clinical imaging. https://core.ac.uk/download/9840194.pdf (accessed on 23 May 2025).
25. Mohd Nor, R. (2010). The organizational implications of medical imaging in the context of Malaysian hospitals. https://core.ac.uk/download/1588563.pdf (accessed on 23 May 2025).

26. Najjar, R. (2023). Redefining radiology: A review of artificial intelligence integration in medical imaging. *Diagnostics, 13*, 2760. https://doi.org/10.3390/diagnostics13172760.

27. Nguyen, R. (2024). Interventional radiology's exploration into artificial intelligence. https://core.ac.uk/download/619706208.pdf (accessed on 23 May 2025).

28. Pasecki, P., Narloch, J., Tkaczewski, K., Wasek, W., Ziecina, P., & Brzozowski, K. (2018). Interventional radiology treatments for iatrogenic severe bleeding during percutaneous coronary interventions. *Polish Journal of Radiology, 83*, e319–e325. https://doi.org/10.5114/pjr.2018.77027.

29. Patel, D. C., Gaba, R. C., Liu, L., & Lokken, R. P. (2019). Tissue plasminogen activator dose and pulmonary artery pressure reduction in catheter directed thrombolysis of sub massive pulmonary embolism. *PLoS One, 14*(2), e0211701. https://doi.org/10.1371/journal.pone.0211701.

30. Pereira, H. V., Teixeira, D. S., Fisher, J., Fleck, S. J., Helms, E., Ide, B. N., & Schoenfeld, B. J. (2025). International consensus on the definition of functional training: Modified e-Delphi method. *Journal of Sports Sciences, 43*(8), 767–775. https://doi.org/10.1080/02640414.2025.2477393.

31. Qian, P., Liu, Y., Ren, J., Xu, X., Zhao, Z., Cao, C., & Yang, L. (2023). [Research progress in diagnostic reference levels in interventional radiology]. *Zhongguo Yi Xue Ke Xue Yuan Xue Bao. Acta Academiae Medicinae Sinicae, 45*(3), 506–511. https://www.semanticscholar.org/paper/d3df958763c995c588d8600dbe270511193cbc07 (accessed on 23 May 2025).

32. Rebonato, A., Mosca, S., Fischer, M., Gerli, S., Orgera, G., Graziosi, L., Maiettini, D., Di Renzo, G. C., Epicoco, G., Krokidis, M., Rossi, M., & Scialpi, M. (2016). Endovascular management of massive post-partum hemorrhage in abnormal placental implantation deliveries. *European Radiology, 26*(6), 1620–1630. https://doi.org/10.1007/s00330-015-4001-z.

33. Rehani, B., Zhang, Y. C., Rehani, M. M., Palkó, A., Lau, L., Lette, M. N., & Dillon, W. P. (2017). Radiology education in Europe: Analysis of results from 22 European countries. *World Journal of Radiology, 9*(2), 55–62. https://doi.org/10.4329/wjr.v9.i2.55.

34. Rohde, S., Weber, W., Berlis, A., Urbach, H., Reimer, P., Schramm, P., German Society of Interventional Radiology and Minimally Invasive Therapy, et al. (2021). Acute endovascular stroke treatment in Germany in 2019. *Clinical Neuroradiology, 31*, 11–19. https://www.semanticscholar.org/paper/aaa2fd54d2c27dabf5abd6667ef299724d4867e8 (accessed on 23 May 2025).

35. Scheschenja, M., Viniol, S., Bastian, M. B., Wessendorf, J., König, A., & Mahnken, A. (2023). Feasibility of GPT-3 and GPT-4 for in-depth patient education prior to interventional radiological procedures: A comparative analysis. *Cardiovascular and Interventional Radiology, 47*, 245–250. https://www.semanticscholar.org/paper/1a3fba1e7239668eb89f4a8bcfc727999a7ab76a (accessed on 23 May 2025).

36. Scollan, M. E., Azimov, N., Garzón, M., & Tulin-Silver, S. (2023). An overview of interventional radiology techniques for the diagnosis and management of vascular anomalies: Part 2. *Pediatric Dermatology, 40*, 767–774. https://www.semanticscholar.org/paper/b5d8373da247492b9a899fc659e2b6be5027f6ab (accessed on 23 May 2025).

37. Seah, J., Boeken, T., Sapoval, M., & Goh, G. (2022). Prime time for artificial intelligence in interventional radiology. *Cardiovascular and Interventional Radiology, 45*, 283–289. https://

www.semanticscholar.org/paper/38747ee6d3acc49686fb34c401e335d1e58a4207 (accessed on 23 May 2025).

38. Taiji, R., Lin, E., Lin, Y. M., Yevich, S., Avritscher, R., Sheth, R. A., Ruiz, J., et al. (2021). Combined angio-CT systems: A roadmap tool for precision therapy in interventional oncology. *Radiology Imaging Cancer, 3*, e210039. https://doi.org/10.1148/rycan.2021210039.

39. Tomassoni, M. T., Braccischi, L., Russo, M., Adduci, F., Calautti, D., Girolami, M., & Spinnato, P. (2024). Image-guided minimally invasive treatment options for degenerative lumbar spine disease: A practical overview of current possibilities. *Diagnostics, 14*(11), 1147. https://doi.org/10.3390/diagnostics14111147.

40. Yancey, K., Ruddy, L., Simmons, C. L., Crawford, D. A., Alzubaidi, S., Naidu, S., & Ozen, M. (2025). Unveiling portal vein anatomy: Clinical impact and significance of variants in transjugular intrahepatic portosystemic shunt creation. *Seminars in Interventional Radiology.* https://www.semanticscholar.org/paper/6699d585a47dfe4359fcb27aac543a87a6ca1c4c (accessed on 23 May 2025).

41. Zhang, R., Zhang, Y., Yang, Z., Chen, J., Wang, Q., Ma, J., Zhang, B., et al. (2022). The safety and efficacy of add-on use of oxytocin in uterine leiomyoma patients undergoing high-intensity focused ultrasound and ultrasound-guided intratumoral ethanol injection: A randomized controlled trial. *Annals of Palliative Medicine, 11*(6), 2033–2042. https://www.semanticscholar.org/paper/bf405f08a4b84e4166e4c346ad581858c9be485a (accessed on 23 May 2025).

42. Zhao, A., Resnick, S., Burton, C. S., & Fadhel, M. (2024). Deciphering the radiation dose summary page in interventional fluoroscopy. *Radiographic, 44*(8), e230197. https://www.semanticscholar.org/paper/44997ec7e08df21f87bc3dea9e1256c7eeffffc3 (accessed on 23 May 2025).

DIGITAL IMAGING AND PACS

10

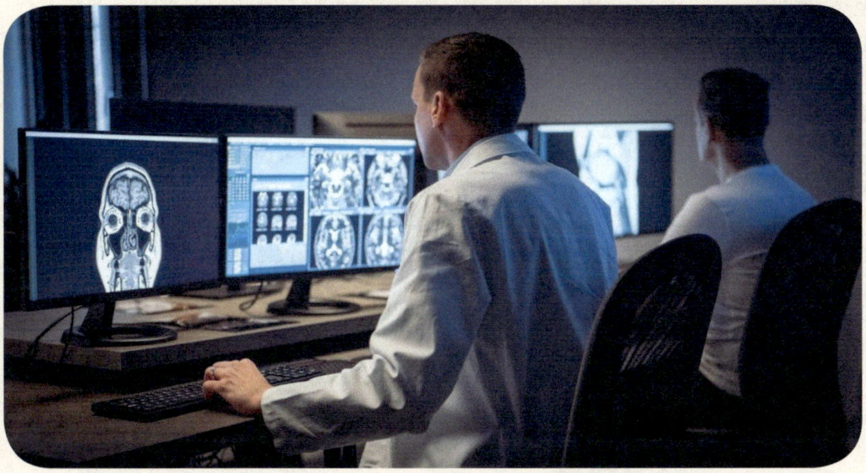

LEARNING OBJECTIVES

After studying this chapter, you will be able to:

1. Understand the historical development and evolution of digital imaging.
2. Identify and describe the key components of Picture Archiving and Communication Systems (PACS).
3. Explore the clinical and operational benefits of implementing digital imaging systems.
4. Analyze the challenges and limitations associated with digital imaging and PACS implementation.
5. Examine emerging future trends in digital imaging.

Introduction

Medical technology keeps changing in unexpected ways, and imaging with data handling is one of the major areas feeling the impact. Digital imaging teamed up with PACS, a system that stores, retrieves, and shares medical images, has become a game changer in clinical routines. Instead of relying on old, clunky films, many hospitals are switching to these digital methods that just work better on many levels. In most cases, this change not only meets the immediate demands of busy healthcare providers but also sets things up nicely for future innovations in patient care. The role of PACS in today's healthcare is hard to overlook. It gives hospitals a smoother way to connect different platforms and get imaging data quickly, which is pretty crucial when fast, accurate diagnoses are needed. Take stomatology, for example the tricky nature of dental decision-making puts a spotlight on how important high-quality images are. Several studies, including one from a Class A tertiary stomatological hospital in China, point out that PACS's ability to integrate and send digital images efficiently has won a lot of support. Dental professionals often mention that, while everyone agrees on what PACS does best, there's still room for some fine-tuning to make things work even better (Wu et al., 2022). RIS, or Radiological Information Systems, steps in as another important part of the digital healthcare mix. Unlike PACS, RIS handles the complete electronic workflow of radiology, bridging across various computer systems in a way that isn't always neat but gets the job done. This kind of linking is key for a smoother digital environment that reduces mistakes while boosting speed in diagnostic tasks. Using standards like DICOM and HL7, RIS helps digital radiology perform at top levels, making information readily available to support on-the-fly decisions. Together, PACS and RIS don't just modernize how things are done; they push healthcare toward more automated processes that generally improve care quality and help cut costs (Babić et al., 2019).

Definition of Digital Imaging

Digital imaging has reshaped things in healthcare and beyond. Nowadays, instead of clinging to old film techniques, capturing, processing, storing, and sharing medical images happens in an almost effortless flow. Methods like digital radiography, CT scans, and MRIs give doctors sharp, clear visuals that help with diagnosis, and that shift isn't just about better resolution, it is also about making images easier to access. A big piece of the puzzle is getting systems to "talk" to each other, and generally speaking, standards like DICOM help ensure that images move smoothly between departments, whether it is in busy emergency rooms or crowded ICUs. Clinics and hospitals have had to adapt as the flood of data keeps growing. Picture Archiving and Communication Systems (PACS) have become the go-to for storing, finding, and sending around these images, effectively ditching old-school storage methods while speeding up the retrieval process so clinicians can obtain what they need more quickly. It is not just about keeping images safe, there's also the need to share them easily across different platforms. Some setups, such as the Java-based Distributed Object Medical Imaging Model (DOMIM), even work to bridge gaps between remote experts, adding extra support for better patient care (Noor et al., 2009). Even with all these improvements, there are still bumps in the road. Issues with data quality and meeting set standards, like when DICOM isn't implemented perfectly, can make it tricky to connect different systems. These hiccups might compromise care, so there's a push to find new ways to check and validate data without burdening users with too many tweaks. For example, building a Web DICOM validation service could be a step toward ensuring things remain consistent and reliable. Overall, keeping high standards is not just a technical challenge but a key part of protecting patient information and streamlining healthcare delivery (Silva et al., 2018) (Figure 10.1).

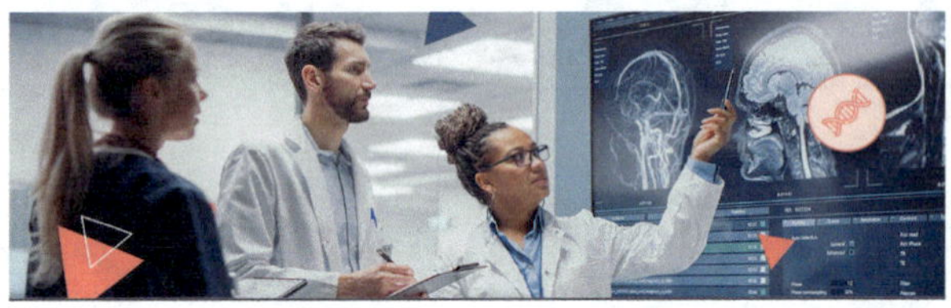

Figure 10.1. Digital Imaging.

Source: https://external-content.duckduckgo.com/iu/?u=https%3A%2F%2Fwww.onixnet.com%2Fwp-content%2Fuploads%2F2023%2F03%2FHow-AI-Powered-Medical-Imaging-is-Transforming-Healthcare.jpg&f=1&nofb=1&ipt=c136fe1fb9215d9557965d0f5b9faba6feaab7962d6c3c4d957284e132f4b949.

Overview of PACS (Picture Archiving and Communication System)

Medical imaging took a new turn once PACS came into play, imaging data now gets stored and retrieved from one central hub, making it a lot easier for radiologists and healthcare individuals to pull up images and reports instantly from different spots. This change means facilities aren't so tied to old-school film and can finally cut down on bulky physical storage. Sure, it all sounds promising, but things aren't without hiccups; manufacturers sometimes combined with the DICOM standard in their own unique fashion, and that leads to interoperability headaches which, in most cases, end up impacting patient care. Software that checks data quality and compliance ends up being a real necessity (Silva et al., 2018).

Then there's the rise of network-based solutions like MIDAS, an open-source, web-based archiving system that handles everything from obtaining data to analyzing and reporting it. MIDAS, with its flexible vibe, lets healthcare professionals store, manage, and even share huge imaging datasets pretty seamlessly. This kind of setup not only nudges researchers into working together more closely but also helps doctors get imaging data quickly, something that often makes a difference for patient outcomes. When you look at how these intuitive systems are shaping up, it is clear that the trend is shifting toward interfaces that are built around the user (Jomier et al., 2010). At its heart, PACS has become a key thread in the fabric of today's digital imaging landscape, shifting the game away from film so clinicians can use digital systems to boost patient care and streamline day-to-day tasks.

That said, its smooth operation depends on manufacturers teaming up to iron out those integration wrinkles and double-check data properly. Overcoming these snags is essential if we're going to unlock all the benefits PACS promises. As medical imaging tools keep evolving, it is pretty evident that systems like PACS, and their ongoing development and integration into everyday workflow, will play a huge role in steering the future of diagnostic imaging and patient management (Figure 10.2).

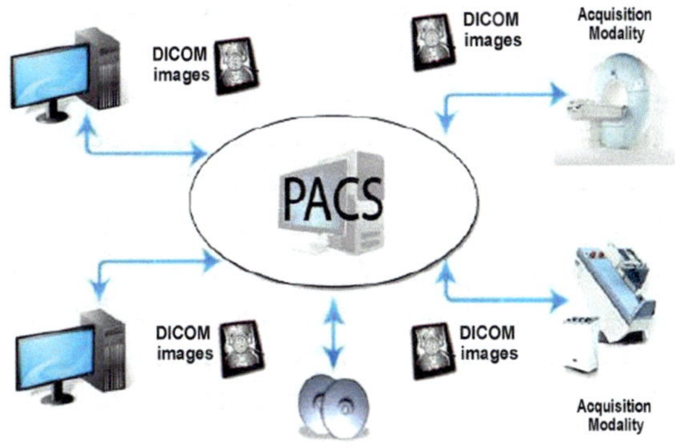

Figure 10.2. Picture archiving and communication system (PACS).

Source: https://cdn.open-pr.com/T/9/T928178402_g.jpg.

Importance of Digital Imaging in Modern Healthcare

Digital imaging is changing how healthcare works today. Hospitals are now using setups like Picture Archiving and Communication Systems (PACS) to smooth out their everyday tasks and boost how accurately they diagnose. Switching to digital storage and sharing of medical images cuts down the time radiologists, indeed, the very backbone of timely intervention, spend hunting for patient details. This way of handling images also has the side benefit of drawing different professionals together, even if it feels a bit unexpected at first glance. Several studies suggest that these benefits go far beyond just operational neatness; they even reshape job roles and social ties within hospitals (Nor et al., 2010). The rules and technical details around digital imaging, believe it or not, play a huge role too. Standards like DICOM and HL7, in most cases, let a range of systems chat with each other smoothly, which, to be fair, creates a more collaborative vibe among staff. By connecting PACS with other electronic health records, patient data stays accessible and in order, something that many clinicians appreciate. As healthcare increasingly leans toward a data-driven style, these frameworks help maintain a steady flow of care, allowing doctors to lean on a full picture of patient information. It is important to note that getting these technologies up and running not only alters the clinical scene but also improves the overall patient experience and outcomes (Hristova et al., 2020). It is also worth noting how digital imaging shifts the social dynamics among healthcare teams. Radiologists, for instance, are now engaging more with both clinical and non-clinical colleagues, a change that, admittedly, isn't always on the radar but makes a big difference. This evolution nudges organizations toward a more team-focused approach, where clear communication can seriously make or break success. When you consider how these systems blend various roles together, it becomes obvious that effective communication among all parties is key. As tech keeps worming its way deeper into healthcare, keeping an eye on these human connections might just be the ticket to significantly better service and outcomes (Nor et al., 2010) (Figure 10.3).

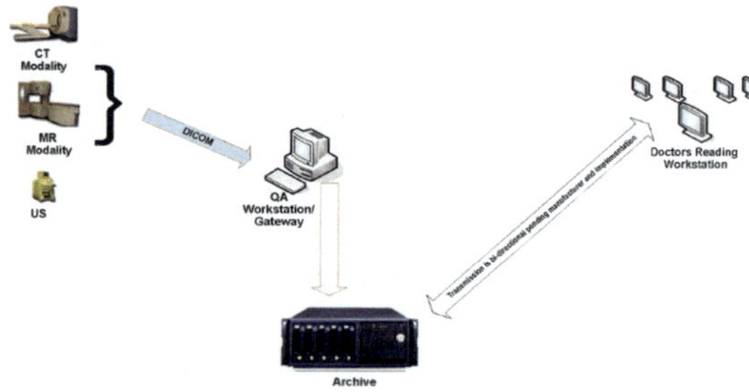

Figure 10.3. A PACS system.

Source: By Dlc00-NJITWILL - Own work, CC0, https://commons.wikimedia.org/w/index.php?curid=10705963.

10.1. History of Digital Imaging

Learning Outcome

1. Trace the evolution from film to digital.
2. Identify key milestones in digital imaging technology.
3. Analyze the impact of digital imaging on medical practices.

Digital imaging changed everything about how we obtain, process, and keep images. In the early days, medical imaging leaned on analog tricks like classic X-rays and film-based approaches, methods that, while pretty groundbreaking, were slow and often fuzzy. Then came digital technology in the late 1900s, and suddenly those limitations started fading away; doors opened for new techniques that just worked differently. CT scans and MRIs, for instance, let us capture details without the clunky constraints of film. This shift upped diagnostic accuracy in ways that changed medicine, making fast, precise info more of a standard than an exception. Standards have been a crucial part of the whole digital imaging story, even if it sounds a bit dry. Instead of a jumble of equipment that couldn't "talk" to each other, protocols were set up so various systems could connect in a practical way. Take the DICOM standard (Digital Imaging and Communications in Medicine) as a prime example, it was a real game changer, letting different imaging devices share data seamlessly. Such regularity smoothed out the process of meshing imaging hardware into healthcare setups, eventually paving the way for Picture Archiving and Communication Systems, or PACS. These tools turned out indispensable for juggling huge piles of image data, helping with storage, quick retrieval and easy sharing, while team efforts from open-source groups and commercial players have kept PACS evolving to always meet the needs of radiologists and other healthcare pros (Nagy et al., 2007). Over time, digital imaging got even smarter. New tools for image analysis started popping up and taking on a bigger role in everyday clinical work. In many cases, pairing imaging with artificial intelligence (AI) and machine learning has given us algorithms that can spot subtle patterns or odd anomalies that might slip by a human observer. This mix of tech isn't just a neat upgrade; it marks the start of a whole new chapter where diagnostics get sharper and patient care more proactive. It is not just about making things more efficient, it's also pushing radiology forward as a field. As imaging technology keeps morphing with emerging trends, a collaborative spirit among developers, healthcare professionals, and researchers is proving critical for sorting out the ever-growing challenges of modern imaging (Nagy et al., 2007).

10.1.1. Evolution from Film to Digital

Moving away from film and switching to digital imaging has reshaped how medical diagnostics and radiology work. Long ago, imaging depended on actual films, a cumbersome process that involved lengthy development, careful interpretation, and frequent issues like slow processing, susceptibility to physical damage, and the general difficulty of sharing images. These film limitations created a real need for something better. When digital imaging came into play, it not only fixed many of these problems but also sparked further innovation in imaging techniques. Before long, hospitals and clinics started adopting systems like Picture Archiving and Communication Systems (PACS) to store, retrieve, and share digital images with a speed and ease that seemed almost revolutionary.

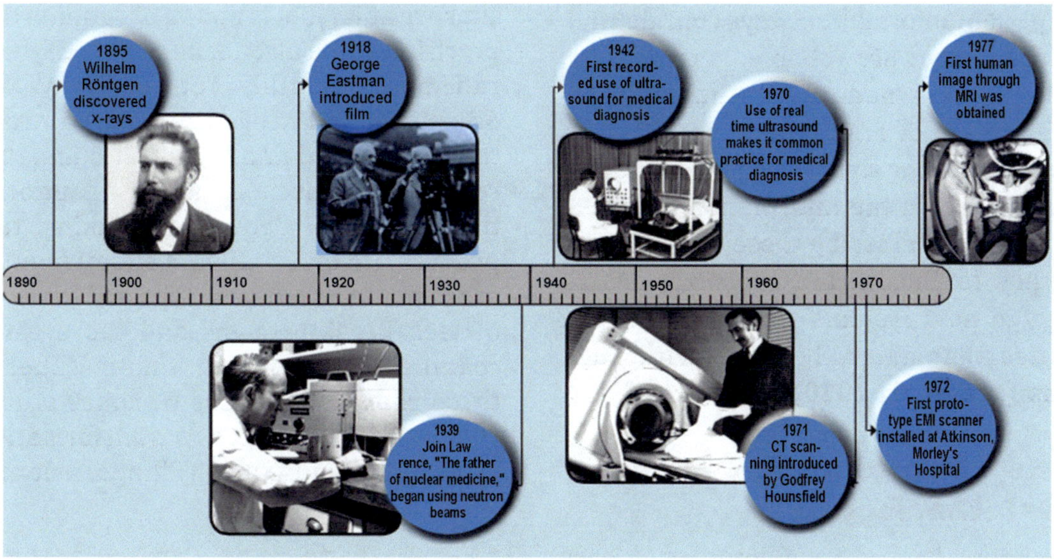

Figure 10.4. Evolution of digital imaging in radiology.

Source: https://www.purview.net/hubfs/Evolution_RadiologyFinal.png.

This change, in many ways, laid the groundwork for a fresh approach to clinical workflows where quick access to patient data helps drive better decisions and improves outcomes (Nagy et al., 2007). As more healthcare centers began to lean on digital solutions, the impact on radiology and imaging became quite evident. Digital tools now hand clinicians the means to work faster and with more precision, generally speaking, while also pushing healthcare teams to learn new digital skills. The integration of PACS has subtly shifted the way radiologists interact with referring clinicians; now, communication is streamlined which helps foster a smoother, more collaborative care process. Radiologists are juggling a dual challenge here: staying updated with technological advances while still ensuring their imaging interpretations remain top-notch. This evolving scenario mirrors a broader trend in healthcare where technology steadily redefines professional roles and relationships in ways that sometimes feel both surprising and natural (Nor et al., 2010). Even though digital imaging offers many operational perks, it brings its own set of challenges that can't be ignored. Switching from film to digital demands significant investments in both technology and the continuous training of staff at every level. On top of that, concerns about data security and the integrity of digital images have risen to the forefront in today's digital health landscape. Ensuring patient information stays confidential, and that the images are reliable, is critical for maintaining trust in medical institutions. Thus, effective adoption of PACS often goes hand in hand with establishing rigorous data governance policies to safeguard the information involved. Recognizing and addressing these multifaceted issues is key for healthcare organizations as they adapt to new systems while tackling the complexities that naturally come with such transitions (Nor et al., 2010) (Figure 10.4).

10.1.2. Key Milestones in Digital Imaging Technology

Digital imaging has come a long way from its humble beginnings. Early on, simple X-ray technology set things in motion, and before you knew it, tools like CT scans and MRI started making serious waves in how doctors figure out what's wrong. As these technologies got better and more commonly used in various fields, there was a growing call to set up clear guidelines. In most cases, these weren't just about checking boxes; they involved leadership training, hands-on competency tests, and ongoing quality checks, all meant to ensure that even innovations like clinical ultrasound (CUS) truly benefit patient care (Strony et al., 2018). Then came a real game changer: picture archiving and communication systems, or PACS. This leap meant the days of managing clunky film were over, replaced by digital storage that made storing and retrieving images a lot smoother. Hospitals quickly realized that switching to PACS not only made radiology more efficient but also boosted teamwork among various professionals. Over time, the need for different imaging technologies to "speak the same language" became obvious, which in turn improved diagnostic accuracy. The flow of information between departments started to feel less forced, helping to streamline patient care even as systems evolved. More recently, the mix of AI with digital imaging has stirred up a fair bit of excitement. AI, getting steadily sharper at its job, is aimed at refining diagnostic precision while also making everyday workflows run more smoothly. Yet, for many healthcare organizations, integrating AI isn't a straight shot, there are social and technical bumps along the road that sometimes make adoption trickier than expected. Generally speaking, the whole process involves a dance between planned implementations and unexpected shifts, a balance of tech breakthroughs and the organization's readiness to embrace them. Understanding these change processes becomes crucial when trying to fully unlock AI's transformative power in imaging landscapes (Ellingsen et al., 2023).

10.1.3. Impact of Digital Imaging on Medical Practices

Hospitals these days are changing in ways you might not expect, all thanks to digital imaging. Picture Archiving and Communication Systems, PACS, for short, let them handle medical pictures a lot quicker and more accurately, which helps with fast diagnosis. Inside each hospital, things like the number of staff and how many resources are available mix with outside rules and regulations to shape how this tech ends up working. One study even found that the Ministry of Health, for example, plays a big role in guiding how things roll out in Malaysian hospitals (Nor et al., 2010). It turns out that the value of digital imaging isn't just about the tech itself, but also about the unique environment in which it's used. At the same time, digital imaging isn't only about new machines, it reshapes what people do. The switch to PACS has shifted how radiographers handle their jobs, even if radiologists and other clinical staff still stick to some of their old routines. This kind of change creates a more connected work scene where sharing information becomes second nature, and even people who aren't directly clinical find themselves working a bit closer with the rest. These changes aren't the same everywhere though; each hospital seems to have its own twist on the story (Nor et al., 2010), showing that using new tech means rethinking old ways of working. Looking at the bigger picture, the rise of digital imaging also points to a growing need for smarter tools to manage stacks of medical data, whether they're patient records or detailed images. In many cases, practical technologies like XML make it easier to handle this information, sometimes even letting doctors check on patients from afar. This ability to work remotely not only boosts access for individuals in crowded cities or isolated areas, but also means care can happen more quickly when it is needed. All of this underlines why ongoing research and new ideas are so important if healthcare is to keep pace with digital innovations (Figure 10.5).

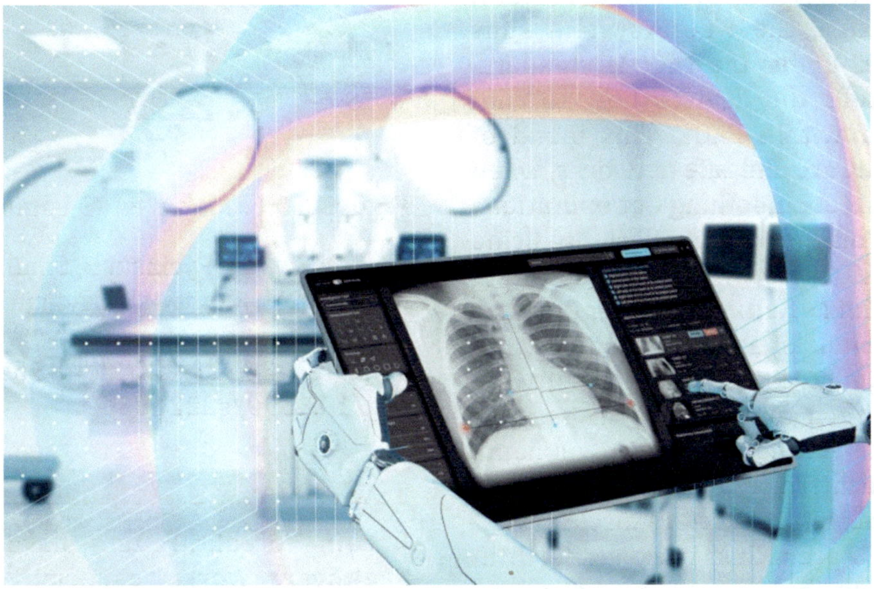

Figure 10.5. Picture Archiving and Communication Systems.

Source: https://www.bgosoftware.com/blog/wp-content/uploads/2024/02/bgo-software-blog-post-size-Role-of-AI-no-title.png.

Test Your Knowledge

1. What were the major differences between traditional film-based imaging and digital imaging in medical diagnostics?
2. What key technological advancements have contributed to the evolution of digital imaging in healthcare?

10.2. Components of PACS

Learning Outcome

1. Understand the various image acquisition devices.
2. Explore storage solutions for digital images.
3. Define workstations and viewing software.

Digital imaging systems lean on a solid setup that, in its own way, boosts radiology's day-to-day performance. It all kicks off with imaging hardware, think digital X-rays, MRIs, and CT scanners, which obtain diagnostic images and turn them into a digital format ready for review. Right after that, a secure, locked network steps in to link these devices with their data hubs. Generally speaking, the whole system runs on a set of rules under the DICOM standard, which sort of tells the devices how to chat with each other within PACS. This blend of trustworthy hardware and safe networks, when put together, aims at smoothing out operations and sharpening diagnosis in modern medicine (Hristova et al., 2020). Viewing stations round out this tech mix. Radiologists and other medical professionals use these screens to check out high-quality images, and the software running them, often quite varied in ease-of-use, can speed up getting patient data on hand. Sometimes these interfaces even foster a sort of collaborative vibe, letting doctors discuss what they see with their peers. Such back-and-forth, in most cases, not only boosts diagnostic accuracy but also helps mesh different perspectives for better patient care (Nor et al., 2010). Then there's data storage, another big piece of the PACS puzzle, handling the ever-growing pile of digital images. These facilities are built to keep vast amounts of imaging data safe while still allowing quick retrieval when a comparison is needed. With robust data-management systems in place, radiologists can easily pull up older images, ensuring continuity in care, no small feat in today's data-heavy world. And by sticking with standards like DICOM, all those imaging tools across various departments can work together, generally speaking, with fewer hiccups. In a nutshell, the way data storage ties in with imaging hardware and viewing stations highlights just how layered and interconnected PACS is in reshaping healthcare delivery (Hristova et al., 2020) (Figure 10.6).

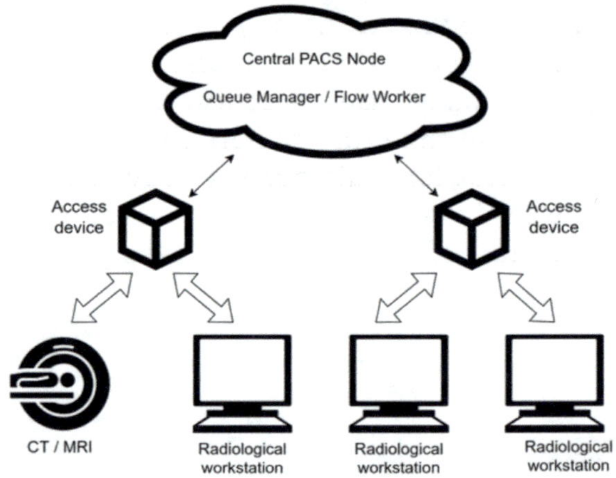

Figure 10.6. Major PACS components.

Source: Kawa J, Pyciński B, Smoliński M, Bożek P, Kwasecki M, Pietrzyk B, Szymański D. Design and Implementation of a Cloud PACS Architecture. *Sensors*. 2022; 22(21):8569. https://doi.org/10.3390/s22218569.

10.2.1. Image Acquisition Devices

Imaging breakthroughs have upended how healthcare works, especially in diagnosing conditions. Devices that capture images now do so in surprisingly varied ways, mixing techniques that yield the kind of clear pictures doctors need for solid diagnoses. Take digital sensors, for example, the ones used in digital mammography have become essential for spotting breast cancer; they come with onboard computer tools for cutting down noise, boosting picture quality, and spotting patterns. Switching from traditional film to digital isn't all smooth sailing either, as managing the huge data sets from these scans creates its own set of challenges. Generally speaking, getting to grips with these devices is key in clinical settings to help ensure patients receive reliable care. Computed radiography has, in most cases, changed the game for medical imaging, turning X-ray pictures into digital files nearly instantly and easing the workflow in busy clinics. Recent projects even hint that educators need to revamp their curriculum guidelines so these new techniques can be woven into existing teaching frameworks. When healthcare professionals learn computed radiography in depth, they tend to handle these devices with a confidence that benefits actual patient care. Overall, this mix of old and new shows a real commitment to preparing future radiologic technologists with the know-how needed to navigate the messy reality of modern imaging. Image acquisition devices, however, do far more than simply capture photos, they're a central part of the larger Picture Archiving and Communication Systems (PACS). When the hardware for image collection and PACS are in sync, top-notch images get not only produced but also quickly transmitted for review and storage. As seen in the advances in digital mammography, better image compression methods become pretty vital when dealing with big chunks of data; whether one opts for nearly lossless or lossy compression, the choice impacts system design. In the end, the push and pull between these devices and PACS highlights why constant innovation and adaptation in medical imaging are so necessary to keep diagnostic accuracy and overall healthcare quality on point (Clarke et al., 1993; Guzman et al., 2002).

10.2.2. Storage Solutions for Digital Images

Digital images have been exploding lately, and because of that, healthcare now needs storage that can keep up, especially in setups like Picture Archiving and Communication Systems (PACS). It's not just about having a massive space for files; getting the right image fast when diagnosing or treating a patient is equally crucial. Web-based apps have stepped into the picture, linking digital databases with storage methods in ways that feel almost effortless. For example, using tools like XML helps manage large swaths of imaging data while keeping security measures and regulations in check. Overall, this way of handling data makes sure that patients get prompt, accurate care, showing just how essential solid storage is for today's digital imaging practices (Lalande et al., 2017). Another angle to consider is the cost, and not just the cost of buying equipment, but also the ongoing expenses of keeping these systems running. As healthcare technology continues to evolve, particularly in places like India, finding affordable options becomes more pressing. Public health systems are increasingly turning to ICT to stretch services farther, especially in remote areas where traditional care just isn't an option. Of course, while advanced storage systems bring a lot to the table, they also come with big upfront price tags for high-end medical machinery. In most cases, their real value goes beyond just holding data; these systems help boost operational speed and improve patient care, which are key factors in today's debates about healthcare technology (Kannan, 2007). And then there's the human side of it all, the move to digital imaging and PACS is also forcing a rethink on how healthcare staff are trained. Effectively using these new tools means professionals have to pick up different skills to manage digital data flows. That makes educational initiatives aimed at ramping up digital literacy among health workers nearly indispensable. By weaving ICT training into everyday professional development, staff can better handle the uniqueness and challenges that come with modern imaging tech. In a nutshell, the success of digital imaging in healthcare depends not just on having robust storage but also on preparing people to work with it (Kannan, 2007) (Figure 10.7).

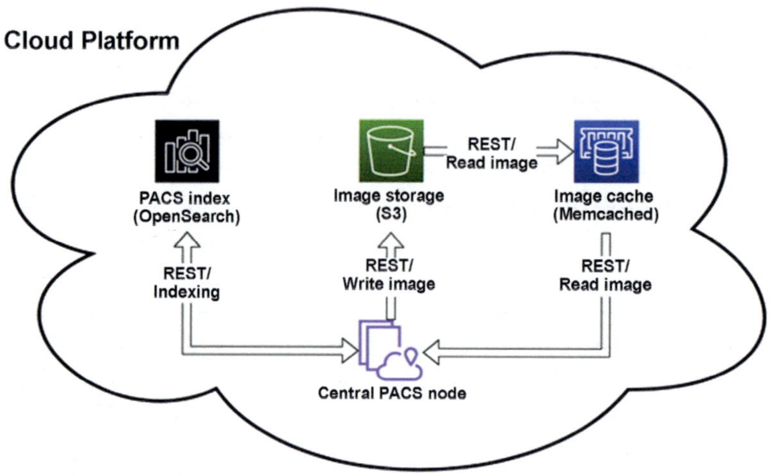

Figure 10.7. PACS storage systems.

Source: Kawa J, Pyciński B, Smoliński M, Bożek P, Kwasecki M, Pietrzyk B, Szymański D. Design and Implementation of a Cloud PACS Architecture. *Sensors*. 2022; 22(21):8569. https://doi.org/10.3390/s22218569.

10.2.3. Workstations and Viewing Software

Robust workstations and advanced viewing tools lie at the heart of Picture Archiving and Communication Systems (PACS) in healthcare. These pieces of tech are often the first stop for radiologists and medical staff who need to look at and analyze images quickly. They trim down the work process, generally boosting diagnostic accuracy while also ramping up patient care speed. The viewer software, which can easily hook up with different imaging machines, plays a key role here. It creates a sort of loose, interconnected network that helps clinicians chat more freely, a factor that, in most cases, is as critical as patient results in sensitive settings. When you dig a bit deeper, it is pretty clear that workstation design substantially shapes user experience and, by extension, the quality of care provided. Consider things like screen clarity, comfy layouts, and software tuned to specific tasks; these aspects can sway a radiologist's ability to catch important details. Many modern setups come with high-res screens that let you see intricate anatomical features vital for a proper diagnosis. In hospitals that have integrated these systems well, research from systems theory shows that the move to digital imaging often nurtures improved interprofessional bonds, which in turn positively impacts patient care. Beyond just making things function, the viewing software also adds an educational layer. Training clinicians to handle these advanced systems is generally seen as paramount if you want to tap into their full potential (Nor et al., 2010).

Often, healthcare facilities face hurdles in getting everyone used to the sometimes-confusing software interfaces, which can hold back PACS from reaching its maximum capacity. As the literature indicates, transitioning to digital not only calls for new tech but also ongoing education and support. Essentially, nurturing a culture of continuous learning turns out to be essential for keeping pace with evolving tools and for boosting overall health outcomes. In practice, this kind of support can lead to more well-informed clinical decisions and help realize the workflow gains promised by these PACS technologies (Scialdone et al., 2002) (Figure 10.8).

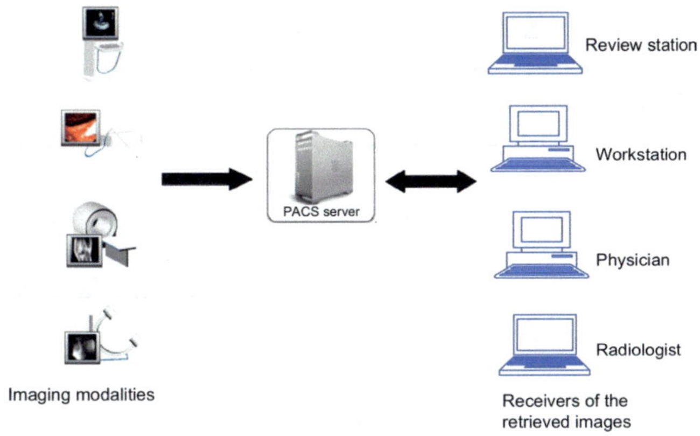

Figure 10.8. PACS and DICOM software and workstations.

Source: https://5.imimg.com/data5/SELLER/Default/2022/3/FO/ZY/EU/77307490/pacs-and-dicom-software-and-workstations.jpg.

Test Your Knowledge

1. What types of image acquisition devices are commonly used in digital medical imaging, and how do they function?
2. What storage solutions are typically employed to manage and archive digital medical images securely and efficiently?

10.3. Benefits of Digital Imaging

Learning Outcome

1. Discuss enhanced image quality and resolution.
2. Understand the improved accessibility and sharing of images.
3. Define the reduction in physical storage space.

Digital imaging has reshaped healthcare. In most cases, it is swept away those old, laborious methods, no more waiting around for film to develop. Hospitals now rely on systems like Picture Archiving and Communications Systems (PACS), which means patient images emerge much faster. Take the case of Reggio Emilia hospital, for example: when they rolled out PACS, their Radiology Department's productivity jumped by about 12%. And this isn't just a number; cutting radiology exam turnaround time by more than 60% means doctors can make diagnoses way sooner. Faster treatment and even shorter patient stays add to an overall boost in how care is delivered. Clearly, the practical benefits of digital imaging make it a key part of today's medical practices (Nitrosi et al., 2007). Image quality, for its part, is a huge deal in diagnosing patients. The rise of digital imaging demands that hospitals equip themselves with high-quality monitors and viewing stations that can handle complex images from various modalities. When the technology falls a bit short, it can hold back that quest for diagnostic excellence, a concern that bodies like IPEM and AAPM have pointed out. Essentially, PACS only works as well as the monitors it relies on, since those screens need to render exact visuals for solid clinical decisions. By sticking to the established criteria for imaging systems, health centers tend to secure a reliable digital process that boosts diagnostic results. So, investing in top-notch imaging tools isn't just about getting a prettier picture; it is about staying true to the goal of improving patient care (Tingberg et al., 2012). There's also a noticeable financial upside with digital imaging and PACS setups. For instance, Reggio Emilia Hospital reported an annual surplus of around $1.9 million after switching over. Often, detailed financial reviews show that reductions in material costs, like film and chemical processing, help drive this positive outcome. Plus, the overall smoother workflow and improved productivity free up resources in a way that makes sense. When hospitals try to balance quality care with tight budgets, digital imaging comes off as a smart, pragmatic move. All these layers of benefits, clinical and fiscal alike, point to digital imaging being more than a simple tech upgrade, it has become a strategic asset in managing healthcare (Nitrosi et al., 2007) (Figure 10.9).

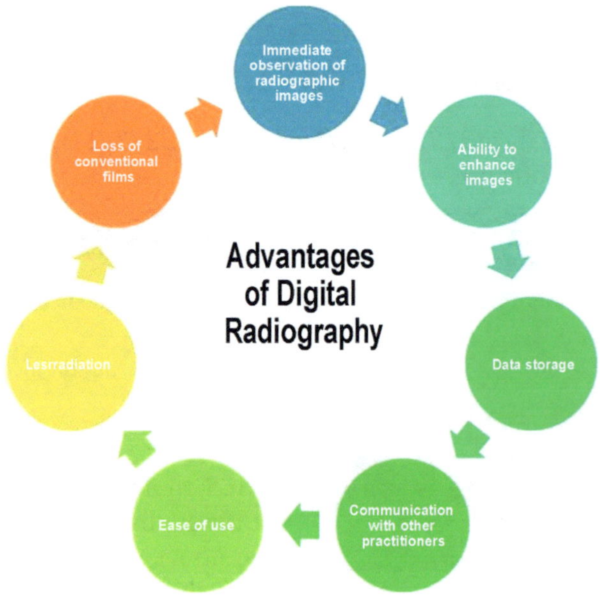

Figure 10.9. Advantage of digital radiography.

Source: https://blogger.googleusercontent.com/img/b/R29vZ2xl/AVvXsEjpkNBbN7q9wp5OvOUrnWkTGhc2I3UYM3BUqzWAaOF-F1FZw8eDEm_RxxwCGcU6ThN5ZTgAX24E3nEQLStTeKAQ1WF8XUT4t9lnI8xI3rrtcICyFhBfkTdEyRoK5T__gN4dFErc0H4d-2yU/s1600/advantage+DR.jpg.

10.3.1. Enhanced Image Quality and Resolution

Image processing is changing the face of digital imaging – especially in nuclear medicine with modalities like PET. Deep learning is now part of the mix, and it has been a game changer for improving diagnostic quality. Sometimes these methods rebuild images from scratch; other times they act more like clever fixes. In many cases, even when data is scarce, these techniques can deliver surprisingly high-quality outcomes. It is not just about making things look better; they help doctors get crucial clinical insights while cutting down on patients' exposure to radiation (Cameron et al., 2022). MRI, for instance, has stepped into a new era thanks to sharper post-processing tools. Nowadays, automated systems for image correction, noise reduction and even resolution tweaks are becoming a regular part of clinical routines. The improvements are not only about getting an excellent soft-tissue contrast but they also help in reading and interpreting the images with more clarity. Deep learning is gradually making its mark in this domain – fixing artefacts and boosting overall image quality. Generally speaking, recent studies indicate that AI is starting to cover gaps that traditional methods left behind, and in many cases, setting a fresh benchmark in clinical practice (Chen et al., 2022). Then there's the big picture: deep learning algorithms are proving their worth by handling massive, complex image datasets which means faster, more accurate analysis. These advancements are having a pretty profound impact on the way diagnoses are made, speeding things up and improving outcomes for patients. Still, we have to keep an eye on how well these AI-based methods work in different, real-world settings. Future advancements must walk the fine line between pushing image quality higher and ensuring that these improvements genuinely help in everyday clinical use, especially in systems like Picture Archiving and Communication Systems (PACS) (Cameron et al., 2022; Chen et al., 2022) (Figure 10.10).

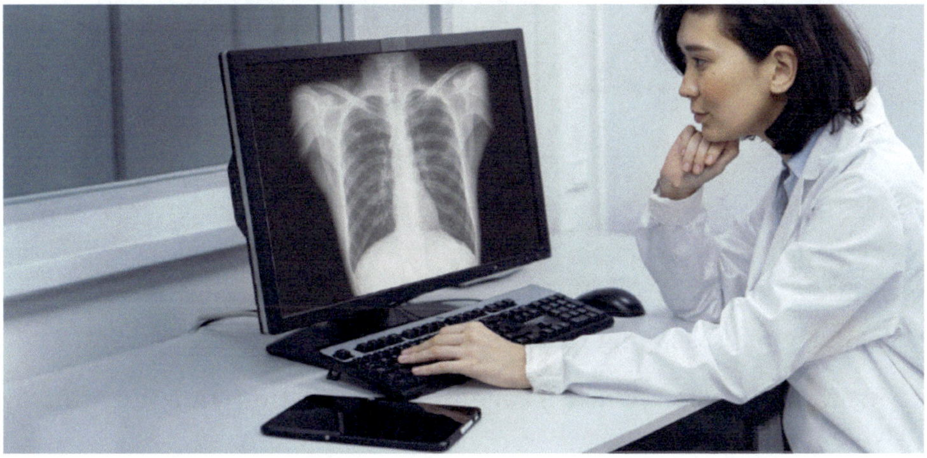

Figure 10.10. Image processing is changing the face of digital imaging.

Source: https://web.allengers.net/uploads/1/NewFolder/Banner%201200x800%20Digital%20 Radiography-01%20-%20Copy%20-%20Copy.jpg.

10.3.2. Improved Accessibility and Sharing of Images

Technology is reshaping modern healthcare in surprising ways. Digital imaging now makes images far easier to get to and share, a change that's boosted patient care. Take Picture Archiving and Communication Systems (PACS), for instance; these systems let healthcare workers quickly obtain, look at, and pass along imaging data. A study done in Hail City even showed that when images emerge fast, patient satisfaction climbs steeply, which generally means that easier image access directly lifts clinical outcomes. Quick access helps cut waiting times and, in most cases, sparks better conversations between radiologists and doctors, so they can decide on the best course of action faster. Overall, having strong imaging systems is key to both smoother operations and happier patients (Alhur et al., 2024). DICOM, or Digital Imaging and Communication in Medicine as it is often called, has also turned the tables on how images are shared across different platforms. In earlier days, DICOM files only worked with specialized viewers locked into specific institutions, limiting how much you could move them around. But now, with innovations like the Padimedical software platform, smartphones can be used to get remote access, and that's pretty revolutionary. Feedback from various practitioners hints that the app isn't just straightforward to use, it also makes sharing high-quality images almost seamless, which in turn refines diagnostic workflows. Accessing imaging files on a mobile makes it easier for healthcare providers to team up and share insights, leading to more prompt clinical decisions (Rahim et al., 2020). This kind of flexibility underscores just how important accessible technology is to today's health systems. Interoperable systems, ones that work smoothly together, are crucial in our increasingly interconnected healthcare world. Easier access and sharing of medical images often mean that responses to patient needs are quicker.

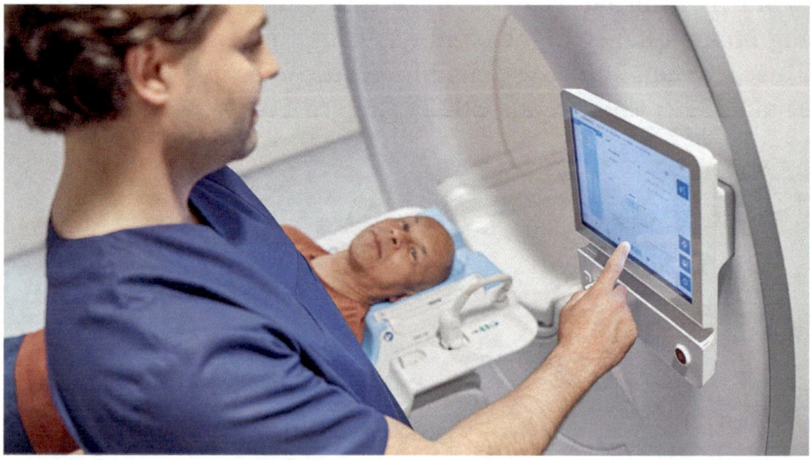

Figure 10.11. Technology is reshaping modern healthcare in surprising ways.

Source: https://www.philips.com/c-dam/corporate/innovation-and-you/global/sep-2022/2-operational-efficiency.jpg.

Observations in Hail City show that clinicians have taken to PACS with open arms, a sign that data-driven decision-making in medicine is identifying on, allowing for real-time assessments and consultations. One might even say that the clear link between effective imaging practices and clinician satisfaction points to higher levels of patient care as technology keeps evolving. As the healthcare scene shifts further, keeping imaging data both accessible and easy to share will always remain a top priority, ultimately paving the way for better health outcomes through smart, innovative digital imaging (Alhur et al., 2024) (Figure 10.11).

10.3.3. Reduction in Physical Storage Space

Digital imaging in medicine has turned things on their head, it is not just about crisper pictures. The old film methods have been mostly replaced by systems like PACS, which let hospitals store and pull up images digitally instead of crowding up space with films and bulky filing cabinets. Hospitals now find they can free up room for more useful resources, while gradually, this digital setup reshapes how images are organized and managed, sometimes leading to better patient care outcomes (Nor et al., 2010). It isn't only about saving space either. With digital tools at play, huge amounts of image data are squeezed down using smart compression methods. Take PACS, for example; it cuts down high-resolution files to smaller sizes, which not only speeds up the retrieval process but also lets institutions keep extensive archives without demanding more physical storage. In most cases, this tech shift even nudges hospitals to care a bit more for the environment by reducing their physical footprint (Ellis et al., 1994). Digital imaging also brings people together in unexpected ways. Centralized digital archives mean that doctors, nurses, and other staff can quickly obtain and share image data, no more sifting through piles of films that lead to repeated work. This ready exchange of information helps spur teamwork where specialists can weigh in on diagnoses and treatment plans. As more hospitals jump on board with these systems, the mix of shared know-how from different places tends to smooth out practices overall, trimming down physical hassles while boosting the quality of care (Nor et al., 2010).

Test Your Knowledge

1. How does digital imaging enhance image quality and resolution compared to traditional film methods?
2. In what ways has digital imaging improved the accessibility and sharing of medical images among healthcare providers?

10.4. Challenges in Digital Imaging and PACS

Learning Outcome

1. Understand the data security and privacy concerns.
2. Explore the integration with existing healthcare systems.
3. Analyze the cost of implementation and maintenance.

Digital imaging hasn't just slid into healthcare without a hitch, tools like Picture Archiving and Communication Systems (PACS) have proven to be a bit of an interesting card. Often, the rollout depends on a jumble of internal and external pressures that end up steering how these systems are used. Take a look at a study from Malaysian hospitals, where it turns out that governance, roles played by bodies such as the Ministry of Health, influences whether and how imaging tech is adopted. In many cases, everyday operations and larger institutional rules mix together in unpredictable ways, reshaping roles and care delivery. All this fuss suggests that a cookie-cutter approach just won't cut it; each facility seems to need its own tailored plan (Nor et al., 2010). Tech challenges add even more layers to the story. Web-based apps have become key players in clinics these days, carving out a fresh niche for telemedicine and eHealth. Innovations like MammoApplet emerge as inventive attempts to boost image viewing and let doctors annotate more easily. Yet, as these digital tools keep advancing, radiologists must keep up with learning, though many places struggle to offer enough continuous education. And then there's the ordeal of managing medical databases; ensuring clinical data remains both accessible and secure ends up spotlighting the messy side of mixing cutting-edge tech with everyday clinical work (Mata et al., 2012). Another snag comes from PACS not always playing nice with other systems. When various tech setups don't sync well, patient data ends up scattered, and smooth care processes take a hit. The real challenge is getting these systems to talk to each other reliably, a must for a seamless flow of information. Without clear, standard protocols, extra costs and delays creep in during any implementation phase. Addressing these communication gaps is crucial, not just for sharper diagnoses but also for keeping daily operations ready and agile. Without a cooperative effort to standardize and integrate tech, all those potential benefits of PACS might just remain out of reach (Nor et al., 2010) (Figure 10.12).

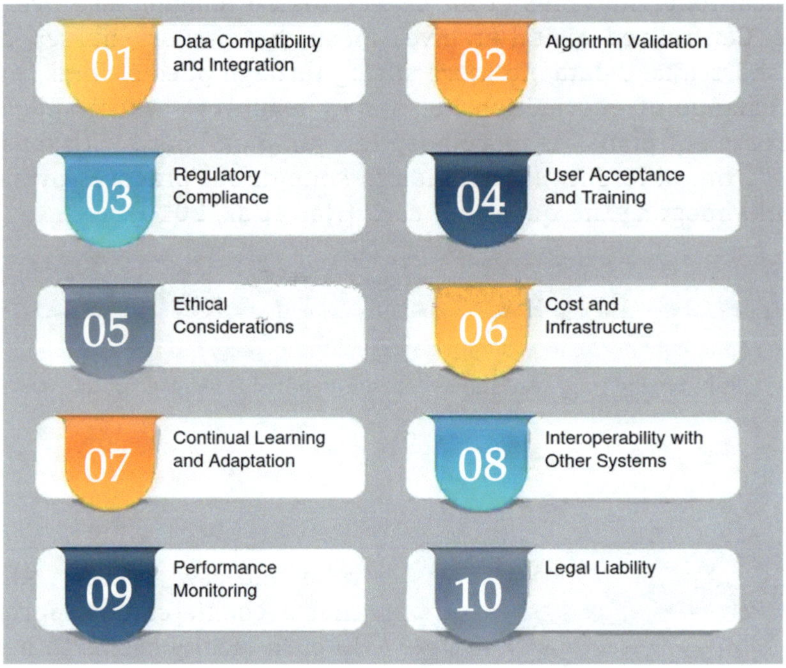
01
Data Compatibility and Integration
02
Algorithm Validation
03
Regulatory Compliance
04
User Acceptance and Training
05
Ethical Considerations
06
Cost and Infrastructure
07
Continual Learning and Adaptation
08
Interoperability with Other Systems
09
Performance Monitoring
10
Legal Liability

Figure 10.12. Challenges in integrating AI with PACS.

Source: https://www.fastercapital.com/content/AI-in-PACS--AI-Integration--The-Next-Frontier-for-PACS.html.

10.4.1. Data Security and Privacy Concerns

Digital imaging and systems like PACS are picking up fast in hospitals and clinics, but with all that convenience comes a heap of security headaches. Nowadays, healthcare organizations send sensitive patient details electronically, a move that can open the door to unwanted access and data breaches, breaches that not only knock privacy off balance but can also throw off the quality of care. Providers need to stick with basics like data encryption, strict access controls, and constant system checks if they're to dodge serious legal fallout and a loss of trust. Generally speaking, without these safeguards, the problems pile up quickly. The spread of Internet of Things devices in healthcare only makes things even more tangled. IoT health devices, or IoTHDs, capture real-time data and form a sprawling web of interconnected gadgets; while they help keep an eye on patients, they also create fresh opportunities for cyber-attacks, especially when their design skips over strong security measures. Recent studies (Affia et al., 2023) hint that grasping how these devices operate is key to gauging their risks and handling them right. In most cases, healthcare centers need to jump on these challenges early, tech is always moving, and so are how vulnerabilities appear. All this shows that keeping patient information safe isn't a one-step fix, it demands a layered, flexible approach. It means building a culture of cybersecurity awareness among staff, adopting advanced tech solutions, and staying hyper-alert to new threats even when things seem okay. Organizations must also keep an eye on changing data privacy rules so they stay compliant and build reliable data governance practices. As security breaches become more common, putting patient privacy front and center is the only way to keep community trust intact. Ultimately, merging digital imaging with vigilant data protection is a moving target that calls for ongoing tweaks and improvements (Nagy et al., 2007).

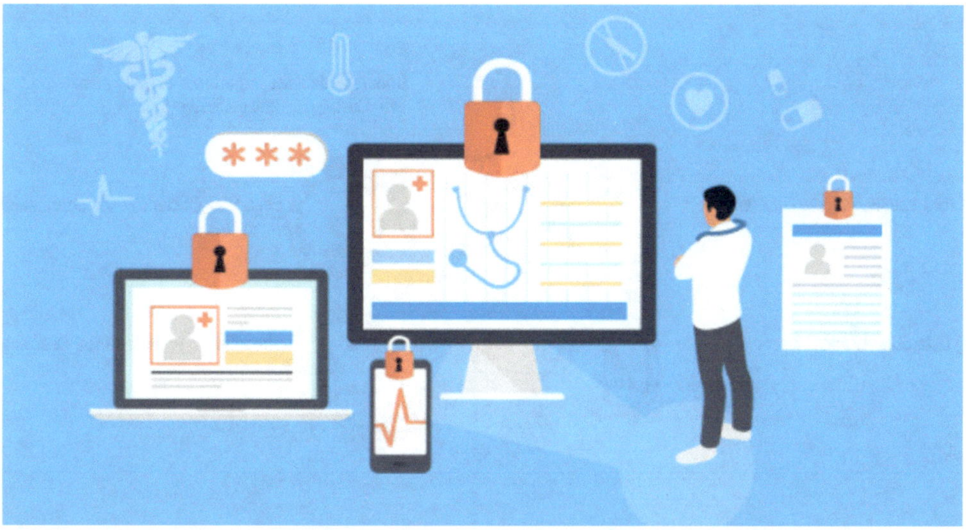

Source: https://media.licdn.com/dms/image/v2/D5612AQHhq2p-UEP2Kw/article-cover_image-shrink_600_2000/article-cover_image-shrink_600_2000/0/1690101133598?e=2147483647&v=beta&t=fO9V271EkyZe825OrEC9egk_fUW3IwjywI4Jbc0xpVI.

10.4.2. Integration with Existing Healthcare Systems

Digital imaging tech wired into healthcare systems makes a big difference for patient care and how smoothly a hospital runs. In many hospitals, picking up Picture Archiving and Communication Systems (PACS) gets shaped by what's happening inside and outside the hospital. Sometimes a tactic one facility digs can ripple over and nudge another's strategy, reminding us that healthcare places have a knack for staying interconnected. It isn't just about plugging in new gadgets, it also shifts how clinical and non-clinical individuals work with each other. One in-depth study even pointed out that rules from organizations like the Ministry of Health play a huge role in steering how digital imaging gets used on the ground (Nor et al., 2010). What drives this integration is the ability of different imaging equipment, from many manufacturers, to talk to one another. The Digital Imaging and Communications in Medicine (DICOM) protocol is generally the go-to standard for making sure these different systems keep in touch. Still, trying to get everything in line with DICOM isn't always a smooth ride; unexpected non-conformities can emerge and lead to data mix-ups. Sometimes, even the way medical staff feed in data only adds fuel to these issues, creating a chain reaction of operational challenges that hurt how well the imaging systems perform. In most cases, using software that double-checks data quality and DICOM compliance becomes a must, because it not only smooths the integration process but also builds a more solid healthcare delivery model (Silva et al., 2018). The impact of blending these technologies stretches way beyond better operations, it also shakes up how healthcare teams gel. Advanced imaging systems have shifted the roles of radiographers and other clinical staff, sparking new, sometimes unexpected ways for professionals to team up. While the bond between radiographers and radiologists tends to hold steady, the rapport between non-clinical personnel and clinicians now feels more intertwined and cooperative. This mix of tech and teamwork isn't just retooling routines; it is changing the very culture inside hospitals. As hospitals adjust to these shifts, it seems clear that grasping how technology and people mesh together will be key in tapping the full potential of digital imaging advances, ultimately helping patient outcomes come out even better (Nor et al., 2010) (Figure 10.13).

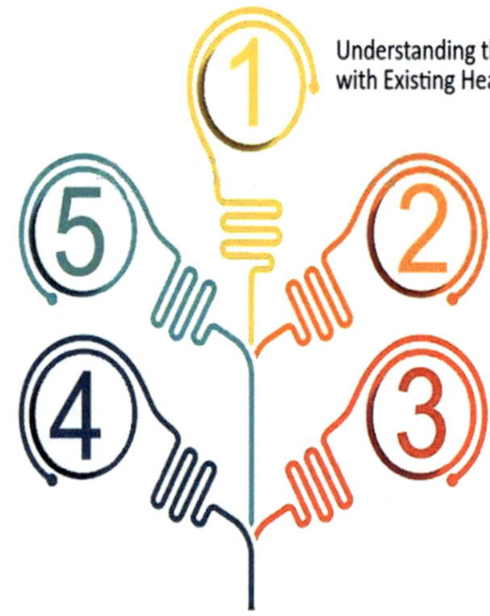
1
Understanding the Importance of Integration with Existing Healthcare Systems
2
Enhancing Efficiency and Coordination
3
Streamlining Workflows and Reducing Errors
4
Ensuring Data Security and Privacy
5
Collaborating with Healthcare IT Experts

Figure 10.13. Integration with existing healthcare systems.

Source: https://fastercapital.com/keyword/existing-healthcare-systems.html.

10.4.3. Cost of Implementation and Maintenance

Shifting to digital imaging with Picture Archiving and Communication Systems brings on a hefty mix of upfront costs and ongoing expenses. It is not just about shelling out for the latest hardware; you're also tied to software licenses and building out the network needed to keep things running. This can hit healthcare facilities pretty hard, especially those in areas where resources are tight. If you look at initiatives pushing for more accessible digital images, you quickly see that the costs, particularly in fields like pediatric radiology where special gear and skills are a must, are nothing to sneeze at. It all might seem like a mountain to climb, but boosting diagnostic speed and patient care means that putting money into both planning and support is essential (Andronikou et al., 2011). Once the system is up and running, it turns out that cost issues don't just stop at installation. Generally speaking, the expenses keep piling up with software updates, technical support, and needed system upgrades that can sneak up on you fast. Staff training also jumps into the mix because getting everyone up to speed on these advanced tools isn't trivial. Malaysian hospitals hinted at how the inner workings of a facility and the pressures from outside shape not just the price tag but also how effective a PACS ends up making an organization overall (Nor et al., 2010). It is a messy, intertwined situation that makes staying on top of things a challenge. Beyond those immediate bills, the long haul of keeping digital imaging systems in shape can reshape how an institution works. As these technologies get woven into everyday routines, even the way medical staff team up can shift noticeably. For example, while radiologists and radiographers might continue working side by side, digital systems can change how decisions or info gets passed around. It goes to show that investing in these systems isn't merely about technology, it is about nurturing new relationships and workflow styles that help the whole setup truly pay off (Nor et al., 2010).

Test Your Knowledge

1. What are some common technical or operational challenges faced when implementing PACS in healthcare facilities?
2. How can issues such as data security and system interoperability impact the effectiveness of digital imaging systems?

10.5. Future Trends in Digital Imaging

Learning Outcome

1. Understand the advancements in imaging technologies.
2. Describe the role of artificial intelligence in image analysis.
3. Explore the potential for telemedicine and remote diagnostics.

Rapid tech shifts are opening new doors in digital imaging, taking PACS in directions you wouldn't have guessed. Schools and various platforms are obtaining onto standards like LTI these days, which means systems designed for images are now expected to work together more naturally. This isn't just about a better user vibe; it even makes sharing vital medical images across fields a lot easier. Then, you've got the buzz around cloud-native setups and blockchain, which seem set to bolster security, data privacy, and how well different systems mesh together. Overall, these moves are key for building a solid, future-ready backbone that still deals with today's hiccups in imaging storage and workflows (Upadhyay, 2025). Machine learning, particularly deep learning, is shaking up how digital imaging aids diagnosis. Tools powered by these advances often find themselves boosting the way images are read, a shift that generally improves accuracy in PACS setups. Many studies even hint at how such tech can simplify processes, cut down on errors, and deliver personalized imaging insights. Some literature, for instance, lays out the ups and downs of diving into these innovations, showing that deep learning can twist itself into various imaging styles. In many cases, as these approaches evolve, the focus may shift toward squeezing out faster and more precise image processing that tackles both current challenges and next-generation demands (Alduhailan et al., 2025).

Looking ahead, blending augmented and virtual reality with digital imaging might just upend how professionals interact with image data. These immersive tools are believed to offer a fresh way to see and understand images, increasing spatial awareness and context in pretty unexpected ways. Toss AI into the mix and you get a naturally flowing, almost intuitive way to handle the heavy-duty data in PACS. Recent chatter in the field underscores efforts to craft more fluid and adaptable ways of delivering training to medical staff, efforts that could not only ease the learning curve but also help lock in crucial imaging skills. Overall, this mix of tech could boost patient care and fine-tune overall efficiency in healthcare settings (Upadhyay, 2025).

10.5.1. Advancements in Imaging Technologies

Advanced imaging tech has shaken up how medical education works, especially in radiology. Gone are the days when classes leaned on static pictures that sometimes left students scratching their heads over tricky anatomical details. Nowadays, cloud-based Picture Archiving and Communication Systems, take PACSBIN, for example, are giving teachers new ways to show things off. One study, generally speaking, found that first-year med students scored about the same whether they looked at scrollable DICOM images or stuck with old-school static CT images, hinting that mixing up methods might just work better for different learning styles (Bitar et al., 2025). New tech isn't just changing our ideas about learning; it's also sparking fresh imaging methods that fit various science fields. I'd say digital holography stands out, it is identifying on because it can obtain real-time, three-dimensional details without the messy, destructive side effects we saw before. Compared to the old methods like traditional microscopy or X-ray diffraction plans, digital holography speeds imaging up and smooths out data processing, making it a real gem for crystallography and material science. This breakthrough shows how stepping up imaging techniques can peel back layers of complexity and offer big perks for things like mineral imaging and microstructure analysis (Kang et al., 2025). The imaging scene still keeps evolving, and how these new advances mix with practical uses will most likely rewrite the future for both classrooms and research labs. Blending digital imaging with clever algorithms, deep learning for instance, opens up exciting doors for better data crunching and visualization. This kind of teamwork not only boosts image reconstruction but also helps smooth over issues like bulky dataset processing and limited field of view. As people continue tinkering with these tools, we're looking at a future where educational aids and research methods are more rounded and effective, holding promise for a wide variety of academic and clinical pursuits (Kang et al., 2025).

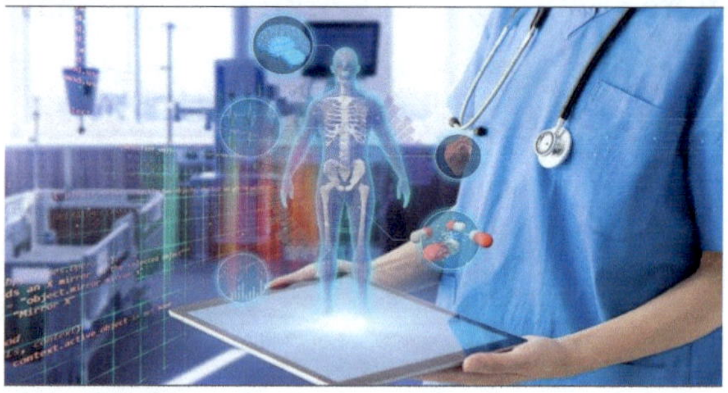

Source: https://catalinaimaging.com/wp-content/uploads/2023/02/AI-data-image.jpeg.

10.5.2. Role of Artificial Intelligence (AI) in Image Analysis

Advanced algorithms are now playing a major role in how doctors look at images, totally reshaping diagnosis while speeding things up in surprising ways. For example, fields like digital pathology now see AI cutting down on screening time and even lifting the overall quality of diagnoses. These tools pick up on tiny details hidden deep within images, helping with tasks like splitting image sections and sorting data with a kind of pinpoint accuracy. That said, all these benefits pretty much hinge on having loads of properly labeled data, which isn't easy to come by since annotating requires both skilled individuals and data experts. Lately, new setups have cropped up, mixing in AutoML with web-based PACS, to make these smart image tools accessible even to medical pros who aren't tech whizzes (Jesus et al., 2024). AI-driven image analysis isn't just shaking up hospitals; it is also lending a hand in diagnosing health issues that often get overlooked, like certain tropical diseases. Take urogenital schistosomiasis as an example, this condition, affecting communities worldwide, now sees its diagnostic process revamped by automated methods. Instead of sticking with the old-school ritual of peering through a microscope to spot Schistosoma haematobium eggs in urine, AI offers a pretty compelling alternative. Researchers have put deep learning models, like YOLOv5 and even YOLOv8, to work so they can automatically flag and locate these eggs in digital images. Even though it means someone still has to do manual labeling of urine samples (a task handled by lab experts), the result is a huge boost in speed and accuracy. Generally speaking, the impressive precision and recall rates these models achieve hint that AI tools might outshine conventional methods (Maturana et al., 2024). Looking at the bigger picture, AI's role in image analysis shows a messy yet undeniably promising potential to change many areas of healthcare. Deploying these advanced algorithms not only sharpens diagnostic capabilities but also eases the load on overworked healthcare teams. The systems we've mentioned don't just streamline detection and sorting; they also open doors for practitioners in resource-limited settings to tap into high-end diagnostic tools. Switching from traditional microscopy to these AI-fueled approaches marks a major shift in medical imaging, a true paradigm change, really. This ongoing tech evolution carries the promise of better health outcomes, ushering in an era where diagnosis is both faster and more precise. In most cases, continuous research and gradual fine-tuning of these systems remain key to a broader rollout in clinical settings and, ultimately, to improving patient care (Jesus et al., 2024; Maturana et al., 2024) (Figure 10.14).

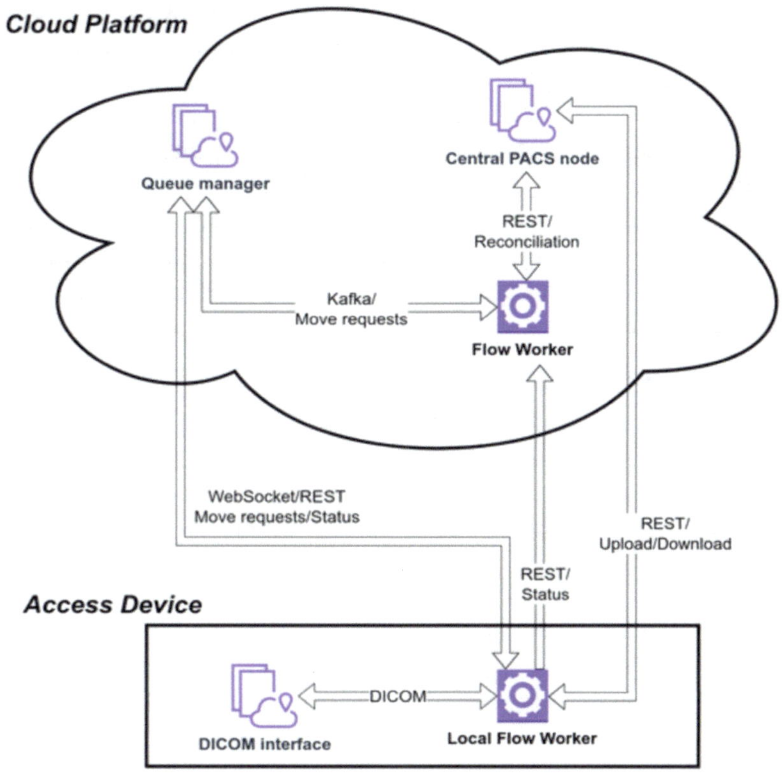

Figure 10.14. Features of the PACS platform.

Source: Kawa J, Pyciński B, Smoliński M, Bożek P, Kwasecki M, Pietrzyk B, Szymański D. Design and Implementation of a Cloud PACS Architecture. *Sensors*. 2022; 22(21):8569. https://doi.org/10.3390/s22218569.

10.5.3. Potential for Telemedicine and Remote Diagnostics

Telemedicine and remote diagnostics are sparking a big change in healthcare, especially when you look at digital imaging and the systems known as PACS. Providers now get real-time access to patient images and data which lets them act quickly, no matter where they are. Cheap computing gear and open-source software (Suhanic et al., 2009) have led to low-cost telemicroscopy solutions that boost diagnostic potential even in places with fewer resources. These tools also encourage teamwork among professionals who, despite being miles apart, can view and discuss vital data together. This type of collaboration tends to sharpen diagnosis accuracy and, generally speaking, creates a vast network of shared experience that enriches clinical practice across many settings. Recent leaps in Health Information Technology have reshaped how diagnoses are handled, and telemedicine plays a crucial role here. As noted in Tuyet et al. (2018), rolling out Laboratory Information Systems in major hospitals has shaken up administrative management and improved both diagnosis and treatment accuracy markedly. New telemedicine gadgets – like mobile health apps and remote monitoring tools – ensure that patient imaging data stays within reach. This smooth integration means that doctors can make decisions faster, which often results in quicker diagnoses and treatment plans tailored to individual needs. In most cases, blending digital imaging with telemedicine not only eases clinical routines but also nudges us toward a more inclusive and equitable healthcare system that steps beyond old boundaries. Remote diagnostics isn't just about immediate medical benefits; it hints at a bigger shift in public health management as well. By collecting and sifting through more diagnostic data on a wide scale, telemedicine could change how we track disease outbreaks and handle health crises. With technology boosting remote communication and easing data sharing, healthcare setups can often ramp up their response and manage resources better when emergencies hit. According to Suhanic et al. (2009), open telemicroscopy workstations support a kind of distributed diagnosis and reporting that shows how working together from afar can offer fast solutions when challenges arise. In short, when digital imaging, telemedicine, and remote diagnostics merge, they set the stage not only for better individual care but also for a more prepared healthcare system ready to take on future public health challenges.

Test Your Knowledge

1. What are some emerging technologies that are expected to revolutionize digital imaging in healthcare in the coming years?
2. How might artificial intelligence (AI) and machine learning influence the future of digital imaging and diagnostics?

Summary

Digital imaging and PACS have shifted how medical diagnostics get done and how care is delivered. We're no longer tied to clunky film, digital methods boost image quality, open up easier access, and streamline processes. Radiologists and clinicians, for example, often mention that these systems just feel more reliable and are simpler to use. Reports come in faster and waiting times shrink, which clearly helps patient care (Alhur et al., 2024). It seems that as healthcare settings lean more into these digital systems, continually tweaking the tech and user experience stays a top priority. The move to digital X-ray imaging has stirred up a new way of thinking about diagnostics, often leveraging innovations such as CT scans to sharpen accuracy. In most cases, there's also an economic angle worth noting; these tools help hospitals cut costs and use resources smarter. And then there's photon-counting CT, a sign that the field is evolving, hinting that more in-depth research might reveal even better ways to improve imaging. At the same time, institutions should take a careful look at how these new processes affect every day work and inter-professional chat (Rayyani et al., 2024). To wrap things up, bringing digital imaging and PACS into the fold isn't just keeping pace with technology, it is a real upgrade for healthcare. Generally speaking, when clinicians get a better feel for the system, patients tend to do better, underscoring the importance of solid implementation. As the medical world changes alongside tech advancements, stakeholders must work hard to boost user acceptance and keep training up-to-date. Future studies should also factor in patient opinions to offer a full picture of digital imaging's effects. Ultimately, this ongoing journey with imaging tech will continue to mold the future of medical practice (Alhur et al., 2024).

Digital imaging and PACS have shaken up modern medicine in ways that are hard to ignore. Switching from old-school film to digital formats means images now get stored, pulled up, and managed without the usual hassle – speeding up the whole diagnostic scene. The new system not only smooths out every day work by making key data instantly available for doctors to act on, but it also makes communication among clinicians feel more natural and quick. You can see how, as noted in Dhami et al. (2008), these shifts have turned patient care on its head, underscoring just how vital digital imaging has become in today's healthcare field. At its core, PACS isn't merely a piece of high-tech equipment; it is more like a catalyst for learning across an organization. Think of it as a tool that invites intuition, interpretation, integration, and yes, even institutionalization, into everyday clinical practice (Sinozic et al., 2014). In most cases, when healthcare pros start using PACS, they end up blending old routines with new skills and artifacts that slowly but surely change how knowledge is gathered at every level of the organization. This messy, ongoing process shows why continuous learning and regular professional training become absolutely crucial, especially as imaging technologies throw more complexity into the mix. Digital imaging also nudges institutions to learn in unexpected ways, handling the unpredictable side of medical innovation. In hospitals, radiologists, technicians, and even administrators end up haggling over how best to use PACS, sometimes in ways that seem spontaneous and even a bit quirky, which then shapes how the system functions day to day. These local, almost organic adaptations end up having surprising effects on the overall learning and effectiveness of the organization (Sinozic et al., 2014). Overall, merging digital imaging with PACS does far more than simply upgrade diagnostic capabilities; it helps build a workplace culture that's constantly adapting and learning, no matter how interesting the tech landscape might get.

KEY TERMS FROM THIS CHAPTER

Clinical ultrasound (CUS)
Data security
Diagnostic imaging
Image compression
Medical technology
Stomatology
Workstation
Communication systems
Deep learning
Digital databases
Medical databases
Modalities
Telemedicine

Critical Thinking Questions

1. **What does PACS stand for in medical imaging?**
   a. Patient Archiving and Communication System
   b. Picture Archiving and Communication System
   c. Patient Assessment and Care Software
   d. Picture Analysis and Coding System
2. **What is the primary purpose of PACS in a healthcare facility?**
   a. To perform surgeries remotely
   b. To enhance the contrast of radiographic images
   c. To store, retrieve, and share digital medical images
   d. To calculate radiation doses
3. **Which of the following is a major benefit of digital imaging over traditional film-based imaging?**
   a. Longer processing time
   b. Lower image quality
   c. Faster image acquisition and easy sharing
   d. Greater storage space required
4. **What is DICOM in relation to digital imaging?**
   a. A PACS manufacturer
   b. A medical imaging test
   c. A standard protocol for handling and transmitting medical images
   d. A type of radiation
5. **How does PACS contribute to patient care?**
   a. By increasing using physical storage
   b. By reducing accessibility to images
   c. By providing quick access to previous imaging studies for comparison
   d. By eliminating the need for radiologists

Short Answer Questions

1. What were some key milestones in the development of digital imaging in medical diagnostics?
2. What are the main components of a Picture Archiving and Communication System (PACS)?
3. How does digital imaging improve workflow, storage, and image accessibility in healthcare settings?
4. What are some challenges healthcare facilities face when implementing digital imaging and PACS?
5. What emerging trends and technologies are expected to shape the future of digital medical imaging?

Answers to Critical Thinking Questions

1. (b); 2. (c); 3. (c); 4. (c); 5. (c)

References

1. Abdul Rahim, E., Abdullah, R., Ahmad Sabri, M. I., Ann Git, et al. (2020). *Padi Medical: Medical Image Sharing Portal with DICOM Viewer–User Experience*. https://core.ac.uk/download/352893369.pdf (accessed on 23 May 2025).
2. Affia, A. O., Finch, H., Jung, W., Samori, I. A., Potter, L., & Palmer, X. L. (2023). IoT health devices: Exploring security risks in the connected landscape. *IoT, 4*(2), 150–182. https://doi.org/10.3390/iot4020009.
3. Alduhailan, A., Kamarudin, N., Sheikh Abdullah, S. N. H., & Dau, A. (2025). Deep learning in biometric authentication: Challenges, recent advancements, and future trends. *Journal of Advances in Information Technology*. https://www.semanticscholar.org/paper/8d0c7c3e4ca99274b969803cb64a2daa1f48e420 (accessed on 23 May 2025).
4. Alhur, A. (2024). Clinician acceptance and adoption of PACS in radiology services: An exploratory study. *Indonesian Journal of Information Systems, 7*(1), 1–12. https://doi.org/10.24002/ijis.v7i1.7614.
5. Andronikou, S., McHugh, K., Abdurahman, N., Khoury, B., Mngomezulu, V., Brant, W. E., Cowan, I., McCulloch, M., & Ford, N. (2011). Pediatric radiology seen from Africa. Part I: Providing diagnostic imaging to a young population. *Pediatric Radiology, 41*(7), 811–825. https://doi.org/10.1007/s00247-011-2081-8.
6. Babić, R. R., Milošević, Z., Đinđić, B., & Stanković-Babić, G. (2019). Radiology information system. In *Compendium of Biomedical Instrumentation*. https://www.semanticscholar.org/paper/264770740fa703b23d5c68fdf84f9ac0e9ab7e9d (accessed on 23 May 2025).
7. Bitar, I., Ghannam, J., Nandalur, K. R., & Al-Katib, S. (2025). Comparative analysis of scrollable DICOM images and static CT images in teaching thoracic imaging anatomy to first-year medical students. *Anatomical Sciences Education*. https://www.semanticscholar.org/paper/b20153049c88858acadde9f49f7837a00c220330 (accessed on 23 May 2025).
8. Chen, Z., Pawar, K., Ekanayake, M., Pain, C., Zhong, S., & Egan, G. F. (2023). Deep learning for image enhancement and correction in magnetic resonance imaging: State-of-the-art and challenges. *Journal of Digital Imaging, 36*(1), 204–230. https://doi.org/10.1007/s10278-022-00721-9.
9. Clarke, L. P. (1993). Digital mammography, cancer screening: Factors important for image compression. In *The 1993 Space and Earth Science Data Compression Workshop*. NASA Goddard Space Flight Center. https://core.ac.uk/download/pdf/42807614.pdf (accessed on 23 May 2025).
10. Dhami, S. (2008). *Strategic Analysis of The Commercialization Potential of a Novel Algorithm*. https://core.ac.uk/download/638896345.pdf (accessed on 23 May 2025).
11. Ellingsen, G., Linstad, L. H., Severinsen, G. H., et al. (2023). *Procurement of Artificial Intelligence for Radiology Practice*. https://core.ac.uk/download/586369760.pdf (accessed on 23 May 2025).
12. Ellis, R. C. (1994). *Global Picture Archiving and Communication Systems (GPACS): An Overview*. https://core.ac.uk/download/617869767.pdf (accessed on 23 May 2025).

13. Guzman, D. N. (2002). *Curriculum Guide to Teach Computed Radiography At El Camino College.* https://core.ac.uk/download/153384852.pdf (accessed on 23 May 2025).

14. Hristova, T. (2020). *Data Infrastructures and Digital Labor: The Case of Teleradiology.* https://core.ac.uk/download/426937685.pdf (accessed on 23 May 2025).

15. Jesus, R., Rodrigues, A., Silva, L. B., & Costa, C. (2024). Streamlining the generation of AI tools on a cloud medical imaging platform. In *2024 IEEE 22nd Mediterranean Electrotechnical Conference (MELECON).* https://www.semanticscholar.org/paper/c6081947880e7803081dcfd33d94c587904c6bb9 (accessed on 23 May 2025).

16. Jomier, J., Bailly, A., Le Gall, M., & Avila, R. (2010). An open-source digital archiving system for medical and scientific research. *Kitware Inc.*, Clifton Park, NY, USA.

17. Kang, W., Zheng, Z., & Huang, H. (2025). Advancements in digital holography for crystalline material characterization: A review (Invited). *Crystal Research and Technology, 60*, 2400264. https://doi.org/10.1002/crat.202400264.

18. Kannan, S. (2007). Technology based health care: An Indian perspective–Opportunities and challenges. *MPRA Paper 13770*, University Library of Munich, Germany.

19. Mata, C., Oliver, A., Torrent, A., & Martí, J. (2012). MammoApplet: An interactive Java applet tool for manual annotation in medical imaging. In *2012 IEEE 12th International Conference on Bioinformatics & Bioengineering (BIBE)* (pp. 34–39). https://doi.org/10.1109/BIBE.2012.6399703.

20. Mohd Nor, R. (2010). *The Organizational Implications of Medical Imaging in The Context of Malaysian Hospitals.* https://core.ac.uk/download/1588563.pdf (accessed on 23 May 2025).

21. Nagy, P. (2007). *Open Source in Imaging Informatics.* https://core.ac.uk/download/pdf/7750510.pdf.

22. Nitrosi, A., Borasi, G., Nicoli, F., Modigliani, G., Botti, A., Bertolini, M., & Notari, P. (2007). A filmless radiology department in a full digital regional hospital: Quantitative evaluation of the increased quality and efficiency. *Journal of Digital Imaging, 20*(2), 140–148. https://doi.org/10.1007/s10278-007-9006-y.

23. Noor, A. S. M., & Saman, M. Y. M. (2009). *Distributed Object Medical Imaging Model.* https://core.ac.uk/download/pdf/87303.pdf.

24. Pain, C. D., Egan, G. F., & Chen, Z. (2022). Deep learning-based image reconstruction and post-processing methods in positron emission tomography for low-dose imaging and resolution enhancement. *European Journal of Nuclear Medicine and Molecular Imaging, 49*, 3098–3118. https://www.semanticscholar.org/paper/30452c455ec6c1b1fbf6ce2ca0d5aa32fd0668a7 (accessed on 23 May 2025).

25. Rayyani, A. A., Shalalni, A. A., Radwan, A. H., Shibli, K. A., Jabin, J. Y., Mokli, M. A. Y., Mabuj, J. M., et al. (2024). Digital X-ray imaging: Emphasis can be placed on developments in digital X-ray technologies and their applications in diagnosis and treatment. *Journal of Positive Psychology and Wellbeing, 6*(4). https://core.ac.uk/download/616775625.pdf (accessed on 23 May 2025).

26. Rubio Maturana, C., Dantas de Oliveira, A., Zarzuela, F., Ruiz, E., Sulleiro, E., Mediavilla, A., Martínez-Vallejo, P., et al. (2024). Development of an automated artificial intelligence-based system for urogenital schistosomiasis diagnosis using digital image analysis techniques and

a robotized microscope. *PLOS Neglected Tropical Diseases, 18*. https://www.semanticscholar.org/paper/8ce0968db78d7deb0fc6a46d3854e0cf291c5ca4 (accessed on 23 May 2025).

27. Scialdone, G. (2002). *Information Technologies for The Healthcare Delivery System*. https://core.ac.uk/download/232138530.pdf.

28. Silva, J. M., Godinho, T. M., Silva, D., & Costa, C. (2018). A community-driven validation service for standard medical imaging objects. *arXiv*. https://doi.org/10.48550/arXiv.1806.08987.

29. Sinozic, T. (2014). *Learning in Clinical Practice: Findings from CT, MRI and PACS*. https://core.ac.uk/download/30608478.pdf.

30. Strony, R., Marin, J. R., Bailitz, J., Dean, A. J., Blaivas, M., Tayal, V., Raio, C., Liu, R., Woods, A., Zwank, M., Fields, M., Abo, A., Wu, S., Kang, T., Liu, T., Leo, M., Smalley, C., Chiricolo, J., Chilstrom, M., & Lewiss, R. E. (2018). Systemwide clinical ultrasound program development: An expert consensus model. *Western Journal of Emergency Medicine, 19*(4), 649–653. https://doi.org/10.5811/westjem.2018.4.37152.

31. Suhanic, W., Crandall, I., & Pennefather, P. (2009). An informatics model for guiding assembly of tele microbiology workstations for malaria collaborative diagnostics using commodity products and open-source software. *Malaria Journal, 8*, 164. https://doi.org/10.1186/1475-2875-8-164.

32. Tingberg, A. (2013). Suspension criteria for image monitors and viewing boxes. *Radiation Protection Dosimetry, 153*(2), 230–235. https://doi.org/10.1093/rpd/ncs302.

33. Upadhyay, S. (2025). Learning tools interoperability: AI-driven integration, security innovations, and future trends in digital education. *International Journal of Science and Advanced Technology, 16*(1). https://doi.org/10.71097/IJSAT.v16.i1.2276.

34. Wu, Z., & Zhang, M. (2022). Application evaluation of picture archiving and communication systems in Chinese stemmatological hospitals. In *Volume 12179*, 121790B–121790B-7. https://www.semanticscholar.org/paper/68a8b45b3fb60cb841392c9e4c997f3937afd446 (accessed on 23 May 2025).

DENTAL AND MAXILLOFACIAL IMAGING

11

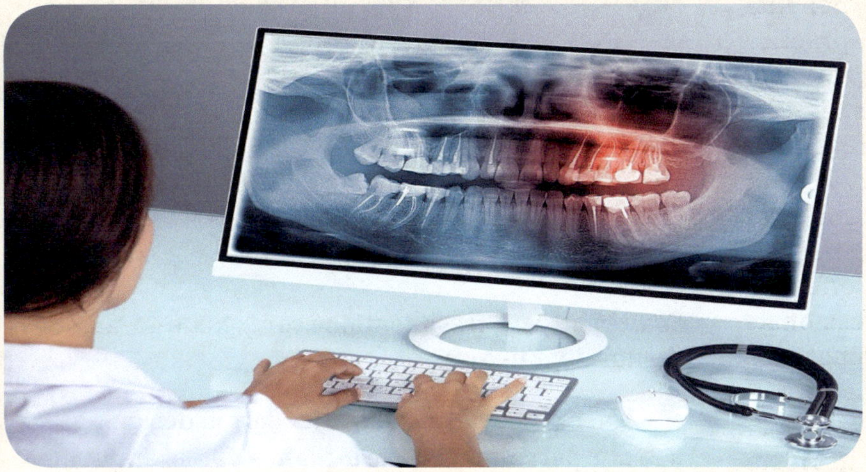

LEARNING OBJECTIVES

After studying this chapter, you will be able to:

1. Identify and describe the various types of dental imaging techniques.
2. Understand the applications of dental imaging in diagnosing.
3. Explore maxillofacial imaging techniques.
4. Examine safety protocols and radiation concerns related to dental and maxillofacial imaging.
5. Investigate future trends and innovations in dental and maxillofacial imaging.

Introduction

Imaging tech has shaken things up in dentistry. Dentists now have fresh tools that help them see details impossible to catch with old flat X-rays. Traditional 2D radiography, for instance, just couldn't capture the twist and turns of complex head and jaw structures, leaving many to puzzle over the images. Enter cone-beam computed tomography (CBCT), a true game-changer that pops up unexpectedly to reveal detailed, volumetric views of the craniofacial area. With CBCT, dental pros get a much clearer picture of how various structures sit together, which generally helps overcome the problems inherent in 2D methods. This move toward 3D imaging marks a turning point in how practitioners understand their patients' conditions, blending modern tech with everyday practice in a way that feels both intuitive and transformative. In orthodontics, switching over to 3D imaging isn't just a neat upgrade, it is quickly becoming standard practice. Instead of relying on static, flat images that can hide important depth cues and positional details, dentists now lean on CBCT to map out complex dental and jaw configurations with an almost uncanny precision. The ability to spin and slice images along multiple planes, mixed in with advances in ultralow-dose radiation, means scans are not only effective but also safe and affordable. In most cases, this extra clarity leads to better treatment planning and smoother follow-ups on orthodontic work. It is a trend that speaks volumes about a broader move toward high-tech imaging solutions, even if the path there is a bit less straightforward than before. The benefits of weaving CBCT into everyday dental practice stretch far beyond making diagnoses. Traditional planar methods often came with issues like magnification errors or even misrepresenting what was going on (Ghali et al., 2017). With 3D imaging, dentists can see the true shape of the maxilla, mandible, and surrounding tissues, a critical detail when figuring out an effective treatment plan. CBCT empowers professionals to tackle complex cases with a fresh, sometimes nuanced perspective, thereby raising the overall standard of care. By tapping into the power of detailed 3D views, dental teams can navigate the nooks and crannies of facial anatomy more confidently, leading to better communication with patients and colleagues alike (Marothiya et al., 2019).

Definition and Scope of Dental Imaging

Various imaging methods mix together to show just how critical dental imaging has become today. Regular radiographs, computed tomography (CT), and even magnetic resonance imaging (MRI) each offer their own slice of insight; in many cases radiography remains the go-to for spotting bone details and decay that are essential for planning treatment. Lately, newer tech – like 3D imaging and cone-beam computed tomography (CBCT) – has shaken up the field, giving extra clarity and precision that matter in tricky implant or orthodontic cases. Overall, this growing mix of imaging tools helps dentists pull together a wide range of useful info for both dental and maxillofacial care. Taking a more holistic look at patient care, dental imaging isn't just about getting a quick peek inside a tooth. It helps check conditions, shape treatment plans, and even monitor progress after procedures.

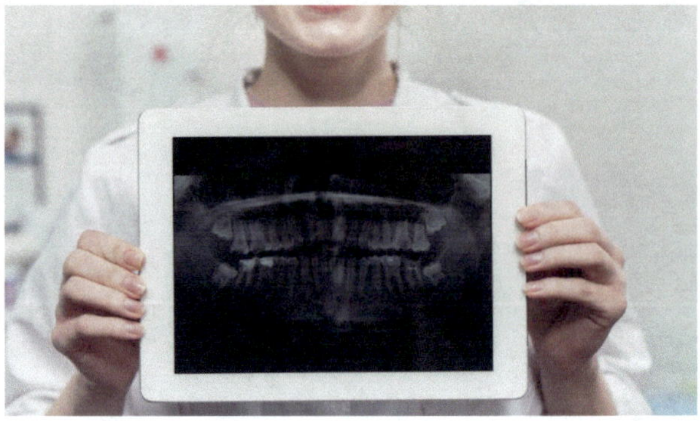

Figure 11.1. Dental X-Rays.

Source: https://freshdentalnc.com/guide-to-the-digital-dental-x-ray/.

Every type of scan plays its part in designing a truly personalized care plan – for example, 3D images can nail implant placements, while MRI sometimes picks up soft tissue issues that standard radiography might miss. Plus, fresh innovations like virtual reality (VR) and augmented reality (AR) have started to appear in training programs, offering immersive experiences that boost the skills of maxillofacial surgery residents. In many ways, blending these various techniques not only sharpens diagnostic accuracy and treatment outcomes but also enriches the learning journey for new practitioners (Abel et al., 2020). Ongoing research and tech breakthroughs keep reshaping what dental imaging means. The COVID-19 pandemic, for instance, kind of showed us that imaging services can be surprisingly nimble, adapting quickly to keep both surgical and diagnostic care rolling along (Kjetil Søreide et al., 2020). Tele-imaging has also popped up as a handy tool for remote consultations and assessments, making care accessible even when patients are far away. This mix of dental imaging with broader public health issues highlights just how flexible healthcare needs to be nowadays. And as these technologies mature, there's potential for entirely new applications that might completely rewrite how we handle dental and maxillofacial care. Ultimately, grasping the full scope of dental imaging stays a key focus in both clinical practice and research (Figure 11.1).

Importance in Diagnosis and Treatment Planning

Today's dental scene has shifted with new imaging methods that let dentists see hidden details beyond what a regular check-up reveals. CBCT as many call it, has become one of those must-have tools when dealing with tricky dental or jaw issues. These scans give individuals a close-up view of things like jaw structure, the arrangement of teeth, and even nearby soft tissues, details that usually get lost in a standard exam. The extra clarity and precision not only boost how accurately a condition can be diagnosed, but they also help shape treatment plans that work better overall. With these sharper images in hand, doctors are often able to spot problems, like endodontic lesions or signs of gum disease, much earlier than before, leading to timely fixes that can sidestep further complications (Calazans et al., 2022). Diagnostic imaging isn't just about naming a disease; it plays a big part in designing treatment plans that fit each patient's needs. In most cases, when a basic exam doesn't cut it, these advanced scans step in to outline just how far a condition has spread and show the sometimes odd relationships between anatomical features. For example, a detailed image can reveal the unusual curves or modifications of tooth roots, which helps dentists avoid mishaps such as leaving behind fragments or even triggering jaw fractures. In situations like periodontal issues, imaging zeros in on where stubborn plaque or calculus is tucked away, guiding more targeted treatments. This deeper understanding, generally speaking, raises the chances for success and boosts decision-making throughout the whole process (Niemiec et al., 2020). And then there's using imaging as a part of ongoing care, which frankly can't be overlooked. Regular radiographs serve as steady checkpoints to monitor if a treatment is working or if a condition is evolving. After gum treatments, for instance, these images let dentists see how tissues are healing and whether plaque control measures are holding up. This kind of feedback not only helps mold treatment plans on the fly, but it also builds a sort of collaborative bond between patient and practitioner, where everyone stays in the loop about what's changing. Ultimately, these advances in dental and jaw imaging arm clinicians with tools that refine their diagnostic sense, elevate treatment planning (even if the process isn't always perfect), and promote a more whole-person approach to care (Calazans et al., 2022; Niemiec et al., 2020).

Overview of Imaging Technologies Used

Over time, imaging in dental and maxillofacial care has truly transformed, offering clinicians sharper diagnostic insights in ways that weren't possible before. One standout tool is CBCT which churns out cool three-dimensional views that let you inspect the details of anatomy. It is pretty key for surgical planning since you get a clear look at the jaw's bony framework and the way teeth sit. In most cases, better imaging seems to bring smoother surgical outcomes with fewer complications. And it is not just about nailing the initial diagnosis, it even helps track how patients heal after surgery. Then there are the good old radiographic techniques, like panoramic radiography, that still hold a major spot in dental imaging. They offer a broad snapshot of the dental arch, which makes noticing issues like impacted teeth, cysts, or tumors a bit easier. Thanks to digital imaging, these classic methods have been upgraded;

images now emerge almost instantly for quick analysis. Digital radiography cuts down on radiation while upping the detail, and it nudges clinicians to make timely decisions, mixing traditional methods with digital advances gives a well-rounded picture that's pretty essential for thoughtful treatment planning. Lately, emerging technologies, particularly artificial intelligence (AI), have started to shake things up even more in dental and maxillofacial imaging. Generally speaking, AI isn't just about making images clearer; it adds a finer touch when spotting problems like cysts or tumors. Some recent studies suggest that these smart algorithms, with their knack for pattern recognition, can boost both preoperative planning and what goes down during surgery, which may lead to better patient outcomes overall. Recent literature even hints that real-time feedback from AI during procedures could ramp up surgical accuracy and efficiency in unexpected ways. When you blend these innovations with traditional imaging techniques, it points toward a future where patient care becomes even more personalized and effective (Annemans et al., 2016; Miragall et al., 2023).

11.1. Types of Dental Imaging Techniques

Learning Outcome

1. Understand the intraoral radiography.
2. Explore the uses and benefits of extraoral radiography.
3. Examine the role of cone beam computed tomography (CBCT).

Dental diagnostics has been on a steady roll lately with many imaging methods that make exams both quicker and more spot-on. Intraoral imaging easily wins attention by snapping pictures right inside the patient's mouth, offering surprising detail, an absolute must in spotting cavities or checking out gum issues. Bitewings and periapical shots get used a lot, largely because they catch early signs of trouble. Lately, though, many clinics are leaning into fancier techniques, like panoramic views and CBCT; these new tools give three-dimensional looks that help set up treatments and surgeries. Advanced imaging in dental offices definitely shapes how patients fare. Take panoramic radiography, for example: it captures the whole mouth in one go and, in most cases, cuts down on exposure time compared to standard intraoral X-rays. This not only boosts the overall comfort during a check-up but also holds up well in diagnostic accuracy. It is handy for checking out impacted teeth, odd jaw lesions, or developmental uniqueness. A recent survey even showed that a good number of dentists now favor panoramic machines, underscoring their widespread use. On top of that, CBCT has brought insane clarity for visualizing craniofacial details, critical for planning implants and other specialized treatments. Overall, these tools prove just how key radiographic techniques are in today's dental and maxillofacial imaging routines. Even though traditional methods set the stage for dental imaging, newer automated systems are shaking things up. Innovations based on machine learning and AI have boosted the ability to pinpoint dental issues with a sharper edge. For instance, Transformer-Based YOLO technologies, yes, the ones that sort of "only look once," are doing a stellar job at categorizing tooth types and flagging pathologies in panoramic views. These approaches mix clever preprocessing with optimization tricks, lending an extra bit of polish to diagnostic images. Integrating such tech not only speeds up the whole process but also helps cut down on human errors. Some tests even showed precision scores close to 99.5%, which pretty much nails the potential of these advancements to work in tandem with classic methods, hinting at a promising future in the field (Puang et al., 2024; Singh et al., 2025).

11.1.1. Intraoral Radiography

In dental clinics, intraoral radiography has become a real game-changer. Technology has improved, and these days you see how imaging methods have shifted. A recent survey among private dentists showed that roughly 90.9%, that's almost all of them, own their own intraoral machines, which pretty much makes the tool essential for identifying issues like dental caries or periodontal problems. This focused type of imaging not only boosts diagnostic accuracy but also cuts down on radiation exposure, a concern that's always in the back of a practitioner's mind. It is interesting to note that many dentists snap between 11 and 20 images each month, a figure that speaks volumes about how embedded this modality is in everyday checkups (Puang et al., 2024). Take a closer look, and the usefulness becomes even more obvious. One retrospective study, for instance, found that intraoral periapical radiographs (IOPAR) were used mainly to diagnose cavities, accounting for 67.05% of all such images. Generally speaking, this double-duty highlights IOPAR as the go-to option for spotting carious lesions. In a somewhat similar vein, these radiographs offer valuable clues for gum disease too, guiding treatment choices while providing high-resolution images of dental structures thanks to sensors being placed super close to the target. In most cases, these tech-driven images give a clear view that's hard to beat, drawing a solid picture of why intraoral radiography sticks around as a staple in modern dentistry (Jadhav et al., 2021).

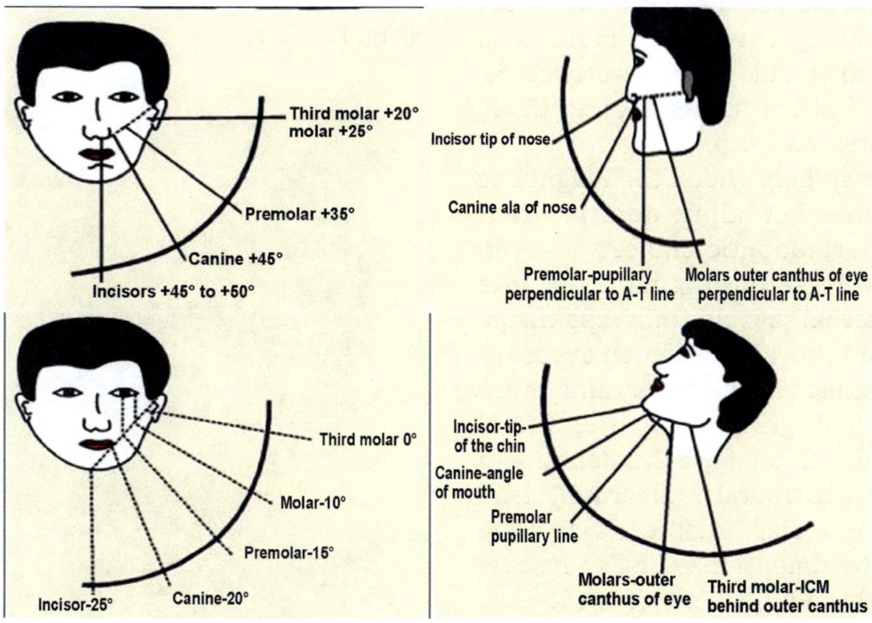

Figure 11.2. Standard conventional radiographic reference points for maxillary and mandibular teeth periapical projections.

Source: Chaitanya NCSK, Padmanabhan V, Islam MS, Hashim NT, Mohammed R, Allam NS, Omar JJ, Zakaria A, Pranathi S and Apoorva M (2024) Enhancing intraoral radiographic technique: introducing "Nallan's Lines." Front. Oral. Health 5:1498117. doi: 10.3389/froh.2024.1498117.

Still, as with anything, there are a few bumps along the way. Practitioners remain cautious about radiation, even though advances have eased some worries. In fact, studies show that over 80% of dentists are quite knowledgeable about radiation hygiene – a reassuring fact in today's fast-evolving tech environment. Even so, clinicians must vigilantly follow safety guidelines to keep exposure low while still getting the detail they need in a diagnosis. Plus, the rise of other imaging techniques means that dentists continually have to brush up on their skills, adapting to new tools while staying true to reliable methods. As dental and maxillofacial imaging steadily evolve, intraoral radiography seems set to keep its pivotal role in patient care (Puang et al., 2024) (Figure 11.2).

11.1.2. Extraoral Radiography

Dental imaging has come a long way, completely changing how dentists figure out jaw and facial issues. Extraoral radiography, for instance, stands out because it gives wide-angle views of the mouth that simple intraoral shots just don't catch. In many cases, this method is crucial for checking out jawbone structure, dental positions, and the tissues around them. Panoramic pictures and cephalometric views, each in its own way, help widen the diagnostic picture, sometimes revealing oddities that may later steer orthodontic choices or even surgical plans. Integrating digital tools into these extraoral techniques not only ups image clarity but also cuts down on radiation exposure for patients, making exams safer and more accurate. Simply put, grasping what extraoral radiography can do is key for solid dental and maxillofacial care. Extraoral radiography isn't only about making a diagnosis; it is also a big part of planning treatment. Take CBCT as a case in point, it has become a kind of must-have partner to older extraoral methods. Generally speaking, CBCT delivers 3D views of the jaw structure, letting clinicians take a detailed look at complex dental relationships that matter in both braces and surgical setups. This kind of imaging has, in most cases, earned praise for its knack in revealing intricate anatomical ties and identifying problems that standard extraoral photos might miss. When weighing the benefits with potential risks, many dental practitioners are increasingly convinced that new digital enhancements in extraoral imaging can boost overall patient care. There's a clear trend moving toward digital extraoral imaging, with ample evidence pointing to a preference for digital over old-school film methods. Almost every modern dental office now leans on digital systems for panoramic shots, a trend that streamlines workflows, simplifies image storage, and makes retrieval way easier. Besides that, shifting to digital aligns with today's evidence-based approach, often yielding more precise diagnoses and improving how professionals interact with patients. As these digital techniques continue to evolve, it remains generally important for dental experts to stay updated on emerging trends and best practices, so they can effectively wield extraoral radiography in their daily clinical routines (Sadhan, 2021; Scarfe et al., 2017) (Figure 11.3).

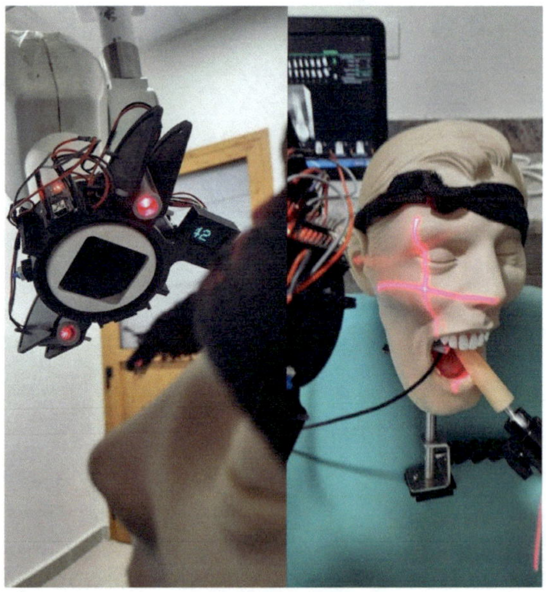

Figure 11.3. Radiograph.

Source: Chaitanya NCSK, Padmanabhan V, Islam MS, Hashim NT, Mohammed R, Allam NS, Omar JJ, Zakaria A, Pranathi S and Apoorva M (2024) Enhancing intraoral radiographic technique: introducing "Nallan's Lines." Front. Oral. Health 5:1498117. doi: 10.3389/froh.2024.1498117.

11.1.3. Cone Beam Computed Tomography (CBCT)

Dental and maxillofacial work now leans on high-res 3D images. CBCT pops up as a handy option, especially when implants or orthodontic tweaks mean you need every bit of precision with spatial details. It doesn't just give you a clear look at bones and tissues; it smooths out planning and surgical moves too. Old-school methods tend to mix up or overlap features, but CBCT pulls together a full, volumetric picture that clears up those issues. In most cases, its knack for recording fine details of both hard and soft parts fills in gaps left by conventional techniques, which is why it is pretty much essential in modern dental practice (Grandoch et al., 2023). It is important for practitioners to get a feel for how CBCT compares to other imaging tools. Studies usually point out that CBCT delivers spot-on geometric and volume data needed for many dental tasks (Figure 11.4).

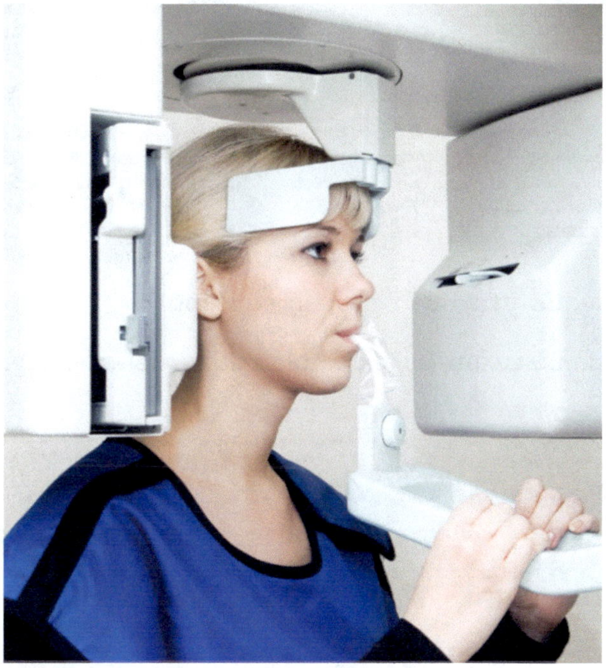

Figure 11.4. Cone beam CT scan.

Source: https://oueisdentistry.ca/wp-content/uploads/2018/04/Cone-Beam-CT-920x1024.jpg.

For example, it is often used in pre-surgical checks to map out key nerve routes and see how different structures relate, spatially speaking. Indeed, techniques like MRI can light up certain areas effectively, yet sometimes they miss some of the finer diagnostic marks. Recent findings even hint that MRI might, on occasion, do a better job at showing particular nerve tracks, though generally speaking, there aren't dramatic differences in overall assessability between the two methods (Grandoch et al., 2023). This underscores why so many rely on CBCT as a baseline tool while still giving credit to MRI's complementary role. CBCT's reach goes well beyond just head and neck imaging. Its applications have grown into other parts of the body, showing off its versatility in unexpected ways. Research has noted that CBCT tends to offer good image quality along with acceptable radiation doses, making it suited for areas outside dentistry too. For instance, clinicians are now tapping into CBCT to image both lower and upper extremities, which has opened doors in orthopedic assessments. Plus, combining CBCT with C-arm technologies has led to breakthroughs in imaging less traditional regions, highlighting its flexible nature. Overall, the continued progress of CBCT not only boosts our diagnostic toolkit but also reinforces the need for advanced imaging options that can keep up with today's ever-changing medical scene (Corazza et al., 2023) (Figure 11.5).

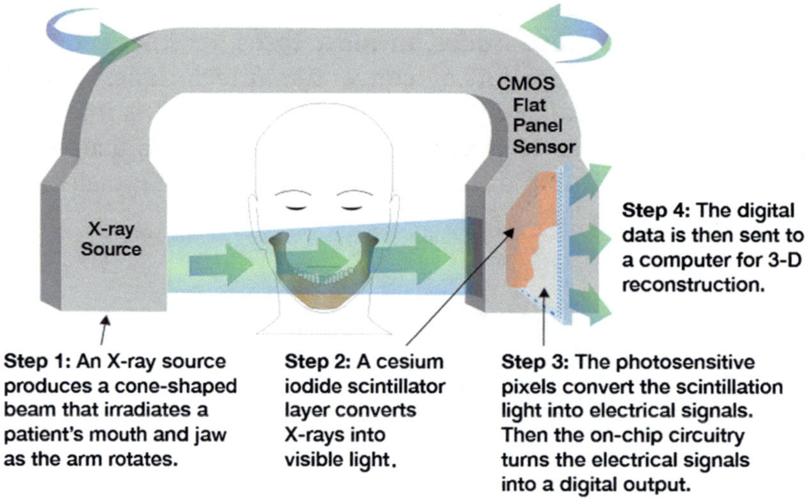

Figure 11.5. Example of dental pan/CBCT system concept.

Source: https://www.hamamatsu.com/us/en/applications/dental-imaging/cone-beam-computed-tomography-CBCT.html.

Test Your Knowledge

1. What are the key differences between intraoral and extraoral radiography in dental imaging?
2. In what clinical situations is intraoral radiography preferred over extraoral radiography, and why?

11.2. Applications in Dentistry

Learning Outcome

1. Understand the role of dental imaging in caries detection and assessment.
2. Define periodontal disease evaluation.
3. Explore the endodontic treatment planning.

New imaging tools are shaking up dentistry these days. Dental MRI now shows its worth in diagnosing head and neck issues, challenging the old reliance on X-rays. It wasn't too long ago that dental MRI was seen as overly complicated and expensive, so many stuck with conventional X-ray methods. Recent tweaks and improvements have boosted its performance, especially when checking soft tissues. New MRI routines even help tackle the tricky challenges in our crowded, anatomy-heavy facial areas. Actual case studies, not just theory, back up its benefits across fields like orthodontics, oral surgery and prosthodontics (Husain et al., 2024). AI is also slowly nudging its way into dental practices. AI, by crunching endless imaging datasets, can flag abnormalities with eye-identifying precision, something that can slip by human judgment in complex cases. In most cases, these smart algorithms add an extra layer of detection where manual reviews might miss a beat. Still, a watchful human eye remains essential to avoid any slip-ups with automated methods. Generally speaking, merging AI with imaging offers a promising route that comes with its own set of ethical questions to iron out. Everyday use of these advanced imaging techniques combined with AI is already changing the game for dental clinics. Dentists and their teams use these clearer imaging methods to get a better look at important structures, which helps with everything from spotting dental decay to planning surgeries. Sometimes, the extra detail means quicker decision-making and smoother workflows in the office. The blend of cutting-edge imaging and smart algorithms is starting to redefine how practitioners approach diagnosis and treatment planning. Ongoing research, and a few adjustments along the way, will be key to harnessing these benefits while keeping ethical issues in check (Husain et al., 2024) (Figure 11.6).

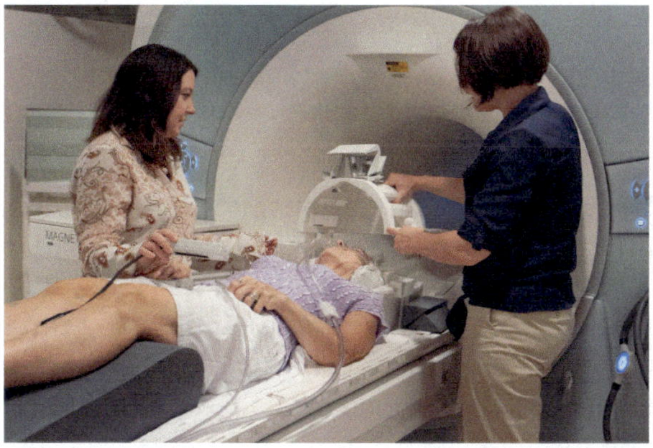

Figure 11.6. Dental MRI.

Source: https://dentalhealthsociety.com/wp-content/uploads/dental-crowns-and-mri.jpg.

11.2.1. Caries Detection and Assessment

Detection and assessment of tooth decay play a huge role in modern dental work, affecting both treatment plans and patient outcomes. Old methods like just checking with the eyes and fingers have been trusted for ages, yet they often suffer from things like operator variability and the fact that judgments can be subjective. Newer imaging techniques, for example CBCT, are now showing promise in boosting exam accuracy. In several cases, CBCT has proven especially good at spotting extra decay hiding beneath composite fillings, pointing to a need for more reliable imaging options, particularly when standard methods just don't cut it in tricky cases. One study looked at how effective CBCT can be by working with extracted human posterior teeth. Researchers drilled different types of cavities on these teeth to mimic secondary decay, then filled each with composite resin and put them through rigorous imaging steps before rating the results on a confidence scale. Intra- and inter-observer assessments generally speaking, demonstrated solid consistency, hinting that CBCT could indeed help improve diagnostic outcomes.

Interestingly, sensitivity and specificity seemed to shift based on the type of restoration; occlusal (O) fillings yielded stronger performance compared to mesial–occlusal–distal (MOD) and distal–occlusal (DO) ones. Such results, in most cases, remind us that leaning solely on CBCT may not always cover every complexity in spotting decay beneath some restorations (Altunkaynak et al., 2017). Better ways to detect decay don't just stop at getting the diagnosis right, they change how treatment is planned and how patients are cared for. A misstep here might lead to unnecessary restorative work on one end or, conversely, missing decay that keeps on worsening on the other. By weaving reliable imaging tools like CBCT into everyday routines, dentists can make more informed decisions that align with evidence-based practices. At the same time, these findings point to a need for further exploration of alternative imaging methods, especially in situations where CBCT's sensitivity or specificity might lag a bit. As dental professionals continue striving for the best patient care, it becomes crucial they understand both the upsides and the limits of each imaging approach so the right tool is chosen for detecting and assessing caries (Khalaf et al., 2014) (Figure 11.7).

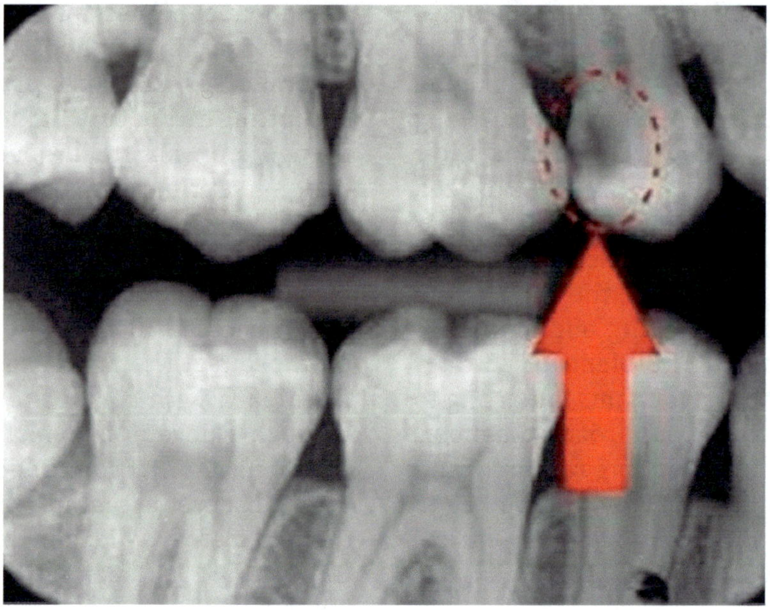

Figure 11.7. Radiograph explanation of tooth carries and normal teeth.

Source: https://peerj.com/articles/cs-1631/.

11.2.2. Periodontal Disease Evaluation

Periodontal disease and dental imaging have a surprisingly tangled relationship. Gum problems can change both the soft and hard tissues in ways that aren't always obvious during a standard checkup. X-rays, like periapical ones, and CBCT, for example, give more than just a flat look; CBCT even shows a 3D picture of the gums and bones, sharpening the diagnosis and guiding treatment planning. Better images mean doctors can often spot damage sooner, which is important for getting patients help early on. Evaluating periodontal disease goes beyond just noticing what's on the surface. It is also about getting to know what's happening underneath and sometimes even how it might tie into issues like heart disease or diabetes. Research generally shows that long-term gum infections might be linked to other health problems, so in most cases a thorough imaging exam isn't just about finding pockets in the gums. It also checks on bone density and the shape of those bones, which are key parts of gum health. In a way, these modern techniques push the approach toward a more complete view, one that covers both local and overall health concerns. New imaging tools have even pushed forward the way dentists tackle complications related to bisphosphonates. As more people use these drugs, the chance of developing jaw problems like osteonecrosis (ONJ) goes up. In such cases, careful imaging, dental X-rays for instance, can help find spots of necrosis and steer treatment decisions. Some studies focusing on bisphosphonate-related jaw issues have pointed out that good imaging is at the heart of successful periodontal evaluations. So, adding advanced imaging to routine check-ups not only boosts diagnostic accuracy but also plays a big role in managing patients on these treatments (Misch et al., 2006; Sebastián et al., 2016) (Figure 11.8).

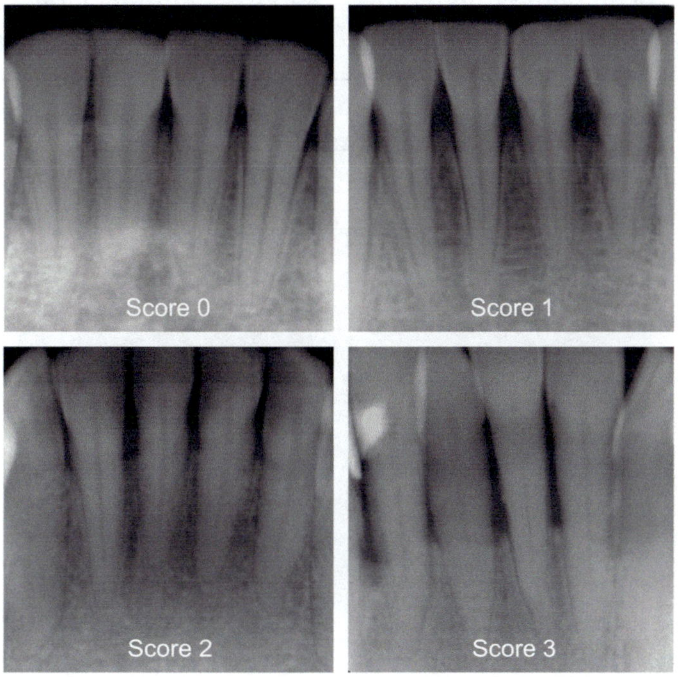

Figure 11.8. Examples of periapical radiographs for all categories: healthy periodontium, periodontal bone loss (PBL) not detectable (Score 0), mild radiographic PBL up to 15% in the coronal third of the tooth (Score 1), moderate radiographic PBL between 15% and 33% of the root length (Score 2), and severe radiographic PBL beyond the coronal third of the tooth (Score 3).

Source: Hoss P, Meyer O, Wölfle UC, Wülk A, Meusburger T, Meier L, Hickel R, Gruhn V, Hesenius M, Kühnisch J, et al. Detection of Periodontal Bone Loss on Periapical Radiographs—A Diagnostic Study Using Different Convolutional Neural Networks. *Journal of Clinical Medicine*. 2023; 12(22):7189. https://doi.org/10.3390/jcm12227189.

11.2.3. Endodontic Treatment Planning

Advanced imaging now plays a key role in planning endodontic treatment to get better patient results. X-rays, along with newer methods like CBCT, give clinicians useful views into tooth structure and what surrounds it. Standard radiography has worked for many years, though it lacks the full picture in cases with several canal systems; CBCT, on the other hand, shows the root canals' layout and nearby lesions with a clarity that boosts diagnostic accuracy. These new imaging methods stress the importance of using specialized techniques to tailor treatment plans to each patient's unique setup, which in most cases increases the clinical results and patient satisfaction. Evaluating possible complications is another angle of endodontic planning where high-resolution images come in handy. They help spot issues like extra or winding canals that might not show up with normal imaging. It is important to get a handle on these details so that the right approach is chosen to access and clean the canals. In many cases imaging also allows for spotting periapical problems early on, letting doctors take steps before things get worse; this added insight makes choosing the right endodontic strategy easier and shows why tech integration is so critical in today's dental practices (Kıvanç Kamburoğlu, 2025). New imaging techniques are also opening doors for a fresh look at endodontics. Microcomputed tomography and ultrasound imaging, for example, are coming up as real-time options without the downside of ionizing radiation. Mixing these advanced tools can help endodontists fine-tune their methods and cut down on mistakes caused by misreading anatomy. Research is still unfolding, and as it does, the future seems geared towards blending modern technology with everyday practice, promising an exciting journey ahead for patient care (Kıvanç Kamburoğlu, 2025) (Figure 11.9).

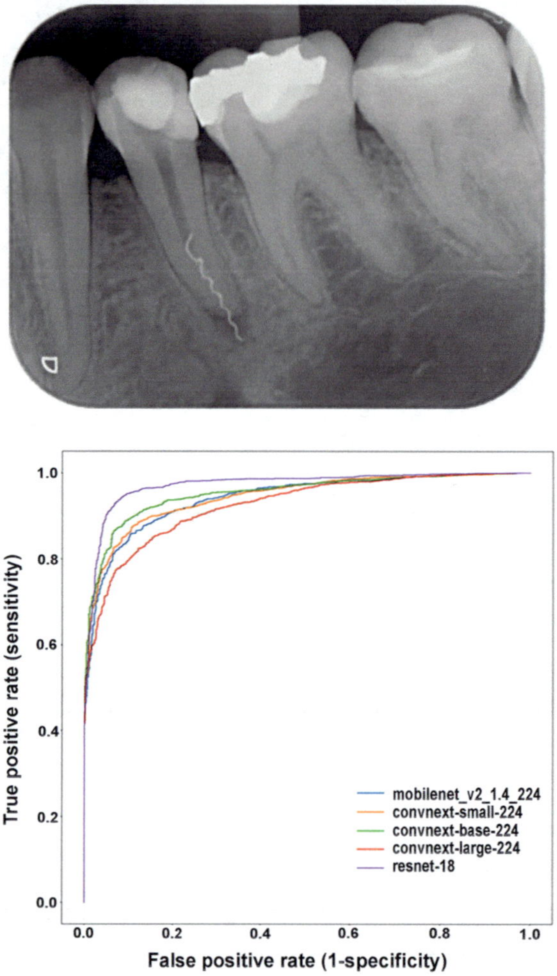

Figure 11.9. AI and analyzing radiographs.

Source: Hoss P, Meyer O, Wölfle UC, Wülk A, Meusburger T, Meier L, Hickel R, Gruhn V, Hesenius M, Kühnisch J, et al. Detection of Periodontal Bone Loss on Periapical Radiographs—A Diagnostic Study Using Different Convolutional Neural Networks. *Journal of Clinical Medicine*. 2023; 12(22):7189. https://doi.org/10.3390/jcm12227189.

Test Your Knowledge

1. How is dental radiography used in the detection and assessment of dental caries?
2. What role does radiography play in evaluating periodontal disease and its progression?

11.3. Maxillofacial Imaging Techniques

Learning Outcome

1. Understand the computed tomography (CT) and magnetic resonance imaging (MRI).
2. Examine the role and advantages of Ultrasound imaging in dental imaging.

Choosing the right imaging method can affect how well maxillofacial issues are spotted. Clinicians need to have a pretty good feel for the different radiographic approaches available. Take panoramic radiography, which gives a wide view of the jaw and nearby structures – it is a handy tool for identifying anomalies and planning treatments, even if it doesn't quite nail the depth perception part. That's where CBCT jumps in; by offering a full 3D picture, it lets practitioners untangle the most complex anatomical details. In orthodontics, where exact measurements of bone and dental structures are absolutely important, this kind of three-dimensional insight can make all the difference. Overall, how these imaging techniques are chosen and used ties directly to improved patient outcomes and more rounded treatment strategies (Mozahab, 2025). Technology is moving fast, and with it, dental imaging is seeing more of AI at work. AI is stepping into maxillofacial diagnostics, generally speaking, by refining how images are read and making clinical workflows a bit smoother. By handling the analysis of radiographic images automatically, these systems can cut down on human error and often lead to diagnoses that are both earlier and more precise. There's also the perk of paving the way for more personalized treatment plans since AI can sift through unique patient details and suggest specific interventions. Still, leaning too hard on AI raises ethical concerns – mainly about keeping real people in charge. Making sure that practitioners stay involved in decision-making helps catch mistakes the AI might make, underscoring the need for a balanced approach in dental imaging. At the same time, as imaging methods get better, our safety practices have to keep up too. The ALARA concept, standing for "as low as reasonably achievable," is a key rule meant to limit radiation exposure, especially for vulnerable groups like kids. Ensuring patient safety during these procedures isn't just ticking a regulatory box; it is also an ethical duty. With new imaging tech coming online, it becomes even more important for practitioners to keep checking the risk-benefit ratio of each method. Digital imaging techniques, which typically use less radiation than old-school approaches, are a good example of how safety and innovation can go hand in hand. These improved methods are proving vital in boosting diagnostic quality while still honoring patient care and safety standards in dental and maxillofacial work (Mozahab, 2025).

11.3.1. Computed Tomography (CT)

Imaging tech has changed the way we look at dental diagnostics, especially in spotting caries. Recent work shows that CBCT can be pretty effective at uncovering secondary decay hiding under composite resin fillings. The numbers – you know, looking at the area under the receiver operating characteristic curve – indicate that detecting occlusal cavities tends to work better than with trickier restorations like mesial-occlusal-distal mixes. Clearly, while CBCT gives us important info about caries beneath fillings, its performance shifts based on how complex a cavity is, so clinicians might sometimes need to check out different imaging options (Altunkaynak et al., 2017). In most cases, knowing both its strong points and its limits is key to smart imaging choices. Beyond detecting decay, CT technology is branching out into other parts of dental and maxillofacial imaging, such as placing dental implants. A new twist comes with piezoelectric surgery, a method that's starting to combined with implant placement and could boost the role of CT in guiding surgeries. When piezoelectric osteotomy teams up with traditional imaging techniques, it offers a clearer look at osseointegration, giving useful clues about bone volume and how tissues react after implant surgery. Some studies using microcomputed tomography even show how different implant designs tweak the healing process, underscoring why capturing detailed images before and after procedures is so important (Fujinaka et al., 2019). Overall, mixing advanced imaging approaches is pretty pivotal for predicting implant success. CT in dental and maxillofacial fields is on a steady climb, echoing the wider push toward precision medicine in dentistry. By using advanced methods like CBCT, clinicians can get a genuine 3D view of anatomical structures, which helps lead to diagnoses and treatment plans that are a lot more accurate. This kind of detail is especially vital in complicated jaw cases where the exact spatial layout can affect surgical outcomes. There's also growing evidence that combining various imaging techniques can boost overall diagnostic accuracy, offering a more rounded look at both hard and soft tissues. As the field moves forward, further research into fine-tuning imaging protocols will remain essential for figuring out the best ways to improve patient care and treatment results in dental practices (Altunkaynak et al., 2017; Fujinaka et al., 2019) (Figure 11.10).

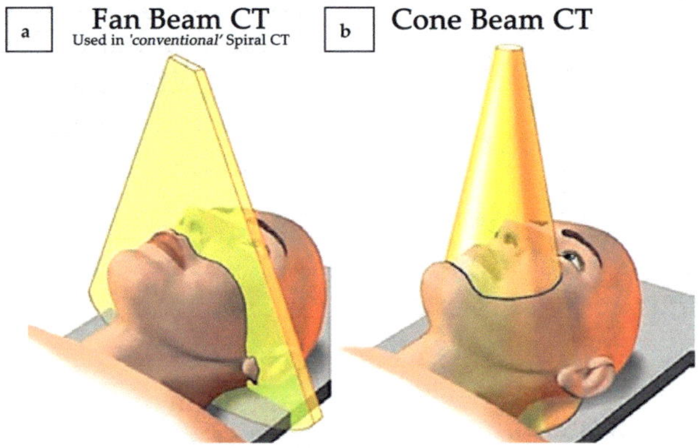

Figure 11.10. Description of the principle of CBCT in comparison to conventional CT. (a) In CBCT, the gantry rotates around the patient just once before the cone-shaped X-ray beam arrives at a flat detector. (b) Multiple linear detectors and a narrowly collimated, fan-shaped beam revolve around the patient in a conventional CT scan to collect multiple image portions per rotation.

Source: Alshomrani F. Cone-Beam Computed Tomography (CBCT)-Based Diagnosis of Dental Bone Defects. *Diagnostics*. 2024; 14(13):1404. https://doi.org/10.3390/diagnostics14131404.

11.3.2. Magnetic Resonance Imaging (MRI)

MRI is now playing a bigger role in dental and facial imaging, changing how we check out soft tissues. For years, X-rays and CT scans held the crown because they're great at examining bones and other hard tissues. But MRI, being non-invasive and free of radiation, comes in as a fresh way to see the softer details, which is pretty handy for spotting problems around the mouth and nearby areas. Lately, new imaging tricks and specially built coils have augmented, delivering sharper pictures that help zoom in on conditions like gum disease or oral tumors. Whether using high-field or low-field systems, doctors can now tackle complex cases more confidently (Sungkaruk et al., 2024). Still, MRI isn't without its bumps, especially when dental implants are involved. Implants made of iron or stainless steel tend to fiddle with the magnetic field and create artifacts that may hide important details. Studies generally speaking point to titanium implants as safer for MRI use, they tend to produce fewer odd distortions, even though tiny ferromagnetic bits can sometimes still sneak in and lower image quality. That's why new techniques to cut down on these artifacts, like adjusting MR settings, trying out advanced scanning sequences, or even using materials like zirconia, are so important. Fine-tuning these approaches helps improve the overall image quality and, in most cases, ramps up patient safety during scans (Sungkaruk et al., 2024). Dental imaging is shifting in unexpected ways, and MRI is stepping up as a strong alternative to old-school X-rays. When dealing with conditions around the jaw and mouth, getting clear images is pretty critical for making the right diagnosis and planning proper treatment. Thanks to recent tech boosts, MRI methods are now often tailored specifically for the head and neck, sidestepping the limitations of more traditional methods. Case studies have shown that dental MRI finds its groove in areas ranging from general dentistry to prosthodontics to oral surgery, sometimes even outshining conventional scans. With dentists, radiologists, and tech experts teaming up more than ever, the future of using dental MRI to boost diagnostic accuracy looks bright, it may well transform standard care practices in the field (Husain et al., 2024) (Figure 11.11).

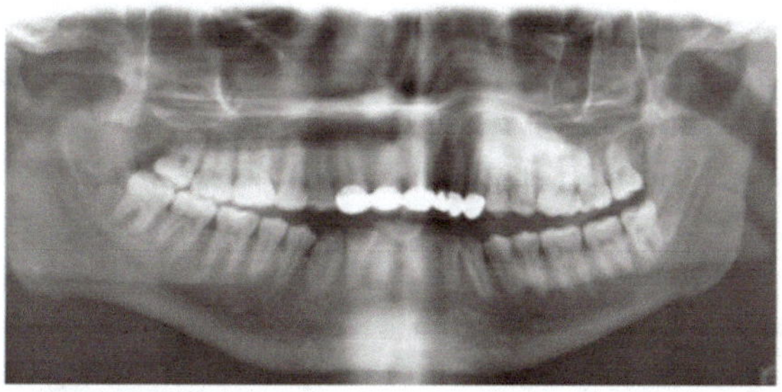

Figure 11.11. Dental analyses.

Source: Alshomrani F. Cone-Beam Computed Tomography (CBCT)-Based Diagnosis of Dental Bone Defects. *Diagnostics*. 2024; 14(13):1404. https://doi.org/10.3390/diagnostics14131404.

11.3.3. Ultrasound Imaging

Dental and maxillofacial practices are shifting gears with new imaging methods these days. Ultrasound, for example, obtains attention, it is noninvasive, works in real time, and checks out soft tissues, blood flow, and subtle anatomical differences without bombarding patients with radiation. Unlike traditional radiography that sticks to bones and other firm structures, ultrasound gives a broader picture, gums, salivary glands, and other soft areas get their moment too. Increasingly, practitioners are saying that sometimes ultrasound can do the job of old-school imaging, leading to personalized treatments and happier patients. Then there's the whole story with improved ultrasound gadgets. New high-res devices dish out images that expose miniscule details in soft tissues, making it easier to spot lesions and oddities, and plan next steps accordingly. In some periodontal checks, ultrasound throws light on things like the periodontal ligament space and nearby soft tissues, offering a refreshed, nuanced take on gum health and disease progression. These outcomes generally reflect earlier findings about the value of good imaging for planning effective treatment (Dileep et al., 2019). So, while it naturally supports standard diagnostics, ultrasound ends up being a key player in more rounded oral assessments. It doesn't stop at diagnostics, ultrasound even branches out into therapy. Take ultrasound-guided procedures like aspiration or injections, which can sharpen the accuracy of treatments in the maxillofacial region. For saltatory issues with the salivary glands, clinicians often use ultrasound to guide needle placement; this minimizes trauma and eases discomfort while keeping treatment effective. Recent studies hint that merging diagnostic and therapeutic uses makes ultrasound a versatile, indispensable asset (Cunha et al., 2016). As the technology evolves, its expanding role is likely to keep raising the standard of dental care and improving patient outcomes (Figure 11.12).

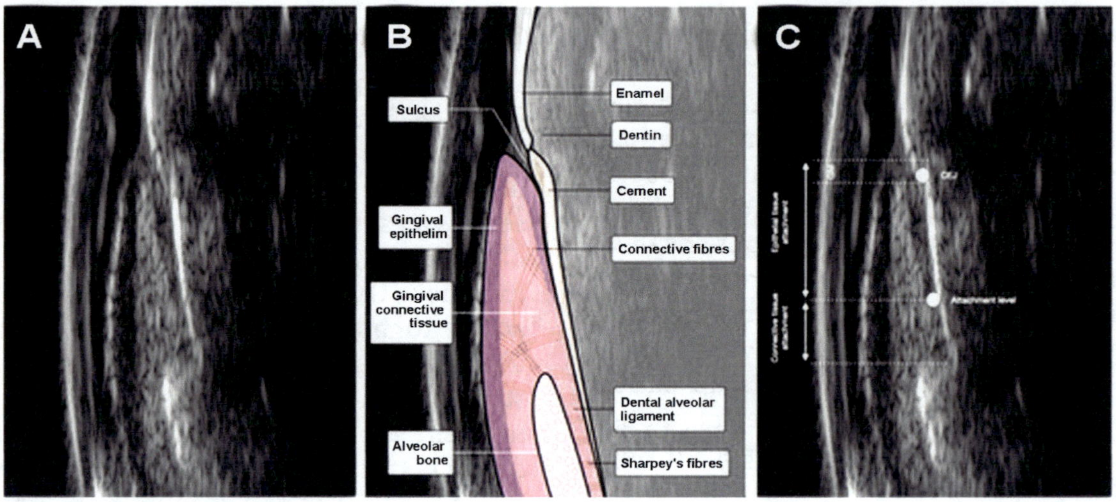

Figure 11.12. Ultrasound in dentistry.

Source: Renaud M, Gette M, Delpierre A, Calle S, Levassort F, Denis F, Rochefort GY. Intraoral Ultrasonography for the Exploration of Periodontal Tissues: A Technological Leap for Oral Diagnosis. *Diagnostics*. 2024; 14(13):1335. https://doi.org/10.3390/diagnostics14131335.

Test Your Knowledge

1. What are some common maxillofacial imaging techniques used to assess facial bones and jaw structures?
2. How does cone beam computed tomography (CBCT) enhance diagnostic accuracy in maxillofacial imaging?

11.4. Safety and Radiation Concerns

Learning Outcome

1. Understand the radiation exposure and risks in dental and jaw imaging.
2. Identify the safety protocols in imaging.
3. Define advances in reducing radiation dose.

Imaging tech in dental and maxillofacial work has changed the game, helping diagnose problems in ways we never thought possible. But with these strides come real concerns about safety and radiation. You know, different methods bring varying levels of radiation; for instance, digital radiography is generally linked too much lower doses than the old film-based X-rays, which means fewer health risks without losing on clarity. In most cases, guidelines push us to stick with the ALARA principle (as-low-as-reasonably-achievable), so that both patients and operators aren't exposed to more than necessary. Then there's the nagging issue of radiation building up over time, a point that matters for vulnerable groups like kids and pregnant women. Imaging can sometimes mean repeated exposures, so it is crucial to adapt the approach to each patient, taking into account their medical background and specific anatomical needs. Dentists ought to use careful risk assessments to justify why a particular imaging technique is needed, and, generally speaking, clear chat with patients about these risks helps secure informed consent, even if it means repeating the basics here and there. It is equally vital that dental professionals keep learning about new tech and updated safety practices. Ongoing training, even if it feels like just another box to check off, can cut down on unnecessary exposure incidents. Bringing together dentists, radiologists, and even medical physicists in a team approach fosters a stronger safety culture. Regular audits of imaging practices, for example, help ensure that safety standards are met while also adapting to fresh clinical insights and innovations. Overall, these combined strategies not only boost patient safety but also prepare the dental workforce to manage radiation issues better, improving clinical outcomes in the process (Figure 11.13).

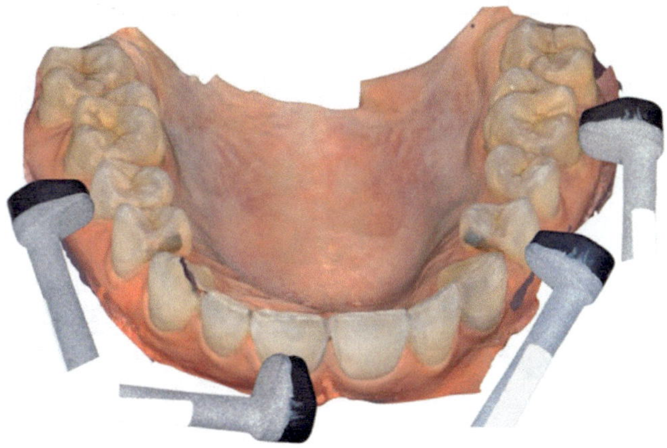

Figure 11.13. Patient safety.

Source: Renaud M, Gette M, Delpierre A, Calle S, Levassort F, Denis F, Rochefort GY. Intraoral Ultrasonography for the Exploration of Periodontal Tissues: A Technological Leap for Oral Diagnosis. *Diagnostics*. 2024; 14(13):1335. https://doi.org/10.3390/diagnostics14131335.

11.4.1. Radiation Exposure and Risks

Radiation exposure in dental and jaw imaging isn't just an issue for immediate patient care, it also shapes how people think about safety. Many individuals simply don't grasp where ionizing radiation comes from or what its risks might be. Take, for instance, a study from Saudi Arabia; more than two-thirds of the participants had no idea that natural sources contribute to ionizing radiation, and quite a few mistakenly assumed that imaging methods like chest X-rays and CT scans give off the same dose (Alburayh et al., 2025). This mix-up, generally speaking, points to the pressing need for better public education and for practitioners to explain the relative risks in everyday language. Different imaging methods can expose patients to very different levels of radiation. Research shows that CBCT is a much safer choice compared to traditional Medical CT scans. For example, while CBCT typically delivers around 100 microsieverts (μSv) per use, a Medical CT scan usually exposes a patient to over 500 μSv. Even though CBCT still provides a high-quality image, its lower radiation dose makes it a preferred option for many dental professionals who, in most cases, want to minimize risk without sacrificing diagnostic quality. On top of that, clearing up the public's misconceptions about radiation risk isn't just about handing out facts, it also involves carefully tailored communication that considers who the audience is. Research indicates that having prior information about radiation can make a big difference in how well individuals understand the risks (Alburayh et al., 2025). Interestingly, demographics like gender and marital status seem to play a role too; for example, males and married individuals often show a more cautious view toward radiological tests and their potential dangers. In most instances, targeted educational efforts that address these specific differences are needed to close the gap between expert advice and everyday understanding about radiation in dental imaging (Figure 11.14).

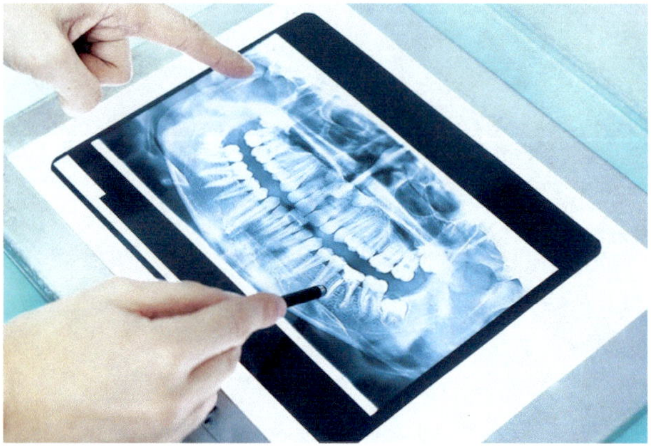

Figure 11.14. Radiation exposure in dental.

Source: https://www.hillandalesmiles.com/wp-content/uploads/dental-x-ray-on-tablet-screen.jpg.webp.

11.4.2. Safety Protocols in Imaging

Dental and maxillofacial imaging safety isn't just about following rules, it is a mix of protecting patients and making sure that diagnoses stay reliable. Cutting down on radiation is a top priority, especially because the tissues in these areas are unusually delicate. CBCT, for example, has shaken up how we think about imaging. It provides high-res images at much lower radiation levels than older methods, and that change is something many have welcomed. Still, keeping things safe means paying attention to details: getting the patient positioned correctly, ensuring equipment is calibrated (and re-calibrated when needed), and checking image quality on a regular basis. In most cases, these steps work together to guard patient health and build trust in the results, even if it means tolerating a couple of extra checks along the way. Another piece of the picture is figuring out the risks that come with these imaging technologies. As dental MRI becomes more common, most experts say it comes with its own uniqueness. While it is great that MRI avoids radiation, it can fall short when imaging hard tissues compared to standard X-rays.

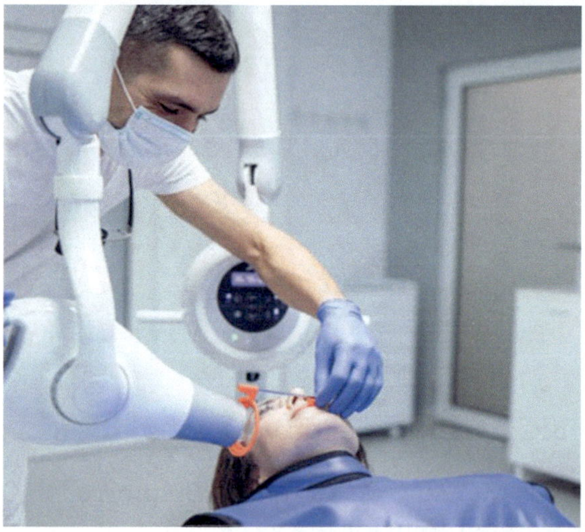

Figure 11.15. Dental and maxillofacial imaging safety.

Source: https://drbooshehri.com/wp-content/uploads/2024/11/The-best-practices-for-patient-safety-in-dental-radiography1.jpg.

That's why, in many cases, it is necessary to create protocols that deal with these limits, like tweaking imaging sequences or using specialized coils, to nail a soft tissue diagnosis in the jaw area. Regular training for healthcare professionals is also key, helping everyone stay on top of these complexities, even if the guidelines sometimes seem to circle back on themselves. Then there's quality control, which, to put it simply, is a must-have in the workflow. Establishing tailored QC programs, particularly for systems like CBCT, often stems from state regulations, accreditation demands, or even manufacturer guidelines in the United States. This typically means that medical physicists get heavily involved, taking on roles that include routine checks of equipment performance, radiation levels, and overall image quality. By putting a solid QC framework in place, imaging centers not only better protect patients but also boost diagnostic accuracy and general outcomes, ultimately fostering a culture of safety in dental imaging practices (Husain et al., 2024; Mihailidis et al., 2024) (Figure 11.15).

11.4.3. Advances in Reducing Radiation Dose

Dental imaging keeps changing, and this shift has, in turn, sparked some cool strides in cutting down on radiation. Dentists are now often leaning on technologies like Cone Beam CT and various digital imaging methods, which puts the spotlight on protecting patients from too much radiation. Recent numbers suggest that digital intraoral X-rays can seriously drop exposure levels while still giving clear, diagnostic images. You might notice that new guidelines for Diagnostic Reference Levels tied to CBCT are now in place, kind of a nod to how we've got to adapt to these fresh techniques. This sort of standard-setting means patients, in most cases, only get what's necessary in radiation (Sadeghi et al., 2025). Plus, mixing in these modern approaches not only lets professionals decide smarter but also bumps up the overall care in dentistry. Researchers have also been poking around with innovative materials and approaches to better shield against radiation. Nanotechnology, for example, is opening up opportunities for lightweight, tailor-made shielding that could outdo the old-school materials. Some studies even hint that these nanostructured materials are more efficient at cutting down on X-ray energy, with estimates pointing to dose reductions between 15 and 35% (Sadeghi et al., 2025). It is interesting since CBCT imaging, which is popping up more and more in clinics, tends to come with higher radiation doses than the standard radiographs most of us know. Overall, this push towards new solutions underscores a genuine commitment to keeping patient safety front and center while also boosting the overall performance of dental imaging techniques. On top of that, newer imaging methods like ultra-low-dose X-ray systems seem ready to shift the landscape of dental and jaw imaging. Some devices built on carbon nanotube-based X-ray sources have, in several tests, shown they deliver excellent quality images with a lot less radiation, often, these devices even score much lower average doses compared to traditional C-arm fluoroscopy, a key win for both patients and medical staff. This kind of progress underscores a gradual, steady move toward imaging systems that put safety first but don't skimp on diagnostic detail. By starting to use these innovations, the dental community might find that sweet balance between effective imaging and keeping radiation exposure as low as possible, all while nudging the field toward a more patient-friendly future.

Test Your Knowledge

1. What measures can be taken to minimize radiation exposure during dental and maxillofacial imaging?
2. Why is the ALARA (As Low As Reasonably Achievable) principle important in dental radiography?

11.5. Future Trends in Dental and Maxillofacial Imaging

Learning Outcome

1. Explore recent advancements in digital imaging advancements.
2. Understand the role of artificial intelligence in diagnostics.
3. Examine the integration of imaging with treatment modalities.

Digital breakthroughs are totally shaking up how we see dental and maxillofacial imaging these days. Instead of sticking with the old-school approaches, clinics are now using high-res 3D scans that give a fuller, sometimes even layered, look at jaw and facial details, this makes treatment planning feel almost custom-tailored. Digital tools have upped diagnostic capabilities in unexpected ways; for example, a closer examination of craniofacial structures now comes as part of routine practice. And, in most cases, as AI weaves its way into the mix, imaging systems seem ready to analyze data and spot subtle abnormalities with surprising precision. These changes hint at a move toward more personalized treatment, where clinicians tailor interventions to fit each patient's scenario. Overall, the blend of modern tech doesn't just refine clinical methods, it also aims to lift overall patient care across various specialties. In the midst of these rapid imaging updates, dental informatics has come into its own. This field mixes together dentistry and IT by leaning on things like electronic health records and even telehealth, which, frankly, boost dental care accessibility. One might even say that soon, digital imagery and informatics will merge further, letting clinicians store, pull up, and share images without the usual hassle. This evolving sphere is full of both hurdles and openings, especially in working together across different specialties and managing vast amounts of data (Hewapathirane et al., 2023). Generally speaking, with an ongoing push for better education and some training tweaks, these digital innovations are on track to reshape everyday workflows in dental practices, ultimately leading to better outcomes for patients and a more practical take on oral health care. Robotics, believe it or not, is starting to turn heads in dental and maxillofacial imaging too. Instead of just being a futuristic fancy, robotic systems are already enhancing how imaging is captured and even how surgical procedures get done. Some devices built for oral surgery now provide high-definition views while helping out with minimally invasive techniques, pretty neat, right? As outlined in Torres et al. (2024), the technical bits, hardware, software, and specialized tools, are all bundled together to give dental professionals a serious boost in both accuracy and performance. Of course, issues like high costs and the need for special training still emerge as obstacles, but overall, the future of robotics seems tied to ongoing tech progress and cross-discipline collaboration. In many cases, this steady march forward could well keep pushing the boundaries of both diagnosis and treatment, making a real impact on patient care.

11.5.1. Digital Imaging Advancements

Digital imaging in dentistry and maxillofacial work has come a long way, it is shaken up how diagnoses and treatments get done. New imaging tech lets healthcare individuals spot details they might have missed before, so they see those tricky anatomical features much clearer. Take high-resolution CBCT for example; it now gives 3D images while generally using less radiation than the old fashioned X-rays. This extra clarity means clinicians can, in most cases, rely on better visuals when planning diagnosis and treatment, which naturally boosts patient care. AI's role here is also worth mentioning, it speeds up and refines how radiographic data get interpreted, turning complex digital shots into actionable clinical ideas that improve outcomes in dentistry (Ahmadi et al., 2024). The boost in imaging capabilities also helps break down barriers between different specialties. With today's advanced systems, professionals like oral surgeons and orthodontists can quickly share detailed visuals without fuss. Sharing the same crisp data makes putting together a treatment plan more straightforward, even if, sometimes, the details get repeated just to be clear. Digital imaging isn't just about crunching numbers or creating detailed scans, it also makes message-passing among specialists a lot smoother, cutting down on misunderstandings and even a few errors. Innovations in telemedicine now allow remote consults based on these shared images, so more patients end up getting access to quality care. In a way, digital imaging has stepped up from being merely a diagnostic tool to a key enabler of integrated healthcare, revamping workflows and patient experiences alike (Torres et al., 2024). Education and training in dental imaging have had to keep pace with these tech leaps. Dental schools and ongoing ed programs are now stressing the need to get hands-on with digital imaging techniques, mirroring the growing demand for comfort with these modern tools. By mixing imaging training into daily curricula, soon-to-be dentists and specialists are being prepped to use these systems effectively in real-world clinics. Given how fast new breakthroughs pop up, continuous learning is pretty much a must, reinforcing just how important digital know-how is in modern dental practice. In most cases, as imaging technology keeps evolving, a mix of solid academic grounding and practical training will be key to shaping tomorrow's landscape in dental diagnostics and patient care (Ahmadi et al., 2024; Torres et al., 2024).

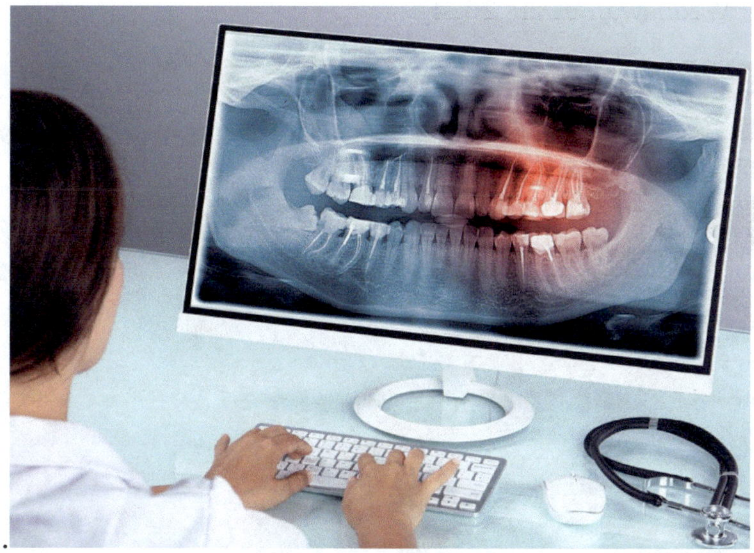

Source: https://www.smilepointdentalvictoria.com/wp-content/uploads/2022/03/Dentist-looking-at-teeth-1200x900.jpg.

11.5.2. Artificial Intelligence (AI) in Diagnostics

AI is shaking up dental diagnostics in ways that keep surprising us. Lately, large language models have started smoothing out exchanges between healthcare pros and patients in unexpected ways. Take ChatGPT from OpenAI, it pulls from publicly available data and bumps up the way dental offices check things out. AI now jumps into clinical decision-making, quickening procedures (especially those tricky ones like oral surgery) and opening doors to fresh research angles in dental and maxillofacial imaging. In most cases, this isn't just about better care; it is about rethinking diagnostics entirely, hinting at a real transformative force in overall healthcare outcomes and efficiency (Ahmadi et al., 2024). Beyond just making conversations easier, AI is proving to be a major player in assessing risks in dental and maxillofacial settings. Machine learning digs into huge, varied datasets, including images, patient histories, and demographics, to spot complex conditions that might otherwise slip by. This skill is particularly crucial when dealing with orofacial trauma, where accurate predictions can guide treatment planning and boost patient outcomes. With its knack for spotting underlying patterns, AI can flag high-risk individuals and even predict complications, adding a helping hand to clinical decisions. Generally speaking, as healthcare leans more toward personalized approaches, blending in AI isn't merely a tech upgrade, it has become a smart strategy for managing patients and using resources more efficiently (Wadhawan et al., 2024). There's now a subtle but steady shift in the healthcare landscape as AI weaves into various diagnostic areas, with dentistry and maxillofacial imaging right at the forefront. This evolving scene opens up chances both to improve diagnostic accuracy and to cut down on evaluation time. As these systems mature, often in unexpectedly clever ways, they're expected to help spot anomalies and plan treatments with a precision that might once have seemed out of reach. Even training for dental professionals gets a boost, helping bridge the gap between what's learned in textbooks and what happens in busy clinics. Ultimately, these AI-led advances aren't just set to rewrite the rules of dental diagnostics; they're laying a groundwork for ongoing, patient-centered improvements, underscoring just how crucial technology has become in broadening and deepening dental care (Ahmadi et al., 2024; Wadhawan et al., 2024).

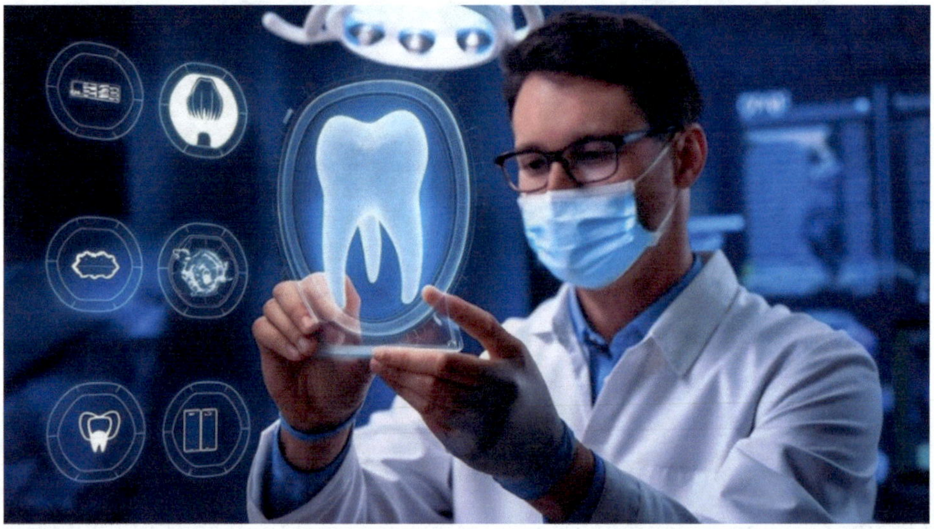

Source: https://miro.medium.com/v2/resize:fit:900/1*pkLwSGvmD2EUG_hGa6V2Og.jpeg.

11.5.3. Integration of Imaging with Treatment Modalities

Imaging has totally changed how dental and jaw surgeries get planned. These days, doctors lean on tools like panoramic X-rays and CT to snag detailed pictures of the mouth and face, pictures that dig into the messy layout of bones and tissues. In surgery, say during a wisdom tooth removal, having these images means the clinical work-up is spot on and backed by solid evidence. It is not just about spotting potential issues; it is also about fine-tuning the procedure to suit each patient, a nod to the move toward personalized care in today's oral and maxillofacial practices (Husain et al.,

2023). Cinematic rendering (CR) is another neat example of innovation in this field. By whipping up life-like three-dimensional visuals, CR gives surgeons a much clearer sense of where lesions sit within the tangle of facial structures. In one case involving the removal of an epidermoid cyst, conventional scans were paired with CR so that doctors could see exactly how the lesion related to its neighbors. That extra bit of perspective helped them plan more carefully, lowered the risk of mistakes, and ultimately led to better outcomes (Husain et al., 2024). And then there's the growing role of AI and machine learning in the mix. Generally speaking, these digital tools step in to boost image analysis, making it easier to predict how surgeries might go. In settings where every tiny detail matters, especially in high-risk procedures, the blend of advanced imaging with smart algorithms helps cut down on inefficiencies and streamlines patient care. As this technology keeps evolving, its merge with treatment methods is nudging dental practices toward a more data-focused, patient-first approach that can enhance both results and satisfaction (Husain et al., 2023).

Test Your Knowledge

1. How is artificial intelligence expected to impact the future of dental and maxillofacial imaging?
2. What are the potential benefits of 3D imaging advancements in dental diagnostics and treatment planning?

Summary

Dental and maxillofacial imaging have shaken up oral healthcare. Old-school methods seem almost outdated now, as newer imaging techniques mix in with smart tools like AI, think of advanced systems such as ChatGPT, and even robotics. The upgrade in diagnostic power has been noticeable, and it often makes conversations between doctors and patients a lot clearer. Precision in everyday clinical work has taken center stage, hinting that better patient results might now be within reach, with tech and imaging working hand in hand. Robotics, too, has started to tweak dental procedures beyond the routine check-up. Sure, there are bumps along the way, costs can be steep and integrating these systems isn't always a walk in the park, but the upside is hard to ignore. Many reports suggest that with robotics cutting down on human error and boosting accuracy, treatments ranging from orthodontics to complicated surgeries are getting a whole lot smoother; in most cases, the shift feels revolutionary, almost like a new era is dawning in dentistry. In wrapping things up, merging advanced imaging with cutting-edge technologies signals a fresh chapter for dental practice. The blend of AI and robotic help not only ups the ante on diagnostics but also improves surgical precision, which means patients might enjoy top-tier care even as the field changes. Ongoing research remains key, addressing hurdles like system integration and training needs will be important, and, generally speaking, a deep understanding of these trends lays the groundwork for better outcomes. Ultimately, moving forward with these innovations may just be the best way to keep pace in an ever-more complex healthcare landscape.

Digital imaging has flipped things around in dental and jaw care. Panoramic X-rays and cone-beam CT scans, for example, give us a wider look at what's going on in the mouth, almost like peeling back layers to spot hidden dental uniqueness. These tools not only help find unusual anomalies but also sharpen orthodontic checks so docs can tailor treatments more effectively. As seen in Mohazab (2025), getting that sharp image isn't just about diagnosis; it also steers us toward safer procedures, especially since younger patients need extra care in radiation. In many cases, it feels as if modern radiology is pushing dental practices to keep up with these fast-changing tech trends. Then there's the game-changing blend of digital imaging with 3D printing. With tools like CT scans and intraoral scanners in play, clinicians can whip up detailed digital models that peel back even the most complex anatomical corners. Further, Kim et al. (2025) even walks through case studies where 3D-printed models help improve surgical moves and give patients a clearer idea of what to expect. Whether it is crafting surgical guides for those tricky spots or modeling out bone harvesting procedures, this mix of imaging and printing makes planning and execution more intuitive. It also creates a sort of hands-on learning vibe, both for the doctor and the patient, as ideas are shared in a more relaxed, almost conversational way. No doubt, embracing these digital advances is more than just riding a trendy wave, it is reshaping how care is delivered. Enhanced imaging and 3D printing aren't simply novel add-ons; they're steadily becoming part of the everyday toolkit, improving everything from precision planning before surgery to smoother steps during operation. Sure, there might be some rough edges as we transition and adapt, but overall, these technologies lower risks and boost patient outcomes. Moving forward, a mix of innovation and ongoing learning will likely steer the future of dental and maxillofacial imaging, ensuring that the quality of care continues to evolve with the times.

KEY TERMS FROM THIS CHAPTER

Artificial intelligence (AI)
Digital radiography
Extraoral radiography
Mesial-occlusal-distal (MOD)
Orthodontics
Panoramic radiography
Prosthodontics
Cone beam computed tomography (CBCT)
Distal-occlusal (DO)
Intraoral periapical radiographs (IOPAR)
Oral surgery
Osteonecrosis (ONJ)
Periodontal disease
Virtual reality (VR)

Critical Thinking Questions

1. **What is the primary purpose of dental radiography (X-rays)?**
   a. To visualize bone fractures
   b. To examine the health of teeth and surrounding structures
   c. To assess blood flow in the gums
   d. To measure the size of the oral cavity
2. **Which type of radiograph is commonly used to assess the overall structure of the jaw and teeth in a single image?**
   a. Panoramic radiograph
   b. Bitewing radiograph
   c. Periapical radiograph
   d. Cephalometric radiograph
3. **What is the primary advantage of Cone Beam CT (CBCT) in dental and maxillofacial imaging?**
   a. It provides detailed images of soft tissues
   b. It offers real-time imaging of the teeth and gums
   c. It allows 3D imaging for detailed bone structures and implants
   d. It eliminates the need for contrast agents
4. **In dental radiology, what is a bitewing radiograph typically used for?**
   a. To check for cavities between the teeth
   b. To examine the temporomandibular joint (TMJ)
   c. To measure the size of the oral cavity
   d. To assess the health of soft tissues
5. **Which of the following is a common concern with dental X-ray imaging?**
   a. High radiation exposure
   b. Inability to visualize cavities
   c. Difficulty in capturing images of teeth roots
   d. Poor image quality

Short Answer Questions

1. What are the different types of dental imaging techniques, and how are they used in diagnosing dental conditions?
2. How is dental imaging applied in various dental specialties such as orthodontics, periodontics, and endodontics?
3. What are maxillofacial imaging techniques, and how do they aid in the diagnosis and treatment planning for facial and jaw conditions?
4. What are the main safety concerns regarding radiation exposure in dental imaging, and how are they mitigated?
5. What are some future trends in dental and maxillofacial imaging, and how might emerging technologies improve patient care?

Answers to Critical Thinking Questions

1. (b); 2. (a); 3. (c); 4. (a); 5. (a)

References

1. Ahmadi, M., Irankhah, E., & Farhadi Nia, M. (2024). Transforming dental diagnostics with artificial intelligence: Advanced integration of ChatGPT and large language models for patient care. *arXiv*. http://arxiv.org/abs/2406.06616 (accessed on 23 May 2025).

2. Alburayh, A. A., Alosaimi, M., Alshumiesy, H., Alzahrani, A., Alkhars, A. S., Doaib, D. M., Alsaleh, M. H., et al. (2025). Assessment of public knowledge and perceptions toward radiation exposure risks in Saudi Arabia: A survey study. *Cureus, 17*. https://www.semanticscholar.org/paper/db930b620f36b25cf93210b4fe6355cc447f0f7b (accessed on 23 May 2025).

3. Al-Haj Husain, A., Bosshard, F. A., Schmidt, V., Stadlinger, B., et al. (2023). Imaging in third molar surgery: A clinical update. https://core.ac.uk/download/611956219.pdf (accessed on 23 May 2025).

4. Al-Haj Husain, A., Hainc, N., Stadlinger, B., Stojicevic, I., et al. (2024a). Advanced imaging and preoperative MR-based cinematic rendering reconstructions for neoplasms in the oral and maxillofacial region. https://core.ac.uk/download/636780806.pdf (accessed on 23 May 2025).

5. Al-Haj Husain, A., Valdec, S., Winklhofer, S., Piccirelli, M., Hainc, N., Kulcsár, Z., Essig, H., et al. (2024b). Dental magnetic resonance imaging: Practical insights and evaluation of benefits and drawbacks in dentistry and oral and maxillofacial surgery. *Swiss Dental Journal, 134*(4), 116–150. https://www.semanticscholar.org/paper/b297e22806ce3489643f821e5c50007bf9b2ea25 (accessed on 23 May 2025).

6. Alshomrani, F. (2024). Cone-beam computed tomography (CBCT)-based diagnosis of dental bone defects. *Diagnostics, 14*. https://www.semanticscholar.org/paper/af760686afe50319dd91b115bea0cf94ca55532e (accessed on 23 May 2025).

7. Altunkaynak, B., Demirel, O., Peker, I., & Yıldızer Keriş, B. (2017). Diagnostic accuracy of cone-beam computed tomography in detecting secondary caries under composite fillings: An *in vitro* study. https://core.ac.uk/download/228070132.pdf.

8. Annemans, L., Gemmel, P., Tack, P., & Victor, J. (2016). 3D-printing techniques in a medical setting: A systematic literature review. https://core.ac.uk/download/84043719.pdf (accessed on 23 May 2025).

9. Bagán Sebastián, J. V., & Gavaldá Esteve, C. (2016). Concept, diagnosis and classification of bisphosphonate-associated osteonecrosis of the jaws: A review of the literature. https://core.ac.uk/download/71060434.pdf (accessed on 23 May 2025).

10. Calazans, M. A. A., Ferreira, F. A. B. S., Alcoforado, M. L. M. G., dos Santos, A., Pontual, A. A., & Madeiro, F. (2022). Automatic classification system for periapical lesions in cone-beam computed tomography. *Sensors, 22*, 6481. https://doi.org/10.3390/s22176481.

11. Corazza, I., Giannetti, E., Bonzi, G., Lomb, A., Paolani, G., Santoro, M., Morrone, M. F., et al. (2023). Using cone beam computed tomography for radiological assessment beyond dento-maxillofacial imaging: A review of the clinical applications in other anatomical districts. *Current Medical Imaging*. https://www.semanticscholar.org/paper/c45c325d611ae500aeaa66f83f90f5d45b73e75f (accessed on 23 May 2025).

12. Cunha, A., Diederich, C., Hsu, I. C., & Mellis, M. (2016). Clinical applications of custom-made vaginal cylinders constructed using three-dimensional printing technology. https://core.ac.uk/download/323074295.pdf.

13. Dileep, A., & Kripal, K. (2019). Role of radiographic evolution: An aid to diagnose periodontal disease. https://core.ac.uk/download/322445031.pdf (accessed on 23 May 2025).

14. Divya, V. C., & Krishnakumar, S. (2024). Ethical aspects and applications of artificial intelligence in maxillofacial imaging. *Journal of Orofacial and Health Sciences*. https://www.semanticscholar.org/paper/11c6d608dbfc300e4c712f36085865b79850d37f (accessed on 23 May 2025).

15. Eastell, R., Rosen, C. J., Black, D. M., Cheung, A. M., Murad, M. H., & Shoback, D. (2019). Pharmacological management of osteoporosis in postmenopausal women: An Endocrine Society clinical practice guideline. *The Journal of Clinical Endocrinology & Metabolism, 104*, 1595–1622. https://doi.org/10.1210/jc.2019-00221.

16. Fujinaka, T. (2019). Comparison of osseointegration in piezoimplants versus cylindrical implants. https://open.bu.edu/bitstream/2144/37058/7/Fujinaka_bu_0017N_14844.pdf (accessed on 23 May 2025).

17. Ghali, S. R., Katti, G., Shahbaz, S., & Katti, C. (2017). Cone beam computed tomography: A boon for maxillofacial imaging. *Journal of Indian Academy of Oral Medicine and Radiology, 29*, 30. https://doi.org/10.4103/jiaomr.jiaomr_89_16.

18. Grandoch, A., Oeser, J., Zöller, J., Grosse Hokamp, N., Lichtenstein, T., & Neugebauer, J. (2023). Morphological studies to identify the nasopalatine and inferior alveolar nerve using a special head and neck MRI coil. *The Journal of Craniofacial Surgery, 34*, 1351–1356. https://www.semanticscholar.org/paper/e30ab7d8feac852b8a0f6531c86f0e4c0d169780 (accessed on 23 May 2025).

19. Haffner, D., Emma, F., Eastwood, D. M., Biosse Duplan, M., Bacchetta, J., Schnabel, D., Wicart, P., et al. (2019). Clinical practice recommendations for the diagnosis and management of X-linked hypophosphatemia. *Nature Reviews Nephrology, 15*, 435–455. https://doi.org/10.1038/s41581-019-0152-5.

20. Hewapathirane, R., & Jayatissa, P. (2023). A review of dental informatics: Current trends and future directions. *arXiv*. http://arxiv.org/abs/2307.03686 (accessed on 23 May 2025).

21. Jadhav, P., Sagar, D. G. V., Kumar, R., Jadhav, P., & Putta, S. (2021). Evaluation of dental radiographic imaging among insured population reporting for dental treatment–A retrospective study. *Scholars Journal of Dental Sciences*. https://www.semanticscholar.org/paper/f96e1e386d1ccea0449a120e65e21b9aebce2407 (accessed on 23 May 2025).

22. Kamburoğlu, K. (2025). Trends in dentomaxillofacial radiology. *World Journal of Radiology, 17.* https://www.semanticscholar.org/paper/f292f8d75f167cb78606eeee7adffca8bae6b591 (accessed on 23 May 2025).

23. Khalaf, K. (2014). Factors affecting the formation, severity and location of white spot lesions during orthodontic treatment with fixed appliances. https://core.ac.uk/download/29151177.pdf (accessed on 23 May 2025).

24. Kim, J., Danielak, M., Lee, D. H., Almaghrabi, B., Andreana, S., Kaenploy, J., Kareem, Y., et al. (2025). Advanced dental surgeries using fused filament fabrication and stereolithography printing: Case reports. *Clinical Advances in Periodontics.* https://www.semanticscholar.org/paper/79fd7e9fa8bc9fe95a008231989b1cf22a8523c4 (accessed on 23 May 2025).

25. Lungu, A. J., Swinkels, W., Claesen, L., Tu, P., Egger, J., & Chen, X. (2020). A review on the applications of virtual reality, augmented reality and mixed reality in surgical simulation: An extension to different kinds of surgery. *Expert Review of Medical Devices, 18*, 47–62. https://doi.org/10.1080/17434440.2021.1860750.

26. Marothiya, S., Patel, V., Jain, D., Agrawal, S., Joshi, S., & Pandey, V. C. (2019). Cone beam computed tomography in orthodontics: A literature review. *International Journal of Applied Dental Sciences, 5*, 233–240.

27. Mihailidis, D. N., Stratis, A., Gingold, E., Carlson, R., DeForest, W., Gray, J., Lally, M. T., et al. (2024). AAPM Task Group Report 261: Comprehensive quality control methodology and management of dental and maxillofacial cone beam computed tomography (CBCT) systems. *Medical Physics*. https://www.semanticscholar.org/paper/97bc73a46d3efde47ef5fea1bc5bf67fdd344b68 (accessed on 23 May 2025).

28. Miragall, M. F., Knoedler, S., Kauke-Navarro, M., et al. (2023). Face the future—Artificial intelligence in oral and maxillofacial surgery. https://core.ac.uk/download/592040362.pdf (accessed on 23 May 2025).

29. Misch, K. A., Sarment, D. P., & Yi, E. S. (2006). Accuracy of cone beam computed tomography for periodontal defect measurements. http://deepblue.lib.umich.edu/bitstream/2027.42/142101/1/jper1261.pdf (accessed on 23 May 2025).

30. Mozahab, A. (2025). Oral and maxillofacial radiology in orthodontics. *World Journal of Biology Pharmacy and Health Sciences*. https://www.semanticscholar.org/paper/f7c850572c85aaacd697af5a542f6ddbd238af39 (accessed on 23 May 2025).

31. Niemiec, B. A., Gawor, J., Nemec, A., Clarke, E., McLeod, K. C., Tutt, C., Gioso, M. A., et al. (2020). World Small Animal Veterinary Association global dental guidelines. *Journal of Small Animal Practice, 61*, 395–403. https://doi.org/10.1111/jsap.13113.

32. Park, H., Han, K., Choi, B., Yoon, H., An, H., Lee, J. S., & Kim, H. (2022). Ultra-low-dose intraoperative X-ray imager for minimally invasive surgery: A pilot imaging study. *Translational Lung Cancer Research, 11*, 588–599. https://www.semanticscholar.org/paper/bb1be554360b05963bcec4c65aef13c9e951629e (accessed on 23 May 2025).

33. Puang, Y. W., Suib, F. H., Chan, B. H. K., Nambiar, P., Subramaniam, R., Azmi, N. N., & Wong, G. R. (2024). Application of radiographic/imaging techniques: A questionnaire study involving private practitioners in Malaysia. *Malaysian Dental Journal, 47*(1), 13–19. https://doi.org/10.4103/MDJ.MDJ_2_24.

34. Sadeghi, S., Saeidi, N., Salehi, A., Attari, K., Irani, M. A. I., Aryanezhad, S. S., Malekzadeh, R., et al. (2025). Advances in radiation protection in oral and dental radiology: Pragmatic approaches and recent innovations. *Frontiers in Biomedical Technologies*. https://www.semanticscholar.org/paper/96a187f1bf1f7964473a2265a73bd0a0f16c2bb9 (accessed on 23 May 2025).

35. Scarfe, W., Azevedo, B., Toghyani, S., & Farman, A. G. (2017). Cone beam computed tomographic imaging in orthodontics. *Australian Dental Journal, 62*(Suppl 1), 33–50. https://www.semanticscholar.org/paper/946cdb6ad0407645c31875deed06434457e6cb70 (accessed on 23 May 2025).

36. Singh, S. B., Laishram, A., Thongam, K., & Singh, K. M. (2025). Automatic detection and classification of dental anomalies and tooth types using transformer-based YOLO with

GA optimization. *IEEE Access, 13*, 59326–59338. https://www.semanticscholar.org/paper/c2abffcb31935d5a97429ffe571f86384a8de38f (accessed on 23 May 2025).

37. Søreide, K., Hallet, J., Matthews, J. B., Schnitzbauer, A. A., Line, P. D., Lai, P. B. S., Gestal Otero, J. J., et al. (2020). Immediate and long-term impact of the COVID-19 pandemic on delivery of surgical services. *British Journal of Surgery, 107*, 1250–1261. https://doi.org/10.1002/bjs.11670.

38. Sungkaruk, P., Rungsiyakull, P., Chaijareenont, P., & Panyarak, W. (2024). Dental implant artifacts in MRI: Compatibility and considerations. *Oral Sciences Reports.* https://www.semanticscholar.org/paper/3d2abf1660932e279687743a86874c0fbb3ce29e (accessed on 23 May 2025).

39. Torres, M. H., Jagarlamudi, V., Eddin, H. S., Argueta, K. A., Maysan, S., & Wajid, M. (2024). The role of robotics in revolutionizing dental practice: A literature review. https://core.ac.uk/download/640070499.pdf (accessed on 23 May 2025).

40. Wadhawan, R., Singh, S. D., Tiwari, A. S., Bora, S. P., Khareliya, D. K., & Tamta, V. P. (2024). Beyond scalpel: Artificial intelligence in risk prediction and managing oro-facial trauma. *South Eastern European Journal of Public Health*, 1258–1277. https://doi.org/10.70135/seejph.vi.2879.

41. Zaman, M. U. (2024). Comparing radiation doses in CBCT and medical CT imaging for dental applications. *Journal of Pharmacy & Bioallied Sciences, 16*, S883–S885. https://www.semanticscholar.org/paper/b13d729fa2513df20fdf5147ea7ef159a113f634 (accessed on 23 May 2025).

PEDIATRIC IMAGING

12

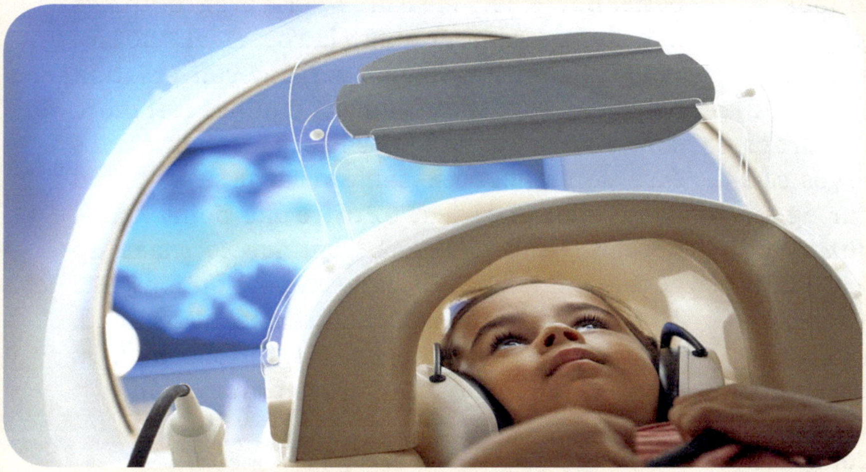

LEARNING OBJECTIVES

After studying this chapter, you will be able to:

1. Identify the various types of pediatric imaging.
2. Understand key safety considerations and protocols specific to imaging in pediatric patients.
3. Explore specialized pediatric imaging techniques.
4. Recognize common pediatric conditions diagnosed.
5. Examine the role of pediatric radiologists.
6. Investigate recent advancements and innovations in advances in pediatric imaging.

Introduction

Addressing the special needs of young patients in medical imaging has become a hot topic in medical circles these days. Pediatric imaging is changing all the time, and now it is mixing in new technology with creative techniques that are designed just for kids. It is important to note that children aren't just little adults – they have different bodies and energy levels that mean we have to look at things in a totally different way. In most cases, the chosen imaging methods should adapt to not only these physical differences, but also to how a child feels emotionally and mentally during the process. This essay, in a rather roundabout way, will dive into the many sides of pediatric imaging, showing both why it is important and how new advances help boost diagnostic precision and make the whole experience better for the patient. Pediatric imaging uses a range of tools, like X-rays, ultrasound, MRI, and CT scans, to uncover everything from broken bones to some pretty complicated genetic puzzles. Each of these options comes with its own set of wins and drawbacks, meaning doctors usually have to think carefully about which one fits best. For example, X-rays can deliver fast images for injuries, while CT scans serve up detailed, cross-sectional views that are key in serious conditions. Generally speaking, choosing the right technique calls on factors such as the level of radiation, the child's age, and the specific signs being looked at. Lately, there's been a push to cut down on radiation danger without losing out on clear, useful images, and this discussion will look at how making smarter choices in imaging tools increases the chances for better results in young patients. Using child-friendly procedures and methods to ease anxiety is also a crucial part of pediatric imaging. A kid's mood or nerves can mess with how well they cooperate during an exam, which in turn can lower the quality of the images produced. That's why many medical professionals are trying different tricks, like child-specific equipment, letting a parent stay nearby, or even using distraction techniques, to help create a more relaxed setting. These approaches underline a growing recognition that sometimes the softer, non-technical aspects play just as big a role in successful imaging as the hardware. In essence, pediatric imaging isn't only about the technical bits; it is equally about care and compassion, which together help to improve the overall healthcare experience for our little ones.

Definition of Pediatric Imaging

Pediatric imaging uses a mix of methods, X-rays, ultrasounds, MRI, and CT scans, to spot and keep an eye on health issues in kids. These tools, which originally came from adult imaging, get tweaked to suit the unique and ever-changing shapes of young bodies. Safety is a big deal here since children tend to be more sensitive to ionizing radiation, so doctors are always trying to balance clear diagnosis with careful risk management. Recent research even points to growing public health worries as the need for imaging increases, making it all the more important to fine-tune protocols and use techniques that fit different age groups just right. Doctors and healthcare teams also play a key role in talking with parents about imaging benefits and risks. Many parents worry about radiation, especially when tests are repeated, and lately there have been efforts to clear things up with easy-to-read handouts (Hwang et al., 2017). In most cases, when caregivers get targeted information, they tend to understand better how safety measures work, even for things like dental radiographs (Lurbe et al., 2016). This shift toward open, everyday conversation helps reassure them and lets families feel more confident about making choices for their child's care, sometimes the same risks get mentioned more than once just to drive the point home. Research and new tech continue to shake up pediatric imaging, too. Non-invasive options, like recent improvements in MRI and ultrasound, now let doctors examine conditions in kids without the heavy downsides of radiation.

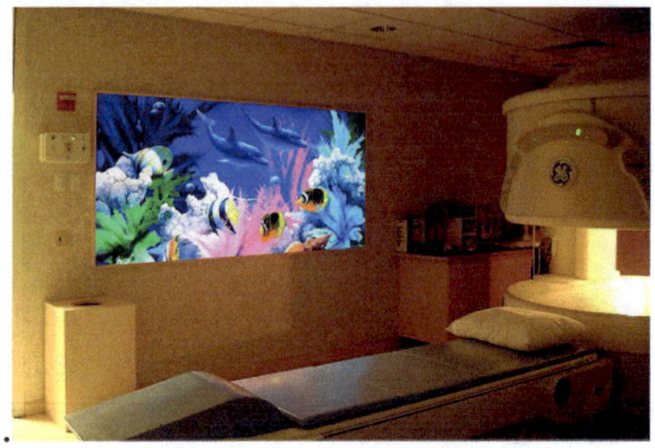

Figure 12.1. Pediatric radiology.

Source: By Glitzy queen00 at English Wikipedia - Transferred from en.wikipedia to Commons by Liftarn using CommonsHelper., Public Domain, https://commons.wikimedia.org/w/index.php?curid=12001366.

For instance, these advances can sometimes offer a full picture while sparing the delicate tissues that are still developing. Kids today come in with more complicated issues, which means that being able to mix precise diagnostic details with lower risks has become essential. As our ideas about kids' health keep evolving, so too does the way we handle pediatric imaging, showing once again that blending innovation with a focus on safety does set a new standard in caring for our younger patients (Hwang et al., 2017) (Figure 12.1).

Importance in Child Healthcare

Imaging tools play a big part in figuring out and keeping an eye on health issues in kids. Since children are still growing, any extra radiation becomes a real worry that needs careful thought. In most cases, it comes down to weighing the upsides against possible downsides. Research shows that even simple steps like handing out easy-to-read inserts can do a lot to help parents understand these risks. Often, when parents are more informed, they feel way more at ease and are ready to let their kids get the scans they need, making treatments work better overall. This mix of clear communication and careful assessment reminds us that easing radiation fears lets families focus more on a childs overall well-being and treatment options. How a risk is seen in kids' imaging depends on how info is passed along to caregivers. A lot of parents don't have all the details about safety rules and the small amounts of radiation common in regular tests. Studies generally note that once parents get simple explanations, say, about dental X-rays, their comfort can jump from around 30% acceptance to nearly 57%. By using the resources and tools offered by healthcare providers, families end up better equipped to make decisions. This improvement not only boosts the immediate care experience but also lays the groundwork for a longer-term trust and collaboration between medical staff and families, which helps make child care more well-rounded. Making sure parents understand why imaging matters in children's health isn't just about throwing facts around, it is about mixing education with honest conversation. It is crucial to strike a balance between knowing why these tests are needed and staying aware of possible risks. Generally speaking, healthcare providers need to share the info openly to build that essential confidence among parents. When radiation concerns are addressed directly and a bit casually, families tend to have a more positive experience overall. In the end, when parents are better clued in, it leads to earlier diagnoses and quicker, more effective treatments. These proactive, everyday steps highlight that informed caregivers are key players in achieving good health outcomes for kids.

Overview of Imaging Modalities

Imaging technology has shaken up pediatric care in recent years. Kids now benefit from tools like X-rays, ultrasound, CT scans, and MRI, each one pulling its own tricks. For example, X-rays and CT scans use ionizing radiation while MRIs rely on magnetic fields to reveal what's inside, all without any incision. Yet not every method is the same; children tend to be more sensitive to radiation, so keeping an eye on these different exposures is super important. In most cases, making the most of these scans means knowing how each works on a child's body, and striking that balance is key to getting the best outcomes in kid-focused imaging. Radiation is on everyone's radar these days, especially when small patients are involved. A number of studies, particularly in nuclear medicine, hint that many patients haven't quite wrapped their heads around the real risks tied to these diagnostic tests. It seems that without a full rundown of what's involved, patients might not truly grasp the benefits versus the risks of a scan. In most cases, a bit of extra education for both families and doctors can help clear up those grey areas. Better conversations about radiation safety can lead to more thoughtful risk management and, ultimately, a safer healthcare experience for children. Besides safety and awareness, the choice of which imaging method to use comes down to the clinical situation. Broken bones often get their first look with an X-ray, while ultrasound might be favored to check out soft tissue issues or monitor a baby's organ development. On the flip side, MRI is usually picked for neurological evaluations, thanks to its sharp soft tissue contrast. Each option comes with its own mix of accessibility, cost, and prep work, which can influence how they're woven into pediatric care. Tailoring the imaging approach to each child's needs helps build a more complete picture for diagnosis and treatment. Regularly rethinking how effective and safe each method is ensures that progress in pediatric imaging keeps up with the unique challenges of working with kids.

12.1. Types of Pediatric Imaging

Learning Outcome

1. Understand the role and applications of X-rays in pediatric imaging.
2. Explore using ultrasound in pediatric imaging.
3. Examine the applications of Magnetic Resonance Imaging (MRI) in pediatric diagnostics.

Technology has reshaped how kids are examined these days. Doctors now mix old and new tricks when checking on children. For instance, the classic X-ray, so widely used for spotting bone breaks, infections, or even birth defects, is still a go-to because it is easy to get and usually does the job well. But then there's the radiation risk, which can be a worry for little ones. That's why, in many cases, physicians end up using alternatives like ultrasound or MRI, especially when they need to see soft tissue details without exposing kids to extra radiation. Take ultrasound, for example. It works by using sound waves to produce images of what's happening inside, making it a handy and non-invasive option. This method not only sidesteps the issue of ionizing radiation but also comes with the perk of real-time imaging and portability. It is often used to check for problems such as developmental dysplasia of the hip, various gastrointestinal issues, or even some heart conditions, and its quick, patient-friendly nature can ease the anxiety of hospital visits. In many ways, the charm of ultrasound lies in its simplicity and adaptability to the lively, ever-changing environment of pediatric care. Then there are the cases where a deeper look is required. Advanced techniques like computed tomography (CT) and nuclear medicine step in for those trickier diagnoses. Generally speaking, CT scans collect detailed cross-sectional images that uncover things like tumors, subtle fractures, or infections that might escape simpler methods, though they too come with some risks. On the flip side, nuclear medicine uses tiny doses of radioactive tracers to give insights into organ function, tracking blood flow or metabolic activity, which proves especially useful when conditions like osteogenesis imperfecta are suspected (Jameson et al., 2013). In most cases, choosing the right blend of imaging techniques based on a child's unique needs is what truly makes pediatric care both dynamic and personalized.

12.1.1. X-Rays

Pediatric care has shifted a lot with new diagnostic tools, yet X-rays still play a central role in imaging. They give doctors a quick look at a child's health, revealing everything from broken bones to early signs of pneumonia, especially when time is critical. The fact that X-rays use ionizing radiation means the benefits have to be carefully balanced against the risks; (Donya et al., 2014) reminds us that making smart choices is key, particularly for children who are more delicate. This kind of thinking nudges healthcare providers to choose imaging methods carefully and stresses the importance of educating both doctors and parents about radiation exposure. Technology marches on, and now AI is making its mark in pediatric imaging by lending a digital boost to traditional X-ray techniques. Machine learning, for instance, speeds up image analysis and often nails the diagnosis, a trend that recent studies generally suggest is promising for spotting pneumonia in kids. Radiologists are teaming up with these smart tools, which signals a shift toward more efficient and reliable imaging. Alzayed (2023) points out that blending classic imaging methods with new tech could improve healthcare delivery for young patients. Even with all these perks, some issues still need attention. One major worry is the risk of overexposure to radiation, kids' developing tissues can be especially vulnerable. Healthcare professionals have to stay on their toes and follow the ALARA (As Low As Reasonably Achievable) principle when ordering scans. Also, access to cutting-edge imaging isn't equal everywhere, so care can be uneven across communities. Its essential that upgrades like AI-enhanced imaging reach all facilities, especially those in underserved areas. Tackling these challenges, it seems, could help create a pediatric imaging landscape that puts safety first while still capitalizing on the benefits of new technology (Figure 12.2).

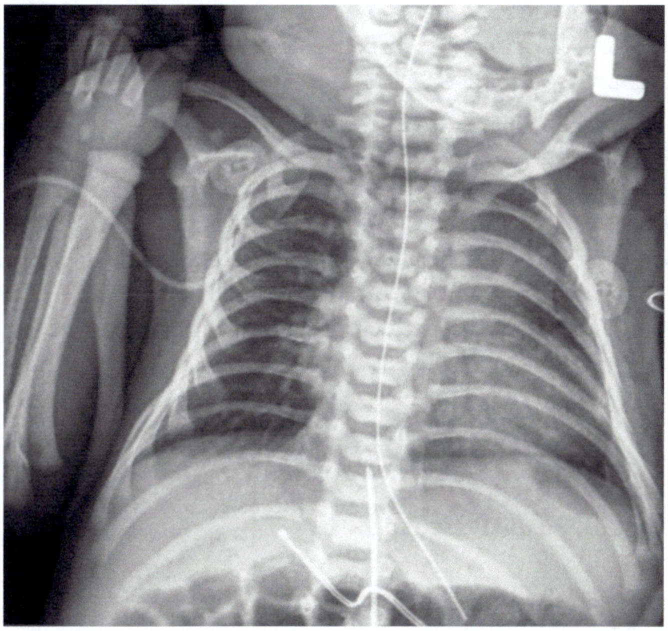

Figure 12.2. A normal pediatric bone X-ray image.

Source: https://www.itnonline.com/sites/default/files/field/image/FDAPediatricXrayGuidance2018.jpg.

12.1.2. Ultrasound

Ultrasound is a go-to method when assessing children's health, giving doctors a live inside look without putting young patients at risk. It is safe, no ionizing radiation here, and that non-invasive approach makes it a natural pick for kids. In many cases, its ability to capture real-time images helps doctors check for issues like appendicitis; a condition that frequently forces kids into emergency surgery. Generally speaking, research shows that ultrasound markers can be around 90%

accurate, which helps in sorting out the simpler cases from those that are far more complicated (Reismann et al., 2019). Overall, having skilled professionals who can decipher these images is key, especially when the symptoms aren't always crystal clear. Ultrasound also works wonders at spotting congenital anomalies, particularly those affecting the brain and other important organs. Identifying these issues early often makes a huge difference by paving the way for timely care. For, instance, congenital cytomegalovirus (cCMV) – a fairly common infection among newborns – can sometimes lead to serious problems like sensorineural hearing loss. Using ultrasound for screening and diagnosis in these cases not only underlines its role in prenatal settings but also shows why it is so valuable, even if we still lack universal screening programs for conditions like cCMV (Lazzarotto et al., 2020). New tech keeps pushing together clearer images and better detection, so even though there's a bit of repetition in its uses, it remains central in both pregnancy and infancy care. Adding to that, the blend of ultrasound with modern devices is reshaping pediatric diagnostics while moving beyond old, rigid methods. Thanks to portable gadgets and smarter imaging software, these exams are now performed in places ranging from small outpatient clinics to bustling emergency departments.

This increased accessibility can speed up both diagnosis and treatment, which is crucial when a kid faces a traumatic injury or sudden abdominal pain. And with AI gradually working its way into the process, making things both quicker and sharper, the need for invasive procedures is reduced, lessening discomfort for patients (Reismann et al., 2019). Ongoing research, with its occasional little uniqueness in presentation, continues to deepen our understanding of pediatric conditions, proving again that ultrasound remains indispensable in today's medical practice (Lazzarotto et al., 2020) (Figure 12.3).

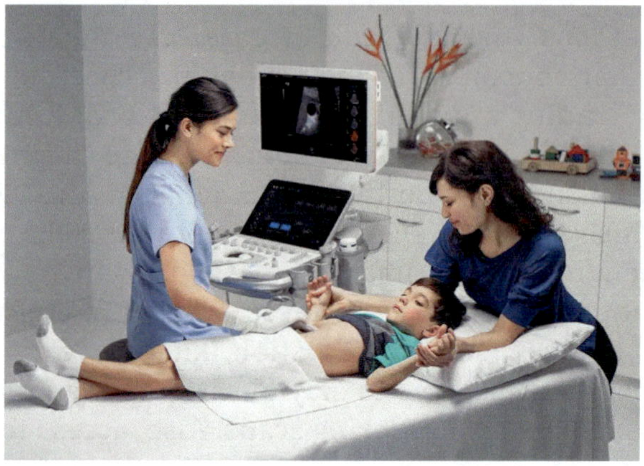

Figure 12.3. Pediatric ultrasound system.

Source: https://marketing.webassets.siemens-healthineers.com/c67e67555aa7dbcf/3008980e9687/v/7fc91627e9df/SHS_US_44939_18_4-3.jpg.

12.1.3. Magnetic Resonance Imaging (MRI)

Imaging tests matter a lot for kids, especially when things get complicated. MRI stands out since it gives clear contrast between tissues, a big help when checking out soft tissue details. In many cases, its major upside is that it skips ionizing radiation, which is crucial because young patients are generally more sensitive to such exposure. This safety point is important, particularly when kids need scans more than once. MRI's knack for capturing detailed anatomical images leads to spot-on diagnoses and quicker interventions, lowering risks tied to overlooked conditions. In pediatric radiology, meeting the unique challenges of young patients often means turning to advanced MRI methods. Diffusion-weighted imaging and dynamic contrast-enhanced MRI, for example, have proven themselves in tracking everything from tumors to metabolic issues. Take nonalcoholic fatty liver disease or biliary atresia: MRI can often zero in on these problems, helping guide treatment in real time. Additionally, some specialized protocols, say, magnetic resonance elastography, give doctors a way to judge how stiff the tissue is, which turns out to be quite handy for identifying hepatic fibrosis or other widespread tissue conditions. Generally speaking, these technical strides show just how much MRI continues to shape better outcomes in pediatric care. As pediatricians and radiologists lean more on MRI to get a complete diagnostic picture, the mix of these advanced techniques underscores its potential. A clear case is pediatric hepatobiliary imaging, where MRI plays a key part in checking out both congenital and structural issues. Techniques like fat quantification and T2 mapping have, in most cases, expanded what we can pull from these scans, leading to improved management of liver-related conditions in children. This multi-angled approach not only boosts patient care but also keeps clinical workflows running more smoothly by dishing out timely, precise info. Consequently, using MRI in imaging kids keeps growing, pushing research and everyday practices toward more effective strategies for uncovering and treating childhood ailments (Arthurs et al., 2019) (Figure 12.4).

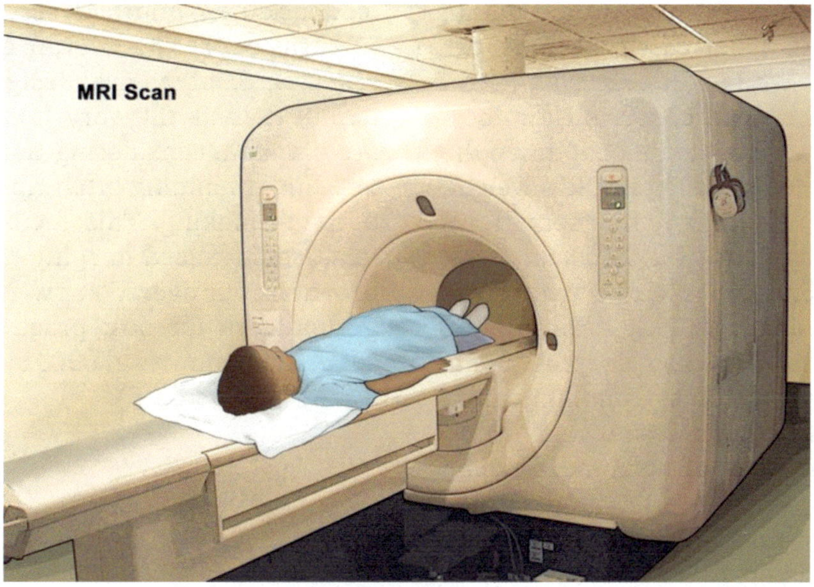

Figure 12.4. Pediatric magnetic resonance imaging.

Source: https://visualsonline.cancer.gov/retrieve.cfm?imageid=10188&dpi=72&fileformat=jpg.

Test Your Knowledge

1. How are X-rays used in pediatric imaging, and what precautions are taken to minimize radiation exposure?
2. What advantages does ultrasound offer in pediatric imaging compared to other imaging techniques?

12.2. Safety Considerations

Learning Outcome

1. Understand the radiation exposure in X-rays.
2. Explore using contrast agents.
3. Describe the guidelines for safe imaging practices.

Pediatric imaging isn't just about taking pictures, it is a tricky business where safety matters. Kids' bodies are growing and respond uniquely to radiation, so even a slight miscalculation can raise the stakes. In most cases, keeping the radiation dose low while still capturing useful images becomes a central concern. New tools appear on the scene, gadgets that cut down the dose and protocols adjusted for a child's weight, which hint at progress in ways that sometimes catch you off guard. It is also important that healthcare providers stay updated with these changes; that means not only training the imaging teams well but also keeping open, sometimes informal, lines of communication with families about what's at risk and what's to be gained. This kind of awareness, when spread around a bit unevenly in everyday practice, ultimately builds a more robust safety net in pediatric imaging. In decision-making for imaging procedures, parents hold a pretty critical role. Their choices tend to mix gut feelings with ethical concerns, so it is essential, generally speaking, to be as clear as possible about both the risks and the process. Studies, though not always perfectly consistent in their findings, seem to show that parents appreciate when the steps of imaging are explained in plain language, from the reasons behind a particular procedure to what outcomes to expect. Getting parents involved isn't just a way to build trust; it also smooths the path to informed consent and better adherence to safety protocols. Many parents even hint that the conversation should cover both emotional and physical aspects, sometimes repeating key points to ensure nothing is lost along the way. Involving them more fully helps bridge that sometimes awkward gap between medical necessity and natural parental worries, paving the way for safer imaging experiences. Sometimes, blending safety into the very design of pediatric imaging trials pays off big time. Aligning trial designs with what parents expect can make a surprising difference in recruitment and compliance rates. A frank, albeit sometimes uneven, discussion of risks tends to ease fears about imaging procedures and makes parents more willing to let their children participate. Strategies that emerge from listening to parent feedback often improve recruitment efforts and, in turn, boost the overall quality of imaging research. Safety in trial design isn't just a minor detail, it is at the very heart of how studies are planned, considering that parents' comfort and understanding often tip the scales in their decision-making. This focus not only pushes forward advanced imaging techniques but also broadens our overall knowledge, setting a solid groundwork for best practices in this critical zone (Benjamin et al., 2018; Duinkerken et al., 2020) (Figure 12.5).

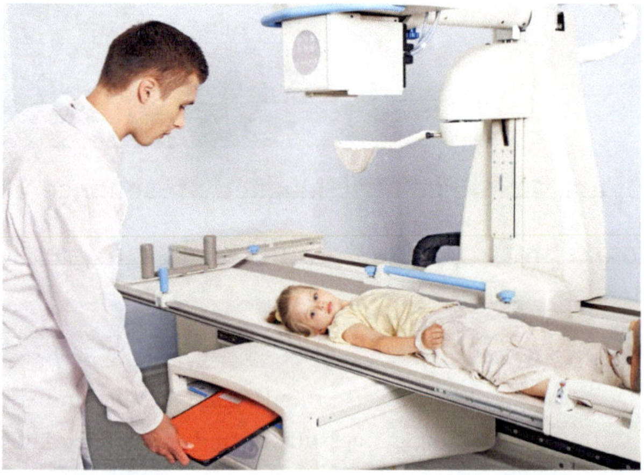

Figure 12.5. Pediatric Imaging Safety Considerations.

Source: https://www.nps.org.au/assets/7e622658cf465735-2bb738403b1a-Doctor_examinig_a_child_in_the_xray_room.jpg.

12.2.1. Radiation Exposure in X-Rays

Pediatric imaging technology is evolving fast, and with that, worries about radiation from X-rays have moved into focus. Kids' tissues, after all, tend to react more strongly to ionizing radiation, which means even small doses can matter a lot. Doctors often find themselves juggling between getting the diagnostic details they need and keeping radiation risks as low as possible. Since children's bodies are more delicate, the reason for ordering an X-ray needs to be looked at carefully, especially in areas like dentistry and orthopedics, where such imaging is common. In most cases, weighing the potential benefits against the possible harms is a key part of making sound medical choices today. Parents, too, are an important part of this conversation. The way risks from ionizing radiation get explained is sometimes pretty mixed up, which can impact how they give consent. Recent work even points out that many caregivers aren't fully clued in on what X-rays might mean for their kids, and often express a real uneasiness about these procedures. That discomfort usually comes from lingering worry over long-term health effects. One study, for example, showed that a simple educational handout made a big difference, after reading the material, many parents felt noticeably more comfortable with dental radiographs (Hwang et al., 2017). Clearly, a bit of clear-cut, everyday language can go a long way in easing concerns and guiding decisions. Even with all the technological advances, strict safety protocols still have to be front and center. On a global scale, experts agree that while X-rays are an indispensable part of modern medicine, it is critical to truly understand how much radiation is involved and what effects it might bring. Best practices aren't just about dialing down the radiation; sometimes they mean considering alternative imaging methods when the situation allows. Generally speaking, the ongoing debates among healthcare professionals stress the importance of carefully balancing risks and benefits. Bringing parents and caregivers into this dialogue only makes the overall approach stronger, reinforcing why evaluating radiation levels should always be a central part of clinical decision-making (Donya et al., 2014) (Figure 12.6).

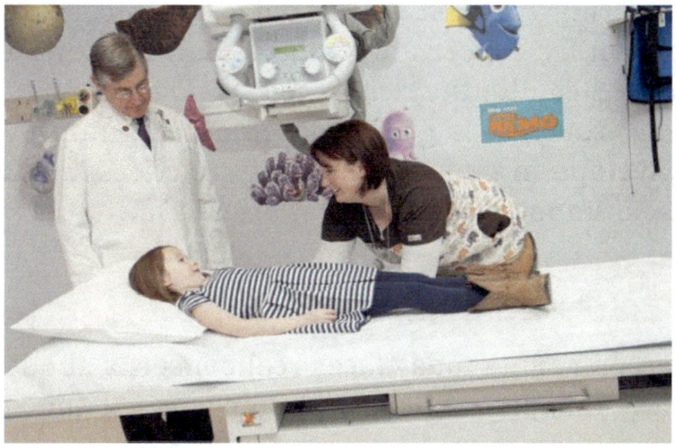

Figure 12.6. Pediatric imaging technology is evolving fast, and with that, worries about radiation from X-rays.

Source: https://med.virginia.edu/radiology/2017/06/15/what-is-an-x-ray-for-kids/.

12.2.2. Use of Contrast Agents

Pediatric imaging with contrast agents brings its own set of challenges and openings, often sparked by the clear physiological differences between kids and adults. Kids aren't just little adults, their organs and systems sometimes react unpredictably. Take, for example, the careful balancing act radiologists face: they need images sharp enough for diagnosis but must also dodge risks like sudden allergic responses or potential long-term issues from iodine-based contrasts. In most cases, weighing the dose against the child's weight and age is key; even a slight miscalculation could tip the balance between clarity and safety. Different imaging methods call for different contrast materials. MRI, for instance, often uses gadolinium-based agents to make tissues pop, while CT scans lean on iodinated contrasts to sketch out blood vessels and organs. Each agent seems to come with its own mix of benefits and worries, meaning that picking one isn't always straightforward. Since many young patients present with tricky challenges, tumors, congenital uniqueness, or similar issues, it becomes pretty critical to know how these agents mingle with varying tissues. Using cutting-edge imaging techniques alongside the right contrast can boost the overall outcome in pediatric radiology. The field is always shifting, with new contrast agents and techniques aiming to iron out old safety concerns from traditional methods. Lately, innovations like low-osmolarity and iso-osmolar contrast agents have started lowering risks, such as contrast-induced kidney problems and allergic reactions, which are of particular concern in children. Some studies even suggest that tweaking the composition of these agents can tip the risk-benefit ratio in a more favorable direction. Ongoing research into optimizing how contrast is given and embracing improved imaging methods promises to keep pushing the envelope in pediatric imaging practices, a reminder of why staying on top of fresh developments is so important (Hwang et al., 2017).

12.2.3. Guidelines for Safe Imaging Practices

Kids' imaging today faces real concerns about radiation, so strict safety rules have become a must. New imaging tools are popping up all the time, clinicians now need to dial back on radiation, keeping in mind that young bodies are simply more sensitive. Studies say that when parents and caregivers get solid, understandable info, they often feel a lot more comfortable letting doctors do the exams (Hwang et al., 2017).

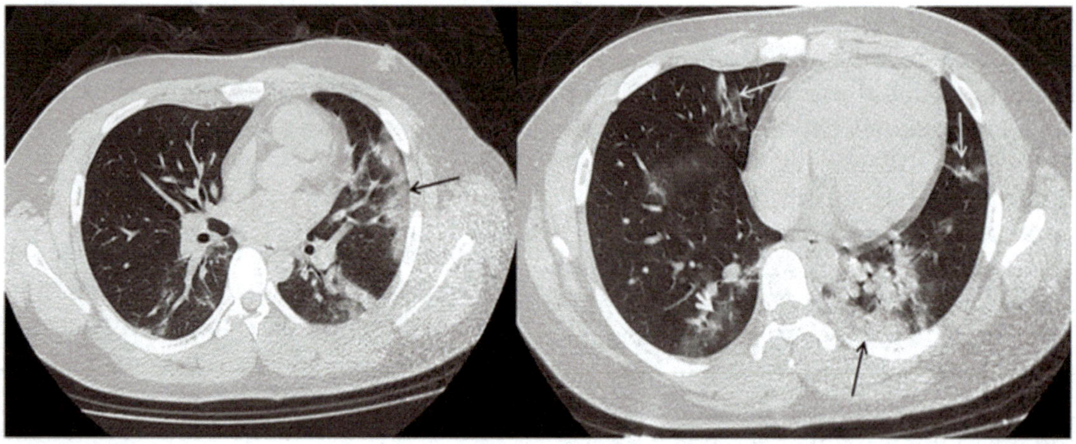

Figure 12.7. 15-year-old boy infected with the original SARS-CoV-2. Initial unenhanced chest CT scans show multiple subpleural consolidations (black thin arrow) accompanied by ground glass opacities (white short arow) in lingual segment of left upper lobe and posterior basal segment of lower left lobe. Streaky opacities (white long arrow) are shown in right middle lobe and lingual segment of left upper lobe. CT findings were assigned CT severity score of 10.

Source: Lin B, Xu X, Shen Z, Huang P, Gao Y, Liu J, Xie Z, Zhao T, Xia J, Lv J, Ren D, Zheng H, Wang X, Hu M, Ruan G and Zhang M (2023) Clinical and radiological characteristics of pediatric COVID-19 before and after the Omicron outbreak: a multi-center study. Front. Pediatr. 11:1172111. doi: 10.3389/fped.2023.1172111.

In many cases, having easy-to-digest resources right in pediatric clinics helps everyone decide with confidence, cutting down unnecessary worries about radiation. At the same time, talking about risks only scratches the surface. Many hospitals are setting up broader, down-to-earth systems to ensure imaging is done safely. It isn't just about outlining radiation hazards; it is about having real, practical procedures in place, take clinical ultrasound (CUS), for instance, where departments need to adopt and stick to their protocols. Most places are rolling out training programs that aim to boost the skills of healthcare workers so they can perform these exams safely and accurately. Then there's the follow-up, think routine quality checks and occasional audits, to keep standards high and patients safe (Strony et al., 2018). Altogether, these measures work together to create an atmosphere where imaging is both effective and secure. In the end, making pediatric imaging safe is a team effort among doctors, parents, and educators alike. Generally speaking, having everyone involved means that safety rules are more likely to be understood and followed across the board. Medical professionals, for their part, have to keep up with new tech and adjust their methods based on the latest research, and that goes a long way in reassuring families about necessary procedures. Ongoing research and education, albeit sometimes a bit messy in the details, play a vital role in ensuring that the benefits of pediatric imaging keep outweighing the risks (Hwang et al., 2017; Strony et al., 2018) (Figure 12.7).

Test Your Knowledge

1. Why is it essential to minimize radiation exposure in pediatric imaging, and what methods are used to achieve this?
2. What role do shielding and alternative imaging techniques, such as ultrasound or MRI, play in ensuring safety during pediatric imaging procedures?

12.3. Pediatric Imaging Techniques

Learning Outcome

1. Understand the role of sedation and anesthesia in imaging.
2. Identify specialized equipment for children.
3. Explore techniques for reducing motion artifacts.

Modern imaging in pediatrics has come a long way with new tech pushing boundaries. Cutting radiation exposure while still getting precise diagnoses is a big deal, approaches like ultrasound and MRI are favored because they skip those risky ionizing rays. Kids' tissues tend to be more sensitive than adult ones, so using these non-invasive methods right from the start is key. In most cases, doctors are opting for these safer options, which not only reduce potential harm but also help boost the overall quality of care. When imaging is needed, the method chosen often comes down to the specific situation. CT scans, for example, are sometimes used when quick results and high-detail images are necessary, say, in instances of trauma or more complex issues. They deliver crisp images fast, giving clinicians the details they need, but the radiation risk remains a significant worry that demands careful thought. Recent initiatives in pediatric radiology are tweaking CT protocols by cutting doses and fine-tuning age-based settings to strike a better balance between clear diagnostics and radiation safety (Downie et al., 2007). There's also a move toward more advanced techniques that open entirely new diagnostic doors. Functional imaging methods, like fMRI and DTI, offer insights far beyond simple anatomy, letting clinicians peek into brain activity and connectivity. This is especially groundbreaking in pediatric care, where spotting developmental shifts and potential problems early can change treatment paths. As these methods evolve, they're likely to reveal more about the subtle changes happening in growing bodies, pointing to an optimistic future focused on sharper precision, reduced risks, and improved health outcomes for kids (Downie et al., 2007).

12.3.1. Sedation and Anesthesia in Imaging

In imaging young patients, sedatives and anesthesia make a big difference in how smoothly the process goes. There are plenty of challenges popping up when trying to keep sedation safe and effective for kids. Sedatives, for example, need to be adjusted to fit each childs age, weight, and prior health history – it is not a one-size-fits-all deal. Interestingly, sedation in kids isn't only the realm of anesthesiologists; doctors in other fields like radiology and emergency care often get involved too. Local rules and training requirements change from place to place, and in most cases, making sure everyone is properly trained and follows evidence-based guidelines is absolutely crucial, especially as the global sedation community works toward more standardized methods (Gozal et al., 2010). Different imaging tests call for different approaches in sedation and anesthesia. Magnetic resonance imaging (MRI), for example, is a crucial tool because it shows off excellent tissue details without using ionizing radiation.

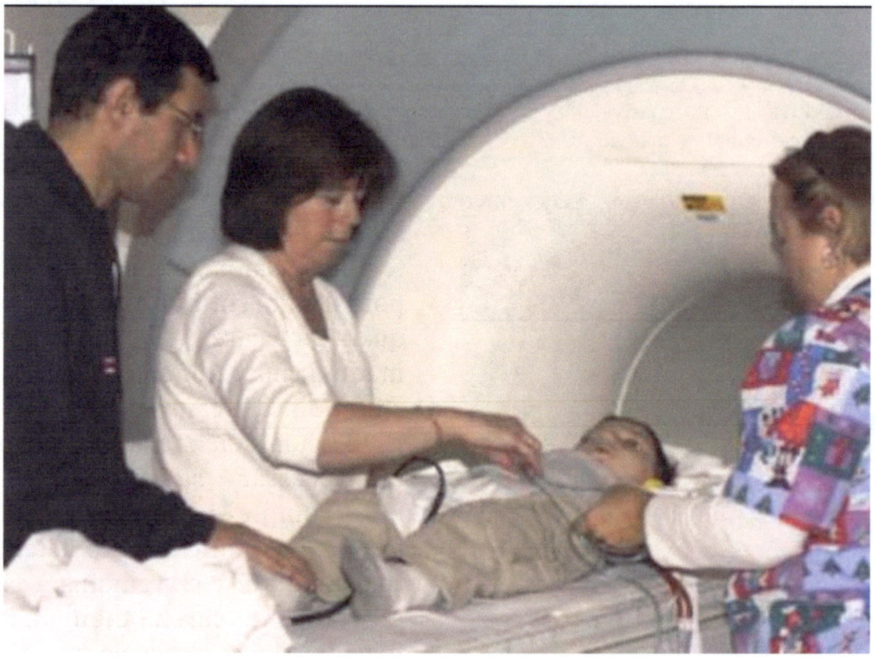

Figure 12.8. Using sedation and general anesthesia in pediatric patients undergoing magnetic resonance imaging examinations.

Source: https://i.ytimg.com/vi/JvncSMS_7nk/hqdefault.jpg.

Yet, using MRI with children can be tricky, as issues like claustrophobia and the need to lie still for long stretches arise. In these situations, sedation becomes key to reducing movement and easing anxiety. In Canada, there's generally a strong emphasis on telling patients and caregivers about such potential risks – a practice that brings ethical concerns into the conversation alongside clinical ones. Health professionals, while juggling these challenges, often find that clear, well-outlined guidelines can boost both patient safety and overall satisfaction (Downie et al., 2007). At the end of the day, a team effort among healthcare providers stands out as the best way to improve sedation and anesthesia practices in pediatric imaging. This cooperative spirit helps ensure that the unique emotional and developmental needs of children aren't lost in the process. Involving a mix of experts, from radiologists and anesthesiologists to nurses, creates an atmosphere where shared experience counts – a factor that is crucial for effective sedation. And, as research continues and guidelines are refined, it is clear that keeping up with new imaging and sedation techniques remains essential. Overall, the combined efforts of medical professionals everywhere can lead to better outcomes in pediatric imaging, benefiting not only the patients but also their families (Downie et al., 2007; Gozal et al., 2010) (Figure 12.8).

12.3.2. Specialized Equipment for Children

Specialized imaging devices made just for kids mark a real turning point in pediatric care. Kids are not just miniature adults – their bodies are unique in size and makeup, and as a result, standard machines often fall short. In everyday practice, many devices struggle with issues like size mismatches, radiation worries, and the simple fact that little ones just can't stay perfectly still. That's why hospitals are now turning to age-appropriate CT scanners and MRI machines built with smaller openings. Often, this kind of dedicated equipment not only boosts the accuracy of diagnoses but also eases discomfort and anxiety, creating a friendlier and more inviting setting for young patients. Keeping safety front and center, especially in terms of radiation exposure, matters in pediatric imaging. In most cases, these specialized machines come equipped with smart, low-dose options that cut down on radiation without sacrificing image quality. It is interesting to see how some devices even have automatic exposure control that tweaks settings based on a kid's size and age – a detail that goes a long way in protecting vulnerable patients. Generally speaking, by fine-tuning these parameters and following careful protocols, healthcare teams manage to keep the balance between clear images and minimal risk, addressing the concerns that many doctors and parents share about conventional methods. It is also important to remember that the experience isn't just about technical safety – the emotional side plays a big role too. Many kids find imaging procedures rather daunting, and a harsh, clinical setting can only add to their anxiety.

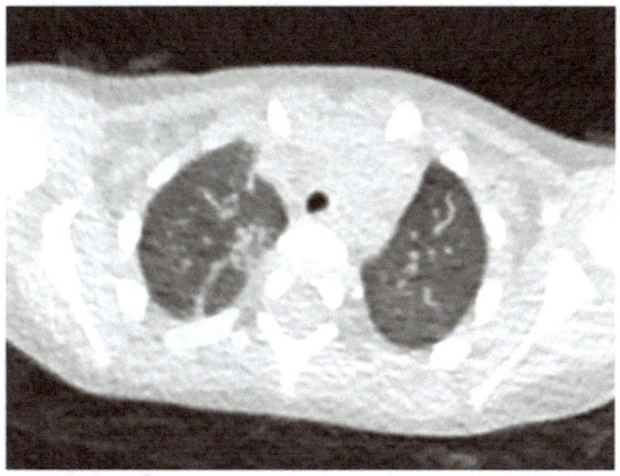

Figure 12.9. 22-month-old boy infected with the Omicron variant of SARS-CoV-2. Unenhanced chest CT scans show consolidation in the apical segment of the right upper lobe. CT findings were as-signed CT severity score of 1.

Source: Lin B, Xu X, Shen Z, Huang P, Gao Y, Liu J, Xie Z, Zhao T, Xia J, Lv J, Ren D, Zheng H, Wang X, Hu M, Ruan G and Zhang M (2023) Clinical and radiological characteristics of pediatric COVID-19 before and after the Omicron outbreak: a multi-center study. Front. Pediatr. 11:1172111. doi: 10.3389/fped.2023.1172111.

By designing equipment with kid-friendly touches – like machines painted in bright colors or even ones with built-in entertainment systems – hospitals help ease nervousness. Staff who know how to engage with children, sometimes even using a light-hearted tone, further reduce the stress of the process. Overall, blending good technology with a warm, comforting atmosphere makes these necessary procedures a lot easier for everyone involved, ultimately leading to better outcomes and more confident families (Figure 12.9).

12.3.3. Techniques for Reducing Motion Artifacts

Pediatric imaging is facing a familiar foe, those pesky motion artifacts, and new methods are emerging that mix old imaging tricks with fresh artificial intelligence (AI) ideas. A burst of innovation now has individuals blending low-dose CT scans with quick, 60-second PET images. These short bursts, surprisingly, yield images nearly as detailed as those from lengthy sessions. In most cases, this means doctors can get a reliable picture without keeping a kid still for too long, and it helps cut down on sedation, which is a boon considering the messiness of motion blur in active youngsters (Zhang et al., 2024). Sometimes it feels almost casual how combining these two modes shakes up the traditional, rigid imaging workflow.

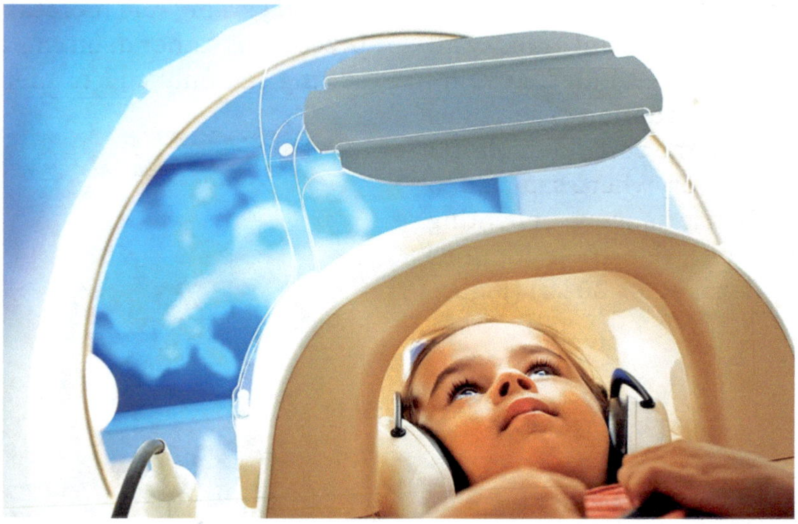

Figure 12.10. Pediatric imaging is facing a familiar foe, those pesky motion artifacts, and new methods are emerging that mix old imaging tricks with fresh artificial intelligence (AI).

Source: https://www.itnonline.com/sites/default/files/field/image/Pediatric_Imaging_MRI_Philips_Ingenia_PR-copy.jpg.

Switching gears a bit, another neat technique is real-time MRI (rt-MRI). This method works at speeds that rival ultrasound, capturing nearly 50 frames per second. Such rapid-fire image acquisition curtails the chances for those unwanted motion errors (Zhang et al., 2024). Generally speaking, the ability to snap so many images so fast leads to a 40% reduction in the need for sedation in children under six, which parents and healthcare teams are quick to welcome. They appreciate how this method not only shows what's possible and what isn't in pediatric imaging but also makes it easier to communicate expectations, even if the process isn't perfect every time

(Hirsch et al., 2023). Overall, these advanced approaches show a steady commitment to improving both image quality and the overall experience for young patients. By interweaving AI and quick-response imaging, the field is gradually shifting away from standard, drawn-out protocols toward a more patient-friendly future. Fewer sedatives, safer procedures, and a gentler atmosphere mean that, in most cases, both the diagnostic accuracy and the care environment get a solid boost. As the technology and techniques continue to evolve, and yes, sometimes with a bit of inconsistency, the prospects for pediatric imaging are looking brighter than ever (Hirsch et al., 2023) (Figure 12.10).

Test Your Knowledge

1. How does using sedation or anesthesia in pediatric imaging procedures differ from adult imaging techniques?
- What factors influence the choice of imaging technique for pediatric patients, particularly in emergency situations?

12.4. Diagnosing Common Pediatric Conditions

Learning Outcome

1. Understand the role of medical imaging in diagnosing respiratory disorders in children.
2. Explore how medical imaging is used to diagnose and assess gastrointestinal issues in pediatric patients.
3. Examine the managing Musculoskeletal Injuries in children.

Pediatric diagnosis hinges on top-notch imaging methods. Kids aren't just little adults, their bodies need imaging that fits their unique growth and structure. X-rays, MRIs, and ultrasounds jump in here, not in some rigid textbook way, but as versatile, on-the-fly tools. In cases when a child shows severe breathing trouble or hints of fluid build-up, an ultrasound can be a game changer, kicking off rapid treatment steps (Chong et al., 2020). Many pediatric experts now generally favor these approaches, and, arguably, a push for more uniform scanning protocols is slowly, but surely, taking shape. In congenital issues, things can get a bit more tangled, too. Take proximal focal femoral deficiency (PFFD) for example; it is that rare situation where the thigh bone is partly or completely underdeveloped in newborns. Early scans, often a prenatal ultrasound, can pick up these anomalies, giving families and doctors a heads-up to plan surgeries or rehab later on (D'Ambrosio et al., 2016). It is like combining puzzle pieces from imaging with a careful clinical check, ensuring that even the trickier congenital cases get the right kind of attention. Then there are everyday challenges like appendicitis or fractures, which demand their own subtle imaging tweaks. Kids don't always show the usual symptoms seen in adults, a fact that calls for age-fit scanning tactics. High-quality ultrasound, for instance, has proven pretty effective at identifying appendicitis among the young; it slashes the need for invasive tests and cuts down on unnecessary radiation exposure (Chong et al., 2020). Overall, as imaging tech keeps marching forward, personalized diagnostic plans are easing worry for both patients and families, making the overall care experience a touch more reassuring and, dare we say, a bit less clinical.

12.4.1. Respiratory Disorders

Respiratory disorders in kids come with unique challenges in diagnosis – after all, a child's breathing system isn't just a mini version of an adult's. In many cases, identifying issues like obstructive sleep-disordered breathing (SDB) early can change the game for treatment outcomes. Recent reviews suggest that mixing hands-on clinical checks with questionnaires and objective tests is pretty crucial for spotting SDB in young patients. Polysomnography (PSG) is often touted as the gold standard; yet its intricate setup and higher price tag mean it is not always practical on a wide scale. At the same time, methods such as respiratory polygraphy offer a more accessible option for monitoring respiration, even if comparison studies in pediatric settings remain somewhat limited. Overall, the push for fresh and innovative diagnostic strategies in respiratory care keeps urging further research and continuous development. In the world of pediatric imaging, Cone Beam Computed Tomography (CBCT) has started to stand out as a promising tool for evaluating upper airway conditions. Its detailed imaging is filling some of the gaps left by traditional techniques, which often struggle with providing the needed spatial resolution and specificity for accurate respiratory assessment. Clinicians can use CBCT to pick up subtle obstructions or abnormal structures that might contribute to breathing issues – findings noted in several recent studies and clinical observations. Generally speaking, its application in conditions like SDB seems to support more targeted interventions and tailored treatment approaches. This technology not only enriches the diagnostic process but also paves the way for improved patient management, hinting at new standards in evaluating pediatric respiratory issues. Looking forward, the management of respiratory disorders in children is set to benefit from integrating advanced imaging with solid, evidence-based practices. Merging state-of-the-art techniques with more traditional methods seems likely to provide a clearer, more holistic view of how these disorders affect young patients. There's growing interest in exploring laboratory biomarkers and radiological findings as potential complements to current diagnostic tools, an area that is, in most cases, ripe for further investigation. Increased investment in research and pediatric clinical trials will be key to standardizing these approaches in everyday practice. By nurturing collaboration among healthcare professionals and making room for innovative ideas, the goal remains to boost the quality of care for children dealing with these challenges, ultimately supporting their long-term well-being. The road ahead is clear: embracing new technological advances will let the pediatric healthcare community dramatically improve how respiratory disorders are diagnosed and managed (Figure 12.11).

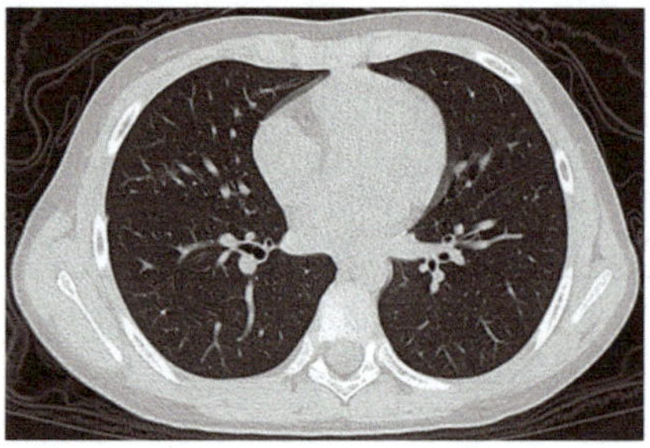

Figure 12.11. 8-year-old boy infected with the Omicron variant of SARS-CoV-2. Unenhanced chest CT scans show ground glass opacity in the right middle lobe. CT findings were assigned CT severity score of 1.

Source: Lin B, Xu X, Shen Z, Huang P, Gao Y, Liu J, Xie Z, Zhao T, Xia J, Lv J, Ren D, Zheng H, Wang X, Hu M, Ruan G and Zhang M (2023) Clinical and radiological characteristics of pediatric COVID-19 before and after the Omicron outbreak: a multi-center study. Front. Pediatr. 11:1172111. doi: 10.3389/fped.2023.1172111.

12.4.2. Gastrointestinal Issues

Figuring out gut problems in kids isn't simple at all and often pushes doctors to use all kinds of imaging tools. Kids can show vague signs when dealing with issues like inflammatory bowel troubles, reflux, or even some birth-related abnormalities in their digestive system, so sometimes a mix of ultrasounds, MRIs, and CT scans is needed just to get a clue what's going on. For example, an MRI, often handy for checking out soft tissues, can help sort out whether the pain is due to swelling or maybe a blockage. And since too much radiation is a big worry in children, non-invasive scans usually take priority to keep them safe while still offering solid info, in many cases, even if the approach ends up feeling a bit all over the place. New developments in scanning methods have given us a better chance at spotting these digestive issues in youngsters. Lately, techniques like contrast ultrasound and even functional MRI (yes, you read that right) are providing more in-depth looks at not only the structure but also how the gut is working. When you're dealing with things like motility troubles, where the gut's movement gets a bit off-kilter, watching how things change in real time can reveal stuff that a single static image might miss. Generally speaking, these tech leaps lead to sharper diagnoses and treatment plans that are more on target; they also remind healthcare providers that staying updated with new imaging tricks is just part of the job. With diagnostic methods changing so fast these days, it is important to settle on a clear, standard approach when imaging young patients with gut issues. Experts sometimes come together to hash out what exactly counts as a condition, take invasive fungal diseases, for instance, which then shapes how pediatric cases are looked at. Even though these classifications usually focus on kids with weak immune systems, the updated terms of "proven" and "probable" invasive fungal diseases show why having a thorough imaging process and clear criteria is key to avoiding mistakes in diagnosis. Bringing together pediatric gastroenterologists, radiologists, and other specialists, often in a somewhat collaborative, hand-in-glove kind of way, can boost the accuracy of these evaluations, making sure that kids get the best care possible (Donnelly et al., 2019) (Figure 12.12).

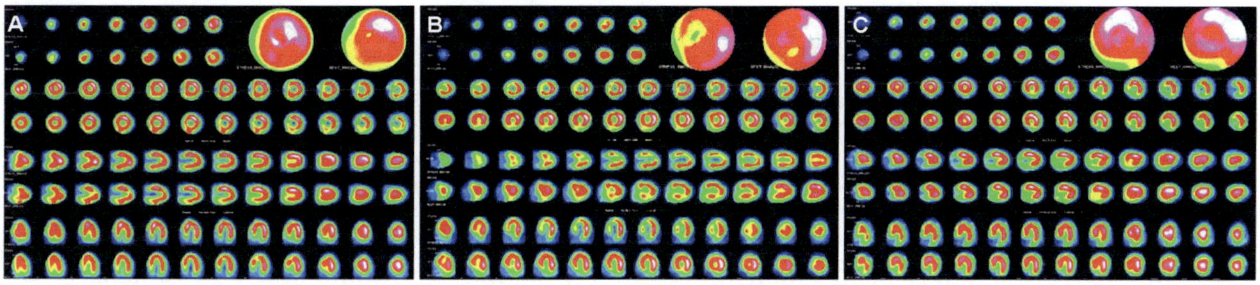

Figure 12.12. Overview of nuclear imaging in pediatric cardiology. CT, computed tomography; PET, positron emission tomography; SPECT, single-photon emission computed tomography.

Source: Venet M, Friedberg MK, Mertens L, Baranger J, Jalal Z, Tlili G and Villemain O (2022) Nuclear Imaging in Pediatric Cardiology: Principles and Applications. Front. Pediatr. 10:909994. doi: 10.3389/fped.2022.909994.

12.4.3. Musculoskeletal Injuries

Kids often get bone and muscle injuries, so it's important to get how their growing bodies differ from adults. Their skeletons are busy growing and behave in ways you wouldn't expect from mature bones. Trauma can hit them differently, and if things aren't spotted or fixed quickly, the results might stick around for a long time. Growing bones might react in unusual or subtle ways to things like breaks or sprains, meaning that when doctors use imaging, it has to be tuned to catch these little details – a tweak that helps avoid misdiagnoses and keeps care on point for young patients (Clark et al., 2013). Looking at these injuries isn't a plain-vanilla process. Doctors usually start with X-rays to check for clear signs of fractures. But really, if there's something off – like a soft tissue issue or a stress fracture that slips past on an X-ray– then MRIs or even ultrasounds come into play. Each tool kind of plays its own role in a layered approach; sometimes, you need a mix to get the full picture. The choice of what imaging to use depends on many things: how old the child is, what exactly went wrong, and the overall clinical snapshot, which helps shape a care plan that feels just right for each kid (Clark et al., 2013). When injuries in kids aren't caught early, the consequences can be pretty serious. Over time, missed or poorly managed injuries might lead to growth hiccups or ongoing issues with how the child functions day-to-day. Research generally shows that understanding exactly how a growing skeleton ties in with injury risk is key for anyone in pediatric care. Spotting injury patterns early – through targeted imaging – opens the door for treatments that work fast and well. Overall, shining a light on these injuries and the role of imaging not only helps prevent long-term issues but also stresses the need to keep the focus right where it belongs – on the kid (Clark et al., 2013) (Figure 12.13).

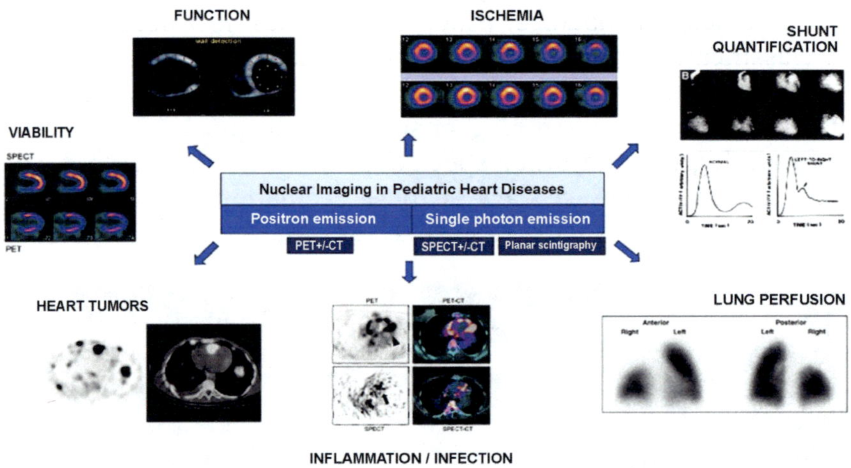

Figure 12.13. Lung perfusion planar scintigraphy. **(A)** Normal lung perfusion scintigraphy. **(B)** Pulmonary perfusion defect in the right upper lobe in patient with pulmonary embolism.

Source: Venet M, Friedberg MK, Mertens L, Baranger J, Jalal Z, Tlili G and Villemain O (2022) Nuclear Imaging in Pediatric Cardiology: Principles and Applications. Front. Pediatr. 10:909994. doi: 10.3389/fped.2022.909994.

Test Your Knowledge

1. How does imaging assist in diagnosing congenital conditions such as heart defects or neural tube defects in infants?
2. What role does imaging play in the diagnosis of respiratory issues like pneumonia or asthma in pediatric patients?

12.5. Role of Pediatric Radiologists

Learning Outcome

1. Understand the training and specialization requirements for pediatric radiologists.
2. Examine the importance of collaboration between pediatric radiologists.
3. Recognize the significance of accurate imaging and diagnosis in ensuring effective treatment for pediatric patients.

Kids' healthcare demands a different kind of imaging altogether, and pediatric radiologists are at the heart of it. They don't just read scans, they get that children's bodies change in ways that aren't found in adults. Often, their approach involves mixing modern tech with a practical sense of how young bodies work, which means they frequently tweak imaging techniques on the fly. It is not simply about fancy equipment; it is about matching the scan to how a child is growing. In many cases, identifying issues early hinges on this flexible, hands-on expertise that these specialists bring to the table. Teamwork plays a huge part in what these radiologists do. They routinely team up with pediatricians, surgeons, and other experts, chiming in with fresh perspectives during case reviews that can evolve into impromptu brainstorming sessions. Ideas often bounce back and forth, with imaging protocols and best practices coming up more than once in conversation, because, honestly, refining these details is key. The collaborative vibe in their circles helps build an overall understanding of a child's situation, and that shared knowledge sometimes even spills over into research efforts. All this joint effort shows that when experts pool their insights, the result is top-notch care for kids. Beyond the day-to-day patient interactions, pediatric radiologists are busy setting the groundwork for evidence-based care practices. Organizations like the European Society of Pediatric Radiology (ESPR) are deep into research that sharpens imaging techniques while keeping radiation exposure low, a big deal since kids are extra sensitive. The ESPR's Strategic Research Agenda paints a picture of how diagnosis, classification, and treatment evaluation should come together, generally speaking. These doctors push for methods that cut down on harmful exposure without losing out on the details needed for a good diagnosis. This drive not only ups patient outcomes but also fills in some of the big gaps in our understanding of pediatric imaging (Arthurs et al., 2019). With that ongoing commitment to excellence, they're pretty much spearheading new standards for care in children's imaging (Ajzen et al., 2007).

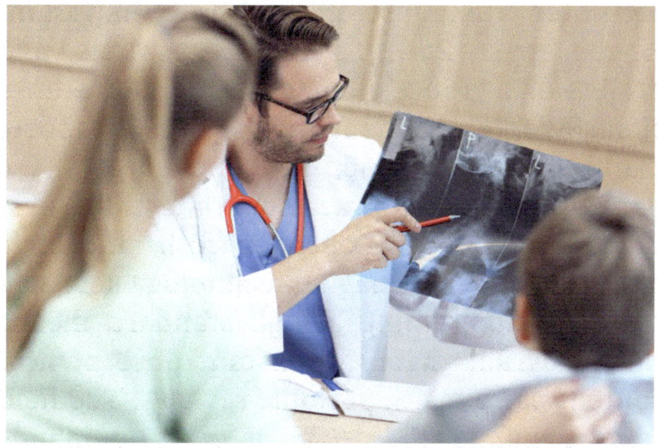

Source: https://pedsondemand.com/wp-content/uploads/2021/07/AdobeStock_225014600.jpeg.

12.5.1. Training and Specialization

Pediatric imaging isn't a one-size-fits-all area – it demands training that's both rigorous and tailored. This imaging isn't just about applying standard radiology principles; it is about picking up on the subtle developmental changes and unique risks that come with different techniques. Research shows that residents and those in further specialization often vary in their abilities, a trend that links back to how different schools cook up their teaching methods. For example, the Brazilian College of Radiology's In-training exam generally finds that residents score higher than their subspecialty peers, hinting at a possible shortfall in the pediatric focus that some advanced tracks offer (Ajzen et al., 2007). Training focused on pediatric imaging is a bit of a mixed bag – a blend of theory and hands-on practice specifically made for kids. Some programs throw in simulations and interactive exercises alongside real-world experiences, letting trainees get a feel for the unique anatomical uniqueness and physiological details of young patients. You have to nail down things like proper positioning and radiation care; it is as much about refining technical skills as it is about genuinely connecting with families. In many cases, regular checks on these abilities seem to boost overall care quality, underscoring why dedicated training setups are pretty important (Ajzen et al., 2007). Schools, hospitals, and professional groups often join forces, sometimes clumsily, other times surprisingly well, to update training rules for pediatric imaging. These partnerships allow practitioners to trade best practices and experiment with fresh, innovative teaching ideas. As imaging technology keeps on shifting, maintaining a high standard means that programs need a constant dose of new content paired with periodic reviews. The field stays dynamic and, in most cases, demands that educational efforts evolve alongside new research and clinical habits. Overall, this ongoing commitment to learning ensures that pediatric radiologists not only master modern imaging tools but also remain sensitive to the ethical and human sides of caring for young patients.

12.5.2. Collaboration with Pediatricians

Working closely together, pediatricians and imaging experts boost how accurately we diagnose issues in kids. In many cases, a child's condition isn't straightforward – its subtleties are best picked up by the doctors who see the little ones every day. These pediatricians notice tiny, sometimes easily-overlooked signs which hint at underlying problems; that firsthand insight then helps radiologists adjust imaging techniques to each child's unique needs. For example, knowing around pediatric common variable immunodeficiency (CVID) guides the team to make smarter imaging choices, especially when complications like granulomatous-lymphocytic interstitial lung disease (GLILD) emerge. When such professionals team up, the results tend to enhance patient care and, generally speaking, lead to better use of clinical resources. In today's fast-changing world of pediatric diagnostics, imaging specialists and pediatricians must chat openly, even if sometimes their conversation jumps from the obvious to the subtle. Pediatricians carry a wealth of firsthand knowledge – from detailed medical histories to knowing just how a child is developing – all of which color the imaging strategy. Working in tandem, these individuals can pick apart imaging results to set up timely interventions that might just change a patient's whole course. Think of techniques like tympanometry or even smartphone-enabled otoscopy: these tools, sometimes used before more intensive imaging, help streamline the process for conditions such as acute otitis media (AOM) (Erkkola-Anttinen et al., 2017). Often, when they hash over imaging plans together, the team stumbles upon new ideas for the next steps, reinforcing a shared drive for top-notch pediatric care. Beyond just reading scans and interpreting tests, this kind of collaboration spills over into education for staff and families alike. Pediatricians, thanks to their close connections with families, can explain why certain imaging tests are needed, making sure parents understand both the perks and the potential bumps along the road. This clear, sometimes informal, dialogue fosters trust, even if the messaging isn't always textbook perfect. Moreover, when doctors from different disciplines join in a meeting, they can easily iron out their different perspectives, aligning on patient management approaches. Such cross-talk may even spark fresh research into updating imaging protocols, gradually improving both standardization and overall care quality. All things considered, a strong, flexible partnership between pediatricians and imaging specialists isn't just a bonus, it is critical for navigating the many modifications of pediatric healthcare.

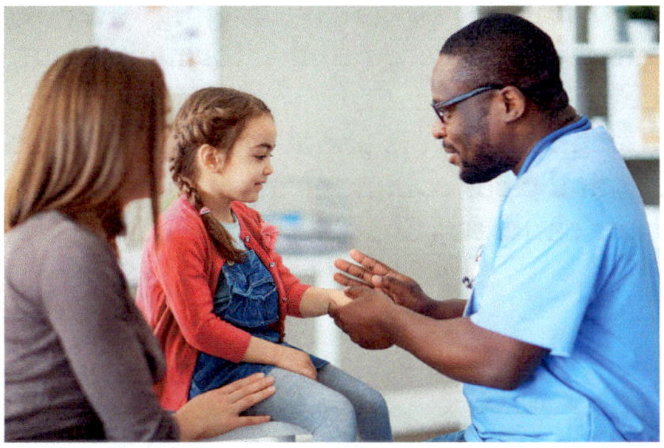

Source: https://webapp2.wright.edu/web1/newsroom/files/2016/11/Pediatrics-Parent-Pediatrician-Partnership.jpg.

12.5.3. Importance of Accurate Diagnosis

Pediatric imaging is always on the move. Diagnosing conditions in kids, especially when facing tough cancers like neuroblastoma, is more critical than ever. MIBG scintigraphy, for example, gives doctors a way to catch tumors and even spot when they've spread, often picking up things that might otherwise be missed. One study, in most cases rather eye-opening, showed that this method is key not only for the initial staging but also for keeping tabs on how treatment is working. By detailing the spread of the disease, MIBG helps nail down treatment choices and, in turn, boosts outcomes for young patients (Otmane et al., 2025). Accurate diagnosis matters in more ways than one. Endocrinology also reaps the benefits of modern imaging when trying to figure out complex child health issues. Advanced 3D MRI, for instance, looks closely at the pituitary gland and helps set a normal baseline, which can then flag any unusual changes. These improvements, generally speaking, sharpen the precision of diagnoses and lead to treatment plans tailored to each child's unique body. As imaging tools continue to improve, mixing these diagnostic techniques into everyday practice becomes increasingly essential for effective healthcare management (Ghorbani et al., 2025). Regular imaging doesn't just guide treatment decisions; it is crucial for tracking disease progress and the body's response to therapy. This is especially true for kids, where prompt and precise interventions can make a difference. Frequent scans let doctors tweak treatments as conditions like neuroblastoma evolve, a point that can affect both immediate care and long-term quality of life. Even as technology keeps pushing forward, reliable diagnostic methods stand as a cornerstone of good pediatric care (Ghorbani et al., 2025).

Test Your Knowledge

1. How does the training and specialization of pediatric radiologists differ from general radiologists, and why is this important in diagnosing pediatric conditions?
2. What is the importance of collaboration between pediatric radiologists and pediatricians in managing the diagnosis and treatment of childhood illnesses?

12.6. Advances in Pediatric Imaging

Learning Outcome

1. Explore recent technological innovations in pediatric imaging.
2. Understand the role of artificial intelligence in enhancing the accuracy and efficiency of pediatric imaging.
3. Investigate future trends and emerging technologies in pediatric imaging.

Pediatric imaging has come a long way over the past few decades, reshaping how diagnoses are made and care is given to kids. Traditional methods like X-rays and ultrasound now pack new technology that offers unexpectedly clear detail. MRI and CT scans, for instance, are now central to spotting everything from birth irregularities to injuries from accidents. A clearer image not only sharpens a doctor's diagnosis but can also cut back on invasive procedures, which, let's face it, can be pretty unsettling for children. Many health professionals keep pushing the envelope so that the experience stays as comfy and effective as possible while still delivering top-notch results. New developments have even birthed equipment designed solely for the little ones. Pediatric imaging machines come with distinct features such as lower radiation doses and smaller imaging fields to suit kids' unique builds. Tools like dual-energy CT and functional MRI (fMRI) now show soft tissues in ways that could easily slip by older methods. A touch of AI has joined the mix too, helping radiologists interpret scans with unexpected precision, thereby lightening the load on overworked staff who now get to spend time focusing more on patient care rather than wrangling with the images. Teamwork is becoming increasingly important as pediatric imaging evolves. Radiologists, pediatricians, and technical experts need to work hand-in-hand to ensure that the imaging process hits the mark for young patients. This kind of collaboration also helps forge safety guidelines, especially on the tricky subject of radiation exposure. Plus, when parents and caregivers understand the ins and outs of pediatric imaging, they feel a bit more empowered and informed about the process. In most cases, the future isn't just about new technology; it is about merging innovation, safety, and clear communication to boost overall care for children (Chepelev et al., 2018) (Figure 12.14).

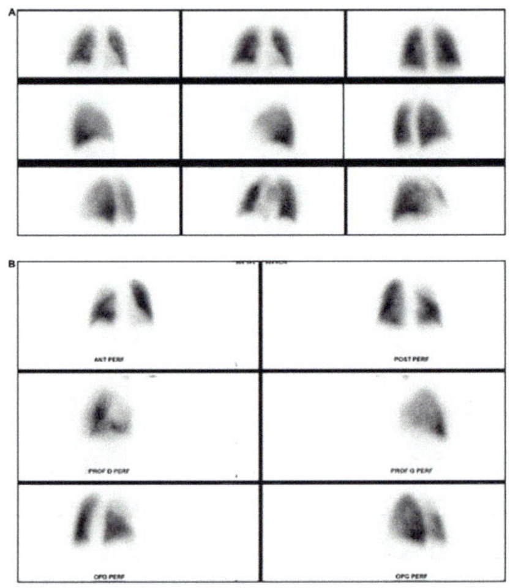

Figure 12.14. Advanced imaging for pediatric patients.

Source: Venet M, Friedberg MK, Mertens L, Baranger J, Jalal Z, Tlili G and Villemain O (2022) Nuclear Imaging in Pediatric Cardiology: Principles and Applications. Front. Pediatr. 10:909994. doi: 10.3389/fped.2022.909994.

12.6.1. Technological Innovations

Imaging technology is changing fast, and it is shaking up how kids get diagnosed. MRI, now a go-to tool for checking conditions like inflammatory bowel disease (IBD), has made its mark. For a generation that might need several scans over the years, using methods that steer clear of ionizing radiation is absolutely key. MRI brings abdominal and pelvic issues into sharper focus while also setting a new benchmark for spotting and tracking perianal conditions in children. With image speeds picking up and resolution getting sharper every day, MRI's role in pediatric care is bound to grow, a shift that's quietly transforming how these problems get managed (Jamieson et al., 2013). Technological progress isn't just about better machines, it goes deeper, touching on the rules that usher these gadgets into everyday clinical use. Recent reports generally suggest that many new devices must pass through rigorous safety checks. In fact, roughly half of these innovations eventually receive the U.S. FDA's nod for clearance, usually via the 510(k) process. This kind of regulatory oversight speeds up the rollout of new tech while keeping safety front and center. As fresh devices hit the market, the collaboration between researchers and industry becomes even more crucial, creating just the kind of environment where innovative solutions can meet the unique demands of pediatric care (Darzi et al., 2016). Advances in imaging also come with efforts to boost the know-how of those using the equipment. Training on the latest tech, especially MRI, is essential to ensure that medical teams can make the most of these tools. Ongoing education plays a big part in keeping up with rapid changes and emerging best practices. Plus, adding AI into the mix helps sharpen how images are read, which in most cases leads to better patient outcomes. As pediatric imaging evolves through this blend of tech and training, healthcare providers are increasingly well-equipped to meet children's specific needs. This mix of innovation and education is set to redefine the future of pediatric radiology, paving the way for more precise and timely care (Jamieson et al., 2013).

12.6.2. Impact of Artificial Intelligence (AI)

Imaging technology has come a long way, making it a lot easier to spot pediatric health issues early on, cancers like osteosarcoma and Ewings sarcoma being prime examples. Even though these cancers don't emerge very often, they still punch hard in child mortality, so quick and spot-on diagnosis isn't just nice to have, it is necessary. MRI, for instance, helps tell the difference between harmful and harmless tumors, though sometimes the images can get a bit muddled because of overlapping features. Interestingly, AI is stepping into this mix, almost ready to turn diagnostic imaging on its head with algorithms that chat about tumor classification and segmentation. As the need for accurate results grows, blending AI with pediatric imaging should, in theory, sharpen how clinicians recognize patterns, potentially cutting down on errors and boosting outcomes (Muñoz García et al., 2024). Recent headways in AI, especially driven by deep learning (in most cases, a real game changer), are redrawing the way we look at image analysis in kid-related diagnostics. Smart algorithms now handle huge amounts of image data, which means diagnoses can come in faster and with greater reliability. It is kind of interesting that tech originally built for completely different fields, say, skin lesion classification, can be refashioned to study bone tumors, hitting accuracy numbers like 91.96% or 93.19% for different conditions. This clever shift, mostly due to AI's knack for learning from a variety of data and adapting to the uniqueness of pediatric images, keeps reminding us that AI might just be that vital tool many have been waiting for (Kavianfar et al., 2021). Beyond just making diagnoses easier, AI in pediatric imaging is shaking up the whole healthcare approach. By smoothing out the diagnostic process, AI gives radiologists a hand while also helping tackle bigger issues like how resources are divvied up in child care. When you have diagnostics that are both quick and reliable, treatments can be prioritized more sensibly, letting healthcare providers spread their resources around a bit better. There's also a kind of back-and-forth here; as AI tools and healthcare professionals start working together more closely, they seem to boost each other's strengths. With pediatric imaging constantly moving forward, it is likely that

AI will become an essential thread in the fabric of clinical routines, ultimately fine-tuning patient management and, hopefully, leading to better outcomes for kids fighting cancer (Muñoz García et al., 2024) (Figure 12.15).

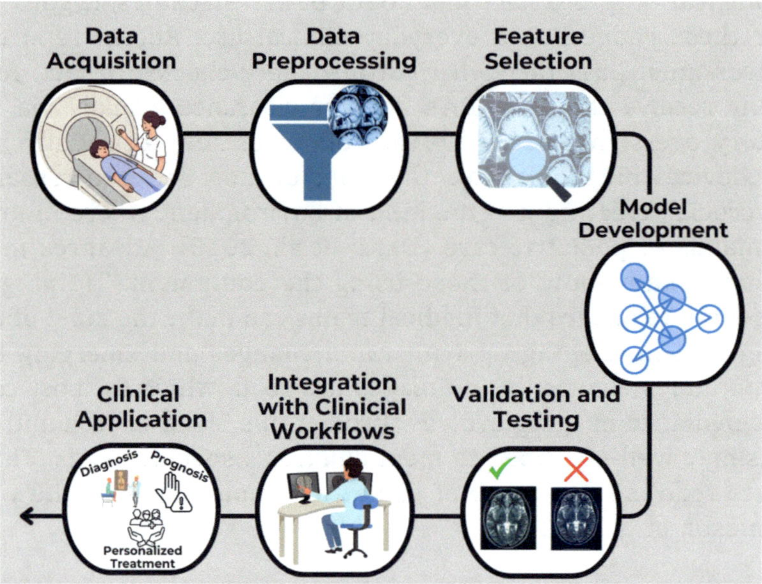

Figure 12.15. Workflow for artificial intelligence based pediatric neuroimaging.

Source: Dalboni da Rocha JL, Lai J, Pandey P, Myat PSM, Loschinskey Z, Bag AK, Sitaram R. Artificial Intelligence for Neuroimaging in Pediatric Cancer. *Cancers*. 2025; 17(4):622. https://doi.org/10.3390/cancers17040622.

12.6.3. Future Trends in Imaging

Pediatric imaging is getting a serious shake-up thanks to emerging technologies that are quietly changing how we diagnose and treat young patients. AI, for instance, now helps sift through enormous piles of imaging data – often much faster and, in many cases, with fewer human errors. You might even say that these smart systems provide doctors with a kind of foresight, offering subtle hints that can lead to earlier, more personalized treatments. It feels as though we're witnessing a gradual move toward precision medicine, where every child's unique needs play a central role in care. Nanotechnology is another player in this evolving scene. Researchers are casually tinkering with materials on a minuscule scale to create contrast agents that highlight the details – kind of like painting with molecules. These targeted agents make it easier to spot things like tumors or inflammation, especially when the usual diagnostic methods struggle with smaller or trickier issues in kids. In most cases, a more accurate delivery of these agents not only enables an earlier catch of potential health problems but also keeps a closer eye on how diseases progress. There's even promising progress toward overcoming barriers such as the blood-brain barrier (BBB), a development that might revolutionize treatments for neurological conditions in pediatric patients. At the same time, as these amazing tools become more common, a host of ethical concerns starts to pop up. When technologies are capable of delving into, and possibly tweaking, a child's biological processes, worries about consent and long-term consequences naturally follow.

Generally speaking, the vulnerability of young patients forces everyone, from clinicians to families, to revisit what ethical responsibility truly means in this brave new age. It is important to keep the conversation going, balancing rapid innovation with a steadfast commitment to a child's well-being, so that advances in imaging never compromise safety or dignity (Omidian and Mfoafo et al., 2023; Whitaker et al., 2018).

Test Your Knowledge

1. What role do advancements in contrast agents play in enhancing the accuracy of pediatric imaging?
2. How do innovations in radiation-reducing techniques impact the safety and effectiveness of pediatric imaging?

Summary

Pediatric imaging has come a long way, yet one thing is clear: our research samples aren't as diverse as they need to be. Recent studies point out that in brain imaging, not every group is getting equal attention, which in turn makes it tricky to apply findings across all kids. Getting this right is key if we want to build health interventions that help everyone. Some recruitment efforts by research teams from different backgrounds show that we've still got work to do in reaching out to underrepresented communities. Building trust using culturally tuned approaches seems to boost enrollment and gives us a fuller picture of child health (Nwana et al., 2025). Tech progress in imaging – think procedures like ureteral stenting – illustrates how new ideas mix with better outcomes for young patients. Data often shows these advanced techniques pull off high success, while the side effects remain within acceptable limits, which makes a solid case for bringing them into clinics. Such improvements open doors to dig deeper into pediatric conditions and craft treatments based on real evidence. As we learn more about how children's bodies differ both functionally and anatomically, our ability to tailor treatments keep on growing. It is important, then, that ongoing studies blend image reviews with thorough clinical checkups to keep care safe and effective (Mazıcan et al., 2025). In short, the future of pediatric imaging depends on mixing diverse perspectives with modern technology. Widening the circle of study participants not only enriches the overall evidence but also makes sure that interventions are fair and work well for every child. New imaging methods and ongoing tech improvements hold a lot of promise for changing pediatric healthcare as we know it. Researchers, practitioners, and everyone involved, need to see that they play a part in boosting diversity and using innovations to their full advantage. This all-around approach should lead to more informed, culturally sensitive care, and set the stage for a healthier future for kids and their families (Mazıcan et al., 2025; Nwana et al., 2025).

Advanced imaging techniques have obtained attention in pediatric care lately. Traumatic brain injuries in kids don't follow a neat recovery plan, the timing of the checkup and the injury's own uniqueness both seem to play a big role. One study looked at moderate to severe TBI, using tensor-based morphometry to watch how brain volumes shifted over time. Some groups of patients showed their own unique structural changes, which generally hints that therapeutic plans might need a personal touch based on how their brains are maturing (Asarnow et al., 2017). In many cases, blending imaging info into clinical decisions helps improve outcomes. Kids dealing with blood-related diseases, such as after treatment for acute lymphoblastic leukemia, find imaging equally valuable. It often spots treatment-related toxicities; the line between hitting cancer hard and causing extra harm can get pretty blurry. A Delphi study with international pediatric oncology groups ended up listing 14 acute toxic effects that matter for clear reporting and to compare different protocols (Schmiegelow et al., 2016). This kind of research, by building consensus, emphasizes that imaging doesn't just point out what's wrong, it also deepens our understanding of the side effects that come with life-saving treatments. Imaging isn't stopping at diagnosis either. It is starting to guide treatments by giving real-time feedback and even helping adjust strategies on the fly (Asarnow et al., 2017). Because children's anatomy and development are so unique, these advanced imaging techniques allow clinicians to fine-tune interventions in unexpected ways. Studies of this sort keep adding evidence that we can optimize safety and effectiveness when every patient's needs are considered. As researchers continue to untangle all the complexities of pediatric health, it looks like imaging will only keep expanding its role in managing conditions from TBI to various leukemias (Schmiegelow et al., 2016).

KEY TERMS FROM THIS CHAPTER

- Acute otitis media (AOM)
- Clinical ultrasound (CUS)
- Emergency surgery
- Muscle injuries
- Pediatric care
- Polysomnography (PSG)
- Vulnerable patients
- Anxiety
- Congenital cytomegalovirus (cCMV)
- European Society of Pediatric Radiology (ESPR)
- Pediatric brain imaging
- Pediatric radiology
- Proximal focal femoral deficiency (PFFD)

Critical Thinking Questions

1. **What is a major consideration when performing imaging procedures on pediatric patients?**
   a. Using the highest possible radiation dose
   b. Avoiding sedation in all cases
   c. Minimizing radiation exposure while maintaining image quality
   d. Avoiding parental involvement
2. **Which imaging modality is often preferred for pediatric brain imaging due to the absence of radiation?**
   a. X-ray
   b. Ultrasound
   c. MRI
   d. CT scan
3. **Why is ultrasound frequently used in pediatric imaging?**
   a. It is expensive and highly detailed
   b. It provides 3D bone images
   c. It is safe, portable, and uses no ionizing radiation
   d. It requires sedation
4. **What is the most commonly used imaging modality for detecting congenital hip dislocation in infants?**
   a. X-ray
   b. CT
   c. MRI
   d. Ultrasound
5. **The ALARA principle, used in pediatric imaging, stands for:**
   a. As Long As Radiation Allows
   b. As Late As Reasonable Aftercare
   c. As Low As Reasonably Achievable
   d. All Levels Are Radiologically Acceptable

Short Answer Questions

1. What are the primary types of pediatric imaging techniques used in diagnosing childhood conditions?
2. How does pediatric imaging differ from adult imaging in terms of technique and equipment?
3. Why is reducing radiation exposure especially critical in pediatric imaging?
4. How does MRI contribute to the diagnosis of pediatric neurological conditions?
5. What are some common pediatric conditions that can be diagnosed using imaging techniques?
6. What role does a pediatric radiologist play in the diagnosis and management of childhood diseases?
7. How have advances in pediatric imaging, such as using low-dose radiation and improved resolution, enhanced diagnostic capabilities?

Answers to Critical Thinking Questions

1. (c); 2. (c); 3. (c); 4. (d); 5. (c)

References

1. Ajzen, S. A., Baptista, L. P. S., Lederman, H. M., et al. (2007). Prova Nacional dos Residentes e Especializandos em Radiologia e Diagnóstico por Imagem no Brasil: Instrumento de avaliação da qualificação do futuro radiologista. https://core.ac.uk/download/268266215.pdf (accessed on 23 May 2025).
2. Alzayed, A. A. (2023). Application of artificial intelligence in pediatric pulmonology: Current scenario and future prospective. https://core.ac.uk/download/573452977.pdf (accessed on 23 May 2025).
3. Aravindh, S., Manigandan, T., Shakila, R., & Kalaiselvi, G. S. N. (2025). A comprehensive overview of upper airway assessment using cone beam computed tomography in the Indian population. *South Eastern European Journal of Public Health*, 1359–1373. https://doi.org/10.70135/seejph.vi.4950.
4. Arthurs, O. J., van Rijn, R. R., Granata, C., Porto, L., Hirsch, F. W., & Rosendahl, K. (2019). European Society of Pediatric Radiology 2019 strategic research agenda: Improving imaging for tomorrow's children. *Pediatric Radiology, 49*(8), 983–989. https://doi.org/10.1007/s00247-019-04406-4.
5. Asarnow, R. F., Babbitt, C., Babikian, T., et al. (2017). Diverging volumetric trajectories following pediatric traumatic brain injury. https://core.ac.uk/download/323079591.pdf.
6. Benjamin, D. K., Bloom, D., Bradley, J., Gamel, B., et al. (2018). Parents' perceived obstacles to pediatric clinical trial participation: Findings from the Clinical Trials Transformation Initiative. https://core.ac.uk/download/323064361.pdf.
7. Borrelli, M., Corcione, A., Cimbalo, C., Annunziata, A., Basilicata, S., Fiorentino, G., & Santamaria, F. (2023). Diagnosis of pediatric obstructive sleep-disordered breathing beyond polysomnography. *Children, 10*(8), 1331. https://doi.org/10.3390/children10081331.
8. Chepelev, L., Wake, N., Ryan, J., Althobaity, W., Gupta, A., Arribas, E., Santiago, L., Ballard, D. H., Wang, K. C., Weadock, W., Ionita, C. N., Mitsouras, D., Morris, J., Matsumoto, J., Christensen, A., Liacouras, P., Rybicki, F. J., Sheikh, A., & RSNA Special Interest Group for 3D Printing. (2018). Radiological Society of North America (RSNA) 3D printing Special Interest Group (SIG): Guidelines for medical 3D printing and appropriateness for clinical scenarios. *3D Printing in Medicine, 4*(1), 11. https://doi.org/10.1186/s41205-018-0030-y.
9. Chong, W. H., & Yang, H. (2020). Critical care ultrasonography and its application for COVID-19. https://core.ac.uk/download/322850187.pdf (accessed on 23 May 2025).
10. Clark, T. J., Cleary, M. A., & Eberman, L. E. (2013). Physeal growth plate fractures: Implications for the pediatric athlete. https://core.ac.uk/download/46946337.pdf (accessed on 23 May 2025).
11. D'Ambrosio, V., Pasquali, G., Squarcella, A., Marcoccia, E., De Filippis, A., Gatto, S., Camilla, A., Pizzuti, A., La Torre, R., & Giancotti, A. (2016). Prenatal diagnosis of proximal focal femoral deficiency: Literature review of prenatal sonographic findings. *Journal of Clinical Ultrasound, 44*(4), 252–259. https://doi.org/10.1002/jcu.22306.
12. Darzi, A., Hughes-Hallett, A., Marcus, A. P., et al. (2016). Regulatory approval of new medical devices: A cross-sectional study. https://core.ac.uk/download/77011535.pdf (accessed on 23 May 2025).

13. Donnelly, J. P., Chen, S. C., Kauffman, C. A., Steinbach, W. J., Baddley, J. W., Verweij, P. E., et al. (2020). Revision and update of the consensus definitions of invasive fungal disease from the European Organization for Research and Treatment of Cancer and the Mycoses Study Group Education and Research Consortium. *Clinical Infectious Diseases, 71*(6), 1367–1376. https://doi.org/10.1093/cid/ciz1008.

14. Donya, M., ElGuindy, A., Firmin, D., et al. (2014). Radiation in medicine: Origins, risks and aspirations. https://core.ac.uk/download/77008838.pdf (accessed on 23 May 2025).

15. Downie, J., Malisza, K., Marshall, J., et al. (2007). A comprehensive analysis of MRI research risks: In support of full disclosure. https://core.ac.uk/download/478607605.pdf (accessed on 23 May 2025).

16. Drey, N., Husson, O., May, K., et al. (2019). Ionizing radiation exposure from medical imaging–A review of patient's (un)awareness. https://core.ac.uk/download/266989986.pdf (accessed on 23 May 2025).

17. Duinkerken, M. S. I., Kelsey; Copeland, J., & Gordon, L. (2020). Jefferson Digital Commons quarterly report: October-December 2019. *Jefferson Digital Commons Reports*, Paper 29. https://jdc.jefferson.edu/jdcreports/29 (accessed on 23 May 2025).

18. Erkkola-Anttinen, N. (2017). Parental role in the diagnostics of acute otitis media in young children. https://core.ac.uk/download/198010819.pdf (accessed on 23 May 2025).

19. Ghorbani, N., Mirfendereski, S., & Moshkenani, N. H. (2025). Determining the normal range of the dimensions and volume of the pituitary gland of children using a 3D magnetic resonance imaging (MRI) protocol in Imam Hossein Hospital of Isfahan in 2021 to 2024. *American Journal of Neurodegenerative Disease, 14*(1), 42–50. https://www.semanticscholar.org/paper/916c6f93355c337b541cd4bae109df91fd0d1a40 (accessed on 23 May 2025).

20. Gozal, D., & Mason, K. P. (2010). Pediatric sedation: A global challenge. https://core.ac.uk/download/pdf/8465035.pdf.

21. Hirsch, W., Frahm, J., Sorge, I., Klee, D., Prenzel, F., Krause, M., Lacher, M., et al. (2023). Real-time MRI: A new tool of radiologic imaging in small children. *European Journal of Pediatrics, 182*, 3405–3417. https://doi.org/10.1007/s00431-023-04996-0.

22. Hwang, H. (2017). Knowledge, attitude and perception on radiation imaging among children's caregivers in the pediatric dental clinic. https://open.bu.edu/bitstream/2144/23797/5/Hwang_bu_0017N_12842.pdf (accessed on 23 May 2025).

23. Jameson, J. R., Albert, C. I., Busse, B., Smith, P. A., & Harris, G. F. (2013). 3D micron-scale imaging of the cortical bone canal network in human osteogenesis imperfecta (OI). In *Medical Imaging 2013: Biomedical Applications in Molecular, Structural, and Functional Imaging* (Vol. 8672, p. 86721L). SPIE. https://doi.org/10.1117/12.2007209.

24. Jamieson, D. H., Shipman, P., & Jacobson, K. (2013). Magnetic resonance imaging of the perineum in pediatric patients with inflammatory bowel disease. *Canadian Journal of Gastroenterology, 27*(8), 476–480. https://doi.org/10.1155/2013/624141.

25. Kavianfar, A., Salimi, M., & Taherkhani, H. (2021). A review of the management of eye diseases using artificial intelligence, machine learning, and deep learning in conjunction with recent research on eye health problems. *Journal of Ophthalmic and Optometric Sciences, 5*(2), 57–72.

26. Lazzarotto, T., Blázquez-Gamero, D., Delforge, M. L., Foulon, I., Luck, S., Modrow, S., & Leruez-Ville, M. (2020). Congenital cytomegalovirus infection: A narrative review of the issues in screening and management from a panel of European experts. *Frontiers in Pediatrics, 8*, 13. https://doi.org/10.3389/fped.2020.00013.

27. Lurbe, E., Agabiti-Rosei, E., Cruickshank, J. K., Dominiczak, A., Erdine, S., Hirth, A., et al. (2016). 2016 European Society of Hypertension guidelines for the management of high blood pressure in children and adolescents. *Journal of Hypertension, 34*(10), 1887–1920. https://doi.org/10.1097/HJH.0000000000001039.

28. Mazıcan, M., Karluka, I., Temiz, A., & Andic, C. (2025). Antegrade ureteral stenting in pediatric patients: Introducing a novel ureteral morphological classification and a new perspective on functional success. *Journal of Clinical Medicine, 14*. https://www.semanticscholar.org/paper/673452ad9143da9c439af6327bdea70a137e12ca (accessed on 23 May 2025).

29. Muñoz García, N. (2024). Artificial intelligence approaches for image segmentation and classification in medical imaging analysis. https://core.ac.uk/download/613979377.pdf (accessed on 23 May 2025).

30. Nwana, O., DeMaster, D., & Vaughn, K. A. (2025). Art of recruiting diverse pediatric samples for randomized clinical trials: A recruiter's perspective. *World Journal of Advanced Research and Reviews, 25*(2), 2295–2308. https://doi.org/10.30574/wjarr.2025.25.2.0528.

31. Omidian, H., & Mfoafo, K. (2023). Exploring the potential of nanotechnology in pediatric healthcare: Advances, challenges, and future directions. *Pharmaceutics, 15*(6), 1583. https://doi.org/10.3390/pharmaceutics15061583.

32. Otmane, M., & Ismaili, N. A. (2025). The pediatric neuroblastoma: Application of MIBG scintigraphy in diagnosis, staging, and follow-up–Analysis of three cases. *Swiss Journal of Radiology and Nuclear Medicine, 17*(1), 1–8. https://doi.org/10.59667/sjoranm.v17i1.14.

33. Reismann, J., Romualdi, A., Kiss, N., Minderjahn, M. I., Kallarackal, J., Schad, M., & Reismann, M. (2019). Diagnosis and classification of pediatric acute appendicitis by artificial intelligence methods: An investigator-independent approach. *PloS One, 14*(9), e0222030. https://doi.org/10.1371/journal.pone.0222030.

34. Schmiegelow, K., Attarbaschi, A., Barzilai, S., Escherich, G., Frandsen, T. L., Halsey, C., et al. (2016). Consensus definitions of 14 severe acute toxic effects for childhood lymphoblastic leukemia treatment: A Delphi consensus. *The Lancet Oncology, 17*(6), e231–e239. https://doi.org/10.1016/S1470-2045(16)30035-3.

35. Strony, R., Marin, J. R., Bailitz, J., Dean, A. J., Blaivas, M., Tayal, V., et al. (2018). Systemwide clinical ultrasound program development: An expert consensus model. *The Western Journal of Emergency Medicine, 19*(4), 649–653. https://doi.org/10.5811/westjem.2018.4.37152.

36. Whitaker, H. N. (2018). Attitudes on medical ethics of criminal neurointerventional treatment (Senior thesis, Liberty University). https://core.ac.uk/download/213462108.pdf (accessed on 23 May 2025).

37. Zhang, Q., Hu, Y., Zhou, C., Zhao, Y., Zhang, N., Zhou, Y., Yang, Y., et al. (2024). Reducing pediatric total-body PET/CT imaging scan time with multimodal artificial intelligence technology. *EJNMMI Physics, 11*. https://doi.org/10.1186/s40658-023-00605-z.

MUSCULOSKELETAL IMAGING

13

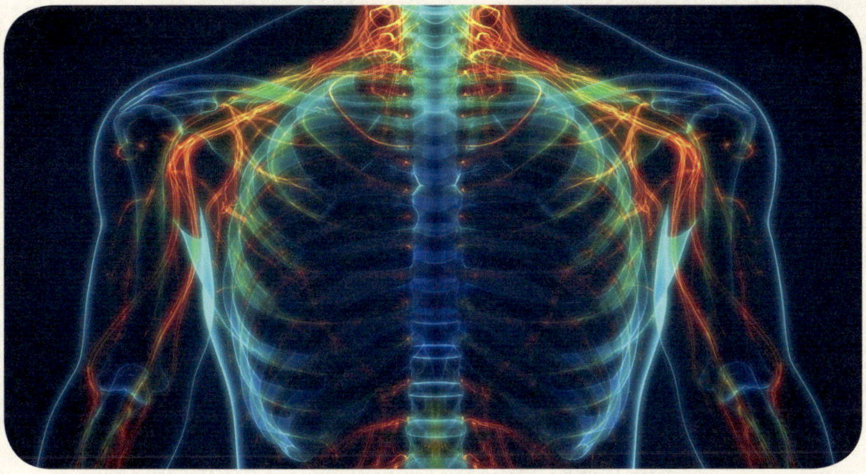

LEARNING OBJECTIVES

After studying this chapter, you will be able to:

1. Examine the identify the indications for musculoskeletal imaging.
2. Examine the advantages and limitations of imaging modalities.
3. Understand the role of imaging in diagnosis.
4. Explore recent advancements in musculoskeletal imaging techniques.
5. Discuss the ethical considerations in musculoskeletal imaging.

Introduction

Medical imaging isn't what it used to be, especially when you look at issues with muscles and bones. New breakthroughs have boosted how well doctors can spot problems, offering more treatment choices along the way. Tools like MRI, CT, and even ultrasound have kind of become everyday items. MRI stands out because it shows soft tissues in such detail that it is great for checking out things like tendon pain, ligament strains, and even cartilage wear. You also get a peek at changes in bone marrow and surrounding tissue, which helps in understanding both wear-and-tear and spots of inflammation. Generally speaking, as new tech comes in, keeping up with these advances is pretty key for great care. Imaging isn't just about taking a look anymore, it is stepping into treatment too. Artificial intelligence (AI) is mixing in with image analyses, offering fresh, sometimes unexpected, ways to read tricky scans. This helps speed up the process and even tailors treatment to the individual, or so it seems. Fusion imaging, where different methods get blended together, gives a fuller picture of musculoskeletal issues, right when degenerative or inflammatory conditions are on the line. In most cases, integrating these advanced techniques with older methods lets clinicians make smarter choices about interventions, and eventually boosts patient outcomes and overall quality of life (Monti et al., 2022). Then there's the rise of dual-energy CT, DECT, that's turning heads. This approach lets doctors tell different tissue types apart almost on the fly, meaning they can get a closer look at problems without having to go invasive. Its uses stretch from cancer care to trauma, and individuals are starting to notice how DECT can be a game changer in musculoskeletal imaging. With tricks like creating virtual non-contrast images (or VNC) and breaking down materials in a new way, DECT not only smooths out diagnostic work but also helps lower radiation exposure. Overall, as imaging keeps evolving with these fresh methods and improvements, its role in healthcare only seems to grow, offering both sharper diagnoses and better ways to treat patients (Alizadeh et al., 2023).

Definition and Importance

Musculoskeletal imaging isn't just about fancy scans; it is a mixed bag of techniques that let us peek into bones, cartilage, and soft tissues in surprising ways. It helps doctors not only figure out what's wrong but also decide on treatment, almost like piecing together a puzzle. For example, ultra-high frequency ultrasound now offers a fresh look at anatomy details once considered lost, pretty cool, right? Reliable image quality is key, especially since it catches hidden conditions that might slip by unnoticed. The way deep penetration and crisp visuals join forces often makes all the difference when assessing and managing these disorders (Liu et al., 2024). Imaging plays a role way beyond that first diagnosis, too, it keeps an eye on disease progress and even how treatments are holding up. Sometimes it gives a quick snapshot, while other times it is more of an ongoing record. When subtle signs like synovitis show up alongside joint troubles, it stresses the need for early scans, especially in cases like psoriasis and psoriatic arthritis. Spotting those barely-there signals early can prompt preventive steps that improve life quality and, over time, even cut down healthcare expenses. In a sense, this proactive streak nudges healthcare providers to work together and tweak their diagnostic playbook for each patient (Zabotti et al., 2023). New tech keeps shaking things up in the field, blending traditional methods with cutting-edge ideas. MRI and CT scans have started hanging out with AI algorithms, which not only quicken the pace but also handle messy data in ways that sometimes feel almost intuitive. These upgrades help smooth out workflow hiccups while still tossing out details doctors rely on. In effect, mixing in these advanced imaging tricks becomes a must for crafting treatment plans that fit. With such enhanced visuals, clinicians end up understanding the musculoskeletal system in a deeper, more personal way, leading to decisions that boost patient outcomes, all while keeping the process refreshingly targeted (Liu et al., 2024) (Figure 13.1).

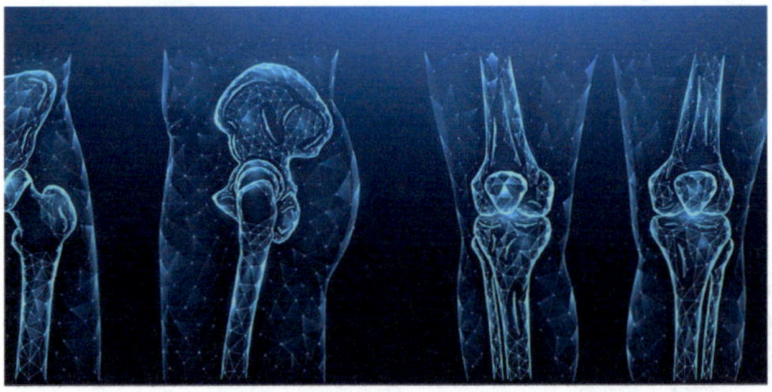

Figure 13.1. Musculoskeletal imaging.

Source: https://www.guthrie.org/sites/default/files/styles/1600x900/public/2021-09/musculoskeletal-imaging.jpg?itok=c-yTmb2F.

Overview of Imaging Modalities

Imaging techniques for musculoskeletal

disorders have taken on a fresh form in today's tech-savvy atmosphere. Advances like MRI and CT scanning now give clinicians a far more detailed look at anatomy, capturing soft tissues such as cartilage and muscle that plain X-rays often miss. It is a leap forward; sometimes even a non-invasive ultrasound approach lets practitioners peek at injuries and joint effusions in real time. By mixing these varied methods, a robust yet flexible assessment framework naturally emerges, boosting both diagnosis and treatment in many cases. Another innovative development is phototherapy, a method that gently shifts how we handle musculoskeletal issues. Generally speaking, this approach uses different kinds of light to encourage healing and modulate cell behavior, which is a refreshing change from traditional methods. Recent studies show it can target problematic cells in bone tumors and inflammation, proving useful in tricky cases like arthritis and bone infections (Zhang et al., 2023).

Researchers are also exploring light-responsive nanosystems that not only improve drug delivery but also bring imaging into the mix, nudging the field closer to true precision medicine. This dual-purpose strategy, with its slight redundancy in goals, seems set to sharpen early diagnosis and intervention techniques. AI is also combined with these advances, reshaping how musculoskeletal diagnostics are done. Techniques such as eXplainable Artificial Intelligence (XAI) help doctors navigate complex data and spot subtle pathological shifts with greater ease. In many cases, deep learning frameworks are now used to classify abnormalities based on imaging data, which naturally builds confidence and efficiency in diagnoses (van der Velden et al., 2022). As healthcare drifts toward more automated, solution-driven approaches, the blend of AI with advanced imaging is bound to improve patient outcomes and streamline decision-making. Overall, the future of musculoskeletal care appears closely tied to this nuanced partnership between smart technology and clinical expertise, paving the way for new therapies and better care.

Historical Development of Musculoskeletal Imaging

Wilhelm Conrad Rontgen's chance discovery of X-rays in 1895 kicked off a new way of looking at what's inside the body. Back then, it wasn't about cutting into a person to see what was wrong, it was a fresh, non-invasive peek at bones and joints. Radiography quickly became that handy tool for spotting fractures and other bone issues, even though it didn't do a great job showing the fine details of soft tissues or the knottier parts of joints. In many ways, that early phase of imaging set the stage for everything that followed, quietly paving a path toward innovations like CT and MRI, which would later change how musculoskeletal disorders get diagnosed and managed (Figure 13.2).

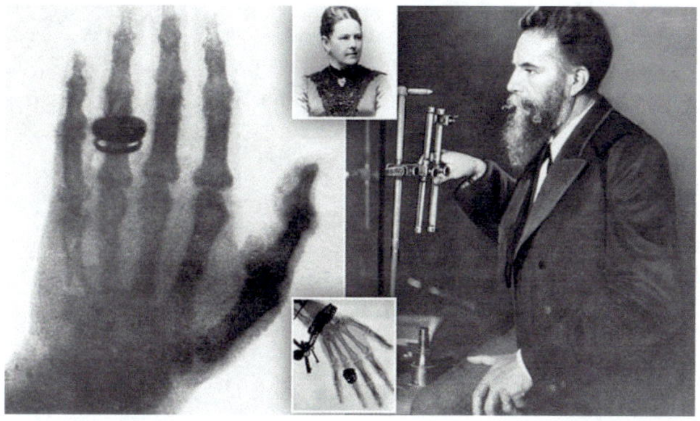

Figure 13.2. Roentgen's first human X-ray of his wife's hand in 1895.

Source: https://i.dailymail.co.uk/1s/2018/12/13/13/7380932-0-image-a-47_1544708060340.jpg.

By the mid-20th century, the imaging scene started to shake things up again. CT scans, which came into play in the 1970s, offered cross-sectional views that made it a lot easier to see complicated fractures and problems inside the joints, being especially useful for trauma cases and pre-surgery checks. Around the same time, MRI made its debut in the late 70s to early 80s, giving doctors spectacular views of ligaments, tendons, and cartilage with a softness in contrast that radiography just couldn't match. This move to less invasive techniques generally bumped up diagnostic accuracy and helped shape better treatment plans. All these leaps and bounds in technology reminded everyone just how important imaging was becoming for untangling musculoskeletal issues, eventually hinting at even newer horizons like AI joining the mix. Today, AI is slowly carving out its own niche in musculoskeletal imaging by crunching huge piles of data and spotting subtle irregularities, even ones that might slip past very experienced radiologists (Najjar, 2023). It is showing up in various forms such as automated image segmentation, computer-aided diagnosis, and even predictive analytics, each element aiming to smooth out workflows and boost detection rates, albeit with a few hiccups along the way. There are still challenges, like ensuring data quality and wrestling with ethical questions about how results are interpreted. Still, the prospect of AI complementing traditional imaging methods signals a pretty big shift toward personalized care and more efficient treatment planning. In most cases, as radiologists and AI developers continue to work together (with the occasional small misstep in process), these advances promise to sharpen diagnostic accuracy and, ultimately, benefit patients a whole lot (Colgate et al., 2020)

13.1. Indications for Musculoskeletal Imaging

Learning Outcome

1. Understand the role of imaging in the evaluation and diagnosis of trauma-related injuries and fractures.
2. Explore imaging techniques used in the assessment of degenerative musculoskeletal diseases.
3. Examine how imaging aids in the detection and monitoring of musculoskeletal tumors and infections.

Understanding musculoskeletal imaging isn't just about the pictures, it is about knowing why we take them in the first place. When someone complains about new pain or a flare-up of long-lasting aches that just won't get better with basic care, doctors often turn to scans. A quick look with X-rays, MRI or CT scans may reveal hidden fractures, awkward joint positions, or early wear-and-tear that a simple exam might miss. Newer imaging methods even give a peek at the soft tissues, so clinicians can sort out things like tendon strains, bursitis, or even ligament tears. In most cases, this kind of insight helps guide treatments that are both timely and tuned to the patient's exact needs, ultimately steering them toward a better outcome. When injury strikes suddenly, like from a fall or a hit, imaging takes on an important role. For example, after an unexpected fracture, a plain radiograph can quickly confirm not only that a break has occurred but also what type of break it is, suggesting whether a non-surgical fix will do or if surgery might be needed. Sometimes when breaks get trickier, say, involving joint surfaces or injuries showing up from multiple angles, a range of scans is used to get a clear picture. And in a couple of cases, what seems like a minor stress fracture might escape standard X-rays, prompting using an MRI to pick up on the finer points. Blending these various techniques means that, ultimately, treatment plans can be finely tuned to help speed up recovery while keeping risks in check. Chronic issues, too, lean heavily on the insights that imaging offers (Tenforde et al., 2022). Conditions like osteoarthritis, rheumatoid arthritis, along with other soft tissue troubles, often call for regular scans to track how the disease is evolving, check out the joint damage, or monitor if a particular treatment is working out. These follow-up images not only help clinch a diagnosis but also guide decisions about interventions, like corticosteroid injections or physical therapy, that can make a difference. When patients see exactly what is going on, they often get a better sense of how to manage their own care. As stated in clinical practice guidelines, using imaging in this considered way generally ups the quality of care, ensuring that interventions happen promptly and fit each individual's circumstances (Glikson et al., 2021).

13.1.1. Trauma and Fractures

Trauma involving bones and joints can be surprisingly tricky. In many cases, when pregnancy is a factor, small shifts – like a surge in blood flow or looser ligaments – can change how fractures need to be handled. Doctors sometimes face a jumble of challenges because these bodily tweaks alter both anatomy and the way medications work. Safe imaging – think MRI or ultrasound – turns critical, even though such scans can sometimes pose risks for a developing fetus. Generally speaking, specialists such as obstetricians and orthopedists must work hand in hand, balancing the care of both mom and baby (Madkhali et al., 2024).

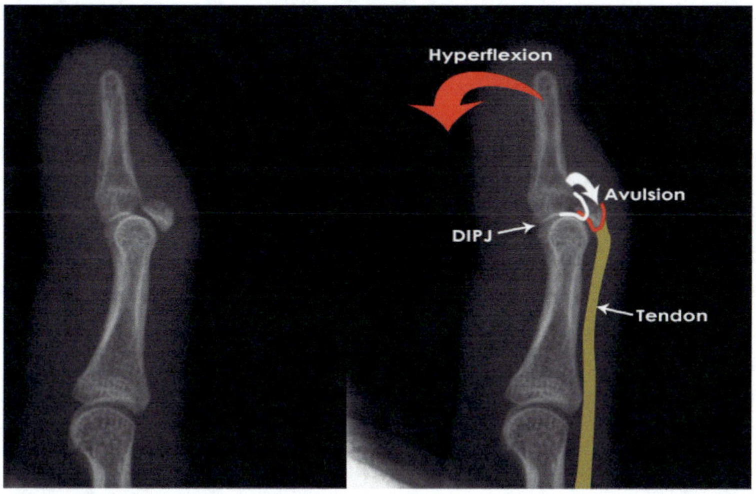

Figure 13.3. Avulsion fracture X-ray.

Source: https://www.radiologymasterclass.co.uk/images/musculoskeletal-images/trauma/avulsion.jpg?mtime=20210304211359&focal=none.

Modern imaging tools now serve as a lifeline in fracture care; ultrasound (US) has emerged as one of those versatile choices. It is increasingly used to assess injuries, particularly among kids and expecting mothers; it offers a fast, non-invasive snapshot that sidesteps the ionizing radiation linked with older techniques. Not only does US help pinpoint problems, it also guides procedures – like aspirations and injections – which can cut down on risks compared to more invasive methods. This clever use of ultrasound generally improves outcomes by lowering complications, steadily marking its growing role in comprehensive fracture care (Tzatzairis et al., 2024). When fractures occur after trauma, identifying the break early becomes key to setting the right treatment course. Quick, accurate imaging lets health professionals decide between simpler fixes – such as splinting or casting – and more involved surgical options. That said, every imaging method carries its own advantages and downsides; advanced scans like CTs and MRIs offer a detailed look not just at the fracture but also at nearby soft tissue injuries. Such in-depth info helps clarify injury severity while shaping plans for surgery and rehabilitation, paving the path for better recovery and a fuller understanding of musculoskeletal trauma (Tzatzairis et al., 2024) (Figure 13.3).

13.1.2. Degenerative Diseases

Degenerative diseases often bring long-lasting pain and disability that tend to lower quality of life in ways that aren't always easy to predict. Take plantar fasciitis, for example, this condition is usually marked by constant heel pain arising from slow, degenerative changes rather than the typical inflammation you might expect. In most cases, modern imaging, ultrasound in particular, has helped us see things differently, revealing features like a thicker plantar fascia and areas that come off as oddly dark or hypoechoic. These scans, by the way, not only boost diagnostic confidence but also offer clues on how well a treatment is working. Clinicians today mix traditional care with newer therapies, leaning on these imaging insights to bridge the gap between an initial hunch and a solid diagnosis (Wen-Tseng et al., 2023). Beyond the immediate physical discomfort, the effects of these degenerative issues ripple into psychological and social spheres, sometimes in ways that complicate patient care. Health professionals, generally speaking, find themselves trying to manage not just the symptoms but also the broader impact on a patient's daily life while keeping them well-informed. Newer imaging techniques, like sonoelastography, for instance, have become invaluable tools that help track how a disease progresses, even as they offer a more detailed view of tissue characteristics. In effect, these tools guide more nuanced treatment choices, even if the process might seem messy at times; as degenerative conditions become more common worldwide, fitting advanced imaging into everyday practice seems essential for better outcomes (Glikson et al., 2021). Research in musculoskeletal imaging continues to evolve, opening up fresh ways to diagnose and treat these conditions. A closer look at the underlying mechanisms, like the changes seen in plantar fasciitis, can nudge us toward both early preventive actions and more targeted therapies. Current evidence generally points to conservative treatments, such as physical therapy paired with extracorporeal shock wave therapy, as often yielding notable improvements in symptoms. Imaging, then, isn't just key during the initial diagnostic phase but is also crucial for monitoring long-term effectiveness, even if the methods occasionally appear a bit unpolished. By combining state-of-the-art visual techniques with a comprehensive understanding of degenerative issues, clinicians can, in most cases, sharpen their decision-making skills and ultimately push for improved health outcomes for patients dealing with these debilitating disorders (Wen-Tseng et al., 2023) (Figure 13.4).

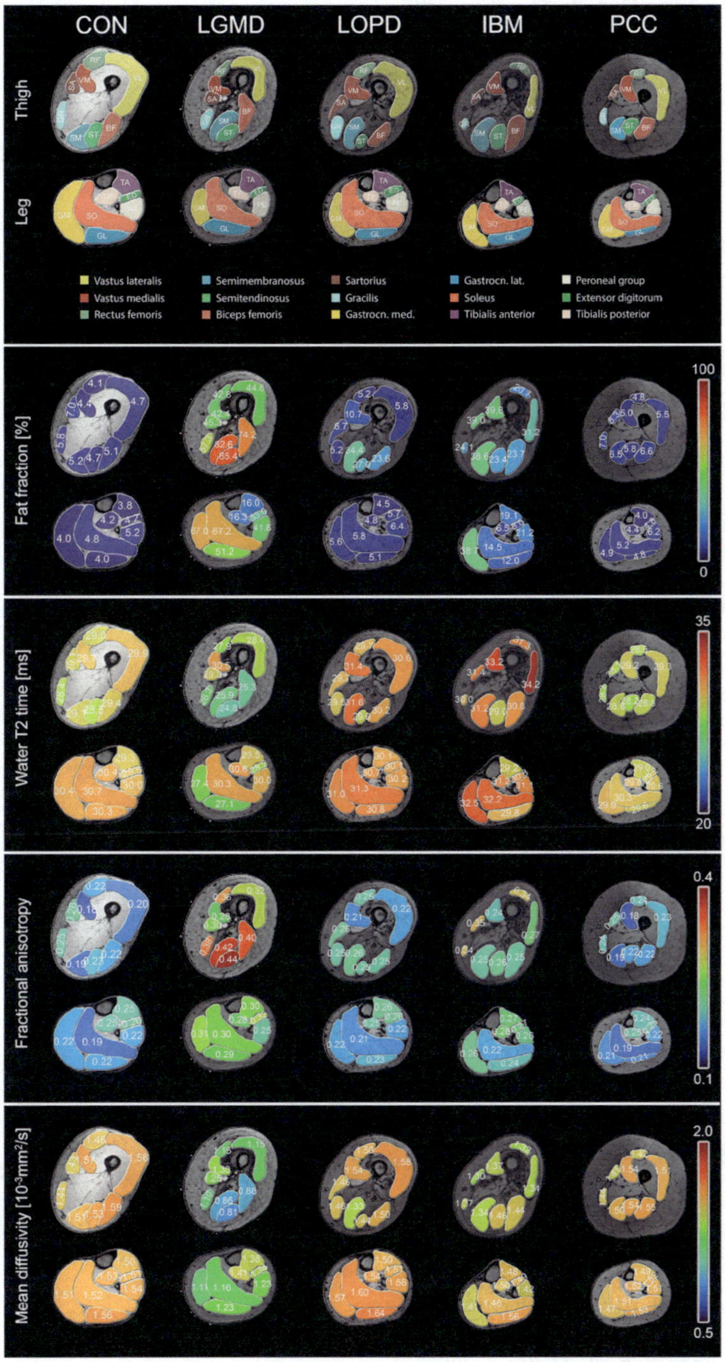

Figure 13.4. MRI of muscle.

Source: Schlaffke L, Rehmann R, Güttsches A-K, Vorgerd M, Meyer-Frießem CH, Dinse HR, Enax-Krumova E, Froeling M, Forsting J. Evaluation of Neuromuscular Diseases and Complaints by Quantitative Muscle MRI. *Journal of Clinical Medicine*. 2024; 13(7):1958. https://doi.org/10.3390/jcm13071958.

13.1.3. Tumors and Infections

Tumors and infections in the musculoskeletal system often mix in a way that makes imaging a real head-scratcher. Bone tumors, especially the nasty ones like osteosarcoma and Ewings sarcoma, can show up alongside infections, so figuring out which is which calls for imaging that goes the extra mile. MRI usually does the trick by mapping out soft tissue lumps and checking how much the nearby bone gets affected; this detail, generally speaking, is key for planning a treatment. It is also worth noting that when infections tag along, the overall outlook can shift, as some studies have shown that infections after procedures like allografts may mess with surgical outcomes and even boost the risk of complications (Aponte-Tinao et al., 2019).

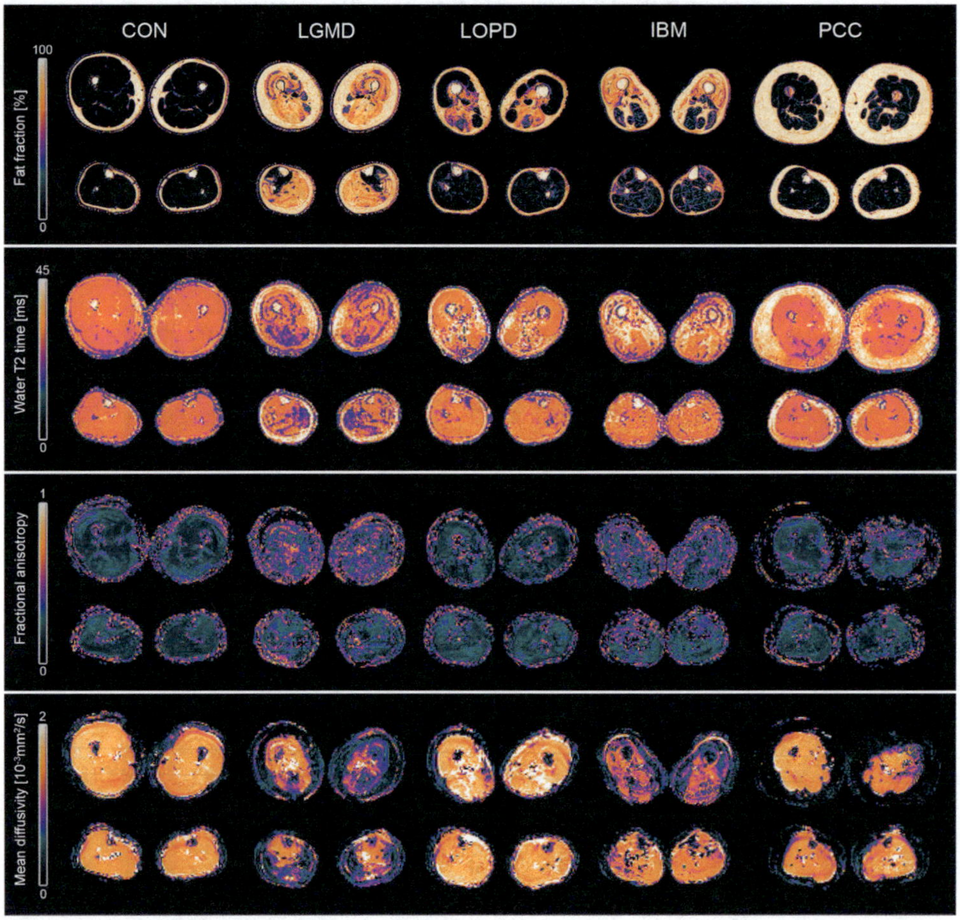

Figure 13.5. Utility of MRI for tissue assessment.

Source: Schlaffke L, Rehmann R, Güttsches A-K, Vorgerd M, Meyer-Frießem CH, Dinse HR, Enax-Krumova E, Froeling M, Forsting J. Evaluation of Neuromuscular Diseases and Complaints by Quantitative Muscle MRI. *Journal of Clinical Medicine*. 2024; 13(7):1958. https://doi.org/10.3390/jcm13071958.

Timing and choice of imaging tests play a critical role in making sense of these messy conditions. CT or PET scans, for example, offer a peek into both metabolic hustle and structural tweaks, thereby improving diagnostic precision. Surgeons often rely on preoperative images to decide whether to aim for a limb-saving operation or, in some cases, go for amputation when an infection is hiding in the mix; then, post-treatment scans help catch any recurrences or unexpected new spots. Also, by revealing shifts in tumor size or related problems like fractures and lingering infections, imaging kind of ties together a multidisciplinary approach that benefits patient care (Aponte-Tinao et al., 2019). Digging into the role of oxidative stress adds another layer to understanding how tumors and infections affect outcomes. Research often points out that oxidative stress, an imbalance where reactive oxygen or nitrogen species overpower the body's antioxidants, gets involved in how tumors start and progress, besides influencing age-related issues. In many patients with musculoskeletal tumors, extra oxidative stress might heighten the chance of identifying infections, making it an area that definitely deserves a closer look. All things considered, targeted antioxidant therapies may someday help improve results for individuals dealing with both challenges, marking this as a promising subject for future research and clinical work (Aponte-Tinao et al., 2019) (Figure 13.5).

Test Your Knowledge

1. What imaging modalities are most commonly used to detect bone fractures after trauma?
2. What are common radiographic signs of degenerative joint diseases like osteoarthritis?

13.2. Advantages and Limitations of Imaging Modalities

Learning Outcome

1. Explain the benefits of X-ray imaging.
2. Understand the limitations of MRI.
3. Identify challenges with CT Scans.

Musculoskeletal issues get looked at with a mix of imaging tests, and each comes with its own ups and downs. MRI, for example, stands out, its knack for capturing soft tissues in sharp detail means it can spot little injuries in cartilage, ligaments, and muscles that might slip past with other techniques. Generally speaking, this imaging tool picks up subtle degenerative changes pretty well, and since it doesn't use ionizing radiation, it's often the go-to for kids or patients who need regular check-ups. That said, MRI comes with a hefty price tag and longer scanning sessions, so sometimes it slows down diagnosis and treatment. Plus, in cases where patients have certain implants or feel uneasy in confined spaces, doctors might have to look for other options. On the other hand, simpler tests like X-rays and CT scans bring their own set of strengths into the mix. X-rays are widely available, inexpensive, and give quick results; they're a solid first step for spotting fractures or other bone issues. CT scans take things a bit further by offering cross-sectional images, which help generate detailed 3D views of tricky bone structures, a real asset when planning surgery. Yet, both X-rays and CT scans use ionizing radiation, posing concerns about repeated exposure, especially for younger individuals or those needing multiple scans over time. Also, while these tests excel in revealing bony details, they just don't match MRI in visualizing soft tissue problems.

In most cases, a combination of these methods is what rounds out a proper look at musculoskeletal conditions. Ultrasound has also carved out its own niche in musculoskeletal imaging lately (Wei et al., 2018). It is prized for giving real-time visuals and letting doctors perform guided interventions on the fly. This tool works well when examining soft tissue areas, say, tendons or muscles, and it is a handy choice when speed is important. Being portable and easy to use, plus lacking ionizing radiation, makes ultrasound attractive in many clinical situations. Still, its performance can depend a lot on the operator's skill, and imaging deeper structures or patients with a higher BMI can be tricky. Occasionally, the presence of gas or even nearby bone can muddy the picture. Despite these kinks, mixing ultrasound with MRI and CT usually offers a more rounded understanding of musculoskeletal pathologies, ultimately boosting diagnostic accuracy (Izquierdo et al., 2021) (Figure 13.6).

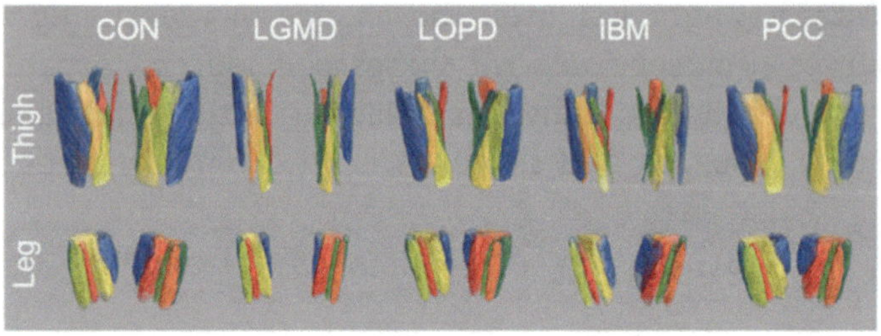

Figure 13.6. Advantages and limitations of imaging modalities.

Source: Schlaffke L, Rehmann R, Güttsches A-K, Vorgerd M, Meyer-Frießem CH, Dinse HR, Enax-Krumova E, Froeling M, Forsting J. Evaluation of Neuromuscular Diseases and Complaints by Quantitative Muscle MRI. *Journal of Clinical Medicine*. 2024; 13(7):1958. https://doi.org/10.3390/jcm13071958.

13.2.1. Benefits of X-Ray Imaging

X-ray imaging has truly reshaped how musculoskeletal issues are handled. It allows the check on our bones by offering a near live peek into skeletal layout, spotting fractures, arthritis signs, and even tumors. A fracture from an accident, for example, might be spotted right away, which in turn can prompt quick action and help dodge later complications.

Besides that, the overall cost tends to be low, making this method a favorite in settings where resources are tight. In conditions like avascular necrosis, things can be a bit more subtle. Generally speaking, although X-rays don't always seal the deal definitively, they still bring solid initial insights. Studies that have pitted X-ray results against MRI findings have noticed that, in most cases, the sensitivity and specificity remain quite robust. In one particular scenario, the accuracy for detecting avascular necrosis of the femoral head clocked in around 82.88%, a figure that supports its value as that first step in diagnosis. Even with their known limits, these scans often lay down the groundwork that guides doctors toward more advanced tests like MRI (Shakir et al., 2024).

The landscape becomes even more dynamic with the infusion of new tech like AI. Deep learning approaches have started to transform how we look at these images by automating tasks such as segmentation and interpretation; models such as U-Net and ViT, for instance, have shown pretty impressive results in picking up fractures and other subtle cues (Panhwar et al., 2024). This boost not only ramps up the efficiency of evaluations but can also flag anomalies that might otherwise slip by unnoticed, making the union of AI with traditional X-ray imaging a real game-changer in both clinical and research settings (Figure 13.7).

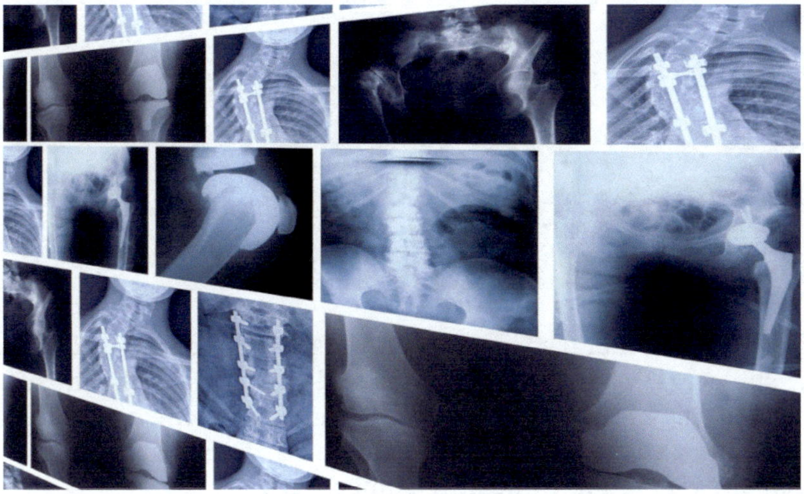

Figure 13.7. X-ray imaging has truly reshaped how musculoskeletal issues.

Source: https://lincolnurgentcare.com/benefits-of-x-rays-in-urgent-care/.

13.2.2. Limitations of Magnetic Resonance Imaging (MRI)

Magnetic resonance imaging, or MRI, is a go-to method for looking at muscles and bones, but it is not without its uniqueness. It struggles in situations like acute fractures, where its contrast isn't as clear-cut compared to, say, computed tomography (CT), which tends to show bone details more crisply in the early stages. Often, this fuzziness in early fracture images can lead to misdiagnosis and slow down treatment, especially for individuals with conditions like osteoporosis, where fractures emerge more frequently and might be easily missed (LeBoff et al., 2022). Further, sometimes MRIs aren't even available in every healthcare setting, making timely patient care even trickier. Then there's the issue of the long scanning times. In a lot of urgent cases, having to sit through a scan that can stretch from 30 minutes to an hour puts patients and healthcare teams under extra pressure. When every minute counts, those lengthy sessions might delay critical decisions in managing musculoskeletal injuries. This slowdown can have serious consequences when handling traumatic injuries or inflammatory conditions where the clock is ticking. Also, factors like claustrophobia or the presence of implants and other metals can further curb MRI's usefulness, sometimes pushing clinicians to opt for other imaging techniques that might not offer the same level of detail (Pesapane et al., 2018). On top of that, MRI sometimes falls short in spotting smaller or evolving issues. In cases where pinpoint accuracy is needed, like when checking for subtle soft tissue abnormalities or lesions, the results might not be as reliable, leading to occasional false negatives. This challenge is even more noticeable among older patients or those juggling multiple health issues, where the blurry lines in diagnosis can complicate decision-making. Given all this, doctors have to be extra careful when interpreting MRI scans, often using additional imaging methods to ensure nothing critical is missed (LeBoff et al., 2022) (Figure 13.8).

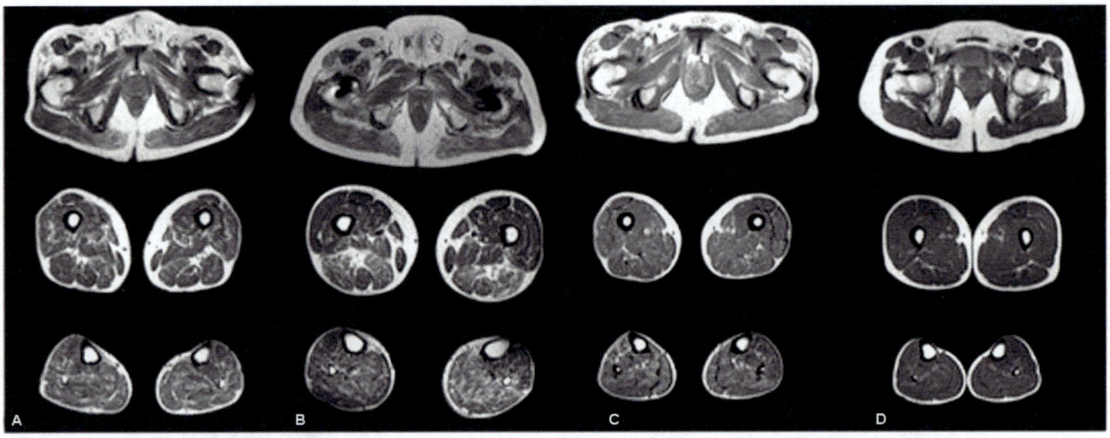

Figure 13.8. Muscle MRI pattern of fatty infiltration in ATTRv patients (#2 in (**A**); #6 in (**B**); #1 in (**C**) and in a healthy subject (**D**). Tensor fascia latae and soleus were the most frequently involved muscles, with relative sparing of the iliopsoas, rectus femoris, gracilis and anterior tibilias muscles (**A**,**B**); in only one case the anterior tibialis presented an asymmetric severe adipose substitution (**C**). No fatty replacement was found in healthy subject (**D**).

Source: Primiano G, Verdolotti T, D'Apolito G, Di Paolantonio A, Guglielmino V, Romano A, Lucioli G, Luigetti M, Servidei S. Muscle MRI as a Useful Biomarker in Hereditary Transthyretin Amyloidosis: A Pilot Study. *Genes*. 2021; 12(11):1786. https://doi.org/10.3390/genes12111786.

13.2.3. Challenges with Computed Tomography (CT) Scans

CT imaging in musculoskeletal care shows both promising insights and noticeable drawbacks. Many appreciate that CT scans can reveal detailed views of bones and joints, yet there's a persistent worry over the radiation exposure, especially for young patients where cumulative doses become a real issue. There's always this tug-of-war between chasing precise diagnoses and facing the risks of ionizing radiation. Sometimes the images don't neatly distinguish between benign and malignant conditions, which can lead to mix-ups and misguided treatments. High-resolution scans, despite their impressive clarity, can sometimes hide those more complicated underlying problems, like elusive joint lesions, that end up prompting extra tests or even mismanaged treatment plans. Overall, it calls for a more careful, if not unpredictable, reevaluation of how these imaging procedures are used when assessing joints and bones. Interpreting CT scans isn't as straightforward as it might appear. Overlapping radiological features often blur the lines between multiple conditions, making it hard to pin down what's going on. For instance, figuring out whether a joint issue is due to an infection or a malignancy can be challenging because both tend to look surprisingly alike on the scan. In many cases, clinicians resort to secondary imaging studies to confirm their suspicions, but these alternatives don't always clear things up either. Research has noted that non-Hodgkin lymphoma can mimic osteomyelitis on radiographic images (Celayir et al., 2025), which means that often a team effort among radiologists, orthopedic surgeons, and oncologists becomes necessary to trim down misinterpretations. On top of that, newer techniques like PET/CT are opening fresh avenues in musculoskeletal evaluation, but they're not without their own uniqueness. Recent studies generally show that innovations such as 68Ga-FAPI PET/CT can sometimes improve diagnostic accuracy, yet they also bring added challenges in interpreting the nuances of tracer uptake and its clinical relevance (Al-Ibraheem et al., 2025). Elevated uptake in various tumors might be mistaken for other degenerative changes, further clouding an already murky picture. This mix-up underscores the need for more robust, standardized protocols in these advanced imaging tools. All things considered, sorting through the complexities of CT scans and newer modalities is key to boosting diagnostic precision and fine-tuning treatment strategies in musculoskeletal care (Figure 13.9).

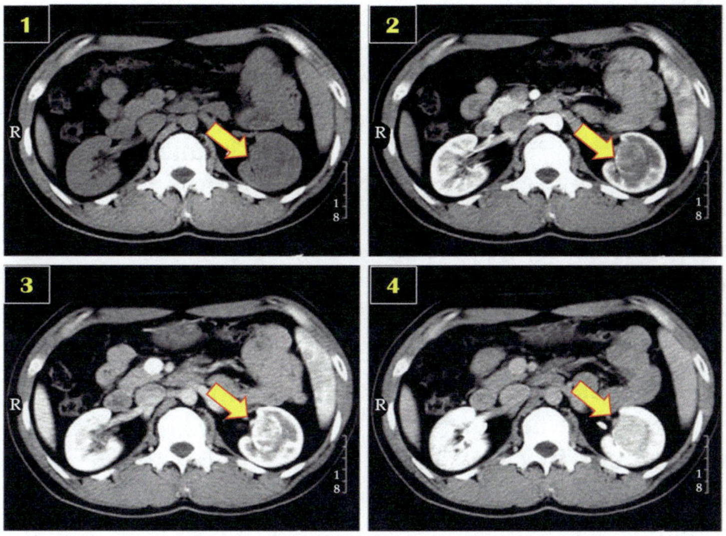

Figure 13.9. Temporal changes in a lesion with contrast-enhanced CT.

Source: Primiano, G., Verdolotti, T., D'Apolito, G., Di Paolantonio, A., Guglielmino, V., Romano, A., Lucioli, G., Luigetti, M., & Servidei, S. (2021). Muscle MRI as a Useful Biomarker in Hereditary Transthyretin Amyloidosis: A Pilot Study. *Genes*, *12*(11), 1786. https://doi.org/10.3390/genes12111786.

Test Your Knowledge

1. What is one key advantage of MRI over X-rays in musculoskeletal imaging?
2. Why might ultrasound be preferred over CT for evaluating soft tissue injuries?
3. What is a common limitation of using X-rays for diagnosing early-stage joint disorders?

13.3. Role of Imaging in Diagnosis

Learning Outcome

1. Develop the ability to identify musculoskeletal pathologies.
2. Understand assessing treatment efficacy in musculoskeletal conditions.
3. Explore the role of imaging in guiding surgical interventions.

Imaging is crucial when doctors try to figure out musculoskeletal puzzles. MRI, ultrasound, and basic X-rays all chip in, each in their own way. X-rays tend to show big, obvious changes and help narrow things down, though they can miss early hints of inflammation and wear, something that's evident in cases like juvenile idiopathic arthritis, where spotting the issue early is key to avoiding permanent joint damage. Nowadays, there's a noticeable shift toward using more advanced scans like MRI, which, generally speaking, picks up on joint details and cartilage shifts much better, helping to steer clinical decisions faster (Hemke et al., 2020). Then you've got Cone Beam Computed Tomography (CBCT), a tool that started off making waves in dental imaging but now shows up all over musculoskeletal diagnostics. Its high spatial resolution mixed with lower radiation makes it particularly handy for checking out small joints and spotting subtle problems. CBCT can, in most cases, give a more detailed view of cartilage issues and joint degeneration than standard radiographs, this extra level of detail not only hones diagnostic accuracy but also paves the way for treatment plans that are more on target, ultimately boosting patient outcomes. As imaging tech continues to evolve, it is important to grasp what each method can do (and its limits) for fine-tuning these strategies (Posadzy et al., 2018). Combining all these imaging techniques creates a fuller picture of a patient's condition. While MRI excels at showing soft tissue details, ultrasound is often the go-to for guiding things like joint injections and offering live feedback. This kind of mixed approach, even with a few uniqueness in phrasing here and there, tends to help doctors better understand disease progress and monitor how treatments are working, which in turn leads to more personalized care. As research slowly unveils more about musculoskeletal issues, leaning into the diverse roles of these imaging tools is bound to shape the way future diagnostic plans and therapeutic strategies come together (Hemke et al., 2020).

13.3.1. Identifying Pathologies

Imaging technology keeps evolving in unexpected ways, shifting how we spot issues in muscles and bones. Musculoskeletal ultrasound, or MSKUS, has been obtaining attention lately because it gives clear, high-res views of soft tissue just under the skin. This tool turns out to be quite handy when checking for things like lateral epicondylitis and other soft tissue hiccups. With its real-time view, docs get to watch changes as they happen and tweak treatments on the fly. In most cases, compared to old-school methods like X-rays, MSKUS offers more precise details, especially when dealing with those messy, complex tissues. It not only helps nail down diagnoses but also makes it easier to follow up on how patients are doing, which can lead to more personalized rehab steps, generally speaking. AI's entry into the musculoskeletal imaging field is kind of a game-changer. These days, AI is being woven into the fabric of diagnosing issues from simple trauma to osteoarthritis and even tumors. AI algorithms now help flag fractures swiftly, a critical step for speedy intervention, even if it means managing cases that might otherwise get overlooked. AIs ability (or sometimes AI's, depending on who's writing) to estimate bone age cuts down on the bumps of inter-observer differences, and that smooths out the radiologist's workload. Instead of replacing human expertise, AI, by and large, serves as that extra set of hands, letting clinicians focus on the trickier parts while routine checks are handled more efficiently. Overall, it's a tool designed to augment, not supplant, the radiologist, especially in a busy era of ever-growing tech demands and patient lists. In detecting musculoskeletal problems, the mix of cutting-edge imaging and emerging technologies creates a curious interplay. Conditions like osteoarthritis and soft-tissue tumors demand precise and sometimes creative imaging techniques, and MSKUS can reveal subtle shifts that regular scans might miss. For instance, a quick glance at an ultrasound display can show tiny changes in tissue that might otherwise slip by unnoticed. At the same time, as AI continues to creep into everyday practice, we're beginning to see more automated reads and interpretations. Generally speaking, this evolution might even refine how outcomes are predicted and how treatment paths are chosen. The blend of innovative imaging tech with its analytical smarts offers clinicians a nearly endless toolbox, one that reshapes both how diseases are diagnosed and how treatments are ultimately planned (Figure 13.10).

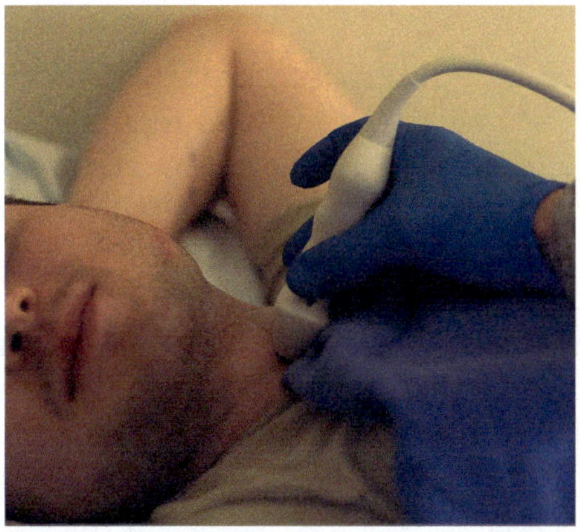

Figure 13.10. Musculoskeletal ultrasound.

Source: By Senior Airman David C. Danford, released - A look beneath the surface, Public Domain, https://commons.wikimedia.org/w/index.php?curid=71875794.

13.3.2. Assessing Treatment Efficacy

Successful care for musculoskeletal problems depends a lot on how we check treatment results, this can change patient outcomes. Even the imaging tools we once used just to diagnose have turned into key ways to watch how therapy is working. Take psoriatic arthritis, for instance; identifying early signs of entheseal inflammation is not only important to avoid joint damage but also helps doctors adjust treatments when needed. Nowadays, ultrasound and MRI, among other methods, give us a clearer look at muscle and joint structures. They help clinicians notice even tiny shifts in how a disease is progressing or responding to treatment. Getting everyone to use common definitions and scoring systems is pretty crucial to keep things consistent in clinical trials and, as Bakewell et al. (2019) points out, to nail down more precise evaluations of new interventions. At the same time, recent advances in imaging have given us a more subtle read on low-grade inflammation, something that can be tricky to spot with older techniques. Techniques like Superb Microvascular Imaging (SMI) have shown they're generally more sensitive at picking up vascular flow related to inflammation than Power Doppler Ultrasound (PDUS). Some studies even suggest that SMI beats PDUS in showing the blood vessel activity in joints that hurt, offering a broader picture of what's going on (Lim et al., 2017). This extra sensitivity can mean earlier interventions, which might shift the disease course and improve patient outcomes. Using these advanced imaging methods lets healthcare providers fine-tune treatment strategies to match an individual's needs based on real-time evaluations, something that's becoming more and more important. Musculoskeletal imaging is always on the move with new technology, so working toward standard practices is key if we want treatment assessments to be effective. The mix of different imaging methods and varied interpretations sometimes makes clinical choices inconsistent, so having validated scoring systems can help compare studies better. By agreeing on definitions and protocols, researchers can more easily figure out how emerging therapies are doing and ensure data from different clinical scenarios match up reliably. This consistency not only strengthens how we interpret imaging findings but also ties in with today's push for personalized musculoskeletal care (Bakewell et al., 2019). In the end, these efforts are pretty fundamental to deepening our understanding of treatment efficacy in a field that's constantly being reshaped by new tech (Figure 13.11).

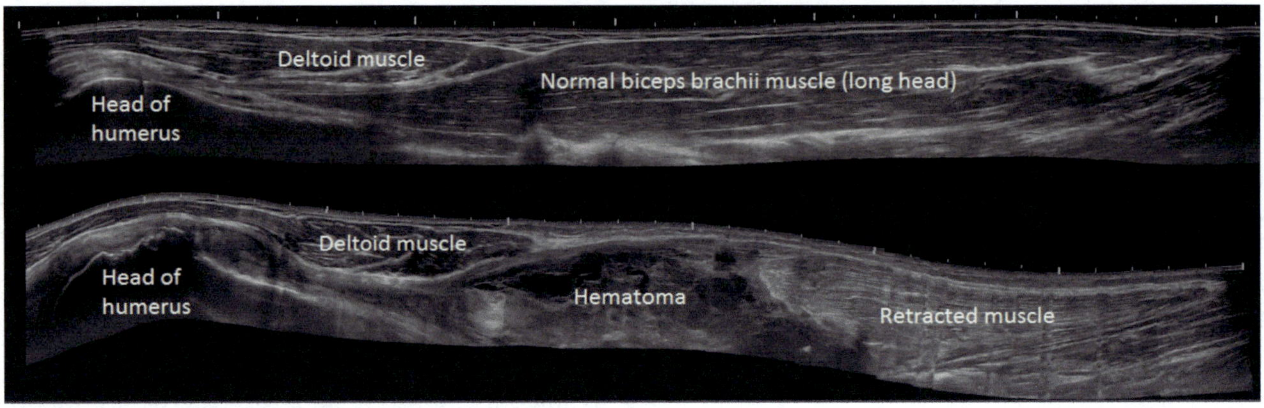

Figure 13.11. Panoramic ultrasonography of a proximal biceps tendon rupture. Top image shows the contralateral normal side, and lower image shows a retracted muscle, with a hematoma filling out the proximal space.

Source: By Mikael Häggström, M.D. Author info- Reusing images- Conflicts of interest: NoneMikael Häggström, M.D. Consent note: Written informed consent was obtained from the individual, including online publication. - Own work, CC0, https://commons.wikimedia.org/w/index.php?curid=80490323.

13.3.3. Guiding Surgical Interventions

Effective communication in musculoskeletal imaging – and how it shapes surgical decisions – is super important for improving patient outcomes. Doctors rely on these scans to figure out what's going on, but sometimes they mix up normal age changes with something more serious, which can spark unnecessary worry and even lead to interventions that aren't needed. One study shows that individuals often mistake harmless changes for major issues, tying their pain to what's just a normal part of aging. Generally speaking, building clear, straightforward ways to talk about these things – drawing on ideas from behavioral science – can help both clinicians and patients deal with the messy realities of musculoskeletal pain. This need for solid, easy-to-understand patient info goes a long way in explaining what imaging means and in calming the anxiety that might otherwise trigger needless surgery (Kirby et al., 2025). New image-guided tools like ultrasound (US) and CT have changed the way surgical decisions are made. These tools deliver live images, letting doctors pinpoint the exact spot where tissues or structures might be causing pain. The move toward these less invasive techniques not only cuts down on risks usually seen in traditional surgery, it also helps lower overall healthcare costs. Techniques such as anesthetic injections or even platelet-rich plasma therapy don't just ease the pain – they also lend a hand in healing soft tissues by initiating the regeneration process. In most cases, these innovations put interventional radiologists right at the forefront of managing issues, since dependable non-invasive options can often let us avoid more drastic surgical moves (Batra et al., 2025). At the end of the day, as musculoskeletal imaging becomes more common, a team effort between imaging experts and surgeons turns out to be key for top-notch patient care. A good team-style approach, built on clear communication, makes sure that surgery happens only when truly needed – only when the benefits outweigh the risks. And as imaging technology keeps evolving, the way we read and explain what's going on in these scans needs to keep up too. By nurturing an environment where different experts freely share their ideas, surgical choices can be made smarter, and patients end up with a broader view of their musculoskeletal health. Embracing this collaborative mindset is essential not just for better clinical outcomes, but for cutting back on the unnecessary operations that weigh down our healthcare system (Kirby et al., 2025).

Test Your Knowledge

1. In what way does MRI contribute to the diagnosis of soft tissue injuries?
2. Why is imaging important for monitoring the progression of musculoskeletal diseases like osteoarthritis?

13.4. Advances in Musculoskeletal Imaging

Learning Outcome

1. Define the technological innovations.
2. Discuss the artificial intelligence in imaging.
3. Explore the future trends and research directions.

Musculoskeletal imaging has come a long way, reshaping how we spot and treat issues with bones, joints, and muscles. Now, instead of a one-size-fits-all check, doctors use a mix of tools that reveal details in surprising ways, taking us beyond simple X-rays. High-resolution MRI, for example, dives deep into anatomy, exposing little changes that sometimes hint at conditions early on; then there's 3D CT, which gives a full, almost tangible spatial picture and proves especially handy when planning surgeries. These new methods boost how accurately problems are diagnosed and, by extension, how treatments are planned, all of which matters for patient care (Almeida et al., 2021). Imaging techniques aren't sticking to old scripts either; they're switching things up, especially in rheumatologic challenges. Take musculoskeletal ultrasound, it has become a favorite for watching over inflammatory troubles like rheumatoid arthritis without needing invasive approaches. Often, this method picks up signs like subclinical synovitis that might not be obvious initially, a detail that can shift the whole outlook on prognosis and treatment. And then, with microvascular imaging identifying even the subtlest blood-vessel shifts that older methods might miss, doctors can try to step in earlier. This blend of techniques underlines just how adaptable and forward-thinking musculoskeletal imaging is in meeting today's clinical needs (Almeida et al., 2021). Peering into the future, combining smart imaging tech with fresh computational methods could well change the game entirely. Machine learning and radiomics are stepping up, sifting through image data to pull out patterns that traditional tools might simply gloss over. In most cases, these approaches help pin down details that aren't immediately obvious, offering a new depth of insight. Moreover, when imaging teams up with genetic and biomarker data, it paves the way for personalized treatments that fit each patient just right. Overall, these developments stress the ongoing need for creative research and constant innovation to keep pushing musculoskeletal diagnostics and therapy forward (Jandan, 2020) (Figure 13.12).

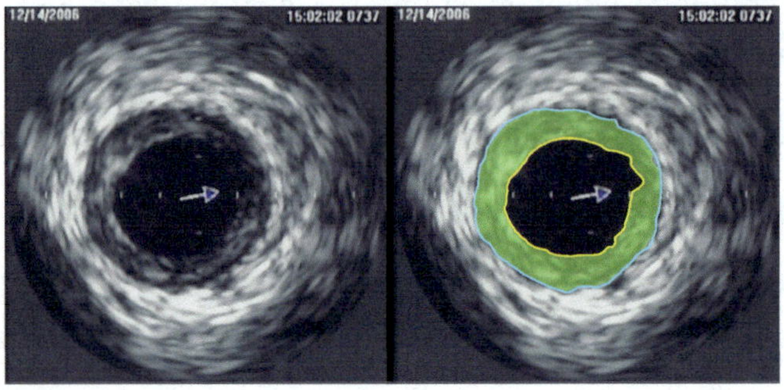

Figure 13.12. Intravascular ultrasound image of a coronary artery (left), with color-coding on the right, delineating the lumen (yellow), external elastic membrane (blue) and the atherosclerotic plaque burden (green).

Source: By The original uploader was Ksheka at English Wikipedia. - Transferred from en.wikipedia to Commons by Stevenfruitsmaak using CommonsHelper., , https://commons.wikimedia.org/w/index.php?curid=5734047.

13.4.1. Technological Innovations

Musculoskeletal imaging has come into its own with the latest tech advances. High-resolution MRIs and CT scans now let doctors get an up-close look at bones, muscles, and soft tissues, often identifying signs of arthritis, fractures, or other injuries sooner than before. These clearer images not only show the anatomy in great detail but also help track how a condition unfolds, which means treatments can be fine-tuned almost in real-time. Generally speaking, this leads to more spot-on diagnoses and treatment plans that feel custom-made, easing the long-term strain of musculoskeletal disorders that affect millions, especially older individuals (Wu et al., 2024). AI is also shaking things up in this field. By crunching massive amounts of imaging data super-fast, AI can pick up on tiny abnormalities that might slip past even the best human eyes. This quick data parsing not only boosts diagnostic precision but also streamlines day-to-day work, freeing clinicians to spend more time on patients rather than paper work. In many cases, AI-driven tools are even starting to predict patient outcomes and help tailor individual treatment plans. Still, as AI becomes more woven into clinical routines, there's a growing need to address concerns about data privacy and the fairness of automated decision-making (Karalis, 2024). Tech breakthroughs and a rising demand for non-invasive tests are pushing further investments in musculoskeletal imaging. Real-time ultrasound, for example, has become a key player in both diagnosing and guiding therapy because it is portable, cost-effective, and can even capture joint movement as it happens. Meanwhile, leaps in imaging software, like 3D reconstructions and even augmented reality features, are giving doctors a fresher, more nuanced view of complex issues. All these innovations, taken together, give orthopedic surgeons, physiotherapists, and other specialists extra tools to craft well-rounded, patient-focused care strategies that tackle the many issues of musculoskeletal disorders.

13.4.2. Artificial Intelligence (AI) in Imaging

AI has been shaking up medical imaging, especially in musculoskeletal diagnostics. We used to rely solely on human interpretation, which could get skewed by factors like tiredness or varying levels of experience. Lately, deep learning methods have stepped into the picture and, generally speaking, turned things on their head. They're great at spotting patterns and can sift through huge piles of data with a kind of precision that's hard to beat. Recent advances show these networks can handle the messy details of medical images, giving clinicians a clearer peek into underlying issues. This shift not only hikes up diagnostic accuracy but also speeds up decision-making, which can mean better outcomes for patients (Lee et al., 2024). Shoulder problems are a perfect example of where things get tricky. In imaging the shoulder, things often end up ambiguous and hard to pin down. Sure, ultrasonography is a neat, non-invasive tool, but sorting out the fine details of shoulder structures isn't always simple. Lately, though, deep learning algorithms have been offered a helping hand by combined themselves to robust image segmentation techniques. For example, models like U-Net have been tried out to see how they can tease apart different shoulder tissues from ultrasound images. In several studies, these approaches showed promising numbers, as seen in metrics like mean Average Precision and Intersection over Union, pointing to a strong potential for refining diagnoses of shoulder injuries (Lee et al., 2024). AI's influence doesn't stop at the shoulder; it stretches across many parts of the body. As more healthcare systems adopt deep learning frameworks, there's generally a growing move toward standardizing diagnostic evaluations. This consistency helps guide less experienced clinicians, since these smart systems can double as decision-support buddies. And as more data gets tossed into the mix, these AI models seem to keep getting sharper in their diagnostic skills. In essence, the blend of AI and imaging looks set to boost the overall effectiveness of healthcare delivery, reminding us that ongoing research and development in the field is absolutely key (Lee et al., 2024) (Figure 13.13).

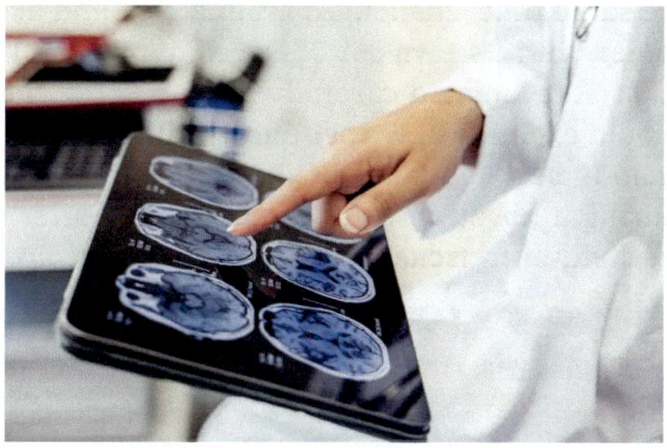

Figure 13.13. Artificial Intelligence (AI) in Imaging.

Source: https://imageio.forbes.com/specials-images/imageserve/67c86f60dfc60d1bb54bfea5//960x0.jpg?height=474&width=711&fit=bounds.

13.4.3. Future Trends and Research Directions

Musculoskeletal imaging is heading into a new era thanks to AI. Nowadays, deep learning helps build smart systems that can catch those tiny anomalies radiologists might easily miss. AI algorithms analyze imaging data in ways that not only boost accuracy and efficiency but also cut down the time needed for reviews. It is important to note that this technology isn't about replacing human expertise, rather, it is combined with routine practice as a supportive partner, creating a more collaborative clinical setting. Researchers, in most cases, now stress the need to test and standardize these methods across different clinical environments to ensure they truly work as intended (Chen et al., 2024). Portable ultrasound devices are also shaking things up. They bring dynamic imaging possibilities outside the confines of big hospitals, sometimes in clinics, sports centers, or even at home. A number of studies suggest that having these devices on hand can enhance decision-making in real time when managing musculoskeletal conditions. As the devices become increasingly sophisticated, it is crucial, generally speaking, for researchers to take a closer look at their long-term effects on patient outcomes and overall healthcare delivery. Comparing these portable options with traditional imaging techniques might well reveal some unexpected insights that could alter current practices (Chen et al., 2024). At the same time, challenges around cost and accessibility keep reminding us that every advancement comes with its own set of issues. While the latest tech promises sharper diagnostic capabilities, it must be evaluated carefully so as not to widen existing gaps in healthcare access. Future studies should examine how cost-effective these new imaging methods are, and explore ways to implement them in settings that are under resourced without compromising quality. Some experts argue that pairing innovation with fairness is key, after all, a balanced approach is what will ultimately drive the field of musculoskeletal imaging forward.

Test Your Knowledge

1. How has 3D imaging improved surgical planning in orthopedic cases?
2. What is the benefit of using artificial intelligence in musculoskeletal image interpretation?

13.5. Ethical Considerations in Imaging

Learning Outcome

1. Understand the importance of obtaining patient consent and privacy.
2. Examine concerns related to radiation exposure concerns.
3. Explore the challenges of cost and accessibility issues.

Technology and healthcare have come together in unexpected ways, shaking up musculoskeletal imaging through using AI. This shift isn't just a new trend, it stirs up important ethical issues, especially when patient care and fairness are on the line. AI now helps decode complex images, making it necessary to keep an eye on biases in these systems that might hurt certain groups. Many believe that, generally speaking, following a kind of unwritten social contract means healthcare pros should actively check for these biases and work to give every ethnic and racial group a fair shot in imaging datasets. Keeping data diverse isn't merely good practice; it is a key part of protecting patient rights in an age where algorithms make more decisions every day, and if we drop the ball here, we risk deepening existing healthcare gaps and undermining trust in the imaging field. AI's growing role in diagnosing and managing musculoskeletal conditions takes ethical concerns a step further than just data fairness. Radiologists and other care providers now need to explain to patients exactly how these smart tools will affect their treatment, a must for proper informed consent. In most cases, this clear communication helps bridge the gap between high-tech imaging and patient understanding. Doctors face a tricky challenge: they must use advanced imaging responsibly while making sure patients know both the upsides and the limitations of AI-driven diagnostics. Adopting a more values-driven mindset reminds everyone that patient well-being should always come before the lure of new technology. In doing so, the imaging community builds trust, which is essential for strong patient-provider relationships and better overall outcomes. The ethical scene gets even more complicated as technology speeds ahead. AI offers the promise of better diagnoses for conditions like osteoporosis and other bone problems, but rapid innovation brings its own set of challenges. Questions about how cost-effective or accessible these new tools are emerge frequently, there's a worry that not everyone will get equal access simply because of socioeconomic differences. From a practical mindset, ensuring fair distribution of these imaging advances could help tackle major health issues more effectively. If everyone benefits from AI-enhanced diagnostics, the healthcare system would do right by its social contract with the public while blending technology with the core mission of improving patient care. All of this underscores the need for ongoing, open conversations about how to ethically weave AI into musculoskeletal imaging as we navigate today's complex medical landscape.

13.5.1. Patient Consent and Privacy

In musculoskeletal imaging, patient consent and privacy matter a whole lot. It isn't just about ticking boxes, sharing sensitive health details for these studies often comes with its own bundle of legal and ethical headaches. Patient data has to be treated with extreme care because a breach isn't a small slip-up; it can hurt patients and break the trust built in our healthcare systems. You might even say that the weak spots in many health systems make the whole situation even messier, pointing us toward a real need for better privacy rules. When providers dig into what patient consent means, they can create an atmosphere where everything feels more open and trustworthy, ensuring patients are not only informed but feel in charge of their own medical decisions. At its core, this way of thinking drives ethical practices in imaging, making it clear that we need more solid frameworks in place to protect personal privacy. Consent procedures today aren't just about being tough; they must also roll with the punches as technology shifts. Many patients find themselves baffled by the complicated language of informed consent, especially when it involves procedures as tricky as musculoskeletal imaging. That's where clinicians step in, untangling the process and explaining exactly what patients are saying "yes" to, risks, benefits, and all. When communication falters, misunderstandings can arise and lead to ethical dilemmas that ultimately chip away at patient independence. Several comparative studies have shown that using plain, friendly language on consent forms, and pairing that with honest, sometimes even ad hoc, discussions between doctors and patients, makes a difference. In most cases, as research on informed consent, privacy, and dignity suggests, nailing these conversations can tie legal rules to ethical practice, helping to nurture an environment that truly values patient choice. The link between patient consent and privacy laws is no small matter in musculoskeletal imaging, it is a mixed bag that calls for proactive, cross-disciplinary action. With digital health technologies evolving so quickly, the risk of data leaks or unauthorized peeks into patient information keeps rising, and that frankly makes everybody more vulnerable.

Legal frameworks, therefore, need to catch up; they must ensure that every consent process isn't just all-inclusive but also enforceable in this whirlwind digital era. One cannot stress enough how crucial it is to have independent oversight groups; these bodies help keep privacy regulations on track, even if their monitoring sometimes seems a bit inconsistent. By pushing adaptive and flexible data security measures, healthcare systems might just be able to lessen the risks tied to sensitive information. Ultimately, balancing patient privacy with the rapid progress of modern medicine remains a tough challenge, one that forces the entire healthcare industry to blend ethical, legal, and tech-savvy approaches into everyday patient care.

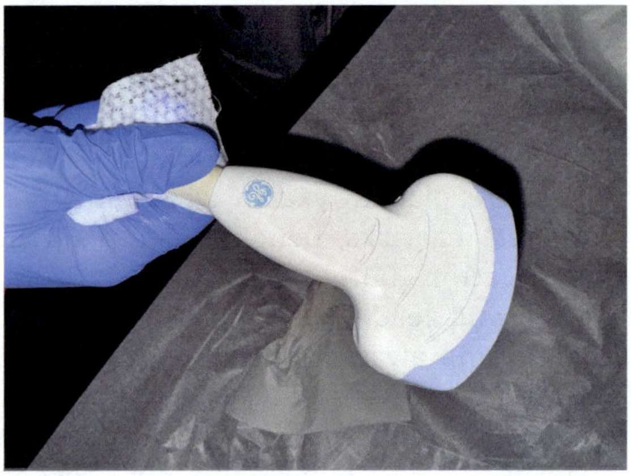

Source: By Harrison Keely - Own work, CC BY 4.0, https://commons.wikimedia.org/w/index.php?curid=149292840.

13.5.2. Radiation Exposure Concerns

Musculoskeletal imaging has come a long way in boosting diagnosis, but it also brings a twist, radiation risks. X-rays, CT scans, and fluoroscopy are everywhere, yet many individuals don't grasp that ionizing radiation matters. A lot of people, it seems, overlook that natural radiation is always around and end up mixing up the doses from different tests. Over two-thirds of participants didn't know much about these natural sources, and many even thought that chest X-rays and CT scans hit you with about the same dose (Alburayh et al., 2025). This shows, generally speaking, that we need new ways to educate patients about the specific dangers tied to each imaging method so they can make smarter choices about their health. Finding the right balance between making an accurate diagnosis and cutting down on radiation isn't easy. Ionizing radiation can lead to serious health issues like cancer and early cell damage, and even low doses can add up over time, especially for people who need frequent imaging for musculoskeletal problems. To make things worse, when radioactive materials from these tests aren't disposed of properly, they can create extra environmental hazards (Adelodun et al., 2025). It is a situation that calls for a thoughtful approach, sticking to safety guidelines, fine-tuning imaging techniques, and sometimes opting for alternatives like ultrasound or MRI when possible to lower the risk. More and more, as awareness of radiation safety grows, it is important to have open, honest talks about both the ups and downs of musculoskeletal imaging. Doctors should speak plainly with patients about why a scan might be needed, what the risks are, even repeating the key points if necessary, and whether there's another way to check things out. One study even noted that when people were given a heads-up about radiation risks, their understanding and perceptions improved.

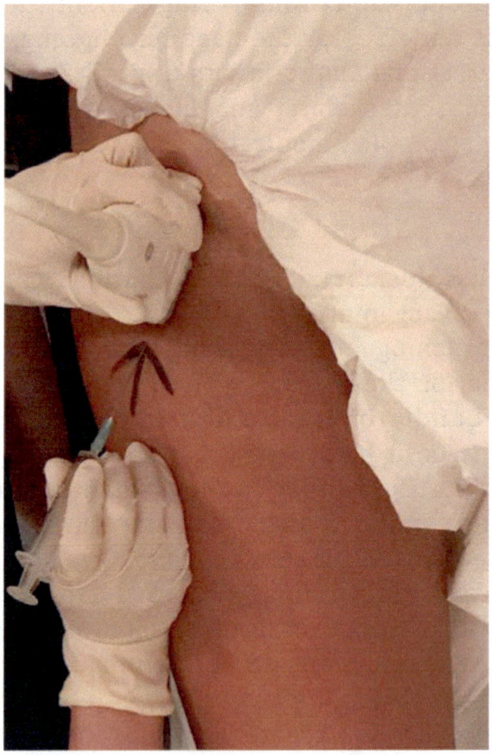

Source: By Phey Ming Yeap, Philip Robinson - (2017). "Ultrasound Diagnostic and Therapeutic Injections of the Hip and Groin." Journal of the Belgian Society of Radiology 101 (S2). DOI:10.5334/jbr-btr.1371. ISSN 2514-8281. Creative Commons Attribution 4.0 International License (CC-BY 4.0), CC BY 4.0, https://commons.wikimedia.org/w/index.php?curid=77482766.

By clearing up common misconceptions, clinicians can help patients feel more involved in making decisions about their care (Alburayh et al., 2025). As imaging technology keeps evolving, ongoing training in radiation safety and more relaxed, honest patient talks will likely boost care quality and help everyone better navigate the complexities of radiation exposure in musculoskeletal assessments.

13.5.3. Cost and Accessibility Issues

Rising prices in musculoskeletal imaging tell a bigger story about overall health spending, and they stir up some real issues with getting care. New imaging tools keep evolving and, generally, their costs tend to climb too. This means that many patients, especially those on tighter budgets or from lower-income backgrounds, end up missing out on these key tests. Providers, facing heavy expenses, may even cut back on offering these essential services. Insurance coverage isn't consistent everywhere, so a lot of individuals find themselves hit with steep out-of-pocket charges for tests that are pretty much a must. Often, this leads to delayed diagnoses and treatment, which only makes conditions worse and drives long-term expenses higher. When you consider how early detection can change patient outcomes and lower overall costs, it becomes clear that making these imaging services affordable is absolutely critical. Money isn't the only barrier here; geography adds its own set of challenges. Individuals living in rural areas or underserved parts of cities often struggle to get advanced scans like MRIs or CTs. Without specialized centers nearby, long travel times and extra expenses can easily discourage someone from getting a needed check-up. And, when limited imaging services are available, the chances of misdiagnosis or delayed care naturally go up, resulting in unnecessary pain and prolonged suffering. In most cases, addressing these spatial inequities means thinking outside the box: locating imaging centers more strategically or even investing in mobile units that bring the service to those who need it most. There's also a strong push from major guideline bodies for imaging to be both accessible and comprehensive. Findings from groups like the ACR and the Arthritis Foundation generally back a range of treatments based on solid evidence, especially in managing osteoarthritis. Yet, these recommendations don't help much if patients can't get the imaging they need for an accurate diagnosis and proper follow-up. As clinicians talk things over with their patients, the availability of these tools has to be front and center in the conversation, particularly for those battling musculoskeletal issues. Ultimately, making sure that imaging services are within reach isn't just a nice-to-have; it is a crucial part of building a responsive, patient-focused healthcare system (Sharon et al., 2020).

Test Your Knowledge

1. Why is informed consent important before conducting any diagnostic imaging procedure?
2. What ethical concerns arise from unnecessary or repeated imaging tests?

Summary

Musculoskeletal imaging has come a long way lately, changing the game for diagnosis and overall patient care. Doctors now lean on modern tools like MRI, CT scans, and even ultrasound, which let them peek at bones, cartilage, and soft tissues in a way that older methods just couldn't match. These tools help catch everything from joint issues to sports injuries sooner rather than later. Machine learning, even if it sometimes seems a bit intrusive, has teamed up with imaging to give clinicians a bit more confidence when making treatment calls. Overall, these shifts aren't just about fancy gadgets; they're paving the way for treatment plans that are more personal and ultimately lead to a better quality of life.

That said, not everything is smooth sailing. There are still hurdles that hold back the full promise of these breakthroughs. Limited access, high costs, and the heavy tech requirements can stall progress, especially in rural or underserved areas. Add in persistent worries over patient data privacy and a lack of agreed-upon imaging protocols, and it is clear that more work must be done. Health leaders need to focus on better training, secure funding, and even tweak policies so that everyone can share in these advances. In most cases, technological progress needs to dance in step with solving these socio-economic challenges. Research and team efforts remain critical for what comes next in musculoskeletal imaging. As experts experiment with new imaging methods or fine-tune existing ones, it is important to keep in mind the full picture: patient outcomes, ethical concerns, and the way care gets delivered. Radiologists, orthopedic specialists, and tech pros, often bringing in each other's perspectives, can create best practices that bridge imaging with everyday treatment. In an atmosphere that welcomes off-the-cuff ideas alongside rigorous study, the community is set to boost both our diagnostic skills and therapies tailored to individual needs. Ongoing exploration, even if a bit messy at times, will help ensure this vital part of medicine keeps up with new technological horizons.

AI is making its mark on musculoskeletal imaging in unexpected ways. Radiologists, who once juggled countless routine checks like fracture spotting and bone age evaluations, now find that AI is easing their workload considerably. In many cases, these smart tools handle repetitive tasks, reducing the natural differences between one observer's reading and another's, and helping speed up decisions when time is of the essence. AI isn't here to replace radiologists; rather, it is there to bolster their expertise, letting them zero in on trickier cases such as osteoarthritis or tumors (Gitto et al., 2024). Generally speaking, understanding these technological shifts is key since they alter clinical routines and the overall delivery of musculoskeletal care. Imaging techniques have come a long way lately, leading to fresh guidelines for soft tissue tumor evaluations. The new European Society of Musculoskeletal Radiology (ESSR) consensus guidelines, born from extensive expert chat, offer some interesting algorithms for staging high-grade sarcomas as well as benign conditions. Sometimes, the guidelines even suggest methods like whole-body MRI for identifying bone metastases or leaning on pulmonary MDCT when dealing with high-grade sarcomas. In most cases, these updates are meant to iron out common diagnostic slip-ups and to pave the way for interventions made on time. It appears that many radiologists agree these standard protocols are just what the field needs (Noebauer-Huhmann et al., 2024).

There's also plenty to be said about keeping things standardized. Having a set framework means exam results can be compared more reliably and helps build those big databases crucial for future research and analysis. By outlining best practices, the new guidelines support radiologists grappling with complex conditions like soft tissue tumors, keeping a steady hand on both diagnosis and future tech development. Overall, merging cutting-edge AI with solid consensus guidelines is clearly shifting the imaging field toward a smarter, more efficient approach that benefits both practitioners and patients alike (Noebauer-Huhmann et al., 2024).

KEY TERMS FROM THIS CHAPTER

- Bone infections
- Degenerative diseases
- eXplainable Artificial Intelligence (XAI)
- Health professionals
- Musculoskeletal care
- Musculoskeletal ultrasound
- Power doppler ultrasound (PDUS)
- Psoriatic arthritis
- Rheumatoid arthritis
- Virtual non-contrast images (VNC)
- Bone marrow
- Ewings sarcoma
- Fracture care
- Ligament tears
- Musculoskeletal tumors
- Osteoarthritis
- Predictive analytics
- Radiographs
- Superb microvascular imaging (SMI)

Critical Thinking Questions

1. **Which of the following imaging modalities is most commonly used for detecting fractures in the bones?**
   a. MRI
   b. Ultrasound
   c. X-ray
   d. PET scan
2. **What is the primary advantage of MRI in musculoskeletal imaging?**
   a. It uses ionizing radiation to provide detailed bone images
   b. It provides high-resolution images of soft tissues like muscles, tendons, and ligaments
   c. It is faster than other imaging techniques
   d. It is commonly used to assess bone density
3. **In musculoskeletal imaging, which of the following is typically assessed using an ultrasound scan?**
   a. Bone fractures
   b. Joint dislocations
   c. Soft tissue injuries such as ligament tears or muscle strains
   d. Tumors in the bone
4. **Which imaging modality is most useful for detecting bone tumors or metastasis?**
   a. X-ray
   b. MRI
   c. CT scan
   d. Bone scintigraphy (Bone scan)
5. **What is the key difference between CT scans and MRI in musculoskeletal imaging?**
   a. CT scans are better for visualizing soft tissue, while MRI is better for bones
   b. CT scans use magnetic fields, while MRI uses ionizing radiation
   c. MRI provides better soft tissue contrast, while CT is better for visualizing bone details
   d. CT scans are generally more expensive than MRI scans

Short Answer Questions

1. What are some common clinical indications for musculoskeletal imaging?
2. When is MRI preferred over X-ray or CT in musculoskeletal assessments?
3. What are the main limitations of ultrasound in musculoskeletal imaging?
4. How does imaging assist in confirming a diagnosis of soft tissue injuries?
5. What recent technological advances have improved musculoskeletal imaging accuracy?
6. How does low-dose imaging technology contribute to safer musculoskeletal diagnostics?
7. Why is it important to consider ethical issues such as radiation exposure and informed consent in musculoskeletal imaging?

Answers to Critical Thinking Questions

1. (c); 2. (b); 3. (c); 4. (d); 5. (c)

References

1. Adelodun, M. O., & Anyanwu, E. C. (2025). Public health risks associated with environmental radiation from improper medical waste disposal. *International Journal of Multidisciplinary Research and Growth Evaluation*. https://www.semanticscholar.org/paper/dc6d18063e00d88248e3ffe66f7760d73f35bf80 (accessed on 23 May 2025).
2. Agarwal, R., Mehrotra, A., Mishra, A., Rana, N. P., Nunkoo, R., & Cho, M. (2024). Four decades of sustainable tourism research: Trends and future research directions. *International Journal of Tourism Research*. https://www.semanticscholar.org/paper/7b7aa4d19eaba11a14570f2209c95292f23d9ca4 (accessed on 23 May 2025).
3. Alburayh, A. A., Alosaimi, M., Alshumiesy, H., Alzahrani, A., Alkhars, A. S., Doaib, D. M., Alsaleh, M. H., et al. (2025). Assessment of public knowledge and perceptions toward radiation exposure risks in Saudi Arabia: A survey study. *Cureus, 17*. https://www.semanticscholar.org/paper/db930b620f36b25cf93210b4fe6355cc447f0f7b (accessed on 23 May 2025).
4. Al-Ibraheem, A., Abdlkadir, A. S., Al-Rasheed, U., Al-Adhami, D., Istatieh, F., Anwar, F., Abdulrahman, M., et al. (2025). First clinical experience of 68Ga-FAPI PET/CT in tertiary cancer center: Identifying pearls and pitfalls. *Diagnostics, 15*. https://www.semanticscholar.org/paper/bae0f8194ecf264bef9191a179eb24599bc46492 (accessed on 23 May 2025).
5. Alizadeh, L. S., Vogl, T., Waldeck, S., Overhoff, D., D'angelo, T., Martin, S., Yel, I., et al. (2023). Dual-energy CT in cardiothoracic imaging: Current developments. *Diagnostics, 13*(X). https://www.semanticscholar.org/paper/d2909346d44ff0e829c691fe1898df0b537a4dc8 (accessed on 23 May 2025).
6. Almeida, D., Costa, E., & Cerqueira, M. (2021). Advances in ultrasound imaging in rheumatology, what do they mean and what challenges do they pose? The example of microvascular imaging. *Journal of Ultrasound in Medicine, 41*. https://www.semanticscholar.org/paper/fd6f11111ffd5f611f4e5586e546c987631112f8 (accessed on 23 May 2025).
7. Aponte-Tinao, L. A., Ayerza, M. A., Albergo, J. I., & Farfalli, G. L. (2019). Do massive allograft reconstructions for tumors of the femur and tibia survive 10 or more years after implantation? *Clinical Orthopedics and Related Research, 478*(3), 517–524. https://doi.org/10.1097/corr.0000000000000806.
8. Bakewell, C., Aydın, S. Z., Ranganath, V. K., Eder, L., & Kaeley, G. S. (2019). Imaging techniques: Options for the diagnosis and monitoring of treatment of enthesitis in psoriatic arthritis. *The Journal of Rheumatology, 47*, 973–982. https://doi.org/10.3899/jrheum.190512.
9. Batra, V., Spalkit, S., Bugata, S. K., Chari, R., & Batta, N. S. (2025). Ultrasound and computed tomography-guided interventions for the hip joint and pelvis: Comprehensive imaging review. *Indian Journal of Musculoskeletal Radiology*. https://www.semanticscholar.org/paper/f0ca66da320ff69040cacefd7c1dff538c7f53e0 (accessed on 23 May 2025).
10. Celayir, A., Afacan, M., Sevgil, B., Ozsahin, M. K., & Botanlioglu, H. (2025). A rare case of non-Hodgkin lymphoma with ankle involvement: Diagnostic and therapeutic challenges. *Cureus, 17*. https://www.semanticscholar.org/paper/276da52a93c48335d98b0d9c50b6ea9e2a2c3821 (accessed on 23 May 2025).
11. Chen, W., Zhang, Y., Wang, X., & Liu, J. (2024). Comparative analysis of imaging modalities for diagnosing musculoskeletal disorders. *Journal of Innovations in Medical Research*. https://

www.semanticscholar.org/paper/b08897c482d81da296f7def6eb1fddc2d2ff9eba (accessed on 23 May 2025).

12. Colgate, V., & Marr, C. M. (2020). Science-in-brief: Risk assessment for reducing injuries of the fetlock bones in Thoroughbred racehorses. *Equine Veterinary Journal, 52*(4), 482–488. https://doi.org/10.1111/evj.13273.

13. Gitto, S., Serpi, F., Albano, D., Risoleo, G., Fusco, S., Messina, C., & Sconfienza, L. (2024). AI applications in musculoskeletal imaging: A narrative review. *European Radiology Experimental, 8*. https://www.semanticscholar.org/paper/d19893b559ab2bf0de46e38bff8d77b9913756fb (accessed on 23 May 2025).

14. Glikson, M., Nielsen, J. C., Kronborg, M. B., Michowitz, Y., Auricchio, A., Barbash, I. M., Barrabés, J. A., et al. (2021). 2021 ESC guidelines on cardiac pacing and cardiac resynchronization therapy. *European Heart Journal, 42*(34), 3427–3520. https://doi.org/10.1093/eurheartj/ehab364.

15. Hemke, R., Herregods, N., Jaremko, J. L., Åström, G., Avenarius, D., Becce, F., Bielecki, D. K., et al. (2020). Imaging assessment of children presenting with suspected or known juvenile idiopathic arthritis: ESSR-ESPR points to consider. *European Radiology, 30*(9), 5237–5249. https://doi.org/10.1007/s00330-020-06807-8.

16. Isaac, A., Akdoğan, A. I., Dalili, D., Saber, N., Drobny, D., Guglielmi, G., Modat, M., et al. (2024). Artificial intelligence applications for imaging metabolic bone diseases. *Seminars in Musculoskeletal Radiology, 28*(5), 610–619. https://www.semanticscholar.org/paper/35e4696f040a19b26ac46a355c7b6c95e5ac0373 (accessed on 23 May 2025).

17. Ismayilova, P. (2024). Exploring the foundations of informed consent, legal capacity, privacy, and dignity in medical law and me. *Juridical Sciences and Education*. https://www.semanticscholar.org/paper/d699d3283490dca874bad8e8b4d4e1c378a790a2 (accessed on 23 May 2025).

18. Izquierdo, M., Merchant, R. A., Morley, J. E., Anker, S. D., Aprahamian, I., Arai, H., Aubertin-Leheudre, M., et al. (2021). International exercise recommendations in older adults (ICFSR): Expert consensus guidelines. *The Journal of Nutrition, Health & Aging, 25*(7), 824–853. https://doi.org/10.1007/s12603-021-1665-8.

19. Jandan, A. A. B. (2020). Radiological assessment of musculoskeletal disorders: Innovations and future directions. *Journal of Namibian Studies: History Politics Culture*. https://www.semanticscholar.org/paper/3bd5411ca2a3f4bf7b49820b9b99f80938bfe411 (accessed on 23 May 2025).

20. Karalis, V. (2024). The integration of artificial intelligence into clinical practice. *Applied Biosciences, 3*(1), 14–44. https://doi.org/10.3390/applbiosci3010002.

21. Kirby, E., MacMillan, A., Brinkley, A., Liew, B. X. W., & Bateman, A. (2025). Evaluating musculoskeletal imaging communication interventions using behavioral science: A scoping review using the COM-B model. *BMJ Open, 15*. https://www.semanticscholar.org/paper/27b5f8088ad82216a57ebee304c769536a1e16ca (accessed on 23 May 2025).

22. Kissi, J., & Annobil, C. (2025). The advantageous impact of telestroke: Global insights and implications for Africa: A scoping review of literature. *Stroke Research and Treatment, 2025*. https://www.semanticscholar.org/paper/2124cc0afbda1b36691f76052d4effa58e32a342 (accessed on 23 May 2025).

23. Kolasinski, S. L., Neogi, T., Hochberg, M. C., Oatis, C. A., Guyatt, G., Block, J. A., Callahan, L. F., et al. (2020). 2019 American College of Rheumatology/Arthritis Foundation guideline for the management of osteoarthritis of the hand, hip, and knee. *Arthritis Care & Research, 72*(2), 149–162. https://doi.org/10.1002/acr.24131.

24. Kolasinski, S. L., Neogi, T., Hochberg, M. C., Oatis, C. A., Guyatt, G., Block, J. A., Callahan, L. F., et al. (2020). 2019 American College of Rheumatology/Arthritis Foundation guideline for the management of osteoarthritis of the hand, hip, and knee. *Arthritis & Rheumatology, 72*(2), 220–233. https://doi.org/10.1002/art.41142.

25. LeBoff, M. S., Greenspan, S. L., Insogna, K., Lewiecki, E. M., Saag, K. G., Singer, A., & Siris, E. S. (2022). The clinician's guide to prevention and treatment of osteoporosis. *Osteoporosis International, 33*(10), 2049–2102. https://doi.org/10.1007/s00198-021-05900-y.

26. Lee, Y. C., Lin, C. Y., Hsiao, C. C., Mo, P. C., Guo, J., & Jan, Y. K. (2024). Using deep learning-based methods for automated segmentation of soft tissues from shoulder ultrasound images. *IEEE Access, 12*, 111481–111492. https://www.semanticscholar.org/paper/495fb3dec66332 6d9c248262c67ff2acd9e9d077 (accessed on 23 May 2025).

27. Liguori, I., Russo, G., Curcio, F., Bulli, G., Aran, L., Della-Morte, D., Gargiulo, G., et al. (2018). Oxidative stress, aging, and diseases. *Clinical Interventions in Aging, 13*, 757–772. https://doi.org/10.2147/cia.s158513.

28. Lim, A., Satchithananda, K., Dick, E., Abraham, S., & Cosgrove, D. O. (2017). Microflow imaging: New Doppler technology to detect low-grade inflammation in patients with arthritis. *European Radiology, 28*, 1046–1053. https://doi.org/10.1007/s00330-017-5016-4.

29. Liu, B., Su, M., Zhang, Z., Sun, L., Yu, Y., & Qiu, W. (2024). A novel coded excitation imaging platform for ultra-high frequency (>100 MHz) ultrasound applications. *IEEE Transactions on Biomedical Engineering, 72*, 1298–1305. https://www.semanticscholar.org/paper/cba28c6ae56917bd1ba90085b4a57edac946eed7 (accessed on 23 May 2025).

30. Madkhali, N. A. M., Alsomali, M. D. Y., Al-Dosari, Y. N. M., ALHarbi, S. T., ALRUWAILI, S. T. F., Alahdal, A. A. M., Almutiri, G. H. D., et al. (2024). A comprehensive multidisciplinary strategy for the management of musculoskeletal fractures throughout pregnancy: Evaluation, treatment, and maternal-fetal considerations. *Journal of Eco Humanism*. https://www.semanticscholar.org/paper/1fadbcf125a68de23b44a434dd67281b5ece527b (accessed on 23 May 2025).

31. Manske, R., Wolfe, C., Page, P., & Voight, M. L. (2025). Diagnostic musculoskeletal ultrasound for the evaluation of the lateral elbow: Implications for rehabilitation providers. *International Journal of Sports Physical Therapy, 20*(1), 137–143. https://www.semanticscholar.org/paper/aa6f2a2c204b57d047f1599da9410c440ceecd51 (accessed on 23 May 2025).

32. Monti, R., Martinese, A., Bonadonna, G., Rocco, M. P., Simonetti, I., Arrigoni, F., Palumbo, P., et al. (2022). Degenerative and inflammatory musculoskeletal disorders: Updates and hot topics in diagnostic and interventional imaging. *European Review for Medical and Pharmacological Sciences, 26*(19), 6958–6971. https://www.semanticscholar.org/paper/3d155dc86c367f67eb78ee79b0c64e9a641744f5 (accessed on 23 May 2025).

33. Najjar, R. (2023). Redefining radiology: A review of artificial intelligence integration in medical imaging. *Diagnostics, 13*(17), 2760. https://doi.org/10.3390/diagnostics13172760.

34. Nittas, V., Ormond, K., Vayena, E., & Blasimme, A. (2025). Realizing the promise of machine learning in precision oncology: Expert perspectives on opportunities and challenges. *BMC*

Cancer, 25. https://www.semanticscholar.org/paper/5eeb4654f65bd7848865dfa20f586b24086b94a8 (accessed on 23 May 2025).

35. Noebauer-Huhmann, I., Vanhoenacker, F. M., Vilanova, J. C., Tagliafico, A., Weber, M. A., Lalam, R., Grieser, T., et al. (2024). Soft tissue tumor imaging in adults: Whole-body staging in sarcoma, non-malignant entities requiring special algorithms, pitfalls and special imaging aspects. Guidelines 2024 from the European Society of Musculoskeletal Radiology (ESSR). *European Radiology*, *35*, 351–359. https://www.semanticscholar.org/paper/75048eec06be70a89002e414f8b4e296e9f64b1b (accessed on 23 May 2025).

36. Panhwar, A. O., Memon, S., Dhomeja, L. D., Memon, N., & Chandio, A. A. (2024). Deep learning-based image segmentation techniques for bone fractures using X-ray images: A systematic review. *VFAST Transactions on Software Engineering*, *12*(4), 99–116. https://doi.org/10.21015/vtse.v12i4.1971.

37. Pesapane, F., Codari, M., & Sardanelli, F. (2018). Artificial intelligence in medical imaging: Threat or opportunity? Radiologists again at the forefront of innovation in medicine. *European Radiology Experimental, 2*. https://doi.org/10.1186/s41747-018-0061-6.

38. Posadzy, M., Desimpel, J., & Vanhoenacker, F. (2018). Cone beam CT of the musculoskeletal system: Clinical applications. *Insights into Imaging, 9*(1), 35–45. https://doi.org/10.1007/s13244-017-0582-1.

39. Santhi, N. N. P. (2025). Patient data privacy challenges in electronic health systems: A juridical analysis of medical information protection in Indonesia. *West Science Law and Human Rights*. https://www.semanticscholar.org/paper/b516945e90890351c5f9d8cd650b3a0c65f0d369 (accessed on 23 May 2025).

40. Shafeeq, H., & Ahmed, S. (2025). Navigating ethical dimensions in algorithmic radiology: A call for action to ensure representation of low-resource contexts. *Indian Journal of Medical Ethics*. https://www.semanticscholar.org/paper/7e1f70a74429e1804c602fdab2bb1a45adb1e100 (accessed on 23 May 2025).

41. Shakir, F. Z., Melwan, R., Mansoor, S., Fahim, S., Kumari, K., Shazma, D. R., & Singh, S. (2024). Diagnostic accuracy of X-ray in diagnosing avascular femoral head, keeping magnetic resonance imaging (MRI) as gold standard. *Biological and Clinical Sciences Research Journal*. https://www.semanticscholar.org/paper/5d6202ac7183f080819061f8c7687451f34e423e (accessed on 23 May 2025).

42. Tenforde, A. S., Borgstrom, H., DeLuca, S., McCormack, M., Singh, M., Soo Hoo, J., & Yun, P. H. (2022). Best practices for extracorporeal shockwave therapy in musculoskeletal medicine: Clinical application and training consideration. *PM&R, 14*, 611–619. https://doi.org/10.1002/pmrj.12790.

43. Tseng, W. C., Chen, Y. C., Lee, T. M., & Chen, W. S. (2023). Plantar fasciitis: An updated review. *Journal of Medical Ultrasound, 31*(4), 268–274. https://doi.org/10.4103/jmu.jmu_2_23.

44. Tzatzairis, T., Skarentzos, K., Grammatikos, C., Karamalis, C., Korakianitis, K., Kourempeles, R., & Drosos, G. (2024). Ultrasound applications in pediatric orthopedics. *Archives of Bone and Joint Surgery, 12*(5), 457–468. https://www.semanticscholar.org/paper/59925c2de86c06c9431d2c10ff413b9a2621bbc3 (accessed on 23 May 2025).

45. van der Velden, B. H. M., Kuijf, H. J., Gilhuijs, K. G. A., & Viergever, M. A. (2022). Explainable

artificial intelligence (XAI) in deep learning-based medical image analysis. *Medical Image Analysis*, *79*, 102470. https://doi.org/10.1016/j.media.2022.102470.

46. Weiß, J., Hoffmann, R., & Clasen, S. (2018). MR-guided liver interventions. *Topics in Magnetic Resonance Imaging, 27*(3), 163–170. https://doi.org/10.1097/rmr.0000000000000146.

47. Wu, A., Cross, M., Elliott, J. M., Culbreth, G. T., Haile, T. G., Steinmetz, J. D., Hagins, H., et al. (2024). Global, regional, and national burden of neck pain, 1990–2020, and projections to 2050: A systematic analysis of the Global Burden of Disease Study 2021. *The Lancet Rheumatology*, *6*, e142–e155. https://doi.org/10.1016/s2665-9913(23)00321-1.

48. Zabotti, A., De Marco, G., Gossec, L., Baraliakos, X., Aletaha, D., Iagnocco, A., et al. (2023). EULAR points to consider for the definition of clinical and imaging features suspicious for progression from psoriasis to psoriatic arthritis. *Annals of the Rheumatic Diseases*, *82*(9), 1162–1170. https://doi.org/10.1136/ard-2023-224148.

49. Zhang, Z., Wang, R., Xue, H., Knoedler, S., Geng, Y., Liao, Y., Alfertshofer, M., et al. (2023). Phototherapy techniques for the management of musculoskeletal disorders: Strategies and recent advances. *Biomaterials Research, 27*. https://doi.org/10.1186/s40824-023-00458-8.

CARDIOVASCULAR IMAGING

14

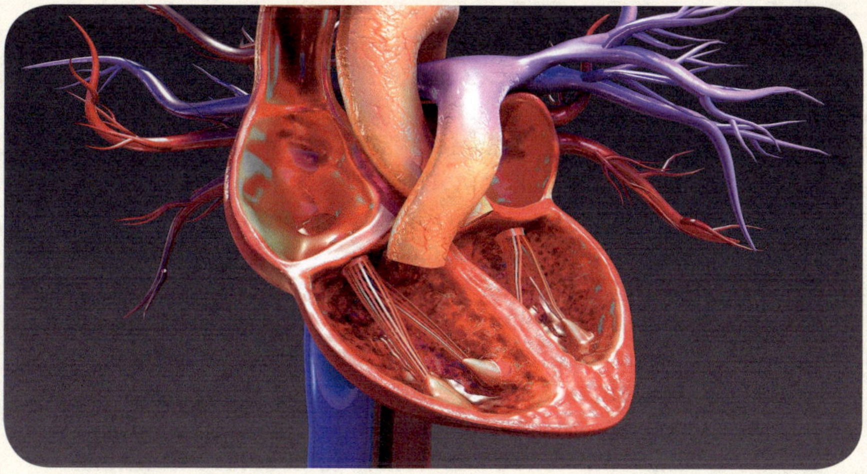

LEARNING OBJECTIVES

After studying this chapter, you will be able to:

1. Identify and differentiate the various types of Cardiovascular Imaging.
2. Understand the principles and applications of echocardiography in diagnosing.
3. Explore emerging technologies in cardiovascular imaging.
4. Examine the clinical implications of cardiovascular imaging.

Introduction

Cardiovascular imaging lays the groundwork for what we know about modern diagnostics and treatments. The field isn't static, new ideas are mixed in with the old, and fresh tech has begun to change the game. Take, for example, mock circulatory loops (MCLs): they mimic the heart and vessels in a hands-on, mechanical way to test out blood flow, and they even bring in 3D anatomical models to help us understand how different cardiovascular devices behave in real life. Over time, these models have slowly improved, which generally means we can simulate patient-specific anatomy a bit better, leading, in most cases, to more effective treatments, as some recent reviews point out (Rocchi et al., 2022). Meanwhile, cardiovascular magnetic resonance (CMR) has become a standout imaging tool largely because it is non-invasive and avoids ionizing radiation. New advancements, like using high-field strength magnets, boost the signal-to-noise ratio in ways that let us see heart structures and functions in much finer detail. As clinicians get more familiar with these tools, they aren't just using CMR for simple images anymore, it is now also about detailed tissue evaluations and managing an array of cardiac issues. The versatility of CMR across various techniques keeps it right up there as an essential part of modern cardiology, making the detection of heart problems more accurate than ever (Situ et al., 2020). The mix of MCLs and CMR shows how the landscape of cardiovascular imaging is changing day by day. Both methods seem to say that sticking to older practices just isn't enough when we're aiming for real-world results; improvements and tweaks are needed to meet the messy challenges of clinical life. A growing emphasis on personalized, patient-centered care pushes for imaging and testing that can capture the unique uniqueness of each body. With ongoing tweaks and plenty of research, our understanding of cardiovascular health, and the way we handle disease, is constantly being redefined, setting new standards for excellence in cardiology.

Definition of Cardiovascular Imaging

Cardiovascular imaging covers many modern techniques that help doctors get a real look at heart problems. In practice, tests like echocardiography, MRI, and CT give clinicians the chance to check out the heart's intricate design and how well it works. You might say it is not just about pictures, the images serve as key clues for spotting issues such as congenital defects, muscle diseases, or valve troubles. New tech improvements have boosted accuracy, making diagnoses more sensitive and specific, which in most cases leads to quicker, personalized treatment plans. Simply put, getting to know these imaging methods matters for everyday patient care. A big part of this imaging scene is its role in identifying both inherited and later-acquired heart conditions. Take congenital heart disease, for example, it is one of the more common birth defects and often needs early detection; imaging helps make that happen. When genetic testing is paired with these visual techniques, doctors have an even better shot at identifying abnormalities early on. Recent guidelines mention that spotting specific gene changes via imaging can shed light on the underlying causes, adding weight to clinical evaluations. Expert recommendations for genetic testing now dovetail with imaging advances, which means treatments can be tailored right from the start. In many ways, fusing imaging with genetic insights is reshaping how we handle heart health. The scope for cardiovascular imaging keeps growing, especially in hereditary issues like cardiomyopathies. Studies show that these advanced scans can catch tiny changes in heart structure, details traditional tests might easily miss. For instance, spotting hypertrophic cardiomyopathy with an echo or an MRI allows clinicians to see thickened walls and any related complications. These techniques aren't just for initial diagnosis either; they help track the disease's progress over time and guide treatment decisions. Plus, combining established genetic testing standards with newer imaging methods has sharpened our ability to predict conditions like HCM, pushing forward more effective care. Overall, merging visual data with genetic info is transforming cardiovascular medicine, making diagnoses and interventions more on point for each patient (Figure 14.1).

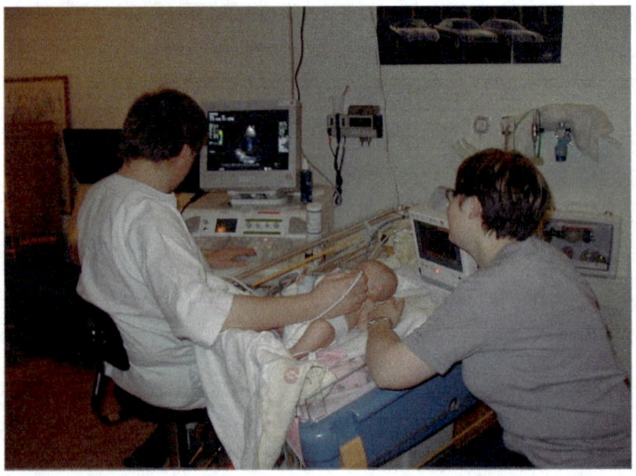

Figure 14.1. Cardiovascular Imaging.

Source: Public Domain, https://commons.wikimedia.org/w/index.php?curid=134675.

Importance in Modern Medicine

Heart imaging has completely reshaped how patients are cared for today. Cardiac MRI, CT angiography (CTA) and similar methods let doctors see the heart's structure and even its rhythm without having to cut in, pretty neat when you think about it. Identifying issues early helps in planning the right interventions, which makes a big difference. As heart problems seem to keep growing worldwide, checking risk factors and tracking disease progress has become, in most cases, a necessity for those in healthcare. In many ways, imaging not only finds the problem but also helps map out treatments and follow up on results, so it is now a key part of overall patient care strategies. It is also interesting how heart imaging now mixes with ideas from other fields like genomics and metabolomics. This blend opens up a more detailed picture of heart conditions that we just didn't have before; for example, using metabolic profiling uncovers some of the subtle biochemical shifts behind the issues, often pointing out markers that could be useful for risk-checking and treatment aims. This kind of combined approach builds on traditional imaging methods and creates a sturdier way to diagnose and manage heart disease, truly a shift from the old ways where imaging worked by itself. There's also a real educational side to all this. Medical programs are now bringing in advanced imaging techniques, giving students hands-on experiences that build critical skills for modern diagnostics. Working with different imaging tools deepens their understanding of the rough-and-tumble nature of heart diseases, something that plays a big role in both research and everyday clinical practice. Learning to interpret these complex images has become almost indispensable in an era when precision medicine is, generally speaking, the goal. By weaving imaging into both the diagnostic and therapeutic parts of patient care, training today is helping shape a new generation of healthcare pros who know how to leverage these innovative techniques, not just for individual patients, but also as a part of wider public health efforts to fight cardiovascular disease (Figure 14.2).

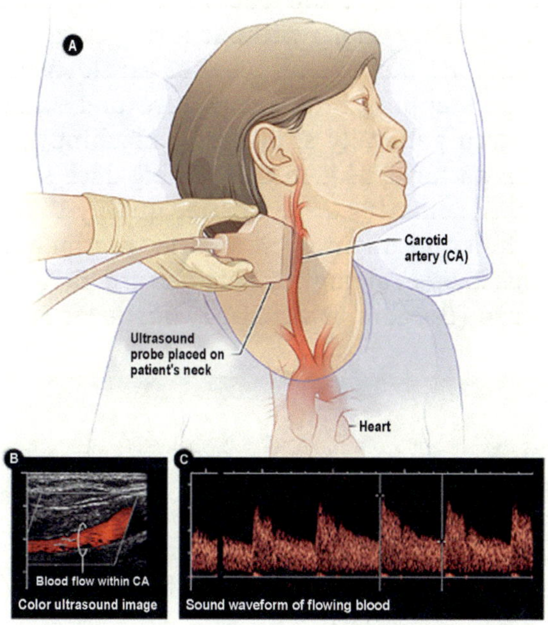

Figure 14.2. Figure A shows how the ultrasound probe (transducer) is placed over the carotid artery. Figure B is a color ultrasound image showing blood flow (the red color in the image) in the carotid artery. Figure C is a waveform image showing the sound of flowing blood in the carotid artery.

Source: By National Heart Lung and Blood Institute (NIH) - National Heart Lung and Blood Institute (NIH), Public Domain, https://commons.wikimedia.org/w/index.php?curid=29587675.

Overview of Imaging Techniques

New imaging breakthroughs have flipped how we take a look at the heart. Nowadays, doctors don't rely on just one method; they use echo, CT scans, and MRI to see what's going on. Echo gives live images of heart movements, CT helps check out the coronary arteries without invasive tricks, and MRI dives into tissue details, each tool bringing its own twist. They usually work side by side rather than stepping on each other's toes, all helping to spot and track heart issues. Mixing different imaging techniques has widened what we can learn about heart health. Take cardiac magnetic resonance, or CMR, for example, it has become a popular non-invasive way to tackle especially tricky heart conditions. In most cases, however, long scan times and pesky motion blur still get in the way. Lately, though, some clever under sampling reconstruction methods have popped up, speeding things along and usually keeping image quality sharp without losing detail. These CMR approaches are now common in hospitals, broadening our overall view of cardiovascular problems. New tech like artificial intelligence (AI) is also stepping into the picture and shaking up heart imaging, in a subtle yet powerful way. Research generally shows that machine learning can cut image reconstruction times by picking up on patterns hidden deep in big data sets. With these techniques, getting an image done can be quicker, sometimes even better quality than before. Our growing insights into the heart's structure and function might even lead to treatments tailored more closely to each patient's needs. And as things keep evolving, innovations are likely to refine how we understand and manage cardiovascular disease (Bergom et al., 2021; Bustin et al., 2020).

14.1. Types of Cardiovascular Imaging

Learning Outcome

1. Understand the principles and applications of echocardiography.
2. Explore using Magnetic Resonance Imaging (MRI) in assessing cardiovascular health.
3. Examine the role of Computed Tomography (CT) in evaluating cardiovascular diseases.

Imaging tech leaps have turned the way doctors examine heart health on its head. Echo, for instance, stays a favorite because, plain and simple, it gives a non-invasive, real-time peek at the heart at work. It uses ultrasound waves to show details like how the chambers do their job, how valves move, and even subtle heart motions; clinicians can then check for issues like heart failure or flawed valves. There's been a push lately with things like 3D views and contrast methods that boost both how well and how precisely these scans work. Research generally shows that mixing AI into echo readings might just sharpen the diagnosis even further, opening doors to more customized plans and better follow-ups for patients (Mrinalini et al., 2022). Magnetic resonance imaging (MRI) also plays a big part in the heart-imaging game, thanks mostly to its knack for capturing high-res images of the heart's structure and motion without any ionizing radiation. It is especially good at checking out details in the heart tissue, so signs of cardiomyopathy, ischemia, or even scarring aren't easily missed. Extra techniques like cardiac motion analysis and perfusion studies add to its value in clinical check-ups. In most cases, recent work hints that machine learning with MRI might speed up diagnoses and offer improved forecasts (Sadegh-Zadeh et al., 2024). As these technological streams merge, MRI's role is bound to expand, making it a must-have tool for deep, comprehensive heart assessments. CTA has also stepped into its own, especially in sizing up coronary artery disease. This method taps into CT scans to generate clear images of blood vessels, pinpointing things like plaque build-ups and blockages that might otherwise slip past notice. Rapid progress in CT tech, take dual-energy imaging or those slick high-res protocols, for example, boosts both diagnostic accuracy and patient safety by keeping radiation levels down. AI is starting to chip in too, helping smooth the entire diagnostic ride and refine risk checks among heart patients. Some recent findings even suggest that pairing CT with other imaging tools could further streamline patient care, letting doctors piece together a fuller picture to make smarter, more informed choices (Mrinalini et al., 2022; Sadegh-Zadeh et al., 2024). Overall, CTA looks set to become even more central in the evolving future of heart diagnostics and care.

14.1.1. Echocardiography

Echocardiography changed everything. This non-invasive method lets us see the heart without any surgical intrusion, it uses high-frequency sound waves bouncing off tissues to craft lively images of the beating heart. Doctors can watch the hearts function in real time; yet, the rapid pace of each beat means some finer details can slip by, so sonographers have to be extra sharp. In most cases, recent boosts from AI have been a game changer, helping to fine-tune image analysis and smooth out diagnostic rough patches, ultimately giving clinicians more reliable tools for evaluations (Zhou et al., 2021). In the field of cancer care, echo snuggles into a crucial role, particularly for those on risky chemo regimens. Treatments with drugs like anthracyclines or HER2-targeted therapies can trigger serious heart issues, left ventricular dysfunction and other problems are not uncommon. That's why baseline exams followed by periodic echo checks are vital for spotting potential trouble early. Guidelines laid out by the British Society of Echocardiography and the British Cardio-Oncology Society almost always stress the need for careful image capture and interpretation. Even if these protocols feel a bit methodical at times, they help ensure that a patient's heart health stays front and center during the ups and downs of cancer treatment (Dobson et al., 2021). Looking ahead, the mix of echocardiography with new digital tools seems set to shake up cardiovascular imaging. AI-driven features now jump in to handle tasks like mapping out heart chambers and automatically assessing function, streamlining the workload for healthcare pros. This tech push not only sharpens diagnostic accuracy but also makes data collection and analysis more orderly, leaning on standardized data for reliable results. In our digitally driven world, this integration offers hope for better outcomes, so, as echo and advanced tech continue to team up, the future of cardiovascular care looks genuinely promising (Zhou et al., 2021) (Figure 14.3).

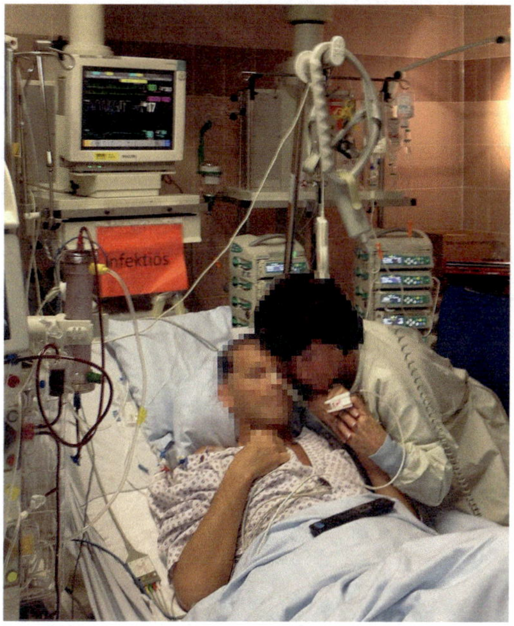

Figure 14.3. Echocardiogram.

Source: By Pittigrilli - Own work, CC BY-SA 4.0, https://commons.wikimedia.org/w/index.php?curid=118649036.

14.1.2. Magnetic Resonance Imaging (MRI)

Medical imaging has come a long way – it is shifted how we spot and treat heart issues. MRI, for example, stands out because it gives crystal-clear pictures without exposing patients to harmful radiation; this is a big help when someone needs multiple scans over time. It shows the heart's inner details so doctors can check both how it works and what its structure is like. Using methods like cine MRI and gathering images of blood flow, clinicians often pick up extra details about the heart muscle, circulation, and even tissue health – details that can shape better care decisions. Beyond just taking pictures, MRI has started mingling with new tech, which has upped its usefulness in watching over heart health. In most cases, current studies show that contrast substances – like gadolinium-based compounds – push the clarity of these scans, giving doctors a more precise look inside. There's also buzz about superparamagnetic iron oxide nanoparticles (IONs), which offer a neat twist for delivering drugs exactly where needed while keeping an eye on patient responses. Altogether, such breakthroughs open doors to fresh treatment ideas, like remote magnetic drug targeting (MDT), which aims to pack more medicine at the spot that needs it while cutting down on side effects, thus helping tackle tough challenges seen in conditions such as acute myocardial infarction (AMI) and atherosclerosis (Yılmaz et al., 2016). MRI's mix with other fields – think three-dimensional printing – shows off its power to transform personalized care. By tapping into MRI data, doctors can whip up custom anatomical models that make preop planning more straightforward and may even lead to better surgical outcomes. The international study by the Bioastronautics and Space Mechatronics Research Groups is a cool example of this cross-over approach, showing how MRI can be a key player in personalizing treatments for various body systems, including the heart (Cornejo et al., 2022). As researchers keep poking into new ways to use MRI, the future of heart imaging looks set to take some unexpected turns, paving fresh paths for better diagnoses, treatments, and overall patient care (Figure 14.4).

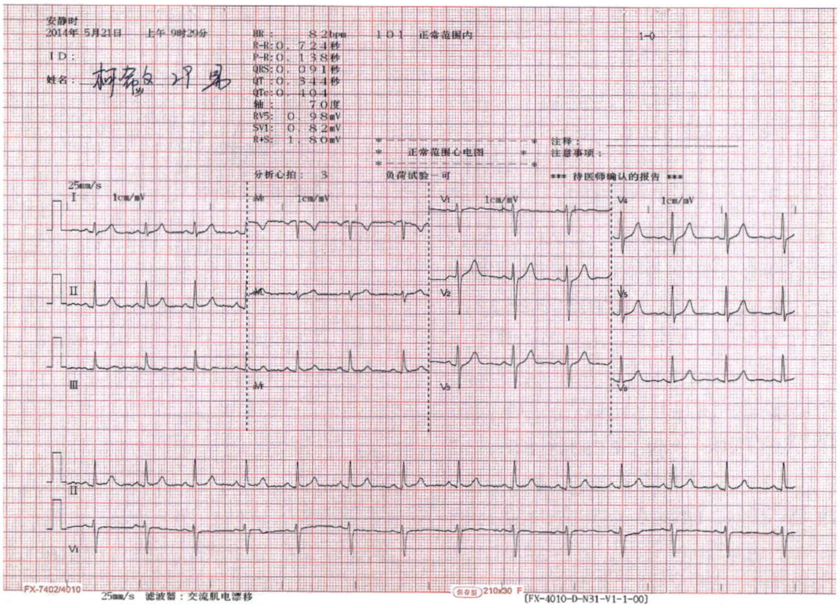

Figure 14.4. ECG.

Source: By Ptrump16 - Own work, CC BY-SA 4.0, https://commons.wikimedia.org/w/index.php?curid=77817932.

14.1.3. Computed Tomography (CT)

Imaging has turned things around for heart disease diagnosis. Computed Tomography (CT) now gives clinicians a way to see heart structures with a clarity that older methods just couldn't match. It is not only about getting a better look, CT also helps reveal tiny anatomical abnormalities.

In cases where the heart's layout is unusually complex, CT scan unexpectedly uncover a clear view of both the main vessels and those feeding the lungs. I remember one instance when CT uncovered several congenital abnormalities, like odd pulmonary venous connections that were later set right with surgery. When doctors mix these CT images with echocardiogram info, they end up with a fuller picture of someone's heart health, paving the way for prompt, spot-on treatment plans (Ahn et al., 2012). Then, there came the era of multi-slice CT which kind of revolutionized everything by offering sharper images while cutting down radiation. The jump to 16-slice CT was, in most cases, a big turning point in everyday practice; it made spotting issues like coronary artery narrowing or heart muscle problems suddenly much more achievable.

These upgrades even led to modifications like 3D imaging, an approach that effortlessly deepens our spatial grasp of cardiac structures. Research pretty much shows that multi-slice CT scan nail down various heart conditions, letting clinicians craft management plans that are, well, tailored to each patient's needs. This boost in diagnostic tricks is crucial for stopping serious heart events by ensuring treatments remain as unique as the patients themselves (Guan et al., 2025). In long-term care and predicting outcomes, CT has come to be seen as indispensable. Its role stretches far beyond that first glance at a problem, it can track the march of cardiovascular disease over time. Studies using CT have often linked imaging findings with major heart events, offering insights that, generally speaking, steer us toward more forward-thinking care. This broader perspective is especially useful for evaluating complex cases like cardiac amyloidosis or even sarcoidosis, where getting that diagnosis exactly right matters a ton. By piecing CT data together with insights from other imaging methods, healthcare providers can craft overall strategies aimed at boosting patient outcomes while, ideally, sidestepping the risks tied to delayed or off-the-mark assessments (Guan et al., 2025) (Figure 14.5).

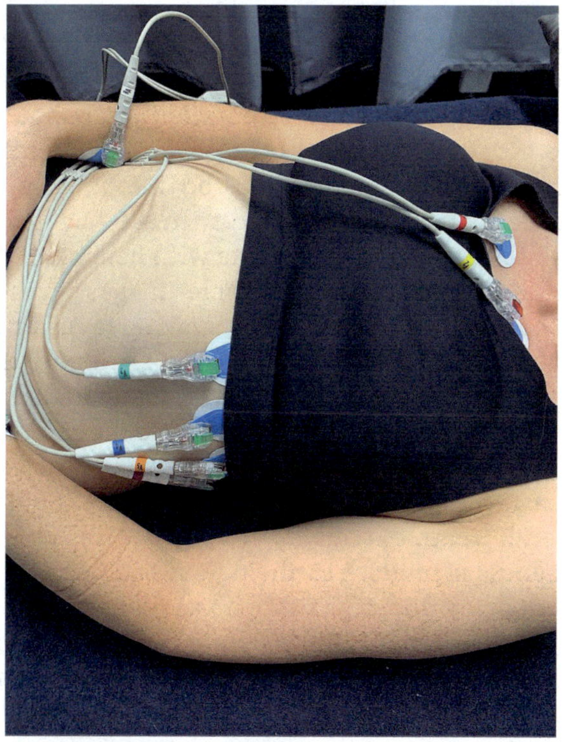

Figure 14.5. Heart scan.

Source: By John orchard - Own work, CC BY-SA 4.0, https://commons.wikimedia.org/w/index.php?curid=91769052.

Test Your Knowledge

1. How does echocardiography contribute to the evaluation of heart function and structure?
2. In what ways does magnetic resonance imaging (MRI) offer advantages over other imaging techniques for cardiovascular conditions?

14.2. Echocardiography

Learning Outcome

1. Understand the principles of ultrasound technology.
2. Differentiate between the various types of echocardiograms (transthoracic, transesophageal).
3. Explore the clinical applications and benefits.

Echocardiography is quickly becoming a staple in heart imaging, especially in spotting and managing a variety of cardiac issues. It works by using high-frequency sound waves that let us take a non-invasive, detailed snapshot of the heart's structure, blood flow, and potential irregularities. Doctors rely on it not only to check for problems like faulty heart valves but also to keep track of patients with heart failure. Its ability to provide real-time images gives it an edge over other methods, making it easier to make timely decisions. Generally speaking, the latest guidelines show that echo assessments can steer treatment strategies and patient outcomes (Vahanian et al., 2021). Overall, weaving echocardiography into everyday care boosts overall treatment quality, it's become absolutely essential in modern cardiology. In settings where identifying the right diagnosis is everything, echocardiography stands out as a real linchpin in heart imaging. It doesn't come in one uniform form; rather, it appears in different forms, like transthoracic echocardiography (TTE) and transesophageal echocardiography (TEE), each crafted to meet specific diagnostic needs. For many outpatients who appreciate comfort and ease, TTE is usually the go-to method. But when the images aren't clear enough or when complex conditions such as atrial fibrillation and intra-cardiac thrombi need to be evaluated, TEE steps in with sharper, more detailed visualization. As noted by the European Society of Cardiology guidelines, choosing the right method plays a huge part in nailing down an accurate diagnosis, so a tailored approach is often the key (Cosentino et al., 2019). Advances like 3D imaging and strain techniques keep reinforcing why echocardiography is so valuable in modern diagnostics. These newer methods enable clinicians to get a closer look at complicated heart structures and assess muscle function with a bit more precision. For example, strain imaging helps doctors examine overall, and even localized, left ventricular performance, which can catch subtle dysfunctions that standard tests might miss. Plus, the rise of portable echo devices has made real-time heart assessments more accessible, even in unpredictable, high-pressure settings like emergency rooms. In most cases, as technology evolves, sticking to established guidelines ensures that healthcare providers use this tool effectively, aligning with best practices in cardiovascular management (Vahanian et al., 2021) (Figure 14.6).

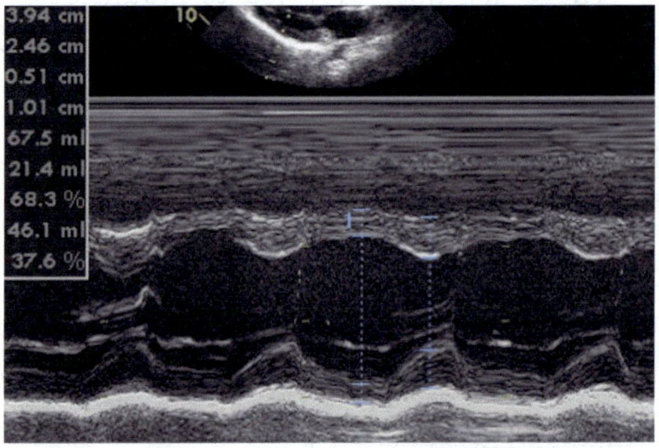

Figure 14.6. Echocardiography (Echo).

Source: Public Domain, https://commons.wikimedia.org/w/index.php?curid=137753.

14.2.1. Principles of Ultrasound Technology

Ultrasound imaging is a major tool in checking out the heart. It works by sending high-frequency sound waves into the body, and these waves bounce off tissues to create live pictures of what's inside. This method is non-invasive and avoids the risks that come with ionizing radiation, making it a safe option for looking at both the heart's structure and its function. A small probe, often called a transducer, sends out these waves, and the echoes are then turned into images of the heart and surrounding blood vessels. This setup helps detect issues like faulty heart valves or congenital defects, and in most cases, it guides a doctor's decisions. Plus, since the device is portable and low cost, it shows up in both routine outpatient checks and emergency care, proving its worth in modern heart diagnostics. A key strength of this technology is its ability to capture motion in real time. Clinicians can see the heart beating and blood flowing almost as it happens (Figure 14.7).

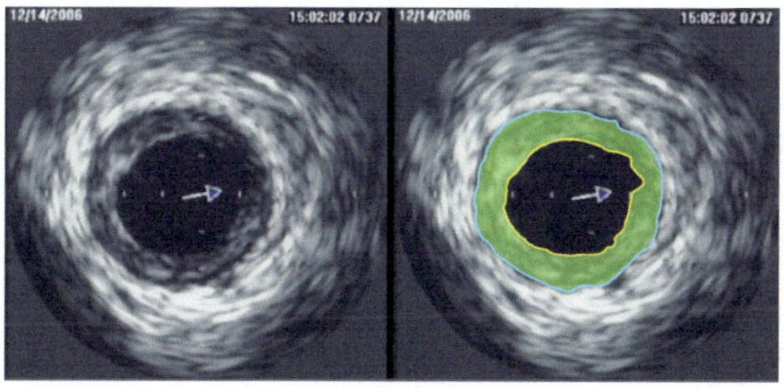

Figure 14.7. A sonographer moves the transducer on the patient's chest, while viewing the echo pictures on a computer.

Source: By The original uploader was Ksheka at English Wikipedia. - Transferred from en.wikipedia to Commons by Stevenfruitsmaak using CommonsHelper., CC BY-SA 2.5, https://commons.wikimedia.org/w/index.php?curid=5734047.

The Doppler effect is central here; by picking up even small changes in frequency as sound reflects off moving blood cells, it offers clues about blood speed and direction. This feature comes in handy when checking for things like aortic narrowing or working out how bad a valve leak is. Color Doppler imaging also steps in to show blood flow patterns in a clear, almost intuitive way. As most guidelines suggest, mixing these ultrasound insights with careful clinical judgment is crucial for the best patient results (Visseren et al., 2021). New improvements are constantly being added to ultrasound technology. Innovations such as three-dimensional echocardiography and strain imaging now let doctors take an even closer look at heart structure and movement.

These advances boost diagnostic accuracy and also open the door to more personalized treatment plans. Still, it is important for healthcare providers to keep up with evolving best practices and guidelines so that care delivery remains top-notch. Thus, while ultrasound continues to be an essential tool in heart imaging, practitioners should remember their responsibility to consider each patient's unique situation and consult public health recommendations when needed (Cosentino et al., 2019). This thoughtful, if sometimes slightly imperfect, approach ultimately refines diagnostic methods and reinforces care centered around the patient (Figure 14.8).

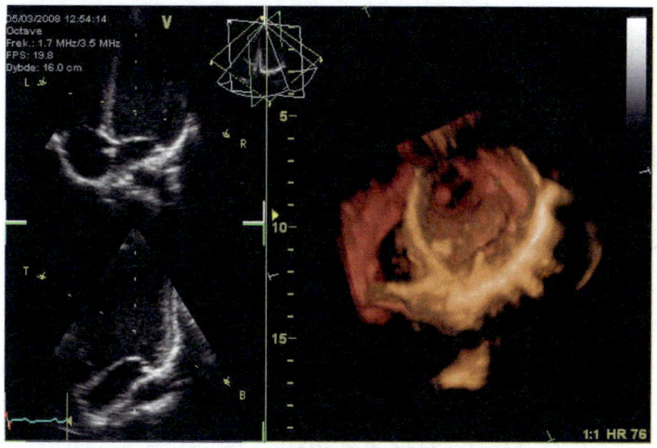

Figure 14.8. The picture created during an echocardiogram of the heart's lower and upper chambers (ventricles and atrium).

Source: By Kjetil Lenes - Own work, CC BY-SA 3.0, https://commons.wikimedia.org/w/index.php?curid=3705964.

14.2.2. Types of Echocardiograms (Transthoracic, Transesophageal)

Echo techniques come in many forms and play a huge role in how we see the heart. Doctors often lean toward transthoracic echo (TTE) because the method simply puts a sensor on the chest to obtain live images of the beating heart. It is non-invasive and lets clinicians quickly check the heart's wall movements, measure ventricle size, and get a general sense of overall function. This ease of access means that, in most cases, TTE is the go-to choice in clinics and even emergency rooms. Still, sometimes issues like a patient's build or lung conditions can mess with the image quality, and that's when another method, transesophageal echo (TEE), comes into play (Figure 14.9).

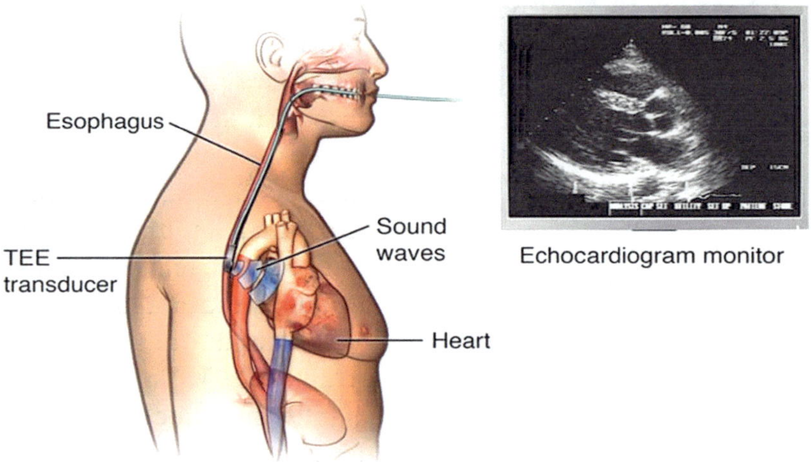

Figure 14.9. Transesophageal echocardiogram (TEE).

Source: https://choc.org/heart/cardiodiagnostics/echocardiogram/.

TEE is especially useful when a detailed view of the heart is needed. By placing the sensor directly in the esophagus, it gets a closer look at the heart, which means less interference from lung tissue and much clearer images of the heart's structure and how it is working. This approach is key for spotting problems like blood clots, valve issues, or congenital defects, especially when regular TTE just doesn't cut it. With its deeper reach, TEE allows for more precise measurements and proves its worth during procedures like cardioversion or surgery, ensuring that all the key parts of the heart are properly assessed (Herwerden et al., 1990). Of course, because TEE is an invasive procedure, it comes with risks that require careful patient selection and extra monitoring. Both TTE and TEE work together to give a complete picture of heart health. Typically, a transthoracic echo serves as the initial screening tool, identifying hints of wall motion irregularities or small fluid accumulations, after which a transesophageal study might follow if more detail is needed (Cianciulli et al., 2018). Each method plays its own part in a broader diagnostic strategy that matches imaging choices to the patient's unique situation. The field of cardiac imaging keeps on evolving, making these techniques sharper and more reliable, which in turn influences treatment decisions. In the end, knowing when to go with TTE or switch to TEE can make a real difference in patient outcomes and boost the overall quality of cardiovascular care (Figure 14.10).

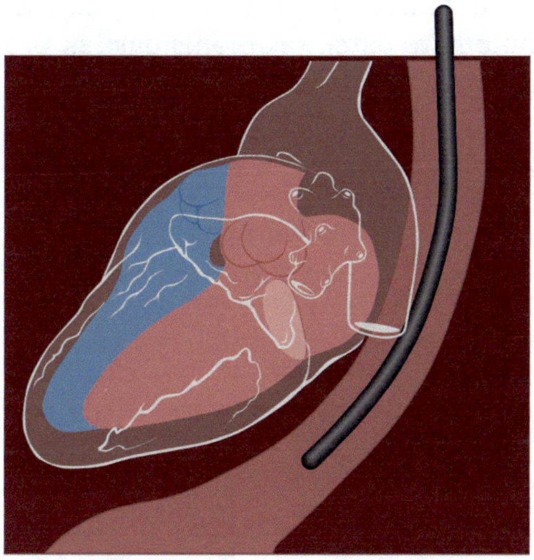

Figure 14.10. Transesophageal echocardiography. (A, B) Transthoracic echocardiography, parasternal long axis view. (C, D) Transesophageal echocardiography set at 61°. (A, C) Red arrows point at thickened and fixed right coronary cusp leaflet of the aortic valve. (B, D) Color Doppler reveals severe regurgitation of the aortic valve.

Source: By Patrick J. Lynch, medical illustrator - Patrick J. Lynch, medical illustrator, CC BY 2.5, https://commons.wikimedia.org/w/index.php?curid=1496615.

14.2.3. Clinical Applications and Benefits

Innovations in imaging have flipped the script on how we look at heart health, it's like a new era in diagnosing and treating cardiovascular conditions. CMR, or cardiovascular magnetic resonance imaging, isn't just a fancy term; it has become a go-to tool, especially when checking things like blood flow in the heart and tissue differences. The move from 1.5T to 3T scanners, generally speaking, gives us crisper images that let doctors peek into cardiac function and viability much more clearly. Research often shows that these sharper images help nail down diagnoses for issues such as ischemic heart disease, which in turn can boost patient outcomes (Hays et al., 2009). Many clinicians are now embracing these novel tools, finding that a deeper, more reliable grasp of heart health opens the door to treatment plans that fit each patient. Autofluorescence imaging (AFI) has also been making unexpected waves. Although mostly known for its work in eye care, AFI is now stepping into the cardiovascular field, sometimes in surprising ways. Its ability to highlight natural light emissions from tissues helps to flag metabolic issues and assess cardiovascular risk factors, almost as if it has become a clever stand-in for more invasive tests. There's even evidence, to some extent, that the glow seen in our skin can serve as a proxy for blood sugar levels and heart risk assessments (Aigner et al., 2020). As these imaging methods continue to grow in support and validation, earlier interventions for those at risk increasingly seem within reach, ultimately bolstering preventive care efforts. Beyond just diagnosing, these emerging imaging techniques seem to be making surgery a bit safer, too. For example, when surgeons, especially those still finding their footing, use AF-guided strategies during thyroid operations, they seem to get a better, quicker read on the differences between parathyroid and thyroid tissues. This extra visual cue helps cut down on errors and complications, a minor but crucial win for patient safety during procedures that even touch on cardiovascular concerns. Overall, as the clinical community keeps testing and fine-tuning these tools, the goal remains clear: using fresh technology to catch problems earlier, provide care that's more on point, and steadily improve how we manage heart health.

Test Your Knowledge

1. What are the fundamental principles behind ultrasound technology used in echocardiography?
2. How do transthoracic and transesophageal echocardiograms differ in terms of their application and imaging capabilities?

14.3. Emerging Technologies in Cardiovascular Imaging

Learning Outcome

1. Explain the 3D imaging and its applications.
2. Discuss the artificial intelligence in image analysis.
3. Explore future trends and innovations.

Cardiovascular imaging is shifting these days, driven by new technology that sharpens both how we diagnose and treat patients. AI now mixes into methods like myocardial perfusion imaging (MPI), in other words, it checks blood flow in the heart, which has tossed out many of the old rules and brought in fresh ways to assess risk for patients with coronary disease. You see, a blend of machine learning techniques and deep learning tools is now digging through complex data coming from all kinds of scans. In most cases, these AI setups help clear up images and cut out noise, so doctors can spot heart issues faster and with more accuracy. Overall, this rising field isn't just smoothing out clinical routines; it is also broadening how we detect conditions like ischemic heart disease, aiming to ease the global challenge of cardiovascular problems (Golub et al., 2025). Robotics in heart procedures is also taking a big leap. Instead of relying mostly on 2D fluoroscopy, effective but sometimes too basic for tough endovascular tasks, new MRI-compatible robots are stepping in. With these systems, imaging has moved into a 3D, radiation-free realm, which generally means way better accuracy in navigation. These smart robots, built to work seamlessly with MRI, use advanced scanning methods that help guide the procedure more reliably, cutting down on the usual pitfalls of manual methods. Meanwhile, early improvements in how doctors and machines interact suggest we might soon see interfaces that allow partial, or even full, robotic control during surgery. This shift opens up a new chapter in endovascular work, as it tackles challenges like high costs and technical complexity while boosting navigational precision (Pescio et al., 2025). The merging of all these fresh technologies into cardiovascular imaging is having a deep impact on everyday clinical practice.

Take AI's role in nuclear medicine, it clearly shows how these tools can transform the game by upping diagnostic precision, consistency, and even speeding up post-processing. Increasingly, physicians are leaning on robust AI systems to fine-tune their decisions, sparking a ripple that bumps up overall patient care standards. With more focus on figuring out risks and predicting outcomes, these advances are letting healthcare teams better customize treatment plans. Of course, upcoming research will need to iron out the technical and clinical wrinkles that appear when integrating these systems into routine use. Simply put, the mix of AI, robotics, and next-level imaging is busy reworking how we approach cardiovascular diagnostics and treatment, marking a pretty decisive shift in the field (Golub et al., 2025; Pescio et al., 2025) (Figure 14.11).

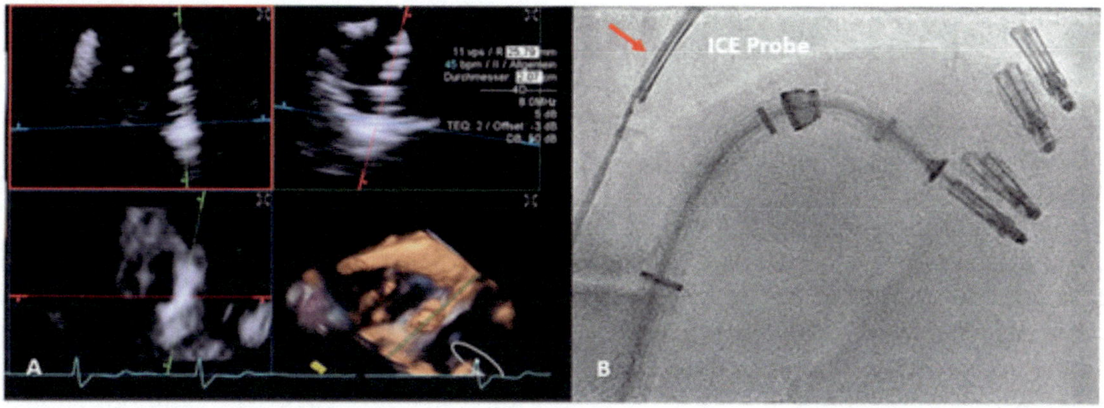

Figure 14.11. ICE application during T-TEER. (**A**) illustrates the live multiplanar reconstruction process used to align the TriClip (Abbott Vascular, Santa Clara, CA, USA) device on the tricuspid valve, for grasping the anterior and septal leaflets. In (**B**), the fluoroscopic position of the intracardiac probe can be observed (red arrow). The proximity of the probe to the device allows us to overcome shadows by obtaining high-quality images. T-TEER: Tricuspid Transcatheter edge-to-edge repair; ICE: intracardiac echocardiography.

Source: De Luca VM, Cammalleri V, Antonelli G, Bombace S, Ruf TF, Gößler TAM, Lurz P, von Bardeleben RS, Grigioni F, Ussia GP. The Other Side of the Coin: Transesophageal Echocardiography Complications following Cardiac Surgery and Transcatheter Structural Heart Interventions. *Journal of Clinical Medicine*. 2024; 13(15):4291. https://doi.org/10.3390/jcm13154291.

14.3.1. 3D imaging and Its Applications

3D imaging has shaken up the field of cardiovascular research and everyday medical work. It is not just about obtaining data, using techniques like CT and MRI, professionals now build detailed 3D models of the heart that capture jaw-dropping complexity. This clearer view means doctors can better understand each patient's unique anatomy and even how diseases play out. In most cases, merging these images with 3D printing has given rise to tailor-made models that serve for everything from planning surgeries to helping students and trainees learn; these printed replicas, for example, make it easier to grasp both congenital and acquired heart conditions (Gharleghi et al., 2021). Beyond showing off pretty pictures, 3D imaging has become a go-to tool in making crucial clinical decisions. Surgeons frequently depend on these precise anatomical models to map out personalized surgical strategies, sometimes even finding that transcatheter procedures are safer and simpler when backed by a physical reference model. Research keeps pointing to the fact that having a real model handy during preoperative briefings and even right in the midst of an operation can make a big difference, especially when dealing with tricky cases like aortic aneurysms or valve replacements, where the heart's complex curves and angles come into play (Wang et al., 2020). In general, this approach not only tends to boost surgical accuracy but also builds a kind of quiet confidence among the teams working on these tough cases. Looking forward, the whole scene of cardiovascular imaging seems poised for even more surprises. There's growing buzz around emerging ideas in bioprinting and tissue engineering, along with cool virtual and mixed reality tools, that could completely remix how we explore and treat heart conditions. The next wave of 3D printing is aiming to recreate models that mimic not just the structure but also the dynamic, almost alive behavior of heart tissues. Generally speaking, this could open up fresh, personalized ways to tackle various heart diseases, even those that have long been a challenge to treat. As ongoing research continues to expand using patient-specific tech, it feels like we're on the brink of a real transformation in both clinical care and medical education (Gharleghi et al., 2021) (Figure 14.12).

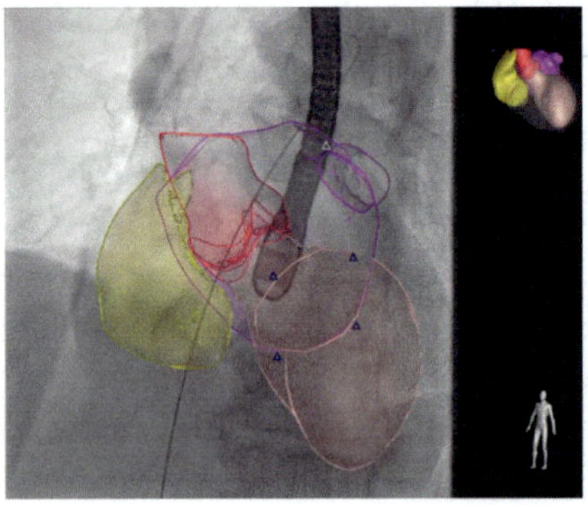

Figure 14.12. The EchoNavigator® (Philips Medical System, Andover, MA, USA) live image guidance. The smart fusion technology simplifies visualization by fusing real-time X-rays and live echo. EchoNavigator may give interventionalists a supportive anatomical understanding and smooth guidance during structural heart disease interventions to reduce the time undergoing TEE. The different colors distinguish various cardiac structures, with the triangles indicating the position of the mitral valve. The right atrium is shown in yellow, the aorta in magenta, the left ventricle in pink, and the left atrium in purple as indicated in the cartoon in the top right. TEE: transesophageal echocardiography.

Source: De Luca VM, Cammalleri V, Antonelli G, Bombace S, Ruf TF, Gößler TAM, Lurz P, von Bardeleben RS, Grigioni F, Ussia GP. The Other Side of the Coin: Transesophageal Echocardiography Complications following Cardiac Surgery and Transcatheter Structural Heart Interventions. *Journal of Clinical Medicine.* 2024; 13(15):4291. https://doi.org/10.3390/jcm13154291.

14.3.2. Artificial Intelligence (AI) in Image Analysis

Artificial intelligence in cardiovascular imaging isn't just another tech upgrade, it changes how we read and use medical data altogether. Tons of imaging information flood in every day, and the old ways of evaluating it can often get swamped, sometimes missing important clues that affect patient care. In most cases, AI steps in with its deep learning tools to comb through this jumble, making sure that no key diagnostic tidbits vanish. Clinicians now lean on these smart models to get a better handle on risk, with coronary artery calcium scoring (CACS) standing out as a clear example. Recent reviews even note that using AI to sharpen CACS is pretty vital for spotting upcoming heart issues and fine-tuning treatment choices (Cecco et al., 2024). Deep learning does more than just speed up analysis; it offers a whole new way to spot trends and connections hidden in vast datasets. Research in the field suggests that it shines when trying to decode the tangled signals in cardiology, challenges traditional rule-based methods often struggle with (Bizopoulos et al., 2021). By breaking down complicated data into bite-sized, actionable insights, this approach helps boost diagnostic accuracy and deepens our overall understanding of cardiovascular diseases. Its layered setup lets us pick up on minor shifts in imaging that might signal early trouble. Such progress matters not only for individual patients but also for the broader public health picture, supporting early detection efforts that can ultimately save lives. In imaging the heart, mixing techniques, like joining CACS with other diagnostic tools, shows just how far AI's potential can reach. New advances in image segmentation and deep-learning reconstructions allow for the simultaneous look at several conditions, offering a fuller picture of a patient's cardiovascular status. This blended approach, courtesy of AI, ramps up diagnosis accuracy and helps in tracking how diseases unfold. And as the healthcare scene keeps on shifting, bringing these AI-driven methods into everyday practice can shake up clinical routines and decision-making processes, boosting the overall standard of cardiac care (Cecco et al., 2024). Ongoing testing and tweaks to these methods hint at a bright future for AI in image analysis, subtly reshaping how doctors deal with heart diagnostics and treatment strategies (Figure 14.13).

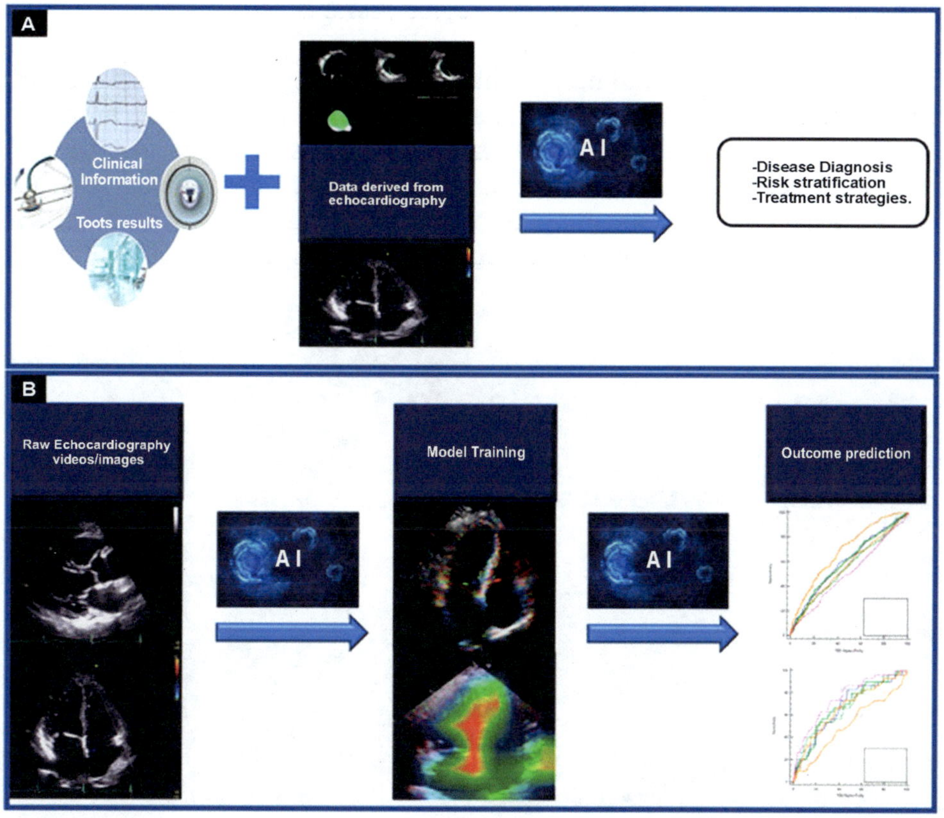

Figure 14.13. Role of artificial intelligence in cardiovascular imaging.

Source: Barry, Timothy, Juan Maria Farina, Chieh-Ju Chao, Chadi Ayoub, Jiwoong Jeong, Bhavik N. Patel, Imon Banerjee, and Reza Arsanjani. 2023. "The Role of Artificial Intelligence in Echocardiography" *Journal of Imaging* 9, no. 2: 50. https://doi.org/10.3390/jimaging9020050.

14.3.3. Future Trends and Innovations

Technology keeps on pushing boundaries and changing how we look at heart imaging. New methods, like AI and machine learning, are now getting woven into our usual imaging practices, helping doctors sift through heavy, messy data to spot those little clues that traditional scans might skip. These tools pick up on tiny patterns that might otherwise be overlooked, so doctors can sometimes catch conditions earlier and more clearly. AI even plays a part in sorting out risk levels for patients, which means treatments can end up being customized a bit more to each person. It is a bit unexpected, but as heart imaging grows with these ideas, the focus might shift from just fixing problems after they occur to nipping them in the bud. Metabolomics has joined the mix, adding a fresh twist to our understanding of heart conditions. By checking out the chemical signatures tied to different heart issues, researchers are uncovering hints about the processes leading to illness. This blending of metabolic clues with imaging data not only deepens our view but also brings out biomarkers that might someday track disease progression. In most cases, diving into systemic chemical changes alongside imaging is revealing surprising details about how our bodies react, which in turn could give doctors a more layered picture of what's going wrong (Pammolli et al., 2005). Over in the European Union, the medical device scene is buzzing with innovation, and heart imaging is definitely reaping the benefits. Traditional scanning methods are now mingling with tech from fields like bioinformatics and nanotechnology, creating gadgets that seemingly streamline the whole process. These new devices can make assessments quicker and more straightforward, possibly lowering long-term costs related to chronic heart issues. The overall impact isn't just clinical, there's a solid economic side to all this progress too. Competition is heating up and, as new interventions are developed, heart imaging continues to lead the way in healthcare innovation, as shown by the rapid evolution of sophisticated diagnostic tools (Yan et al., 2017).

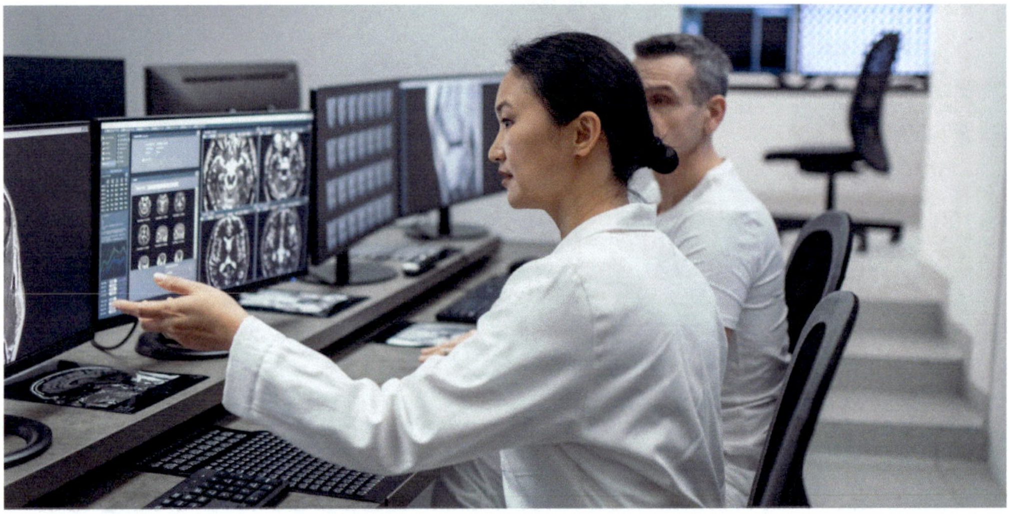

Source: https://www.dicomdirector.com/wp-content/uploads/2022/04/radiologists-review-medical-imaging-2250x1125.jpg.

Test Your Knowledge

1. How is artificial intelligence enhancing image analysis in cardiovascular imaging?
2. What role does 3D and 4D imaging play in advancing cardiovascular diagnostics?

14.4. Clinical Implications of Cardiovascular Imaging

Learning Outcome

1. Identify the impact on patient management and treatment.
2. Evaluate the cost-effectiveness and healthcare outcomes.
3. Discuss ethical considerations in imaging practices.

Cardiovascular imaging has changed how we handle heart conditions. New technologies like CMR and computed tomography (CT) have boosted the way we make diagnoses. These tools let us check out the heart's structure, how it is functioning, and even some details about the tissue, all without needing invasive procedures. CMR, for example, can pick up late gadolinium enhancement (LGE), which is pretty key when trying to figure out things like acute myocarditis; it even gives doctors clues about the chance of future problems. Knowing what these images imply helps clinicians adjust treatment plans and, overall, make patient care smarter, as many systematic reviews have shown (Georgiopoulos et al., 2021).

The push for more personalized care has also put cardiovascular imaging center stage in sorting risks out. Sometimes, the details from an image, like the severity of a condition, point out who might be more prone to complications; this means doctors can shape preventive measures and treatments in a more tailored way. That kind of customized approach not only cuts down on the dangers tied to heart issues but also bumps up overall care by encouraging a more proactive stance. It is hard to stress enough how mixing imaging results with a patient's full background gives healthcare individuals the extra edge in making solid, evidence-based choices. In many cases, showcasing the part imaging plays in clinics underscores its key role in comprehensive patient care and backs ongoing innovations in the field (Wichman, 2020). Beyond helping patients at the moment, cardiovascular imaging is also tweaking clinical guidelines and protocols, changing our whole take on diagnosing and treating heart disease. As new imaging methods pop up, they force us to reconsider the old ways of looking at things. For instance, findings from these advanced tools have started to shape guidelines that call for tighter monitoring and management of issues like coronary artery disease and heart failure. By making imaging a cornerstone of patient checks, healthcare systems can fine-tune how they spot and handle emerging heart problems. In the end, constantly weaving in fresh imaging methods not only improves outcomes, it deepens our overall understanding of heart health, hinting at a future where diagnosing and treating go hand in hand more seamlessly than ever before (Georgiopoulos et al., 2021) (Figure 14.14).

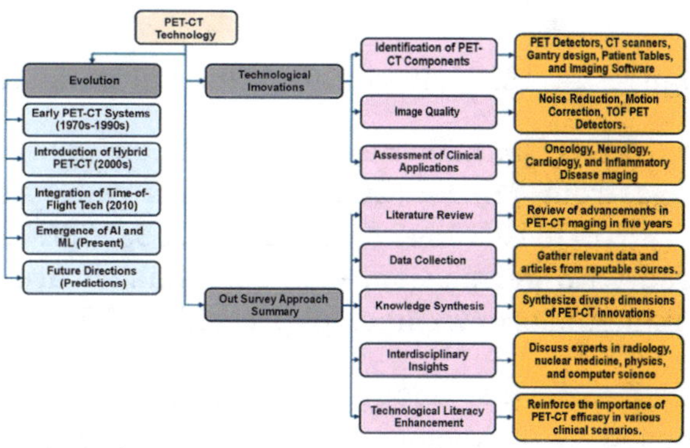

Figure 14.14. PET CT.

Source: Hussain, Dildar, Naseem Abbas, and Jawad Khan. 2024. "Recent Breakthroughs in PET-CT Multimodality Imaging: Innovations and Clinical Impact" *Bioengineering* 11, no. 12: 1213. https://doi.org/10.3390/bioengineering11121213.

14.4.1. Impact on Patient Management and Treatment

Technology keeps shifting how we handle patient care, especially in imaging the heart. AI now brings tools that let clinicians spot heart problems earlier than before. Take echoes or cardiac MRI, for example: these methods, boosted by smart algorithms, offer clearer, more usable info. By using these AI perks, doctors can look at imaging data with a precision you'd rarely expect, which means treatment plans get tailored specifically to each patient. This kind of personalized care, generally speaking, makes sure interventions not only come on time but also work better to meet each patient's needs, ultimately leading to improved outcomes overall in cardiovascular care (Chaudhary et al., 2024).

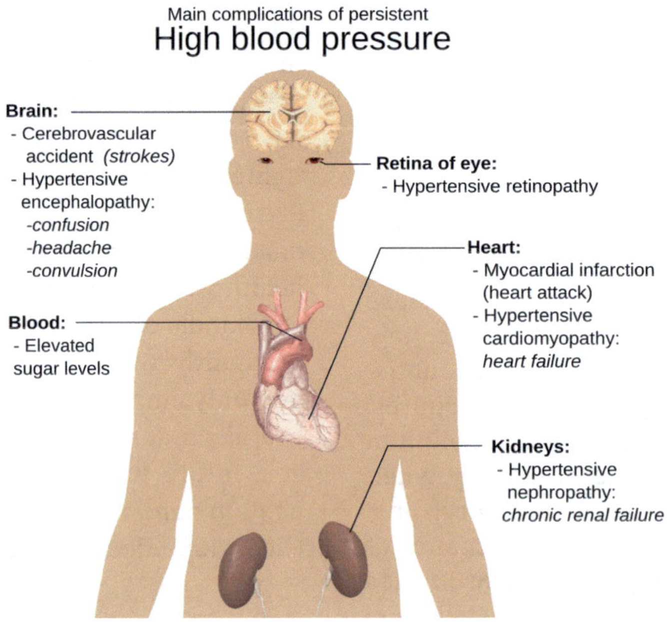

Figure 14.15. Main complications of persistent high blood pressure.

Source: By Mikael Häggström. When using this image in external works, it may be cited as: Häggström, Mikael (2014). "Medical gallery of Mikael Häggström 2014." WikiJournal of Medicine 1 (2). DOI:10.15347/wjm/2014.008. ISSN 2002-4436. Public Domain.or By Mikael Häggström, used with permission. - All used images are in public domain., Public Domain, https://commons.wikimedia.org/w/index.php?curid=5678966.

It isn't just about diagnosis either; AI also plays a role in fine-tuning how treatments are chosen. With advanced algorithms that crunch through loads of patient data, clinicians can usually pinpoint which groups are at higher risk, sometimes even spotting trends that might otherwise slip by. By comparing past treatment results with current patient conditions, AI-driven analysis helps guide decisions about medications and other therapies. In most cases, this personalized risk assessment paves the way for treatments that align more closely with what each patient needs, making the whole process a bit more straightforward (Kńska et al., 2024). This influence even reaches into the operating room. Real-time decision tools powered by AI analytics let doctors navigate challenging procedures with a mix of gut instinct and hard data, even in high-pressure, life-saving situations. This blend of immediacy and accuracy, albeit with a few rough edges in this brand-new approach, helps cut down on errors and boosts overall efficiency. In effect, these tech breakthroughs are setting up a new era in cardiovascular care where evolving innovations and everyday medical decisions work hand-in-hand toward better, safer outcomes (Szyma Kńska et al., 2024) (Figure 14.15).

14.4.2. Cost-Effectiveness and Healthcare Outcomes

Cardiovascular imaging is pushing healthcare in new directions. Heart failure rates are rising fast, and with that, it is not enough to know a test works unless we can see it pays off. Many new diagnostic and monitoring systems have hit the scene lately, but many of these innovations haven't taken off because the high trial costs stall practical use. In many cases, without rock-solid proof of worth, doctors and facilities tend to hold back, leaving patients with less access to the kind of enhanced diagnostics that could boost outcomes (Rosano et al., 2019). The way care is delivered matters too. The Patient-Centered Medical Home model has become a key route for better heart care by knitting together coordinated treatment and genuine patient involvement. Evaluators typically lean on measures that mix how money is spent with how clinically sound an approach is (Rosenthal et al., 2012). By aligning financial rewards with outcomes that truly center on patients, healthcare systems can get a better read on what these imaging advances offer. This kind of collaborative, almost team-like effort helps track improvements, and it paves the way for newer techniques to be weighed both in dollars and in results. Today's healthcare is getting more tangled, and digital tools add another layer of complexity. Mobile technology gives patients a chance to take charge of their heart health, but it also throws a wrench into data integration and the consistent read of diverse health info. In most cases, tech developers and healthcare individuals need to work closely together to ease telemedicine into the routine care. Given tightening budgets, these digital moves must show they're both cost-savvy and clinically sound. As Rosenthal et al. (2019) point out, fresh reimbursement models might just be the clever solution to support advanced imaging innovations while keeping quality care on track.

14.4.3. Ethical Considerations in Imaging Practices

Advanced imaging in cardiovascular care has shifted how clinicians work, but it also stirs up some tricky ethical issues that you just can't ignore. New AI tools now help with diagnoses, yet their inner workings often remain a bit mysterious, making it hard to pin down who's at fault when things go wrong. Doctors sometimes find themselves in a bind, having to trust analyses that can be as opaque as they are high-tech, which might lead to mixed signals in patient care. There's a growing call for Explainable AI in imaging, clinicians need clear, understandable results to build trust and keep ethical standards in check. In most cases, even though AI shows a lot of promise for better outcomes, its ethical side demands close attention to prevent any slip-ups in care or trust erosion (Tulsani et al., 2023). Patient consent and data privacy jump in as equally tangled issues in this evolving imaging landscape. With these technologies becoming the norm, it is now up to every physician to ensure patients truly get what they're agreeing to, especially when machine learning digs into their personal data. Patients need a clear picture of how their imaging data will be used, the risks involved, and what the implications might be for their health down the road. Protecting privacy isn't a side note; it calls for strict data rules, particularly when dealing with sensitive heart-related records. Building secure data systems and communicating openly about patient rights isn't just bureaucratic red tape, it is essential for trust and ethical care, even if it sometimes feels a bit over the top (Adertinto et al., 2024). Then there's the whole issue of bias creeping into imaging technologies. Sometimes, the data feeding these AI systems carries hidden biases that can skew diagnostic accuracy for certain groups, unintentionally fueling health disparities. Researchers and clinicians alike have to double-check that the data sets they rely on aren't just a narrow slice of the population but cover a diverse range of backgrounds. Running ongoing evaluations to catch any slanted outcomes is vital, this helps keep the decisions made by these systems fair and reliable. Ultimately, doing ethical work in cardiovascular imaging is all about committing to equity, using proactive measures to spot and mitigate bias, so every patient gets solid, unbiased care (Adertinto et al., 2024; Tulsani et al., 2023).

Test Your Knowledge

1. How does cardiovascular imaging aid in the early detection of heart diseases?
2. In what ways can imaging results influence treatment planning for cardiovascular conditions?

Summary

Advances in heart imaging have changed the game lately, doctors are now able to see the heart in motion using tools like echocardiography, MRI, and CT. As tech keeps moving forward, this means issues can now be spotted earlier and treatments can be shaped more personally for each patient. Often it is the combination of different imaging methods that gives clinicians a fuller picture, not just relying on one type alone. In many ways this progress shows that looking at heart health from several angles is key to better patient care. Imaging isn't just about figuring out what's wrong, it also keeps tabs on how well treatments work. For instance, consider a young patient with peripheral T-cell lymphoma who underwent a lengthy lysis therapy and eventually showed a big drop in the clot in the right atrium. By using multiple imaging techniques at once, doctors got a pretty accurate look that guided their clinical decisions. Cases like this keep popping up, proving that imaging is more than a one-shot diagnostic tool; it plays a central role in managing complicated heart conditions. This stresses why ongoing research and further breakthroughs in this area are so necessary. Looking ahead, the future of cardiovascular imaging holds tremendous promise for boosting both clinical practice and patient outcomes. Research efforts, backed by organizations such as the Medical Research Council and the Wellcome Trust), signal a strong commitment to pushing this field forward. Such support is essential for sparking fresh ideas and widening using imaging technologies in heart care. As these techniques continue to evolve, the combined strength of various imaging methods will be key to untangling the many layers of cardiovascular diseases. In the final analysis, the path forward isn't just about cutting-edge machines; it is about a whole new vision for timely, accurate, and holistic patient care (Lorenz et al., 2007).

Cardiovascular imaging has come a long way and now plays a bigger role in spotting heart issues. We used to rely mainly on echocardiograms and X-rays, but now techniques like cardiac MRI, and CT scans offer a non-invasive look inside the heart's workings. Newer tools shake up the old routine, giving doctors clearer views that help guide treatment. Generally speaking, guidelines suggest weaving these methods into daily practice to boost diagnostic precision and improve patient care outcomes. Health professionals need to grasp these changes if they're to make solid decisions that match today's shifting imaging standards (Mach et al., 2019). At the heart of this progress is a careful, evidence-supported approach that puts patients first. Years of clinical research show which imaging methods hit the mark, while also hinting at some ethical side-notes. Even though guidelines lay out a broad framework for doing things right, they never replace a clinician's need to judge each patient's unique situation. In many cases, reading imaging results requires keeping an eye on broader clinical aims along with public health advice, even when these differ from one group to another (Cosentino et al., 2019). Keeping current with the latest imaging techniques is crucial for anyone in healthcare these days. As technology in this field keeps evolving, professionals are constantly nudged to adapt and try new approaches. When imaging methods get more advanced, practitioners must stay tuned to current guidelines and ethical norms to choose the right strategies. This constant learning not only leads to better clinical outcomes but also builds a safer, more effective care environment, which reinforces the core goals of modern cardiovascular imaging practices (Mach et al., 2019).

KEY TERMS FROM THIS CHAPTER

- 3D anatomical models
- Atherosclerosis
- Congenital heart disease
- CT angiography (CTA)
- Genetic testing
- Iron oxide nanoparticles (IONs)
- Myocardial perfusion imaging
- Transthoracic echocardiography (TTE)
- Acute myocardial infarction (AMI)
- Cardiovascular magnetic resonance (CMR)
- Coronary artery disease
- Echocardiography
- Heart health
- Mock circulatory loops (MCLs)
- Transesophageal echocardiography (TEE)
- Vascular imaging

Critical Thinking Questions

1. **Which imaging modality is commonly used to assess the coronary arteries and heart function during a heart attack?**
   a. X-ray
   b. CT Angiography (CTA)
   c. MRI
   d. Ultrasound
2. **What is the main purpose of echocardiography in cardiovascular imaging?**
   a. To measure heart muscle thickness
   b. To visualize heart valves and blood flow
   c. To provide detailed images of coronary arteries
   d. To assess bone health
3. **Which of the following imaging techniques is commonly used for evaluating myocardial infarction (heart attack) and assessing heart function?**
   a. Magnetic Resonance Imaging (MRI)
   b. Electrocardiography (ECG)
   c. Positron Emission Tomography (PET)
   d. Chest X-ray
4. **In cardiovascular imaging, what is the role of a coronary angiogram?**
   a. To visualize the heart's electrical activity
   b. To assess the size and shape of the heart
   c. To detect blockages in the coronary arteries
   d. To measure blood flow in the lungs
5. **What is a major advantage of Magnetic Resonance Imaging (MRI) in cardiovascular imaging?**
   a. It is non-invasive and uses no ionizing radiation
   b. It is less expensive than other imaging modalities
   c. It provides real-time imaging for heart surgeries
   d. It is the best tool for detecting coronary artery disease

Short Answer Questions

1. What are the primary differences between echocardiography and other cardiovascular imaging techniques?
2. How does echocardiography help in the diagnosis of heart conditions?
3. What are the advantages of using magnetic resonance imaging (MRI) in cardiovascular imaging?
4. How do emerging technologies like 3D imaging enhance cardiovascular diagnostics?
5. What clinical conditions benefit most from using cardiovascular imaging techniques?
6. What are the potential risks associated with cardiovascular imaging, and how can they be mitigated?

Answers to Critical Thinking Questions

1. (b); 2. (b); 3. (c); 4. (c); 5. (a)

References

1. Adertinto, N., Adertinto, N., David-Olawade, A. C., & David-Olawade, A. C. (2024). Advancements and applications of artificial intelligence in cardiology: Current trends and future prospects. https://core.ac.uk/download/603653360.pdf (accessed on 23 May 2025).

2. Ahn, J., Park, S. H., Kim, D., Kim, T., Jo, S., Lee, H., & Cho, A. (2012). Role of echocardiography in sinus venosus atrial septal defect combined with systemic and pulmonary vascular disease. *Journal of Cardiovascular Ultrasound, 20*(1), 49–51. https://doi.org/10.4250/jcu.2012.20.1.49.

3. Aigner, F., Pratschke, J., Schumann, T., et al. (2020). Recent advances and the potential for clinical use of autofluorescence detection of extra-ophthalmic tissues. https://core.ac.uk/download/323257980.pdf (accessed on 23 May 2025).

4. Akin, I., Baumann, S., Becher, T., et al. (2014). The value of multimodality imaging for detection, characterization and management of a wall adhering structure in the right atrium. https://core.ac.uk/download/46603006.pdf (accessed on 23 May 2025).

5. Bergom, C., Bradley, J. A., Ng, A. K., Samson, P., Robinson, C. G., Lopez-Mattei, J., & Mitchell, J. D. (2021). Past, present, and future of radiation-induced cardiotoxicity: Refinements in targeting, surveillance, and risk stratification. *JACC: Cardio Oncology, 3*(3), 343–359. https://doi.org/10.1016/j.jaccao.2021.06.007.

6. Bizopoulos, P., & Koutsouris, D. (2021). Deep learning in cardiology. http://arxiv.org/abs/1902.11122 (accessed on 23 May 2025).

7. Bustin, A., Fuin, N., Botnar, R. M., & Prieto, C. (2020). From compressed-sensing to artificial intelligence-based cardiac MRI reconstruction. *Frontiers in Cardiovascular Medicine, 7*, Article 17. https://doi.org/10.3389/fcvm.2020.00017.

8. Cardiovascular Medicine Professional Committee of Medical Genetics Branch of Chinese Medical Association, Cardiology Group of Pediatric Surgery Branch of Chinese Medical Association, He, G., Qi, M., & Yang, D. (2024). Specification for genetic diagnosis of congenital heart disease. *Zhonghua Yi Xue Yi Chuan Xue Za Zhi = Chinese Journal of Medical Genetics, 41*(6), 641–650. https://www.semanticscholar.org/paper/0d573fe6a2980c68a8b7e896ba8bb293b5b02dbb (accessed on 23 May 2025).

9. Chaudhary, I., & Anwar, H. (2024). The impact of artificial intelligence on cardiovascular disease diagnosis: A review. *Pakistan Journal of Medical and Health Sciences*. https://www.semanticscholar.org/paper/a4e96e2247ad9801749c739d6004da11ee9f9502 (accessed on 23 May 2025).

10. Cianciulli, T. F., & Saccheri, M. C. (2018). *Actinic Papillary Fibroelastoma of the Left Ventricle*. https://core.ac.uk/download/322439588.pdf (accessed on 23 May 2025).

11. Cornejo, J., Cornejo, J., Vargas, M., Helguero, C. G., Andrade, R. M., Torres, S., Asensio-Salazar, J., et al. (2022). Anatomical engineering and 3D printing for surgery and medical devices: International review and future exponential innovations. *BioMed Research International, 2022*, 1–28. https://doi.org/10.1155/2022/6797745.

12. Cosentino, F., Grant, P. J., Aboyans, V., Bailey, C. J., Ceriello, A., Delgado, V., Federici, M., et al. (2019). 2019 ESC guidelines on diabetes, pre-diabetes, and cardiovascular diseases developed in collaboration with the EASD. *European Heart Journal, 41*, 255–323. https://doi.org/10.1093/eurheartj/ehz486.

13. Dobson, R., Ghosh, A. K., Ky, B., Marwick, T. H., Stout, M., Harkness, A., Steeds, R. P., et al. (2021). BSE and BCOS guideline for transthoracic echocardiographic assessment of adult cancer patients receiving anthracyclines and/or trastuzumab. *JACC: Cardio Oncology, 3*, 1–16. https://doi.org/10.1016/j.jaccao.2021.01.011.

14. Gennari, A. G., Rossi, A., De Cecco, C. N., van Assen, M., Sartoretti, T., Giannopoulos, A. A., Schwyzer, M., Huellner, M. W., & Messerli, M. (2024). Artificial intelligence in coronary artery calcium score: Rationale, different approaches, and outcomes. *The International Journal of Cardiovascular Imaging, 40*(5), 951–966. https://doi.org/10.1007/s10554-024-03080-4.

15. Georgiopoulos, G., Figliozzi, S., Sanguineti, F., Aquaro, G. D., Di Bella, G., Stamatelopoulos, K., Chiribiri, A., et al. (2021). Prognostic impact of late gadolinium enhancement by cardiovascular magnetic resonance in myocarditis. *Circulation: Cardiovascular Imaging, 14*. https://doi.org/10.1161/circimaging.120.011492.

16. Gharleghi, R., Dessalles, C. A., Lal, R., McCraith, S., Sarathy, K., Jepson, N., Otton, J., et al. (2021). 3D printing for cardiovascular applications: From end-to-end processes to emerging developments. *Annals of Biomedical Engineering, 49*, 1598–1618. https://doi.org/10.1007/s10439-021-02784-1.

17. Golub, I. S., Thummala, A. R., Morad, T., Dhaliwal, J., Elisarraras, F., Karlsberg, R. P., & Cho, G. W. (2025). Artificial intelligence in nuclear cardiac imaging: Novel advances, emerging techniques, and recent clinical trials. *Journal of Clinical Medicine, 14*. https://www.semanticscholar.org/paper/ad5f9cc5b538c9b30df9ca0c29da1f45fbeed2c9 (accessed on 23 May 2025).

18. Hays, A. G., Schär, M., & Kelle, S. (2009). Clinical applications for cardiovascular magnetic resonance imaging at 3 teslas. *Current Cardiology Reviews, 5*(3), 237–242. https://doi.org/10.2174/157340309788970351.

19. Herwerden, L. A. van. (1990). Epicardial echocardiography. https://core.ac.uk/download/19889823.pdf (accessed on 23 May 2025).

20. Lorenz, C. H., Fieno, D. S., Di Cesare, E., Grothues, F., Sandstede, J., Selvanayagam, J., Francis, J. M., et al. (2007). Effects of steady state free precession parameters on cardiac mass, function, and volumes. https://core.ac.uk/download/30698183.pdf (accessed on 23 May 2025).

21. Mach, F., Baigent, C., Catapano, A. L., Koskinas, K. C., Casula, M., Badimón, L., Chapman, M. J., et al. (2019). 2019 ESC/EAS guidelines for the management of dyslipidaemias: Lipid modification to reduce cardiovascular risk. *European Heart Journal, 41*, 111–188. https://doi.org/10.1093/eurheartj/ehz455.

22. Pammolli, F., Riccaboni, M., Oglialoro, C., Magazzini, L., Baio, G., & Salerno, N. (2005). Medical devices competitiveness and impact on public health expenditure. *Enterprise Directorate-General, European Commission*.

23. Pescio, M., Kundrat, D., & Dagnino, G. (2025). Endovascular robotics: Technical advances and future directions. *Minimally Invasive Therapy & Allied Technologies*, 1–14. https://doi.org/10.1080/13645706.2025.2454237.

24. Rocchi, M., Ingram, M., Claus, P., D'hooge, J., Meyns, B., & Fresiello, L. (2023). Use of 3D anatomical models in mock circulatory loops for cardiac medical device testing. *Artificial Organs, 47*(2), 260–272. https://doi.org/10.1111/aor.14433.

25. Rosano, G. M. C., Spoletini, I., & Vitale, C. (2019). Who approves/pays for additional monitoring?

European Heart Journal Supplements: Journal of the European Society of Cardiology, 21(Suppl M), M64–M67. https://doi.org/10.1093/eurheartj/suz228.

26. Rosenthal, M. B., Abrams, M. K., Bitton, A., & the Patient-Centered Medical Home Evaluators' Collaborative. (2012). Recommended core measures for evaluating the patient-centered medical home: Cost, utilization, and clinical quality. The Commonwealth Fund.

27. Sadegh-Zadeh, S. A., Khezerlouy-Aghdam, N., Sakha, H., Toufan, M., Behravan, M., Vahedi, A., Rahimi, M., Hosseini, H., Khanjani, S., Bayat, B., Ali, S. A., Hajizadeh, R., Eshraghi, A., Ghidary, S. S., & Saadat, M. (2024). Precision diagnostics in cardiac tumors: Integrating echocardiography and pathology with advanced machine learning on limited data. *Informatics in Medicine Unlocked, Article 101544*. https://doi.org/10.1016/j.imu.2024.101544.

28. Santos, E. D. S., Kuhn, G. D. C., Almeida, A. G. C. de, Pimentel, J. V. A., Figueiredo Neto, N. V., Melo, B. C., et al. (2025). Genetic, clinical, and sociodemographic profile in individuals with diagnosis or family history of hypertrophic cardiomyopathy: Insights from a prospective cohort. *medRxiv*. https://doi.org/10.1101/2025.01.24.25321106.

29. Situ, Y., Birch, S. C. M., Moreyra, C., & Holloway, C. J. (2020). Cardiovascular magnetic resonance imaging for structural heart disease. *Cardiovascular Diagnosis and Therapy, 10*(2), 361–375. https://doi.org/10.21037/cdt.2019.06.02.

30. Suri, J. S., Bhagawati, M., Paul, S., Protogerou, A. D., Sfikakis, P. P., Kitas, G. D., Khanna, N. N., Ruzsa, Z., Sharma, A. M., Saxena, S., Faa, G., Laird, J. R., Johri, A. M., Kalra, M. K., Paraskevas, K. I., & Saba, L. (2022). A powerful paradigm for cardiovascular risk stratification using multiclass, multi-label, and ensemble-based machine learning paradigms: A narrative review. *Diagnostics, 12*(3), 722. https://doi.org/10.3390/diagnostics12030722.

31. Szymańska, K., Szmyt, K., Krasnoborska, J., Samojedny, S., Superson, M., Walczak, K., Wilk-Trytko, K., Zarębska, J., & Duplaga, T. A. (2024). Revolutionizing cardiovascular treatments with the use of AI: Current status and future prospects. *Quality in Sport, 19*, Article 53072. https://doi.org/10.12775/QS.2024.19.53072.

32. Tulsani, V., Sahatiya, P., Parmar, J., & Parmar, J. (2023). XAI applications in medical imaging: A survey of methods and challenges. *International Journal on Recent and Innovation Trends in Computing and Communication, 11*(9), 181–186. https://doi.org/10.17762/ijritcc.v11i9.8332.

33. Vahanian, A., Beyersdorf, F., Praz, F., Milojevic, M., Baldus, S., Bauersachs, J., Capodanno, D., et al. (2021). 2021 ESC/EACTS guidelines for the management of valvular heart disease. *European Heart Journal, 43*(7), 561–632. https://doi.org/10.1093/eurheartj/ehab395.

34. Visseren, F. L. J., Mach, F., Smulders, Y. M., Carballo, D., Koskinas, K. C., Bäck, M., Bénétos, A., et al. (2021). 2021 ESC guidelines on cardiovascular disease prevention in clinical practice. *European Heart Journal, 42*, 3227–3337. https://doi.org/10.1093/eurheartj/ehab484.

35. Wang, C., Zhang, L., Tao, Q., Xi, Z., Sun, L., Wu, H., & Li, D. M. (2020). 3D printing in adult cardiovascular surgery and interventions: A systematic review. *Journal of Thoracic Disease, 12*(7), 3227–3237. https://doi.org/10.21037/jtd-20-455.

36. Wichmann, D. (2020). Autopsy findings and venous thromboembolism in patients with COVID-19. *Annals of Internal Medicine, 173*, 1030. https://doi.org/10.7326/l20-1206.

37. Yan, D., Afifi, L., Jeon, C., Trivedi, M., Chang, H. W., Lee, K., & Liao, W. (2017). The metabolomics of psoriatic disease. *Psoriasis (Auckland, N.Z.), 7*, 1–15. https://doi.org/10.2147/PTT.S118348.

38. Yılmaz, A., Bietenbeck, M., Florian, A. R., Faber, C., & Sechtem, U. (2016). Remote magnetic targeting of iron oxide nanoparticles for cardiovascular diagnosis and therapeutic drug delivery: Where are we now? *International Journal of Nanomedicine, 11*, 3191–3203. https://doi.org/10.2147/ijn.s110542.

39. Zhou, J., Du, M., Chang, S., & Chen, Z. (2021). Artificial intelligence in echocardiography: Detection, functional evaluation, and disease diagnosis. *Cardiovascular Ultrasound, 19*. https://doi.org/10.1186/s12947-021-00261-2.

NEUROIMAGING

15

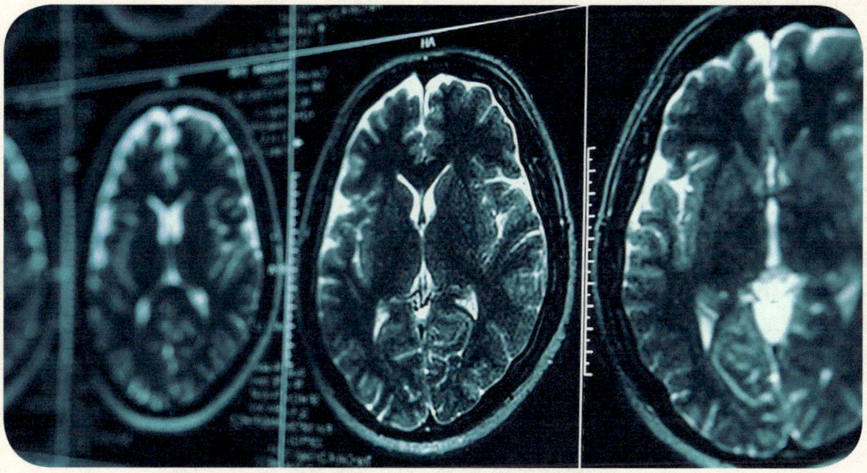

LEARNING OBJECTIVES

After studying this chapter, you will be able to:

1. Trace the historical development and milestones in the field of neuroimaging.
2. Differentiate between various neuroimaging techniques.
3. Explore the clinical and research applications of neuroimaging.
4. Assess the strengths and limitations of current neuroimaging modalities.
5. Identify emerging trends and future directions in neuroimaging technologies.

Introduction

Technology is advancing fast, and we're now looking at ways to peer into the brain that weren't imaginable just a few years back. Neuroimaging lets us see the brain's inner workings in a pretty direct way, offering a glimpse into those intricate systems. Tools like functional magnetic resonance imaging (fMRI) and positron emission tomography (PET) aren't just about mapping structure, they let us follow cognitive processes as they happen. Machine learning is now mixing in to sift through neural data, opening up surprising routes to discovery in both research and clinical settings. All this lays a foundation for diverse uses, especially in studying tough neurological disorders. Then there's a cool breakthrough called image reconstruction from brain signals (IRBS). It uses deep learning with large neuroimaging datasets to visualize mental images from brain activity, pretty interesting, right? This innovation doesn't just answer academic questions; it also has a shot at practical clinical application in psychiatry. Generally speaking, IRBS pushes us to reconsider ideas about consciousness, perception, and what thought is. Of course, one can't ignore the limitations and ethical issues, like data privacy and whether we're reading the signals correctly, which are key for ensuring the technology is used responsibly (Lu, 2023). Another exciting direction is estimating brain age with neuroimaging. Researchers have begun applying machine-learning models to brain scans, which helps create frameworks for figuring out an individual's brain age. This measurement, in many cases, shows promise in diagnosing neurological conditions and crafting personalized treatment plans. The potential impact on neuropsychiatry is huge; these age estimations might trigger early interventions to slow cognitive decline. A handful of studies point to a broad range of clinical applications, echoing how brain age estimation can tie into larger goals for neuropsychiatric care. Still, ongoing research is needed to overcome current challenges and explore the full possibilities of neuroimaging (Sone et al., 2022).

Definition of Neuroimaging

Neuroscience has taken some unexpected turns lately as new ways to watch the brain in action keep emerging. Neuroimaging – you know, tools that let us peek at brain structure and activity – has become one of those game-changers. Sometimes, you'll hear about magnetic resonance imaging (MRI) that shows how the brain is built, while other times it is functional techniques like fMRI or even PET scanning that capture bursts of neuronal work during different tasks. All of these approaches, in one way or another, have reshaped what we think we know about the brain, linking specific regions to mental functions and nudging forward our understanding of neurological issues. Researchers, as they dig deeper into how these imaging methods tick, are starting to see more profound ripple effects on psychology and cognitive science. In most cases, by following the subtle shifts in brain activity tied to emotions or even attention and memory, scientists gain a layered view of how our feelings mix with thought processes – even if the picture is a bit messy sometimes. When studies blend neuroimaging with traditional ideas in psychology, you end up with a richer, sometimes more redundant, take on normal versus abnormal brain states. Seeing the neural dance in real time isn't just cool; it paves the way for treatments that are more finely tuned to actual brain behavior. The story doesn't stop there, though.

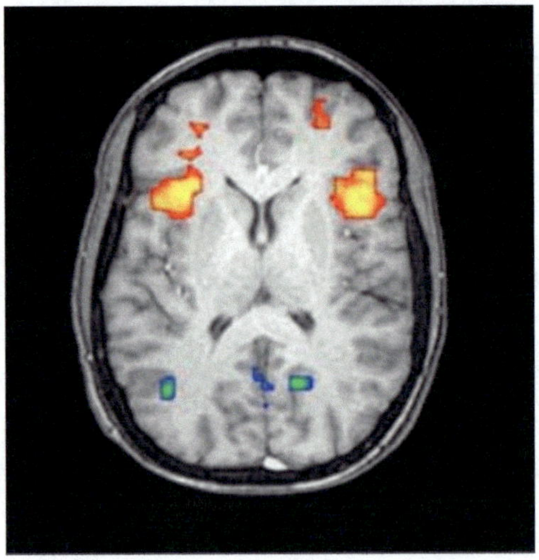

Figure 15.1. Axial MRI slice at the level of the basal ganglia, showing fMRI BOLD signal changes overlaid in red (increase) and blue (decrease) tones.

Source: https://upload.wikimedia.org/wikipedia/en/d/d1/FMRIscan.jpg.

There's been a quiet revolution, if you will, in the way scientists explore mental experiences using imaging. For example, a growing curiosity about how brain regions react to different triggers has pushed neuroimaging beyond just mapping structures. Recent studies hint that these advanced techniques let us observe how tiny areas in the brain respond to varied stimuli, which in turn shape our emotional responses. This blend of neuroscience, psychology, and even a pinch of philosophy, generally speaking, encourages a cross-disciplinary look at mental processes. And as this field meanders forward, the promise for neuroimaging to untangle the brain's intricate workings remains vast, hinting at fresh theoretical insights and practical steps for mental health treatments (Figure 15.1).

Importance of Neuroimaging in Neuroscience

For years, the complexity of the brain has kept both researchers and clinicians on their toes. People have had to get creative, especially when trying to wrap their heads around conditions like autism spectrum disorder (ASD). Nowadays, thanks to new neuroimaging methods, scientists can peek into the brain's inner workings, spotting both its physical build and how it fires up. It is pretty interesting that doctors can even notice unusual connectivity in little ones, sometimes as young as six months, which, in turn, gives clues about the developmental paths of ASD. And it isn't just for diagnosing; these scans help sort out different autism groups, factoring in both genetic hints and environmental bits. In most cases, understanding these brain signals could eventually tie certain treatments to the right subgroups, improving care and outcomes for affected children (Muhle et al., 2018). Our understanding of brain function has also shifted as cognitive neuroscience has grown, today it is less about one isolated brain area and more about the chatter between networks. Imaging studies show that both the brain's wiring and how actively different parts connect play a huge role in how cognitive abilities hold up with age. You see, when regions of the brain interact well, skills like memory and language tend to stick around better; too much cross-talk between networks, however, might end up causing problems. Generally speaking, these findings reveal just how valuable neuroimaging is for mapping out the effects of aging on mental performance and even hint at ways to soften age-related decline (Antonenko et al., 2013). And then there's the clinical side of things, neuroimaging isn't only about early development or aging. Techniques like fMRI have become central to showing how the brain responds during treatments, such as non-invasive brain stimulation. By tracking shifts in connectivity during specific tasks, researchers can gather clues on how these changes influence overall performance. This kind of info is pure gold when designing rehab programs for people bouncing back from strokes or traumatic brain injuries (TBI). As imaging technology pushes forward, its role in bridging theoretical research with everyday patient care grows even more crucial, steadily nudging clinical practices toward more effective and tailored therapies (Antonenko et al., 2013).

15.1. History of Neuroimaging

Learning Outcome

1. Examine the early techniques and developments that laid the foundation for neuroimaging.
2. Identify key milestones in the advancement of neuroimaging technology.
3. Analyze the evolution of neuroimaging applications in both clinical and research settings.

Neuroimaging took an unexpected turn long ago. Instead of offering deep insights, early methods like X-rays and angiography only pointed at the obvious abnormalities. Then in the 1970s, CT scans popped up, slicing the brain into cross-sectional images that made spotting hemorrhages or tumors way easier. The real shake-up happened in the 1980s when MRI arrived, suddenly we had high-resolution images without worrying about harmful radiation. Later on, fMRI stepped in, tracking blood flow in a way that let us peek at brain activity in real time; this shift from static pictures to live mapping laid the groundwork for studying our thinking processes. As these tools matured, their applications spread in unexpected ways. Techniques like PET began revealing details about cerebral metabolism and even the subtle buzz of neurotransmitters, broadening what we knew about neuropsychiatric conditions. Sometimes PET was even paired with MRI in hybrid systems that mixed their strengths for a fuller picture. With neuroimaging becoming more accessible, people from areas like psychology, neuroscience, and even market research, started getting curious. In many cases, this richer look into the brain's complex workings has helped uncover clues about disorders like Alzheimer's, schizophrenia, and ASDs, influencing clinical practices and research setups along the way. However, these technological leaps aren't without their ethical bumps. As our ability to capture and analyze brain data grows, so do debates about mental privacy, cognitive freedom, and even consent, concerns that our most private thoughts could be misused. There's a growing blur between what's for clinical help and what's for commercial gain, pushing the need for stronger ethical safeguards. Generally speaking, as neuroethics makes its way into the public conversation, it reminds us that balancing scientific progress with protecting individual rights is a must. In navigating this unfolding journey of neuroimaging, it is clear that every advance should honor our freedom and privacy (Ienca et al., 2017) (Figure 15.2).

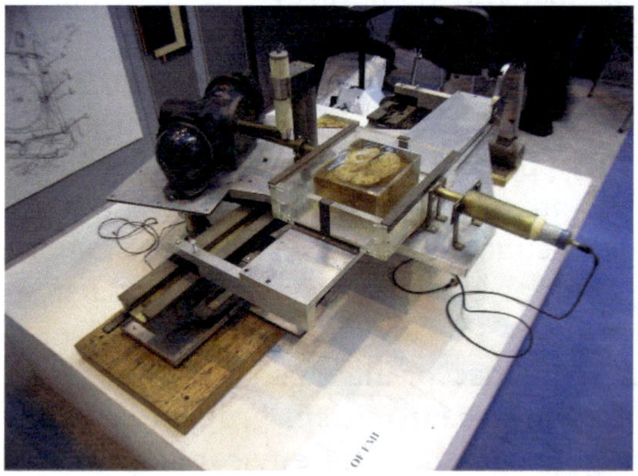

Figure 15.2. The prototype computerized tomography (CT) scanner.

Source: By No machine-readable author provided. Gdh~commonswiki assumed (based on copyright claims). - No machine-readable source provided. Own work assumed (based on copyright claims)., CC BY-SA 3.0, https://commons.wikimedia.org/w/index.php?curid=1006700.

15.1.1. Early Techniques and Developments

Recent brain imaging breakthroughs come from mixing new technology with fresh ideas about how our minds work. Magnetoencephalography, or MEG, popped up in the late 1900s as a neat way to listen in on the brain's magnetic buzz from its electrical signals. It can capture activity down to the millisecond and pick up details on a scale of 2–5 mm. Early MEG setups, however, were pretty tied down by their reliance on SQUIDs, those superconducting quantum interference devices that need cryogenic cooling, which made scanning certain individuals, like infants or people with smaller heads, kind of problematic. This snag, generally speaking, pointed to a broader need for imaging tools that are both sharper and easier to use (Brookes et al., 2022). Switching focus, electrical impedance tomography (EIT) has quietly stepped into the limelight with its own twist. Instead of measuring magnetic fields directly, EIT takes a look at how electrical current shifts between electrodes on the body's surface, offering an indirect peek at how tissue properties are spread out.

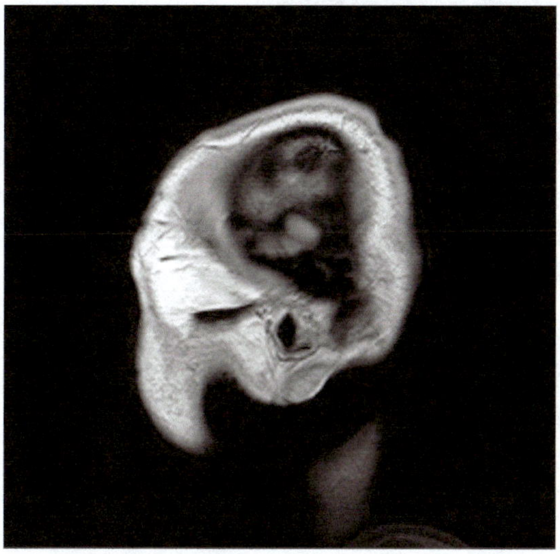

Figure 15.3. MRI of the brain.

Source: By Dwayne Reed at English Wikipedia, CC BY-SA 3.0, https://commons.wikimedia.org/w/index.php?curid=4390827.

In most cases, this method holds exciting promise for tackling issues like epilepsy, stroke, and cerebral edema since it lets clinicians see brain conditions in real-time. Still, there are bumps along the way: accurately mapping the intricate maze of our anatomy isn't straightforward, which keeps the technique from reaching its full potential just yet (Ke et al., 2022). Building on those earlier methods, recent innovations have begun ironing out many of the old problems. For instance, optically pumped magnetometers (OPMs) are now being used in MEG systems and are showing real promise, they don't need those tricky cryogenic conditions and can even be arranged into sensor arrays that snugly fit a participant's head. This not only improves signal quality but also cuts down on motion issues, making studies with children or movement-impaired patients far more feasible. In most cases, this shift feels like a pivotal moment in neuroimaging, opening up more natural experiment styles while gradually peeling back the layers of our brain's complex workings (Brookes et al., 2022) (Figure 15.3).

15.1.2. Milestones in Neuroimaging Technology

This journey has reshaped neuroscience in ways that matter for clinics and research alike. Back in the 1920s, cerebral angiography first gave us a sneak peek into the brain, and then, quite dramatically, the 1970s brought computed tomography (CT) into play, which changed the game for how we view brain structure and function. In the 1980s, MRI stepped in with crisp, high-resolution images that not only highlighted anatomy but also hinted at function. This shift, in most cases, laid a rough, yet promising, path toward techniques like fMRI that let scientists peek at real-time brain activity. These landmark developments, to put it plainly, have been the backbone of progress in both diagnosing and understanding what goes on in our brains, pushing forward our grasp of neuroanatomy and disease processes. AI's entrance into the neuroimaging lab is another big leap. Advanced algorithms now sift through images, hunting for patterns and oddities, which means clinicians can often catch issues faster and more accurately. The technology, capable of processing enormous amounts of data in a heartbeat, is especially good at spotting those minor, hard-to-detect shifts linked to neurological troubles. Take fMRI studies, for instance; researchers are combined with these tools as they dig deeper into neural networks to understand psychiatric conditions. Generally speaking, while AI holds promise for tailoring medicine to individuals, it also forces us to pause and think about ethics, data privacy, and how to avoid biases (Varnosfaderani et al., 2024). At the same time, fresh strides in neuroimaging are giving regenerative a serious boost, especially in the realm of stem cell research. As imaging gets sharper, researchers can now get a better read on the success of new treatments for neurological disorders. Whether it is human pluripotent stem cells or multipotent mesenchymal stem cells at work, the evidence suggests these cells might repair damage from spinal injuries to degenerative brain conditions. In many cases, neuroimaging has become the essential tool for tracking how these treatments affect brain structure and function, often repeatedly proving its worth. As the field moves forward, it seems only natural that researchers not only chase technological breakthroughs but also carefully consider how to bring these innovations into everyday clinical use, setting the stage for exciting future developments in neurotherapy (Hoang et al., 2022) (Figure 15.4).

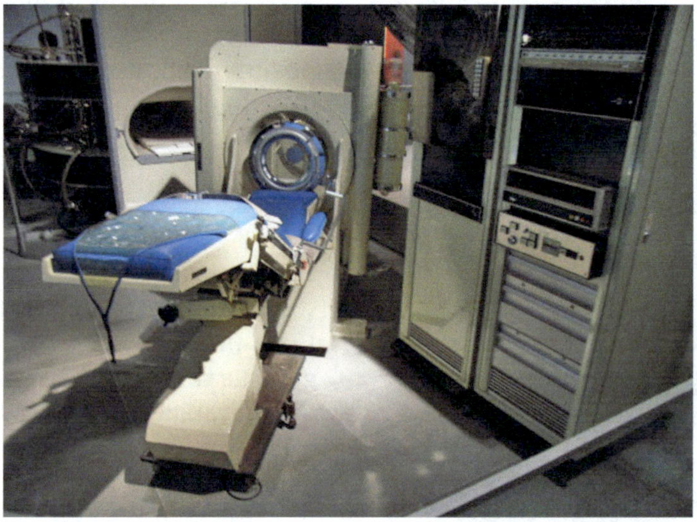

Figure 15.4. A historic EMI-Scanner Mark I, alongside the minicomputer used to process the CT image data.

Source: By Philipcosson at English Wikipedia - English Wikipedia: en:File:Emi1010.jpg., Public Domain, https://commons.wikimedia.org/w/index.php?curid=1006690.

15.1.3. Evolution of Neuroimaging Applications

Neuroimaging has flipped our view of the brain, its structure and activity, in ways we once couldn't imagine. In the beginning, tools like CT and routine MRI offered only static images, which didn't quite capture the brain's lively inner workings. Then, before we knew it, real-time scans emerged; functional neuroimaging let researchers watch brain activity unfold. fMRI, for example, opened doors to studying thought processes and emotions that had long slipped under the radar. Over time, blending insights from areas like artificial intelligence (AI) and biomechanics helped us piece together a richer picture of motor behavior and cognition, nudging us toward more balanced models of brain function and behavior (Arabameri, 2024). New advances in neuroimaging have sparked breakthroughs in fields like clinical psychology and neurology, too. High-tech scans now do more than just take pictures, they even let us peek into therapeutic realms, such as hypnotherapy, where the subtle shifts in brain states during hypnosis can be seen pretty clearly. Several studies suggest that hypnosis tweaks activity in certain areas, hinting at how it might steer clinical results. In most cases, figuring out these changes with modern imaging is opening up new paths for better treatments. As these tools evolve, it seems likely that their sharpened capabilities will become key players in boosting the success of psychosomatic therapies (Barbosa et al., 2024). Looking ahead, neuroimaging stands at a crossroads of significant promise and tough challenges. The new models and techniques are set to deliver deeper insights into how our brains tick, which could well lead to innovative treatment strategies and ways to keep diseases at bay. Yet, some theoretical and practical hurdles still remain, meaning that careful checks are needed to trust what the scans tell us. At the same time, as more fields mix their ideas, future work should keep in mind the socio-cultural angles that affect what we see in neuroimaging results. Ethical issues, especially about data privacy and the careful use of such advanced tools, also need to stay in focus. Teaming up across disciplines, daring to try fresh approaches, and keeping ethics first will, generally speaking, be essential for moving neuroimaging forward in a responsible, effective way (Arabameri, 2024).

Test Your Knowledge

1. What are some key milestones in the development of neuroimaging technology?
2. How have neuroimaging applications evolved to improve the diagnosis of neurological disorders?

15.2. Types of Neuroimaging Techniques

Learning Outcome

1. Define the structural imaging (e.g., MRI, CT).
2. Describe the functional imaging (e.g., fMRI, PET).
3. Understand the electrophysiological techniques (e.g., EEG, MEG).

Neuroimaging has changed our view of how the brain works. MRI, for example, gives us detailed pictures of brain structure, while its offshoot fMRI watches how blood oxygen levels shift, hinting at which parts of the brain kick into gear during different tasks. Researchers love it because it lets them catch brain regions lighting up when we do various things. That said, fMRI isn't perfect, it can get thrown off by even slight head movements and its signals are rather indirect. In most cases, scientists tend to mix it with other methods to get a more rounded picture of neural activity. Ultimately, MRI and fMRI have become go-to tools, opening doors to a deeper look at the brain's complex routines. PET is another big name in the field, coming at things from a different angle by focusing on metabolic activity. Using radiolabeled tracers to bring biochemical processes into view, it has become essential in labs and clinics alike. This approach helps in spotting things like shifts in glucose metabolism and tracking how neurotransmitter receptors bind – crucial clues in diagnosing neurodegenerative conditions (Bayeleva, 2021). Of course, PET's spatial resolution is generally lower than that of MRI, and the need for radioactive tracers sometimes makes it a bit tricky on safety and accessibility fronts. Still, by complementing the structural insights of MRI and fMRI with functional data, PET stays a critical part of our neuroimaging toolkit, deepening our grasp of intricate neurological disorders. Then there's the combo of EEG and MEG, which zoom in on the timing of brain activity. EEG picks up electrical signals via electrodes on the scalp; it is brilliant for identifying fast, fleeting events, even if it sometimes stumbles when pinpointing exact locations. MEG, on the other hand, senses the tiny magnetic fields produced by neurons, offering both excellent timing and a better idea of where the action is. This mix lets researchers figure out not just when things happen, but also where they originate, an edge that proves especially handy in cognitive studies. Together, these methods bridge the gap between static images and real-time monitoring, enriching our understanding of neural dynamics (Xu et al., 2023) (Figure 15.5).

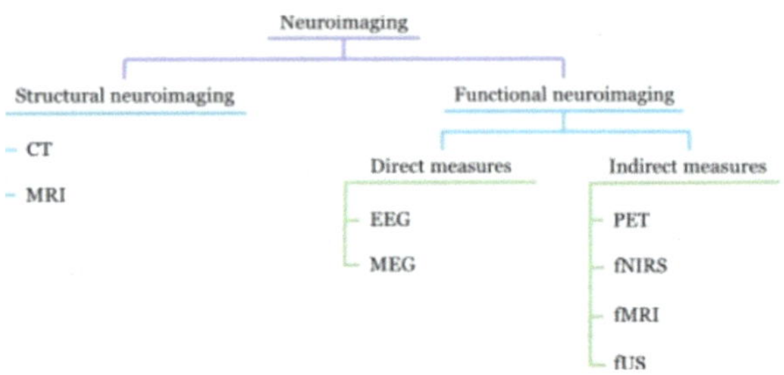

Figure 15.5. Neuroimaging techniques.

Source: https://ars.els-cdn.com/content/image/3-s2.0-B9780128244470000182-f12-49-9780128244470.jpg.

15.2.1. Structural Imaging (e.g., MRI, CT)

Neuroimaging progress has changed how we catch and manage brain issues, especially those tricky tumors found in kids. CT scans and MRIs still help doctors see brain abnormalities pretty well, but they're mostly stuck looking at structures; they miss a lot in telling one tumor apart from another. The old methods, in many cases, focus solely on the brain's outline, yet struggle in detailing the type or grade of a tumor. That's where new imaging techniques jump in, methods that dig deeper into how these tumors behave. For instance, advanced MRI tricks like diffusion-weighted imaging (DWI) and MR spectroscopy offer extra bits of info about tumor metabolism and overall function, which in turn helps tailor early interventions and improves patient outcomes (Nikam et al., 2022). Neuroimaging isn't standing still. Nowadays, there's a noticeable shift towards blending structural scans with functional imaging. Take second-generation psychiatric neuroimaging as an example, it mixes regular MRI with techniques that capture brain activity to better understand mental health conditions. This approach lets researchers peek at both the physical changes in brain structure and those hidden neurobiological processes behind various disorders.

By integrating these higher-tech methods, richer data comes to light, and that data then helps in shaping therapies that suit each patient. Clearly, it appears that the future of brain imaging will lean on these mixed-mode approaches, closing the gap between pinpointing a problem and applying a treatment (Schmidt et al., 2016). Recognizing that psychiatric disorders have their own uniqueness has pushed us to refine our imaging protocols so they guide clinical care more effectively. Looking back at early techniques, which mostly just focused on what the brain looked like, it is now obvious that methods capturing dynamic changes over time are essential. Emerging tools like diffusion tensor imaging (DTI) and resting-state fMRI throw light on the ways neurons connect and how brain activity flows, underscoring how structure and function play off each other. This broader view is key in addressing mental health conditions more completely, thereby paving the way for better diagnoses and therapies. As researchers continue to explore these advanced imaging techniques, the possibility of turning these insights into everyday clinical practice feels more real than ever (Rahul et al., 2022) (Figure 15.6).

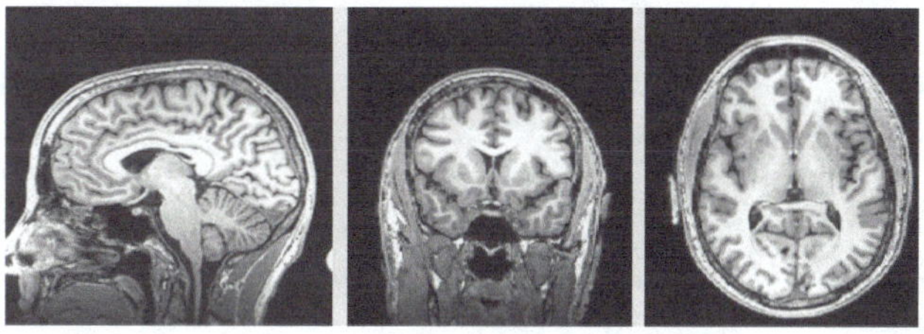

Figure 15.6. Structural MRI imaging.

Source: https://fmri.ucsd.edu/images/T1_v3.png.

15.2.2. Functional Imaging (e.g., fMRI, PET)

Functional imaging has turned things around in how we dig into the brain's busy workings. Instead of following a strict order, imagine this: fMRI picks up on blood flow shifts that light up brain regions in action, while PET, using radioactive tracers, checks out the brain's metabolic buzz. It is almost like getting both a still snapshot and an ongoing movie at once, which gives us a window into neural circuits and connectivity during different tasks. Overall, this mix makes these techniques invaluable in both research labs and everyday clinical practice. In clinical settings, these imaging tools have offered pivotal insights that are shaping our understanding of neurological conditions. For example, methods like FDG PET and resting-state fMRI help spot characteristic patterns in conditions such as Parkinsons disease. In most cases, being able to sing out these patterns not only flags the disease but also helps identify Parkinson's from its atypical type, yes, it can be a bit confusing sometimes. Some research even weaves in network analysis via graph theory to dig deeper into how brain connectivity shifts occur, and this gradual progress nudges us closer toward precision medicine, where tailored treatment becomes more feasible. Meanwhile, as these imaging technologies keep evolving, they're often combined with other methods to create a more well-rounded view of brain health. A variety of techniques, including the classic fMRI and PET, plus newer ones like single-photon emission computed tomography (SPECT) and diffuse optical imaging (DOI), come together, sometimes in unexpected ways, to tackle the complex nature of disorders like brain tumors and others. Sure, there are still challenges, such as figuring out the best way to fuse data from these different scans or relying on machine learning to automate analysis; nevertheless, steady advancements remain essential for better early detection and improving patient outcomes, underscoring the indispensable role of functional imaging in the future of neuroimaging (Nakano et al., 2025) (Figure 15.7).

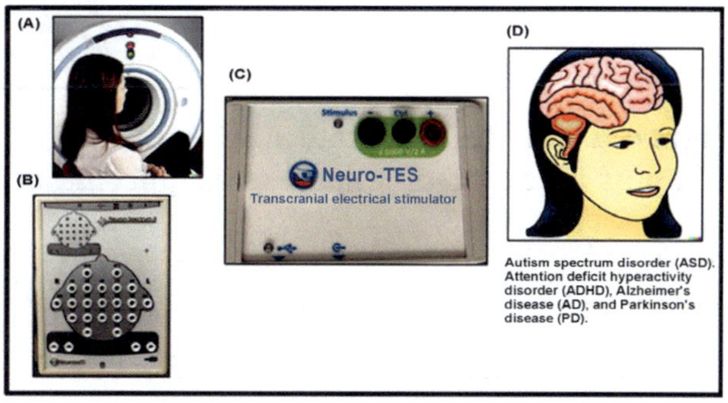

Figure 15.7. Neuroimaging.

Source: Yen C, Lin C-L, Chiang M-C. Exploring the Frontiers of Neuroimaging: A Review of Recent Advances in Understanding Brain Functioning and Disorders. *Life*. 2023; 13(7):1472. https://doi.org/10.3390/life13071472.

15.2.3. Electrophysiological Techniques (e.g., EEG, MEG)

Neuroimaging has come a long way in showing us how the brain works in almost real time. Direct measurements of electrical activity help us peek into those fleeting neural moments. Take EEG, for example. It is a method that reads neuron signals using electrodes on the scalp to help us see how the brain behaves during tasks. Still, EEG doesn't always give a clear picture of where things are happening because the skull messes up the signals. This shortfall nudges researchers to try out other methods that mix well with EEG and give a broader view of brain function (Figure 15.8).

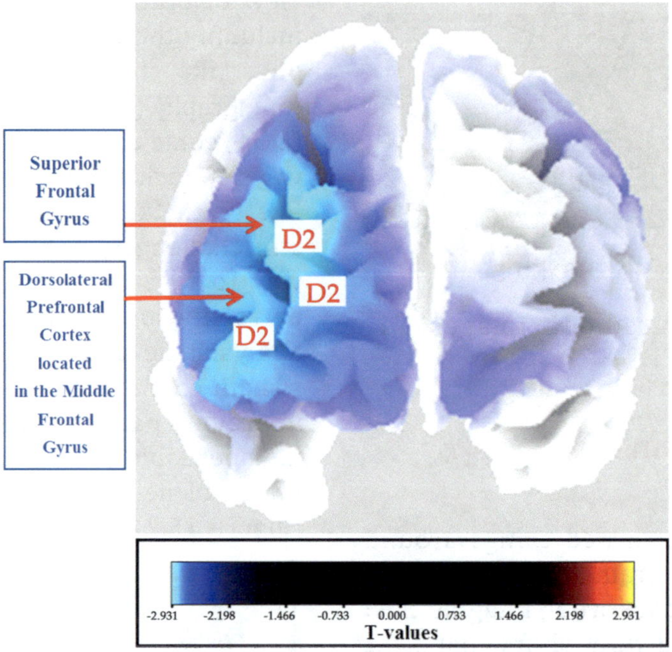

Figure 15.8. Resting state EEG neuroimaging findings illustrating dopamine D2 post-synaptic receptor blockade in female schizophrenia on medicated with atypical antipsychotics.

Source: https://www.researchgate.net/figure/Resting-state-EEG-neuroimaging-findings-illustrating-dopamine-D2-post-synaptic-receptor_fig2_285370953.

Magnetoencephalography, or MEG, offers a fresh spin by using the tiny magnetic fields generated by neurons to chart a more detailed map of brain activity. MEG ties together fast timing, often in the millisecond range, with a spatial detail that can be as sharp as 2 to 5 mm, something EEG just can't match. Traditional MEG systems, for the most part, rely on cryogenic sensors that, while sensitive, are also pretty clunky and require heavy magnetic shielding. Lately, there's been buzz about optically-pumped magnetometers (OPMs). These sensors boost signal pickup and spatial clarity without needing cryogenic cooling, which means more flexible and dynamic studies can be done. Of course, the new OPM-MEG tech is not without its uniqueness. Some current designs still use only a handful of sensors, making it tricky to capture the full story of brain activity. Recent work, in most cases, hints at pathways toward more complete, whole-head coverage. Combining OPMs into wearable setups, even if it is a bit rough around the edges at first, could let subjects move naturally while researchers gather richer data. In the end, these strides may deepen our grasp of both typical and atypical brain functions, marking OPM-MEG as a pivotal tool for what comes next in neuroimaging research) (Brookes et al., 2022; Hill et al., 2020) (Figure 15.9).

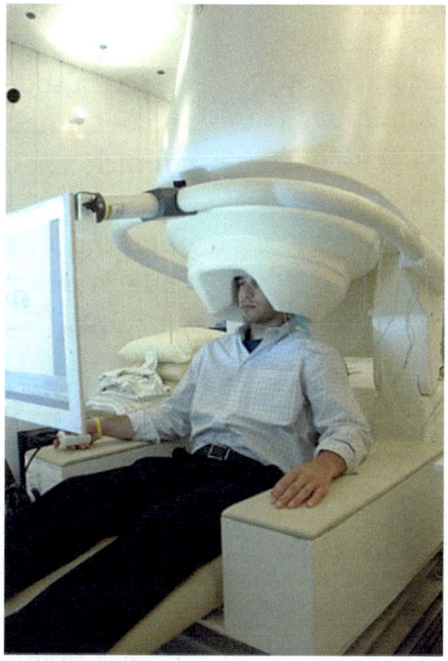

Figure 15.9. Magnetoencephalography (MEG).

Source: https://en.wikipedia.org/wiki/Magnetoencephalography.

Test Your Knowledge

1. How does functional magnetic resonance imaging (fMRI) differ from structural MRI in neuroimaging?
2. What is the role of positron emission tomography (PET) in neuroimaging?

15.3. Applications of Neuroimaging

Learning Outcome

1. Understand the role of neuroimaging in clinical diagnosis and treatment planning.
2. Explore using neuroimaging in cognitive neuroscience research.
3. Examine the applications of neuroimaging in diagnosing and managing psychiatric disorders.

Neuroimaging has come a long way – it is not just deepening our grasp of how the brain works but also pushing clinical practices forward in unexpected ways. Researchers now often mix techniques like functional magnetic resonance imaging (fMRI) with functional near-infrared spectroscopy (fNIRs) to face some pretty messy neurological challenges. This combo gives both crisp spatial details and quick timing that help map brain activity during all sorts of cognitive and clinical tasks. In many cases, this kind of synergy has been key to probing disorders like stroke and Alzheimer's, and we even see these methods used both at the same moment and separately, which sharpens location accuracy and checks treatment effectiveness. All of this is slowly setting a kind of blueprint for where neuroimaging might go next (Yang et al., 2025). Then there's continuous wave-diffuse optical tomography (CW-DOT) – a method that shakes things up in non-invasive brain analysis. It manages to pull off high spatial resolution that even traditional fNIRS struggles to achieve – thanks to its advanced hardware and some pretty clever reconstruction algorithms. A number of literature reviews point to its success in detailed brain mapping, which not only backs up clinical diagnoses but also fuels cognitive neuroscience research. Sure, there are still bumps in the road, like needing more standardized protocols and a bit more quantitative precision.

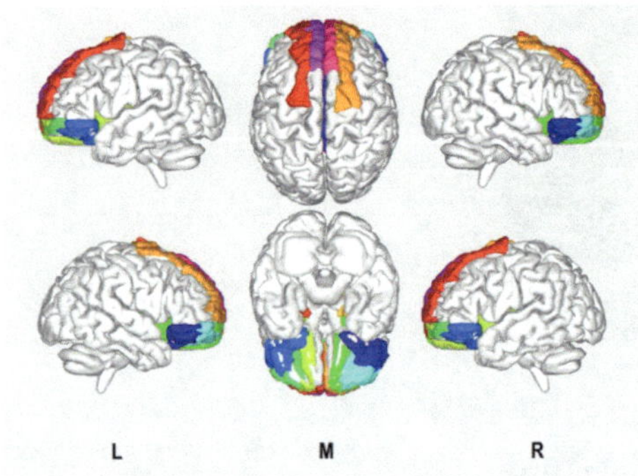

Figure 15.10. Major brain regions associated with anorexia nervosa.

Source: Chen, X., Ai, C., Liu, Z. *et al.* Neuroimaging studies of resting-state functional magnetic resonance imaging in eating disorders. *BMC Med Imaging* **24**, 265 (2024). https://doi.org/10.1186/s12880-024-01432-z.

Addressing those issues is, generally speaking, crucial to fully leveraging CW-DOT's potential and confirming its role as a robust tool in the ever-evolving field of brain imaging (Guan et al., 2025). And there's more beyond just diagnosis. Neuroimaging is increasingly stepping into the realm of behavioral neuroscience. Researchers, for instance, are now embracing hyper scanning – looking at the brain activity of multiple people at once during interactive tasks – which sheds light on how social cognition plays out. This approach, sometimes repeated in various studies to good effect, helps uncover the neural threads that connect us during social interactions, paving the way for richer models of human behavior. Plus, as machine learning techniques get woven into imaging data analysis, we might soon be able to crack complex data sets and even pinpoint biomarkers for psychological conditions. Overall, these cross-disciplinary moves underline the vast and transformative potential of neuroimaging in broadening our understanding of the human brain and its many functions (Figure 15.10).

15.3.1. Clinical Diagnosis and Treatment Planning

Modern neuroimaging advances have shaken up how neurologists figure out diagnoses and plan care. Nowadays, these methods let doctors see not just the brain's shape but also how it works, making it easier, for example, to tell frontotemporal dementia (FTD) apart from Alzheimer's disease (AD). Machine learning tools often sift through neuroimages to catch patterns that standard exams might miss; in most cases, this twist helps form treatment plans as unique as each patient's neurobiology (Dattola et al., 2025). Scans like Positron Emission Tomography (PET) and Single Photon Emission Computed Tomography (SPECT) are real workhorses, they not only kick off the diagnostic process but also guide decisions for surgery and treatment follow-ups. These techniques use radioactive tracers to peek into brain metabolism and neuron activity, offering clues when structural pictures alone don't cut it. Generally speaking, uncovering extra issues like co-morbid conditions lets clinicians piece together a more rounded, personalized approach to care (Rahman, 2024).

Of course, rolling out these neuroimaging tricks isn't without its hiccups. Even if machine learning shows promise, putting it to work in everyday clinical routines is a tall order, larger, more varied datasets and standard protocols are still needed (Dattola et al., 2025). Plus, the real world of patient symptoms can be messy, with overlapping signs that complicate matters.

While these new tools are opening doors to better insights, ongoing research and tweaks remain vital to sharpen treatment plans and boost patient care in neurology (Figure 15.11).

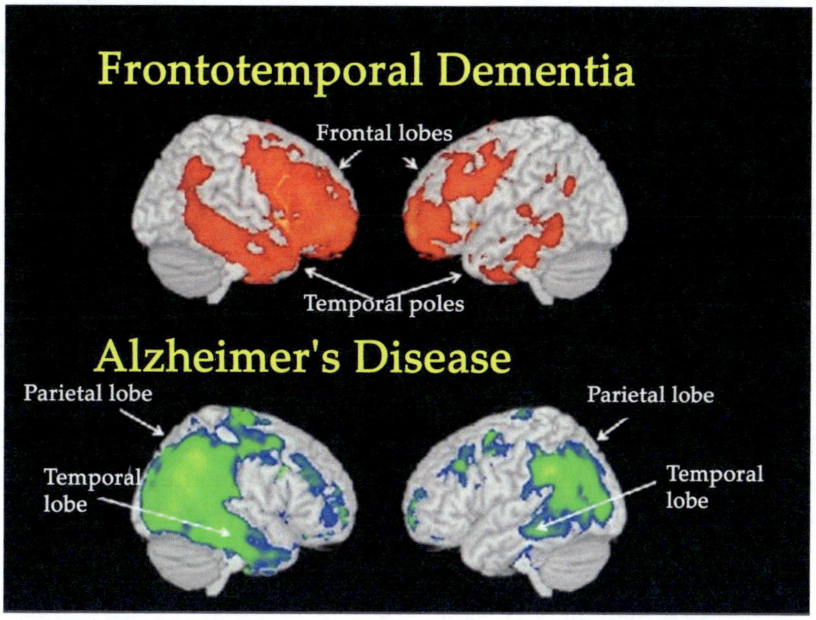

Figure 15.11. Frontotemporal dementia (FTD) versus Alzheimer's disease.

Source: https://i.pinimg.com/originals/c7/da/86/c7da864e7bd9d5bac3bf695e13a6d26f.jpg.

15.3.2. Research in Cognitive Neuroscience

Neuroimaging has changed things up in how we look at the brain, it's no secret that such technology now lets us peek at brain structures and functions in ways that were once hard to imagine. One can see how this breakthrough helps scientists get a handle on neurodegenerative issues like Alzheimer's Disease (AD); after all, when you can spot biomarkers early, you're in a better spot to kick off treatments before severe damage sets in. Techniques like PET and MRI allow researchers to notice amyloid plaques and tau tangles, the telltale signs of AD, sometimes long before major cognitive problems emerge (Wang et al., 2024). Using neuroimaging as part of cognitive evaluations has become a real game changer, opening doors to treatment plans that are increasingly tailored to each patient. Machine learning has now joined the party by diving into neuroimaging data, and it is done some impressive work identifying early signs of Alzheimer's. By sifting through huge piles of scan data, these algorithms can pick up on subtle patterns that traditional methods might just miss. In many cases, studies show that the smart mix of ML can separate individuals with mild cognitive impairment, full-blown AD, and even those with a healthy brain, which bumps up the accuracy of diagnoses (Wang et al., 2024). This knack for parsing complex data not only sharpens diagnostic precision but also deepens our understanding of how the disease creeps along, affecting brain functions in sometimes puzzling ways. Cognitive neuroscience itself is shifting gears as it blends neuroimaging with genetic studies and brand-new therapeutic ideas. Recent work has even started to mix in observations from neuroimaging, genes, and environmental factors to shed light on how Alzheimer's takes hold (Wang et al., 2024). Some researchers are even looking at the gut-brain axis, where the microbes in our systems might nudge neuroinflammation and, in turn, impact cognitive health, another twist in the AD puzzle. All these bits and pieces coming together hint at not just improved early diagnostics but also smarter, more interconnected intervention methods. Even if it sometimes feels a bit all over the place, the drive to mix different fields seems essential to push forward our fight against neurodegeneration.

15.3.3. Neuroimaging in Psychiatric Disorders

Lately, breakthroughs in brain imaging have shifted how we diagnose and treat mental health issues. fMRI, for instance, lets researchers peek into how the brain functions, a stark contrast to the old methods that leaned too much on personal impressions. Mixing these brain data images with insights drawn from casual patient chats (capturing emotional cues, really) opens a door to more straightforward testing. In most cases, rather than sticking with subjective guesses, this blend might pinpoint conditions more precisely and even fine-tune treatments by zeroing in on specific brain pathways, ultimately shaking up psychiatric care (Li, 2025). Biomarkers from these scans are carving out unexpected paths in understanding mental health. Resting-state fMRI picks up on the brain's natural chatter, and those shifts in connectivity, as captured in ongoing research, reveal things about disorders like depression and schizophrenia. When experts apply graph-based connectivity methods – sometimes with surprising clarity – they uncover irregular patterns that may serve as trustworthy hints for both diagnosis and treatment planning. Generally speaking, this fresh approach jives with the rise of psych radiology, an evolving field that rethinks diagnosis and therapy based on the rich details hidden in neuroimaging data (Fallahi et al., 2024). Then there's the curious mix of language processing and brain scanning technologies. With tools like ChatGPT used in the flow of interactive patient interviews, subtle emotional data, often brushed aside in older surveys, gets its due attention when measured alongside imaging results. This combo seems to produce notably accurate predictions, often outpacing the traditional, checklist-like methods. In essence, tailoring treatment to an individual's unique brain and emotional profile could soon be a real game changer in psychiatric care, making outcomes more personal and effective (Li, 2025) (Figure 15.12).

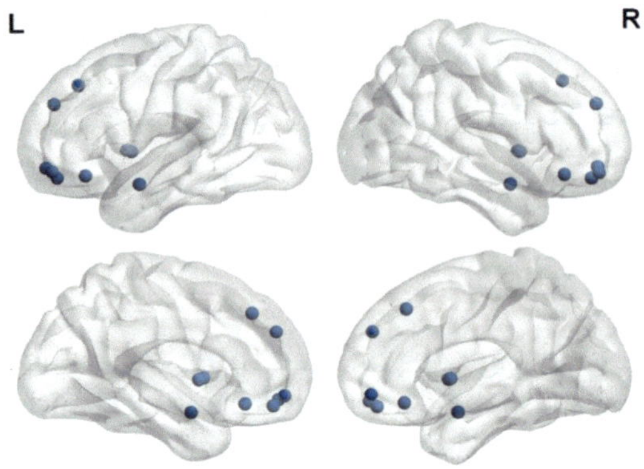

Figure 15.12. Specific brain regions associated with bulimia nervosa.

Source: Chen, X., Ai, C., Liu, Z. *et al.* Neuroimaging studies of resting-state functional magnetic resonance imaging in eating disorders. *BMC Med Imaging* **24**, 265 (2024). https://doi.org/10.1186/s12880-024-01432-z.

Test Your Knowledge

1. What are the key applications of neuroimaging in assessing brain function during surgeries or treatments?
2. How does neuroimaging contribute to the study of brain connectivity and network analysis?

15.4. Advantages and Limitations of Neuroimaging

Learning Outcome

1. Evaluate the advantages of neuroimaging in diagnosing.
2. Identify the limitations of neuroimaging techniques.

15.4.1. Advantages of Neuroimaging

Brain scanning has come a long way, changing how we see and handle brain issues in clinics. New imaging tools let doctors catch problems sooner, often before symptoms fully develop. fMRI, for example, gives us a look at active brain regions in real-time, which helps tailor treatments on the spot. It is especially useful when early help can make a big difference, like in kids facing neurodevelopmental challenges. Using a blend of different scanning methods, clinicians can track even small changes in brain activity to see if a treatment is working. Techniques like OPM-MEG, despite some old hurdles with clarity and detail, push these insights even further (Brookes et al., 2022). Many of these methods are non-invasive, which means they don't put patients at risk and work well across all sorts of groups, kids, seniors, you name it. MRI and PET scans, for instance, often don't need a lot of prep, so they fit neatly into regular check-ups. This ease of use generally leads to earlier diagnoses and smoother follow-up, which is crucial when dealing with conditions that slowly change over time. In most cases, even breakthroughs like nanotech-enhanced imaging agents are giving us tougher contrast and sharper detail, refining how we spot trouble spots. The field is steadily moving forward, hinting at even more sensitive tools soon (Teleanu et al., 2019). Neuroimaging isn't just about making diagnoses, though, it also opens doors to understanding thoughts, feelings, and behaviors more deeply. Researchers mix various brain scanning techniques with computer models to unravel how neural circuits work. This mix can clarify the messy details behind disorders such as schizophrenia and depression, sometimes even suggesting new ways to treat them. Often, by tracking specific brain markers, the path is paved toward personalized care that targets the root issues rather than just the symptoms (Brookes et al., 2022) (Figure 15.13).

Study	Effects
Auvichayapat et al. (2022)	The main objective of this chapter is to investigate the lasting effects of tDCS on the treatment of patients with ASD. The study utilized a randomized controlled trial design, with the control group receiving sham stimulation and the experimental group receiving tDCS treatment. The study evaluated the efficacy of treatment at 6 and 12 months post-treatment. The findings suggest that compared to the control group, the experimental group who received tDCS demonstrated significant improvements in symptoms of autism, language, and social interaction 6 and 12 months after treatment.
D'Urso et al. (2021)	Research focuses on cerebellar transcranial direct current stimulation's efficacy, feasibility, and safety in children with autism spectrum disorders. The study also explored unexpected results, such as the impact of tic disorders and epilepsy in these children.

Study	Effects
Kang et al. (2023)	The main objective of this article is to explore the potential impact of tDCS on ASD by examining differences in EEG microstates between typically developing children and those with ASD. Moreover, the study aimed to compare EEG microstates and scores on the Autism Behavior Checklist before and after tDCS in children with ASD who were given either experimental or sham stimulation. The results indicate that tDCS could be a promising intervention for ASD.
Prillinger et al. (2021)	The main objective of this chapter is to outline the study protocol for a double-blind, randomized, and sham-controlled clinical trial that seeks to examine the impact of repeated tDCS sessions on adolescents who have ASD. The chapter includes comprehensive information on the study design, criteria for participant selection, intervention procedures, outcome measures, and statistical analysis approach.
Qiu et al. (2021)	This chapter centers on investigating the impact of tDCS on the left dorsolateral prefrontal cortex on cognitive and behavioral functioning among children with ASD. Specifically, the study aims to determine whether tDCS can enhance social communication, executive function, and behavior among children diagnosed with ASD.
Sun et al. (2022)	This chapter aims to evaluate the effects of tDCS, one of the first-line treatments, on neuronal activity in children with autism. Specifically, the study explored the impact of tDCS on the MMN (mismatch negativity) response characteristics of brain-dysregulated stimuli in children with autism, which is related to the perception and language development of children with autism. The study used quantitative electroencephalography (QEEG) technology to measure brain electrical activity and compared tDCS with sham stimulation (sham) to assess its effect on MMN responses.

Figure 15.13. Some evidence suggests that tDCS may be beneficial in improving social communication deficits in individuals with ASD.

Source: Yen C, Lin C-L, Chiang M-C. Exploring the Frontiers of Neuroimaging: A Review of Recent Advances in Understanding Brain Functioning and Disorders. *Life*. 2023; 13(7):1472. https://doi.org/10.3390/life1307147*215.4.1.1 Non-invasive nature of many techniques.*

Brain imaging has taken an unexpected turn recently, no longer do we need to resort to invasive measures to get a glimpse of what's happening inside our skulls. Researchers now use tools like fMRI and MEG to record signals right from the space outside our heads. It is kind of interesting how capturing brain activity live can shift our understanding of how neurons fire over time and space, especially in cognitive neuroscience (Brookes et al., 2022). Sometimes the idea of reading brain signals without surgery just feels like a breath of fresh air compared to the old, riskier methods. MEG, in particular, draws the eye because of its speed in tracking those rapid neural pulses. Older MEG systems, which relied on cryogenic sensors, often made participants feel uncomfortable and forced them to keep their heads overly still. Lately, however, the shift to using OPMs has opened up a new chapter. OPM-MEG setups let people move about more naturally during tests, boosting how "real" the results feel and broadening studies to groups like infants or others who struggle with traditional rigs (Hill et al., 2020).

The best part is that these non-invasive techniques are making high-quality neuroimaging accessible to a wider range of individuals. When participants can move freely and feel at ease, it is easier to gather genuine responses, which matters when studying young children or patients with neurological challenges. Plus, the tweakability of OPM-MEG, adjusting sensor arrangements to fit one's unique head shape, leads to clearer, more reliable signals. In most cases, this level of adaptability is a huge plus for long-term research and interventions, as it safeguards both participant comfort and data quality. Overall, these advances hint at a future where exploring the brain's intricacies won't come at the cost of anyone's well-being (Brookes et al., 2022).

15.4.1.1. Ability to Visualize Brain Activity in Real-Time

Neuroimaging keeps evolving, letting us catch brain activity as it happens. Older approaches just couldn't keep up with the quick flickers of signals, so they often fell short in clinical use. Now, techniques like optoacoustic imaging have stepped in, they let us dive deep into tissues to spot both blood flow details and calcium pulses, all while delivering a three-dimensional view. It is kind of neat that this method overcomes the old snag of hemoglobin soaking up visible light. Researchers even used genetically encoded calcium indicators in mouse models to show, in many cases, that stimulus-triggered calcium shifts can be seen at depths and clarity we hadn't expected. These shifts, generally speaking, are changing the way we peer into our brain's workings (Degtyaruk et al., 2019).

Mobile neuroimaging in clinics is a real game-changer for pain assessment. Traditional systems were too stiff for on-the-spot use in acute cases, and that made them less than ideal. Enter the CLARAi framework, it uses functional near-infrared spectroscopy to track brain activity during episodes of induced pain. With the help of AI, these systems can sort hemodynamic signals into pain and no-pain groups, which opens the door to more tailored treatment plans.

There's even talk about mixing in augmented reality so that doctors might see a live, tangible snapshot of brain function during an appointment; this could soon reshape how we look at pain objectively (Xiao-Hu et al., 2019). Blending advanced neuroimaging with everyday clinical practice offers more than just a boost for research, it paves the way for practical treatments. A major perk of watching brain activity in real time is that it gives us clues about disorders like epilepsy, depression, and anxiety. This kind of live imaging helps doctors notice shifts in cerebral patterns, which sometimes allows them to adjust treatments on the fly. As these techniques continue to improve, the idea of merging neuroimaging with other biomedical fields becomes more and more plausible, hinting at a future where personalized medicine takes off. In most cases, pushing real-time visualization isn't just an academic pursuit; it is a step toward transforming modern healthcare (Degtyaruk et al., 2019; Xiao-Hu et al., 2019) (Figure 15.14).

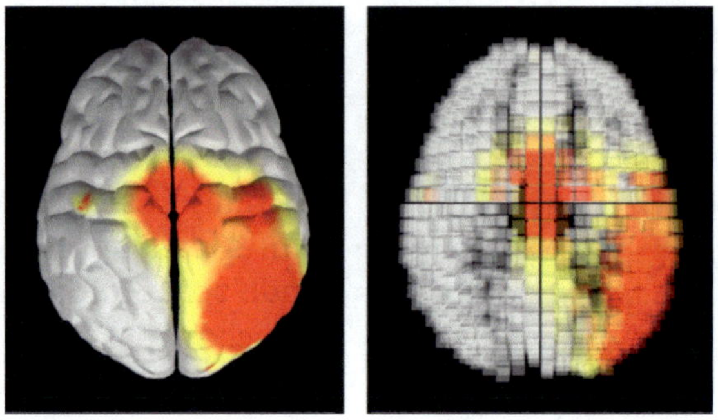

Study	Effects
Barham et al. (2022)	This research aims to explore the possibility of using tDCS to enhance executive function, with a focus on planning and working memory, in adults diagnosed with ADHD. Through conducting five consecutive sessions of neuropsychological tests, the study aims to compare the effectiveness of active tDCS and sham stimulation. The study concludes that tDCS can be an effective method to modulate cognitive functions in adults diagnosed with ADHD.
Dubreuil-Vall et al. (2021)	The study finds that anodal tDCS targeting the left dorsolateral prefrontal cortex modulates cognitive and physiological measures in the Eriksen flanker task in a state-dependent manner, suggesting that tDCS has a positive effect on cognition in ADHD. Furthermore, the study highlights the importance of event-related potentials as cross-sectional biomarkers for executive performance and their implications for developing personalized treatments for ADHD.
Guimaraes et al. (2021)	The study utilizes a randomized, triple-blind, sham-controlled crossover design to assess the therapeutic effects, as well as the safety and feasibility of tDCS treatment. Multiple neuropsychological tests, including the Wechsler Intelligence Scale and the Neuropsychological Assessment Battery, will be administered to assess patient performance before and after tDCS treatment. The study's outcomes may facilitate the development of alternative, non-pharmaceutical treatments for enhancing cognitive and behavioral performance in patients diagnosed with ADHD.
Nejati et al. (2021)	This research aimed to investigate the impact of tDCS on inhibitory control in children with ADHD and assess whether the severity of ADHD symptoms influenced the effectiveness of tDCS. The study involved two groups of children with ADHD, one with severe and the other with mild symptoms, who underwent anodal or sham tDCS over the right dorsolateral prefrontal cortex while performing inhibitory control tasks.

Figure 15.14. There is some evidence to suggest that tDCS may be beneficial in reducing symptoms of ADHD.

Source: Yen C, Lin C-L, Chiang M-C. Exploring the Frontiers of Neuroimaging: A Review of Recent Advances in Understanding Brain Functioning and Disorders. *Life*. 2023; 13(7):1472. https://doi.org/10.3390/life13071472.

15.4.1.2. Contribution to Personalized Medicine

Neuroimaging has kicked off a new era in personalized medicine that lets doctors fine-tune treatments for each individual. Clinicians dig into brain scans to spot subtle cues in structure and function that tie into various diseases. This way of working not only ups the accuracy of diagnoses but also opens the door to therapies that are more likely to hit the mark. Deep learning models working on these images are getting pretty clever, picking up connections that older methods might miss. In many cases, this kind of innovation backs a move toward tailoring treatment based on each brain's uniqueness, ultimately boosting predictions in everyday clinical care (Zhou et al., 2021). The reach of neuroimaging goes deep into challenging areas like disorders of consciousness (DoC). New imaging techniques have changed the way outcomes are predicted, as doctors mix brain scans with electrophsiological assessments to uncover hidden layers of awareness in patients who seem entirely unresponsive. This ability to detect what some call cognitive motor dissociation (CMD) gives a much richer understanding of brain function and, generally speaking, nudges treatment choices in new directions. Research shows that spotting intact neural networks can shift recovery paths, stirring hope for rehabilitation plans that feel more custom-tailored. Overall, blending neuroimaging with individualized care marks a forward-thinking step in handling DoC, where sharper imaging guides bespoke therapeutic moves that lift the quality of patient care (Edlow et al., 2020). Emerging neuroimaging tools carry the promise to reshape personalized medicine by sparking fresh pharmacological and electrophysiological therapies. As advanced scans reveal more about the inner workings behind various neurological disorders, scientists and doctors find themselves better poised to design treatments aimed at jump-starting damaged neural circuits. These new methods not only boost recovery prospects for patients suffering severe brain injuries but also allow for a sort of on-the-ground evaluation of how well a therapy works for each unique neurobiological profile. In most cases, as imaging technology keeps climbing, mixing big data analytics with scan details may drop insights we never expected. Such breakthroughs point to a significant shift toward medical interventions customized around brain imaging markers, hopefully leading to improved outcomes within the personalized medicine framework (Zhou et al., 2021).

15.4.2. Limitations of Neuroimaging

Neuroimaging has opened up whole new ways of seeing how the brain works, though it isn't without its issues. Traditional methods like EEG, for example, bring along discomfort and a fair bit of procedural hassle. Modern EEG systems are usually pretty dependable, but they still rely on those wet electrodes that many find unwieldy and that demand specialized know-how for proper setup. Dry electrode systems seem like a promising alternative for easier use, yet we're still waiting on a full head-to-head evaluation with the traditional wet ones. When you look at these emerging options, there's a clear need to balance everyday usability with keeping signal quality high, which directly shapes how broadly we can apply neuroimaging results across different groups and research scenarios (Flumeri et al., 2019). Beyond just the usability challenges, interpreting neuroimaging data brings its own set of headaches. Brain activity is inherently complex, and trying to pick out distinct neural signals from a tangle of images can be quite the task. Everyone's brain is a little different, and that, combined with the built-in noise of these methods, often muddies the waters. Take transcranial magnetic stimulation (TMS) – individual differences in brain anatomy and the varying effects on neural networks can lead to results that don't match up neatly between studies, our current approaches force us to sift through data very carefully when assessing the potential of treatments like TMS, particularly for conditions such as Obsessive-Compulsive Disorder (OCD) (Cocchi et al., 2018). All of this points to the need for stronger experimental designs and more comprehensive methods in neuroimaging. Technological hiccups can also sap the reliability and overall effectiveness of neuroimaging techniques. Sure, tools like fMRI and PET scans have, in most cases, revolutionized neuroscience, but they still wrestle with limits, like not delivering enough detail in either space or time. For instance, fMRI plays a great role in showing where brain activity happens, yet it falls short on nailing down the exact timing. This split focus makes it tricky to pin down clear cause-and-effect links between what's happening in the brain and how we behave. Also, the demanding nature of some imaging protocols can stress out participants, which may slightly skew the results. To shore up the validity of these studies, researchers need to address these shortcomings with better tech integration and more rigorous experimental controls. Only by confronting these issues head on can the field move toward applications that are both more accurate and more relevant in clinical practice (Flumeri et al., 2019) (Figure 15.15).

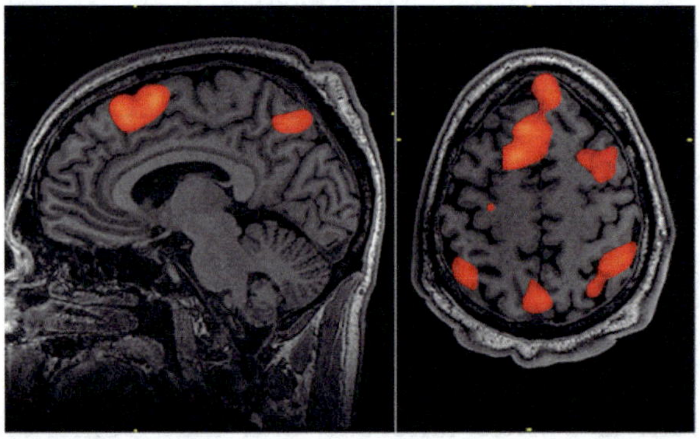

Figure 15.15. Neuroimaging has opened up whole new ways of seeing how the brain works.

Source: https://miro.medium.com/v2/resize:fit:1400/0*Wm5SxicojqfrKw8a.

15.4.2.1. Cost and Accessibility of Advanced Techniques

Advancements in neuroimaging continue to impress, yet uneven access to these modern techniques brings a host of challenges for both research labs and everyday clinical practice. The hefty price tag that comes with cutting-edge equipment is a major hurdle, buying, running, and keeping up with high-performance MRI scanners and elaborate software for data crunching usually demands a serious financial commitment. Smaller facilities or those in low-resource areas often find these costs overwhelming, which in most cases means that many patients might not get quick and dependable diagnostic help for conditions like Alzheimer's disease, as some current studies on machine learning-based early detection have noted (Moya, 2024). Then there's the rising expense of analyzing the large volumes of neuroimaging data. While preprocessing pipelines are crucial for ensuring data quality, their resource demands often bog down even well-designed algorithms. Recent work on MRI preprocessing has shown that, ironically, even smart algorithms struggle under the weight of heavy computing needs, especially in labs that can't afford the latest hardware (Mé et al., 2024). This situation leaves smaller studies or those in underfunded environments unable to fully capitalize on these techniques, which weakens their overall research impact in the field. Addressing these issues calls for a joint effort from both the scientific community and funding organizations. There's a clear need for cooperative projects that push the development of more cost-effective imaging solutions, along with training programs to boost technical know-how. By also combined machine learning improvements into the mix, it might be possible to lighten the computational load while sharpening diagnostic accuracy (Moy, 2024). Ultimately, creating a research setting that welcomes institutions of all sizes, and even those struggling with limited resources, could widen the benefits of neuroimaging techniques, enhancing early detection and intervention strategies for neurodegenerative diseases.

15.4.2.2. Interpretation Challenges and Potential for Misdiagnosis

Neuroimaging has come a long way in helping us diagnose and understand tricky brain conditions. Deep learning is now in the mix, and suddenly reading these scans isn't always so cut and dry. These fancy algorithms can nail it when spotting issues like AD, yet they aren't without flaws. Sometimes the detailed patterns they find end up being mistaken for real pathology, which can lead to a misdiagnosis. And then there's the issue of relying too much on these so-called black-box techniques; doing so might hide the true neurobiological picture and leave clinicians without a clear path to address the core causes of cognitive decline. Overall, while advanced machine learning shows a lot of promise, it also brings its own set of challenges when interpreting neuroimaging data (Jo et al., 2019). Another wrinkle comes from trying to analyze brain connectivity using fMRI scans. Breaking these connections into what we call functional or effective types demands some tough computational methods, often ones built on graph theory. Still, in most cases those subtle nuances in connectivity can send us in different directions when we try to figure out cognitive or neurological disorders. Everyone's brain is a little unique, and factors like age or medication only add to the mix. A number of researchers have noted that when fMRI analyses zero in mainly on resting-state connectivity, they might overlook those important shifts that occur during active tasks. Relying on just one mode of analysis can, therefore, skew diagnostic accuracy, highlighting the need for more comprehensive approaches that consider several angles and factors (Farahani et al., 2019). Even with all these leaps in neuroimaging, misdiagnosis remains a serious concern that deserves a closer look. Several studies generally show that diagnostic precision can suffer because of biases woven into how algorithms are trained or simply due to the types of neuroimaging data chosen. For instance, errors can emerge when multimodal data aren't blended well or when features that should have been in the mix accidentally get left out. Such pitfalls point to the necessity of a multidimensional strategy, both in clinical practice and in research. It seems crucial for neuroimaging experts, neurologists, and data analysts to work together, fine-tuning methods and boosting clarity. By keeping the conversation open across disciplines about these complexities, we can significantly drop the chances of misdiagnosis and help ensure that patients get more accurate, effective (Farahani et al., 2019).

15.4.2.3. Ethical Considerations in Neuroimaging Research

Neuroimaging's advances have opened up a host of ethical puzzles that need careful thought. Researchers diving into the maze of brain workings might not always realize that participants often don't fully grasp what's at stake when their scans are taken. Some individuals may even get anxious when they hear about unexpected findings, say, unusual brain features or a hint that they might be prone to mental health issues. This means scientists have to keep things clear and upfront about what the study involves and what kinds of results might turn up, building a steady sense of trust along the way. Brain scans aren't merely images; they can reveal some very personal details about someone's thoughts and feelings. With the whole big data trend shaking up neuroscience, worries over breaches or misuse of sensitive data keep mounting. A slip in managing or storing this information might compromise individual privacy, and in most cases, that outcome could undermine public trust in the research effort (Ritchie et al., 2018). Researchers are thus pushed to set up solid, sometimes even stringent, data protocols to safeguard identities and personal tidbits, ensuring that things aren't left open for misuse. Then there's the challenge of including underrepresented groups, which layers on an extra dose of complexity. Studies looking at differences, like those noting sex differences in brain structure, offer huge insights into mental disorders and aging, yet they also run the risk of reinforcing stereotypes or even deepening existing inequities. In most instances, researchers must tread carefully and avoid exploiting these groups just to push science forward. By genuinely embracing a diverse mix of participants, the field can capture a richer picture of human experiences, ultimately strengthening ethical practices in neuroscience research (Patricios et al., 2023).

Test Your Knowledge

1. What are the main advantages of using neuroimaging techniques in diagnosing brain disorders?
2. What are some limitations of neuroimaging in detecting early-stage neurological conditions?

15.5. Future Directions in Neuroimaging

Learning Outcome

1. Explore upcoming technological advancements in neuroimaging.
2. Understand the integration of neuroimaging with other diagnostic modalities to enhance clinical outcomes.
3. Analyze the potential impact of neuroimaging advancements on the understanding and treatment of brain disorders.

Neuroimaging is on the cusp of some pretty big changes, technology is sneaking into every nook and cranny of the field. Lately, mixing AI with machine learning has totally shifted how we crack complex brain scans. These smart tools let researchers map brain networks with a clarity we haven't seen before, which in most cases means better diagnosis for all kinds of mental health issues. New imaging methods are showing promise in uncovering the delicate neural signals behind conditions like depression and anxiety, hinting at a future where mental healthcare is a lot more tailored. Then there's the whole new world of neurostimulation and neuromodulation techniques that could flip traditional treatment on its head, making care both personal and effective. Recent studies even suggest that we're looking at a real turning point, a shift toward a subtler, more focused understanding of the brain that could target specific neurobiological uniqueness in patients (Sinha et al., 2025). Another interesting track in this space zeroes in on the BBB and its links to various neurological issues. Some latest findings indicate that when the BBB isn't working right, it might be behind conditions like schizophrenia, giving doctors a potential marker for diagnosis. Techniques such as arterial spin labeling (ASL) now allow researchers to watch BBB permeability and track neuroinflammation live, as it happens. By getting to the bottom of how the BBB functions (or falters), scientists can start piecing together new treatment plans that deal with these problems head-on. This kind of work not only deepens our grasp of brain disorders but also opens the door for interventions that aim to restore the BBB's integrity on a more personal level. As neuroimaging in this domain progresses, it is likely to unlock fresh avenues for both diagnosis and treatment (Zhang et al., 2025). Then there's the ethical side of all these fast-changing advances in brain imaging. As our ability to peer into brain function and structure grows, so do the hard questions about privacy, consent, and even data misuse. Plus, when these new imaging techniques start shaping clinical decisions, concerns over who gets access and whether benefits are spread evenly keep cropping up. It seems crucial that researchers, tech experts, and clinicians come together to set guidelines that preserve ethical standards while still encouraging innovation. Looking ahead, making sure ethics stays front and center might just be the key to ensuring neuroimaging benefits as many people as possible. Tackling these challenges thoughtfully could mean that the future of brain imaging not only pushes science forward but also improves patient care responsibly (Figure 15.16).

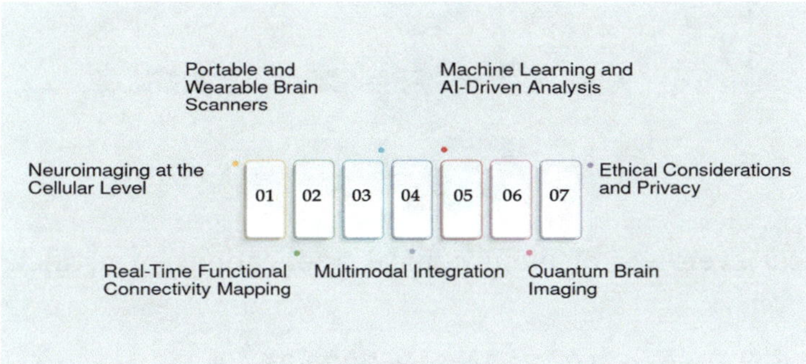

Figure 15.16. Future directions in brain imaging technology.

Source: https://fastercapital.com/topics/introduction-to-brain-imaging-technology.html.

15.5.1. Technological Advancements on the Horizon

Neuroimaging is taking center stage in our rapidly changing world, and these advances are shaking up lots of fields like neuroscience and clinical psychology. Machine learning and AI are now in the mix, and they're changing how we look at neuroimaging data, as if giving it a fresh pair of eyes. These newer methods help spot subtle patterns and even improve our predictions, which generally means better diagnoses and treatment plans. Then there's blockchain, stepping in to boost data trust and security, a big plus when you're worried about patient privacy and data leaks. Overall, as these tech tools evolve (and they surely will), they're set to completely transform neuroimaging and widen our view of the brain's many aspects. Technology isn't just tweaking the way we do things; it is reshaping the very backbone of neuroimaging facilities. Take energy storage batteries, for example, often highlighted in discussions about modern energy systems. These batteries help keep a steady, reliable power flow, which means fewer unexpected shutdowns and less data loss while scans are happening. Reliability like this is a real deal-breaker, especially when imaging techniques demand continuous, high-precision operation. Pairing these batteries with smart grid technology further refines resource management, making sure energy use adapts to the ups and downs of imaging needs.

As healthcare slowly embraces these upgrades, the whole neuroimaging scene is bound to run smoother and more effectively. In tackling neuroimaging challenges, future approaches might blend upgraded imaging tech with real-time data analytics. Imagine using high-resolution functional MRI (fMRI) or next-level PET scans, it is likely these innovations will dig deeper into how our neural networks work. In most cases, as research becomes more collaborative across disciplines, both hardware and software are set for improvements. With algorithm-driven learning and artificial neural networks joining the party, researchers will have even better tools to not only sharpen imaging accuracy but also to predict neurological conditions based on data. All these strides promise a neuroimaging field that can better address mental health disorders while paving the way for treatment strategies that are as innovative as they are practical (Figure 15.17).

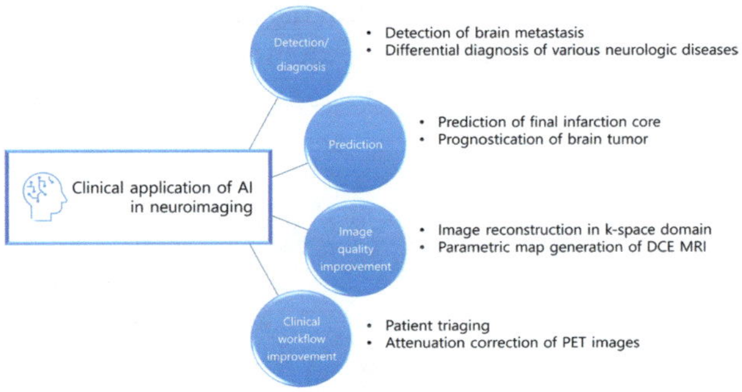

Figure 15.17. Graphical overview of main clinical applications of artificial intelligence (AI) in neuroimaging.

Source: https://www.i-mri.org/pdf/10.13104/imri.2022.26.1.1.

15.5.2. Integration of Neuroimaging with Other Modalities

Neurodegenerative disorders aren't simple to pin down, they call for some pretty sophisticated testing, which, in most cases, is becoming more doable by mixing various neuroimaging methods. MRI, PET, and SPECT, for instance, are now used in unexpected combinations to give us a layered look at the brain's condition. Each method gives its own slice of the story, and that patchwork of details turns out to be especially useful for tricky cases like Parkinson's disease and its atypical siblings. In many instances, this mix helps spot key markers that line up with different stages and symptoms, nudging treatment plans closer to what each patient needs. Given the wide variety, sometimes interestingly different symptoms and underlying issues, depending on one combined framework is crucial (Saeed et al., 2020). In anxiety disorders, things take a slightly different turn. Research now often weaves neuroimaging with genetic clues and clinical observations, which overall beefs up both how we study and treat anxiety. A good example is the ENIGMA-Anxiety Working Group, where researchers from more than a handful of countries team up to tackle old problems like tiny sample sizes and mismatched methods. By pooling over 100 distinct samples, this collaborative effort builds a richer picture of what fuels anxiety. This isn't just about crunching bigger numbers; it also makes it easier to compare results across different studies and come up with conclusions that feel solid enough to make a difference (Hoogendam et al., 2020). On the flip side, blending neuroimaging with other types of assessments might just be what drives personalized medicine forward in mental health and brain disorders. Take, for example, how pairing imaging data with behavioral tests opens a new window into the link between brain activity, emotion, and thinking, a mix that leads to a fuller view of patient well-being. Such multimodal work can even spotlight biomarkers that hint at who might respond better to certain treatments, thereby chipping away at the gap between lab-based data and everyday clinical practice. As this field moves forward, developing more automated tools for juggling and interpreting these data streams will be key, if not a game changer. Ultimately, these integrated approaches may spark major leaps in both our science and how we care for patients, ushering in what might be a transformative era for neuroimaging in research and healthcare delivery (Bas et al., 2020; Saeed et al., 2020) (Figure 15.18).

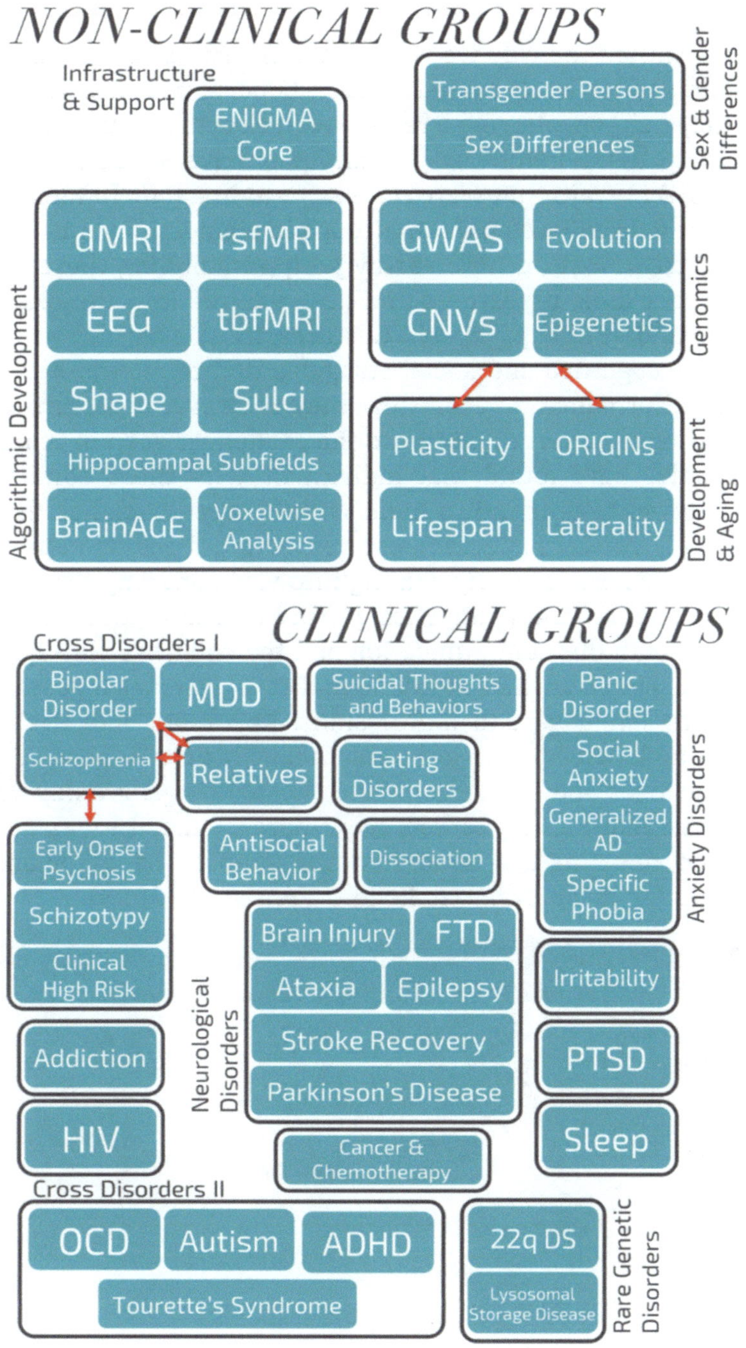

Figure 15.18. The ENIGMA brain research.

Source: Thompson, P.M., Jahanshad, N., Ching, C.R.K. *et al.* ENIGMA and global neuroscience: A decade of large-scale studies of the brain in health and disease across more than 40 countries. *Transl Psychiatry* **10**, 100 (2020). https://doi.org/10.1038/s41398-020-0705-1.

15.5.3. Potential Impact on Understanding Brain Disorders

Brain imaging tools have shifted the way we view brain disorders, it is a game changer for figuring out how the brain's build and its work come together. Experts now use stuff like fMRI and EEG to catch brain signals as they happen, offering a real-time peek into neural activity that older methods just couldn't match. Lately, these noninvasive techniques have let us look at conditions such as schizophrenia, ASD, and AD in ways that were once hard to imagine. In most cases, this direct look into the brain's wiring not only exposes hidden hiccups in connectivity and activity but also nudges us toward more tailored treatments, a noteworthy jump in handling these complex ailments (Yen et al., 2023). Taking a closer look at gestures and how they tie into the brain brings a fresh spin, especially when trying to understand psychosis. Gestures, those everyday nonverbal signals we use, can spill secrets about the cognitive and social struggles tied to mental health issues. Sometimes, when people's gesture performance or even how they interpret a gesture goes awry, it hints at deeper neurobiological glitches, a sort of mirror to the challenges seen in schizophrenia and related issues. A handful of studies have found that individuals with these conditions often show odd gesture patterns, which seem to go hand in hand with lowered social skills and cognitive twists. As researchers increasingly connect specific gestures with particular neural circuits, the idea of spotting biomarkers for psychosis is slowly coming into view, opening doors for creative therapies (Walther et al., 2016). Mixing neuroimaging with gesture research adds another layer to our grasp of how brain circuits back both our communication and the cognitive slip-ups in various disorders. By watching which regions light up when someone makes or watches a gesture, scientists get clues about the networks fusing language and motor skills. Key spots, like the inferior frontal gyrus and sections of the parietal lobes, appear to be real heavy hitters in gesture processing, a finding that extends into broader ideas about core cognitive shortcomings. Frankly, as imaging technology keeps getting better, we're likely going to see even more nuanced looks at how nonverbal cues weave into brain function, boosting our understanding of social behavior and paving the way for more effective treatments for these brain challenges (Yen et al., 2023).

Test Your Knowledge

1. What potential does functional neuroimaging hold for understanding brain plasticity and recovery in neurological disorders?
2. How could the integration of multiple neuroimaging modalities enhance diagnostic capabilities and treatment planning in the future?

Summary

Brain imaging has changed our view of the brain in ways that aren't always expected. Recent tech advances are shifting our understanding considerably, and it is interesting to see how the brain's wiring links up with our behavior, especially with conditions like Body Dysmorphic Disorder (BDD). Some scans show that areas like the orbitofrontal cortex and amygdala tend to be unusually active, hinting at the deeper biological roots of certain psychological issues. This kind of evidence nudges us toward mixing different treatment methods, using both talk therapies and meds, to better tackle mental health challenges (Çınaroğlu, 2025). And as we dig further into neuroimaging, new layers of insight keep unfolding, each one sparking a fresh idea about treatment. Looking closer, there's growing chatter around adult neurogenesis, which simply puts a spotlight on the brain's awesome ability to rewire itself. Studies now show that new cells emerge in places like the sub granular zone of the dentate gyrus, and that, in most cases, suggests the brain is constantly adapting to what's happening around it, boosting both cognitive flexibility and emotional resilience. With today's imaging gear, researchers can literally catch these changes as they occur, showing us, in real-time, how shifts in neural circuitry happen (Gideon et al., 2024). This evolving picture underscores why teaming up researchers from different fields, like those focused on imaging and those in behavioral psychology, can offer a deeper, more rounded take on brain function in both health and disease. Altogether, neuroimaging acts as a fresh lens on how brain function meshes with behavior. It not only helps pinpoint intricate details in conditions such as BDD but also guides us in formulating therapies that match the brain's true nature. As imaging tech gets even more detailed, it promises to shine an even brighter light on these disorders and lead to more effective treatment options. Plus, folding in discoveries about neurogenesis creates a neat bridge between neuroscience and psychological practice. Generally speaking, going forward, a careful mix of ethical awareness, open-mindedness, and cross-disciplinary work will be key to unlocking neuroimaging's full potential in modern neuroscience (Çınaroğlu, 2025; Gideon et al., 2024).

Neuroimaging has shifted how we see the brain, it is no longer a mysterious black box. Techniques like fMRI and PET let us catch the brain in action almost like tuning into a live broadcast, which has pushed our grasp of brain structure and function into much sharper focus. This ever-growing stash of insights has helped us pick out tricky issues like neurodegenerative conditions and mental health challenges. As these imaging tools get even better, it is becoming clear that researchers have to somehow patch together and summarize all this information, especially when trying to nail down how our brain's wiring ties to behavior (Fitria, 2023). It isn't just about peering into the brain either; what we see often sparks new ways to treat it. Take neuroplasticity, knowing that the brain can rewire itself means doctors can craft rehabilitation programs that fit each person's recovery, even if it sounds a bit out-of-the-box. Merging what you see on a scan with therapeutic ideas creates a broader way to handle cognitive issues and, in most cases, boost patient outcomes. This mix of imaging and treatment keeps pushing the need for individuals in the field to explain complicated details in a clear, everyday manner (Kim et al., 2022). On the flip side, making sense of neuroimaging data can be pretty tricky, mainly because each brain seems to have its own uniqueness. Age, genetic factors, and even what surrounds us all mess with what we consider "normal," so it is a real challenge to come up with one-size-fits-all benchmarks. As more studies pile up, researchers find it necessary, sometimes even a bit messy, to sift through the data and boil it down to the essentials. Ultimately, getting these ideas straight not only helps scientists and clinicians work together better but also makes it easier for everyone to join the conversation about how our brains work (Kim et al., 2022).

KEY TERMS FROM THIS CHAPTER

Autism spectrum disorder (ASD)
Brain mapping
Electrical impedance tomography (EIT)
Epilepsy
Magnetoencephalography (MEG)
Neurodegenerative diseases
Neuroscience
Psychology
Brain interact well
Diffusion Tensor Imaging (DTI)
Electroencephalography (EEG)
Image reconstruction from brain signals (IRBS)
Neural networks
Neuroinflammation
Positron Emission Tomography (PET)
Structural imaging

Critical Thinking Questions

1. **Which of the following imaging modalities is most commonly used for detecting acute hemorrhages in the brain?**
   a. MRI
   b. PET scan
   c. CT scan
   d. X-ray
2. **What is the primary advantage of MRI in neuroimaging?**
   a. Quick detection of bone fractures
   b. Visualization of blood flow in real-time
   c. High-resolution images of brain structures and soft tissues
   d. Detection of radioisotope activity
3. **Functional MRI (fMRI) is primarily used to:**
   a. Detect skull fractures
   b. Observe metabolic processes in the brain
   c. Map brain activity by detecting changes in blood flow
   d. Evaluate spinal cord compression
4. **Which neuroimaging technique uses radioactive tracers to study brain metabolism and function?**
   a. CT scan
   b. fMRI
   c. PET scan
   d. X-ray
5. **What is the main use of diffusion tensor imaging (DTI), a specialized form of MRI?**
   a. To detect tumors in the spinal cord
   b. To map white matter tracts in the brain
   c. To assess cerebrospinal fluid levels
   d. To detect bone deformities

Short Answer Questions

1. What was one of the earliest methods used in the history of neuroimaging?
2. How do structural and functional neuroimaging techniques differ?
3. Name two clinical applications of neuroimaging in diagnosing brain disorders.
4. What is one major advantage of MRI over CT in neuroimaging?
5. What limitation is commonly associated with functional MRI (fMRI)?
6. How might artificial intelligence shape the future of neuroimaging?

Answers to Critical Thinking Questions

1. (c); 2. (c); 3. (c); 4. (c); 5. (b)

References

1. Alex, G. S., Oke, O. O., Ekokojde, J. W., Gbayisomore, T. J., Anene-Ogbe, M. C., Glory, F., et al. (2024). Adult neurogenesis: A review of current perspectives and implications for neuroscience research. *Journal of Neuroscience and Neurological Disorders, 8*(2), 106–114. https://dx.doi.org/10.29328/journal.jnnd.1001102.
2. Ali, B. M., Alfallj, T. H., Alqathaniyyin, M. M., Ashoor, M. M., Alqurashi, R. M., Alrashidi, A. Q., Futayni, T. Y., Alhussain, R. M., Alzhrani, A. S., & Alobidi, R. A. (2024). *4*(10), 521–527.
3. Ali, K. (2023). A review of emotions, behavior and cognition. *Journal of Biomedical and Sustainable Healthcare Applications*. https://www.semanticscholar.org/paper/27fdbc3848a3b33d8a9648ed3ac78db70fb5d843 (accessed on 23 May 2025).
4. Antonenko, D., & Flöel, A. (2013). Healthy aging by staying selectively connected: A mini-review. *Gerontology, 60*(1), 3–9. https://doi.org/10.1159/000354376.
5. Arabameri, E. (2024). The evolution of motor behavior: Lessons from past research and future prospects. *Health Nexus, 2*(4), 134–151. https://doi.org/10.61838/kman.hn.2.4.16.
6. Barbosa, F. C., Tadine, R. M., Rezende, J. D. P., Lopes, G., Attie, A., Machado, S., & Barbosa, E. S. (2024). Neuroscience of hypnosis: A neurophysiological view of hypnotherapy. *Revita de Gestão Social e Ambiental*. https://www.semanticscholar.org/paper/c729c92d4026a1f05e7691fa211887eb86fb21d2 (accessed on 23 May 2025).
7. Bas-Hoogendam, J. M., Groenewold, N. A., Aghajani, M., Freitag, G. F., Harrewijn, A., Hilbert, K., Jahanshad, N., et al. (2020). ENIGMA-anxiety working group: Rationale for and organization of large-scale neuroimaging studies of anxiety disorders. *Human Brain Mapping, 43*(1), 83–112. https://doi.org/10.1002/hbm.25100.
8. Bayeleva, T. (2021). Applications in cognitive neuroscience: Electroencephalography-based prediction of treatment response in schizophrenia and the effect of authenticity on emotion perception (MPhil thesis). Queensland Brain Institute, The University of Queensland. https://doi.org/10.14264/7504094.
9. Berrios Moya, J. A. (2024). Addressing the gaps in early dementia detection: A path towards enhanced diagnostic models through machine learning. *ArXiv*. https://www.semanticscholar.org/paper/289eb82cef1ab46fbf8ed8635d2820bbd11aab17 (accessed on 23 May 2025).
10. Brookes, M. J., Leggett, J., Rea, M., Hill, R. M., Holmes, N., Boto, E., & Bowtell, R. (2022). Magnetoencephalography with optically pumped magnetometers (OPM-MEG): The next generation of functional neuroimaging. *Trends in Neurosciences, 45*(8), 621–634. https://doi.org/10.1016/j.tins.2022.05.008.
11. Çınaroğlu, M. (2025). Neural mechanisms and cognitive-behavioral interventions in body dysmorphic disorder: A neurobehavioral perspective. *JNBS, 12*(1), 32–34.
12. Cocchi, L., Zalesky, A., Nott, Z., Whybird, G., Fitzgerald, P. B., & Breakspear, M. (2018). Transcranial magnetic stimulation in obsessive-compulsive disorder: A focus on network mechanisms and state dependence. *NeuroImage Clinical, 19*, 661–674. https://doi.org/10.1016/j.nicl.2018.05.029.
13. Cryan, J. F., O'Riordan, K. J., Cowan, C. S. M., Sandhu, K. V., Bastiaanssen, T. F. S., Boehme, M., Codagnone, M. G., et al. (2019). The microbiota-gut-brain axis. *Physiological Reviews, 99*(4), 1877–2013. https://doi.org/10.1152/physrev.00018.2018.

14. Dattola, S., Ielo, A., Varone, G., Cacciola, A., Quartarone, A., & Bonanno, L. (2025). Frontotemporal dementia: A systematic review of artificial intelligence approaches in differential diagnosis. *Frontiers in Aging Neuroscience, 17*, 1547727. https://doi.org/10.3389/fnagi.2025.1547727.

15. Degtyaruk, O., Mc Larney, B., Deán-Ben, X. L., Shoham, S., & Razansky, D. (2019). Optoacoustic calcium imaging of deep brain activity in an intracardially perfused mouse brain model. *Photonics, 6*(2), 67. https://doi.org/10.3390/photonics6020067.

16. Di Flumeri, G., Aricò, P., Borghini, G., Sciaraffa, N., Florio, A., & Babiloni, F. (2019). The dry revolution: Evaluation of three different EEG dry electrode types in terms of signal spectral features, mental states classification and usability. *Sensors, 19*(6), 1365. https://doi.org/10.3390/s19061365.

17. Dugré, M., Chatelain, Y., & Glatard, T. (2024). An analysis of performance bottlenecks in MRI preprocessing. *GigaScience, 14*. https://www.semanticscholar.org/paper/a488274db8430d8ba543e510672068e2d3abab9c (accessed on 23 May 2025).

18. Edlow, B. L., Claassen, J., Schiff, N. D., & Greer, D. M. (2020). Recovery from disorders of consciousness: Mechanisms, prognosis and emerging therapies. *Nature Reviews Neurology, 17*(3), 135–156. https://doi.org/10.1038/s41582-020-00428-x.

19. Fallahi, A., Tavakoli, H., Hoseini-Tabatabaei, N., RostamiRostami, R., Soltanian Zadeh, H., & Nazem-Zadeh, M. (2024). Application of functional connectivity analysis in TMS treatment evaluation for patients with mental disorder. *Frontiers in Biomedical Technologies*. https://www.semanticscholar.org/paper/7ac84c6b6f45c7b9afeabd06aee2afb83d8ce915 (accessed on 23 May 2025).

20. Farahani, F. V., Karwowski, W., & Lighthall, N. R. (2019). Application of graph theory for identifying connectivity patterns in human brain networks: A systematic review. *Frontiers in Neuroscience, 13*, 585. https://doi.org/10.3389/fnins.2019.00585.

21. Fitria, T. N. (2023). Using manual and automatic summarization: What should students consider in writing a summary? *English Language and Education Spectrum*. https://www.semanticscholar.org/paper/da604863564235dc8ad4a4e5322a11f30c979ed5 (accessed on 23 May 2025).

22. Guan, S., Li, Y., Gao, Y., Luo, Y., Zhao, H., Yang, D., & Li, R. (2025). Continuous wave-diffuse optical tomography (CW-DOT) in human brain mapping: A review. *Sensors, 25*(7), 2040. https://doi.org/10.3390/s25072040.

23. Hill, R. M., Boto, E., Rea, M., Holmes, N., Leggett, J., Coles, L. A., Papastavrou, M., et al. (2020). Multi-channel whole-head OPM-MEG: Helmet design and a comparison with a conventional system. *NeuroImage, 219*, 116995. https://doi.org/10.1016/j.neuroimage.2020.116995.

24. Hoang, D. M., Pham, P. T., Bach, T. Q., Ngo, A. T., Nguyen, Q. T., Phan, T. T. K., Giang, N. H., et al. (2022). Stem cell-based therapy for human diseases. *Signal Transduction and Targeted Therapy, 7*, Article 183. https://doi.org/10.1038/s41392-022-01134-4.

25. Hu, X. S., Nascimento, T. D., Bender, M. C., Hall, T., Petty, S., O'Malley, S. S., Ellwood, R. P., et al. (2019). Feasibility of a real-time clinical augmented reality and artificial intelligence framework for pain detection and localization from the brain. *Journal of Medical Internet Research, 21*, e13594. https://doi.org/10.2196/13594.

26. Ienca, M., & Andorno, R. (2017). Towards new human rights in the age of neuroscience and

neurotechnology. *Life Sciences Society and Policy, 13*. https://doi.org/10.1186/s40504-017-0050-1.

27. Jo, T., Nho, K., & Saykin, A. J. (2019). Deep learning in Alzheimer's disease: Diagnostic classification and prognostic prediction using neuroimaging data. *Frontiers in Aging Neuroscience, 11*. https://doi.org/10.3389/fnagi.2019.00220.
28. Ke, X. Y., Hou, W., Huang, Q., Hou, X., Bao, X., Kong, W. X., Li, C., et al. (2022). Advances in electrical impedance tomography-based brain imaging. *Military Medical Research, 9*. https://doi.org/10.1186/s40779-022-00370-7.
29. Kim, J. S., Amendola, A., Barg, A., Baumhauer, J., Brodsky, J., Cushman, D., Gonzalez, T. A., et al. (2022). Summary report of the Arthritis Foundation and the American Orthopedic Foot & Ankle Society's symposium on targets for osteoarthritis research: Part 1: Epidemiology, pathophysiology, and current imaging approaches. *Foot & Ankle Orthopedics, 7*. https://www.semanticscholar.org/paper/83192de89ef522b92876a27da4a8d2178bd7e4d4 (accessed on 23 May 2025).
30. Li, R. (2025). Integrative diagnosis of psychiatric conditions using ChatGPT and fMRI data. *BMC Psychiatry, 25*. https://www.semanticscholar.org/paper/826ff32d3eb1cc8694b8fcc0bbd86e666c3c1fd2 (accessed on 23 May 2025).
31. Lu, Z. (2023). Visualizing the mind's eye: A future perspective on applications of image reconstruction from brain signals to psychiatry. *Psych Radiology, 3*, kkad022. https://doi.org/10.1093/psyrad/kkad022.
32. Maleki Varnosfaderani, S., & Forouzanfar, M. (2024). The role of AI in hospitals and clinics: Transforming healthcare in the 21st century. *Bioengineering, 11*(4), 337. https://doi.org/10.3390/bioengineering11040337.
33. Muhle, R., Reed, H. E., Stratigos, K., & Veenstra-VanderWeele, J. (2018). The emerging clinical neuroscience of autism spectrum disorder. *JAMA Psychiatry, 75*(5), 514. https://doi.org/10.1001/jamapsychiatry.2017.4685.
34. Nakano, Y., Niethammer, M., & Eidelberg, D. (2025). Imaging of disease-related networks in Parkinson's disease. *Cold Spring Harbor Perspectives in Medicine*. https://www.semanticscholar.org/paper/312ab7dfa986c8d95e78c194ea5177f6fc53179b (accessed on 23 May 2025).
35. Nikam, R. M., Yue, X., Kaur, G., Kandula, V., Khair, A., Kecskemethy, H., Averill, L., et al. (2022). Advanced neuroimaging approaches to pediatric brain tumors. *Cancers, 14*. https://www.semanticscholar.org/paper/6a8adca7cc4167d79360b9788550cc1e4124f782 (accessed on 23 May 2025).
36. Patricios, J., Schneider, K., Dvořák, J., Ahmed, O. H., Blauwet, C., Cantu, R. C., Davis, G. A., et al. (2023). Consensus statement on concussion in sport: The 6th International Conference on Concussion in Sport–Amsterdam. *British Journal of Sports Medicine, 57*(11), 695–711. https://doi.org/10.1136/bjsports-2023-106898.
37. Rahman, A. (2024). Positron-emission tomography (PET) and single-photon-emission computed tomography (SPECT) diagnosis of neurological disorders. *Bangladesh Journal of Medicine, 36*(1), 3–14. https://doi.org/10.3329/bjm.v36i1.78589.
38. Redouani, A., Ikmel, G., Zared, K., ÄŒyras, G., & El Amrani El Idrissi, N. (2024). A comprehensive review of integrated energy storage batteries in renewable energy stations: Technological

advancements, challenges and future trends. *Insights into Regional Development, 6*(3), 40–52.

39. Ritchie, S. J., Cox, S. R., Shen, X., Lombardo, M., Reus, L. M., Alloza, C., Harris, M. A., et al. (2018). Sex differences in the adult human brain: Evidence from 5216 UK Biobank participants. *Cerebral Cortex, 28*(8), 2959–2975. https://doi.org/10.1093/cercor/bhy109.
40. Saeed, U., Lang, A. E., & Masellis, M. (2020). Neuroimaging advances in Parkinson's disease and atypical parkinsonian syndromes. *Frontiers in Neurology, 11*, 572976. https://doi.org/10.3389/fneur.2020.572976.
41. Schmidt, A., & Borgwardt, S. (2016). Editorial: Third-generation neuroimaging: Translating research into clinical utility. *Frontiers in Psychiatry, 7*. https://www.semanticscholar.org/paper/37bed0ac32336032e4da836c7add6af079b0d1ec (accessed on 23 May 2025).
42. Sinha, R., & Kumar Sahu, K. (2025). Advancements in neuroscience for healthcare: Recent innovations and breakthroughs in mental health treatment. *Journal of Neonatal Surgery, 14*(1S), 403–407. https://www.jneonatalsurg.com/index.php/jns/article/view/1556 (accessed on 23 May 2025).
43. Sone, D., & Beheshti, I. (2022). Neuroimaging-based brain age estimation: A promising personalized biomarker in neuropsychiatry. *Journal of Personalized Medicine, 12*(10). https://www.semanticscholar.org/paper/a87df116cc6e06330acd94fae81dd39d9e20596b (accessed on 23 May 2025).
44. Teleanu, D. M., Chircov, C., Grumezescu, A. M., Volceanov, A., & Teleanu, R. I. (2019). Contrast agents' delivery: An up-to-date review of nano diagnostics in neuroimaging. *Nanomaterials, 9*(4), 542. https://doi.org/10.3390/nano9040542.
45. Varghese, A., Thilak, K., & Thomas, S. M. (2024). Technological advancements, digital transformation, and future trends in blood transfusion services. *International Journal of Advances in Medicine, 11*(2), 147–152. https://doi.org/10.18203/2349-3933.ijam20240368.
46. Walther, S., & Mittal, V. A. (2016). Why we should take a closer look at gestures. *Schizophrenia Bulletin, 42*(2), 259–261. https://doi.org/10.1093/schbul/sbv229.
47. Wang, H., Shi, C., Jiang, L., Liu, X., Tang, R., & Tang, M. (2024). Neuroimaging techniques, gene therapy, and gut microbiota: Frontier advances and integrated applications in Alzheimer's disease research. *Frontiers in Aging Neuroscience, 16*. https://www.semanticscholar.org/paper/e60f66bed869705c0fc3323796891805ee35f6cc (accessed on 23 May 2025).
48. Ward, T., & Roantree, M. (2024). An intelligence emotions, behavior and cognition. *Journal of Biomedical and Sustainable Healthcare Applications, 3*(2). https://doi.org/10.53759/0088/JBSHA202303016.
49. Xu, M., Ouyang, Y., & Yuan, Z. (2023). Deep learning aided neuroimaging and brain regulation. *Sensors (Basel, Switzerland), 23*. https://www.semanticscholar.org/paper/ca7eb4e3a202db2300f2b34a6c528e1054cfdeb0 (accessed on 23 May 2025).
50. Yang, L., & Wang, Z. (2025). Applications and advances of combined fMRI-fNIRs techniques in brain functional research. *Frontiers in Neurology, 16*. https://www.semanticscholar.org/paper/db5608655f4f77c84bb1aa41b8f3a539633a7990 (accessed on 23 May 2025).
51. Yen, C., Lin, C. L., & Chiang, M. C. (2023). Exploring the frontiers of neuroimaging: A review of recent advances in understanding brain functioning and disorders. *Life, 13*(7), 1472. https://doi.org/10.3390/life13071472.

52. Zhang, F., Zhang, J., Wang, X., Han, M., Fei, Y., & Wang, J. (2025). Blood–brain barrier disruption in schizophrenia: Insights, mechanisms, and future directions. *International Journal of Molecular Sciences, 26*(1). https://www.semanticscholar.org/paper/a72847dc662078acb459bf550fafa95a45f00841 (accessed on 23 May 2025).

53. Zhou, S. K., Greenspan, H., Davatzikos, C., Duncan, J. S., van Ginneken, B., Madabhushi, A., Prince, J. L., et al. (2021). A review of deep learning in medical imaging: Imaging traits, technology trends, case studies with progress highlights, and future promises. *Proceedings of the IEEE, 109*(5), 820–838. https://doi.org/10.1109/jproc.2021.3054390.

INDEX

D

E

K

L

M

N

O

P

Q

R